ICD-10-CM AND ICD-10-PCS
Coding Handbook

ICD-10-CM AND ICD-10-PCS Coding Handbook without Answers

2021 Revised Edition

NELLY LEON-CHISEN, RHIA

CENTRAL OFFICE ON ICD-10-CM AND ICD-10-PCS
OF THE
AMERICAN HOSPITAL ASSOCIATION

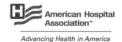
American Hospital Association™

Advancing Health in America

HEALTH FORUM, INC.
An American Hospital Association Company
Chicago

Printed in the United States of America—08/2020

COVER DESIGN: Mellissa Dempsey

INTERIOR DESIGN AND TYPOGRAPHY: Fine Print, Ltd.

COMPOSITION: Westchester Publishing Services

NEW ILLUSTRATIONS FOR THE 2012 AND SUBSEQUENT EDITIONS: Christoph Blumrich

PAPERBACK ISBN: 978-1-55648-454-4, Item Number 148076

DIGITAL ISBN: 978-1-55648-455-1, Item Number P148076

To my husband, Penku (Jorge) Chisen,
who supported and encouraged me
with his patience and understanding
throughout the long and arduous months
it took to complete this handbook

Contents

List of Tables and Figures. ix

About the Author and Contributors. xii

Acknowledgments. xiii

How to Use This Handbook xv

FORMAT AND CONVENTIONS AND CURRENT CODING PRACTICES FOR ICD-10-CM AND ICD-10-PCS

1 Introduction to the ICD-10-CM Classification 3

2 ICD-10-CM Conventions 13

3 Uniform Hospital Discharge Data Set 23

4 The Medical Record as a Source Document 35

5 Basic ICD-10-CM Coding Steps 41

6 Basic ICD-10-CM Coding Guidelines 47

7 Introduction to the ICD-10-PCS Classification. 61

8 Basic ICD-10-PCS Coding Steps 77

9 ICD-10-PCS Root Operations in the Medical and Surgical Section 85

10 ICD-10-PCS Medical- and Surgical-Related, Ancillary,
and New Technology Procedure Sections. 101

11 Z Codes and External Cause of Morbidity Codes. 121

CODING OF SIGNS AND SYMPTOMS

12 Symptoms, Signs, and Ill-Defined Conditions 135

CODING OF INFECTIOUS AND PARASITIC DISEASES, ENDOCRINE DISEASES AND METABOLIC DISORDERS, AND MENTAL DISORDERS

13 Infectious and Parasitic Diseases 143

14 Endocrine, Nutritional, and Metabolic Diseases 159

15 Mental Disorders 173

CODING OF DISEASES OF THE BLOOD AND BLOOD-FORMING ORGANS, CERTAIN DISORDERS INVOLVING THE IMMUNE MECHANISM, AND DISEASES OF THE NERVOUS SYSTEM

16 Diseases of the Blood and Blood-Forming Organs
and Certain Disorders Involving the Immune Mechanism 193

17 Diseases of the Nervous System and Sense Organs 203

CODING OF DISEASES OF THE RESPIRATORY, DIGESTIVE, AND GENITOURINARY SYSTEMS

18 Diseases of the Respiratory System 223

19 Diseases of the Digestive System 245

20 Diseases of the Genitourinary System 263

CODING OF DISEASES OF THE SKIN AND DISEASES OF THE MUSCULOSKELETAL SYSTEM

21 Diseases of the Skin and Subcutaneous Tissue 289

22 Diseases of the Musculoskeletal System and Connective Tissue 299

CODING OF PREGNANCY AND CHILDBIRTH COMPLICATIONS, ABORTION, CONGENITAL ANOMALIES, AND PERINATAL CONDITIONS

23 Complications of Pregnancy, Childbirth, and the Puerperium 321

24 Abortion and Ectopic Pregnancy 355

25 Congenital Anomalies 367

26 Perinatal Conditions 375

CODING OF CIRCULATORY SYSTEM DISEASES AND NEOPLASTIC DISEASES

27 Diseases of the Circulatory System 393

28 Neoplasms 457

CODING OF INJURIES, BURNS, POISONING, AND COMPLICATIONS OF CARE

29 Injuries 487

30 Burns 519

31 Poisoning, Toxic Effects, Adverse Effects, and Underdosing of Drugs 527

32 Complications of Surgery and Medical Care 537

Final Review Exercise 559

Appendix A Coding and Reimbursement 577

Appendix B Reporting of the Present on Admission Indicator 585

Appendix C Case Summary Exercises
(An expanded table of contents can be found on page 593.) 593

Index 723

List of Tables and Figures

FIGURE 1.1   Table of Contents from ICD-10-CM 5

FIGURE 7.1   Sample Excerpt of ICD-10-PCS Table 63

FIGURE 7.2   Structure of Codes in the Medical and Surgical Section 64

FIGURE 7.3   Examples of Body Part Values 65

TABLE 7.1   ICD-10-PCS Sections and Their Corresponding Character Values 66

TABLE 7.2   Medical and Surgical Section Body Systems and Values 67

TABLE 7.3   ICD-10-PCS Root Operations and Their Corresponding Values 68

FIGURE 7.4   Excerpt from Table Showing Bilateral Body Part 70

TABLE 7.4   Medical and Surgical Section Approaches 72

FIGURE 7.5   Illustrations of Medical and Surgical Section Approaches 74–75

FIGURE 7.6   Excerpt from the Device Aggregation Table 76

FIGURE 8.1   Excerpt of 0FT Table from ICD-10-PCS 81

FIGURE 8.2   Excerpt of 0Y6 Table from ICD-10-PCS 82

FIGURE 9.1   Table Excerpt Demonstrating Location of Root Operation Definition 86

TABLE 9.1   Root Operations to Take Out Some or All of a Body Part 89

TABLE 9.2   Root Operations to Take Out Solids/Fluids/Gases from a Body Part 91

TABLE 9.3   Root Operations Involving Cutting or Separation Only 92

TABLE 9.4   Root Operations to Put In/Put Back or Move Some/All of a Body Part 93

TABLE 9.5   Root Operations to Alter the Diameter or Route of a Tubular Body Part 94

TABLE 9.6   Root Operations That Always Involve a Device 95

TABLE 9.7   Root Operations That Involve Examination Only 97

TABLE 9.8   Root Operations That Include Other Repairs 98

TABLE 9.9   Root Operations That Include Other Objectives 99

TABLE 10.1   Medical- and Surgical-Related Sections 102

FIGURE 10.1   Structure of Codes in the Placement Section 102

TABLE 10.2   Placement Section Root Operation Values and Definitions 103

FIGURE 10.2   Structure of Codes in the Administration Section 105

FIGURE 10.3   Structure of Codes in the Measurement and Monitoring Section 106

FIGURE 10.4   Structure of Codes in the Extracorporeal or Systemic Assistance
and Performance Section 107

FIGURE 10.5   Structure of Codes in the Extracorporeal or Systemic Therapies Section 108

FIGURE 10.6   Structure of Codes in the Osteopathic Section 110

FIGURE 10.7   Structure of Codes in the Other Procedures Section 111

FIGURE 10.8   Structure of Codes in the Imaging Section 113

FIGURE 10.9   Structure of Codes in the Nuclear Medicine Section 114

FIGURE 10.10   Structure of Codes in the Radiation Therapy Section 115

FIGURE 10.11   Structure of Codes in the Physical Rehabilitation and
Diagnostic Audiology Section 117

TABLE 10.3   Physical Rehabilitation and Diagnostic Audiology
Root Types 118

FIGURE 10.12   Structure of Codes in the New Technology Section 119

TABLE 13.1   Gram-Negative and Gram-Positive Bacteria 150

FIGURE 14.1   Major Organs of the Endocrine System 160

FIGURE 15.1   Side View of the Brain 174

TABLE 15.1   Root Type Values in the Mental Health Section 187

TABLE 15.2   Root Type Values in the Substance Abuse Treatment Section 188

FIGURE 16.1   Four Major Types of Blood Cells 200

FIGURE 17.1   The Nervous System 204

FIGURE 17.2   The Eye 215

TABLE 17.1   Coding of Glaucoma 218

FIGURE 17.3   The Ear 219

FIGURE 18.1   The Respiratory System 224

FIGURE 19.1   The Digestive System 246

FIGURE 19.2   Excerpt from ICD-10-PCS Table for Hepatobiliary System Extirpation 254

FIGURE 19.3   Illustrations of Bariatric Surgery 259

FIGURE 20.1   The Urinary System 264

TABLE 20.1   Hypertensive Chronic Kidney Disease and Hypertensive
Heart and Chronic Kidney Disease and the Applicable CKD Stages 269

FIGURE 20.2   The Male Reproductive System 276

FIGURE 20.3   Common Sites of Endometriosis Implantation 277

FIGURE 20.4   The Female Reproductive System 278

FIGURE 20.5   Breast Reconstruction Surgery 282

FIGURE 21.1   The Skin and Subcutaneous Tissue 291

FIGURE 22.1   The Human Skeleton 301

FIGURE 22.2   The Spinal Column 303

TABLE 22.1   Components of Each Column of the Spine 310

FIGURE 22.3   Structure of the Spine Involved in Spinal Fusion 311

FIGURE 22.4   Columns of the Spine, Lateral View 312

FIGURE 22.5   Types of Spinal Fusion Surgeries 313

TABLE 22.2   Common Fusion and Refusion ICD-10-PCS Qualifiers 314

FIGURE 23.1   Primary Organs of the Female Reproductive System 323

FIGURE 23.2   Examples of Fetal Presentations 336

FIGURE 23.3   Structure of Codes in the Obstetrics Section 342

FIGURE 23.4   Root Operations in the Obstetrics Section 342

FIGURE 24.1   Excerpt from ICD-10-PCS Table for Abortion Procedures. 361

FIGURE 27.1   Major Vessels of the Arterial System 394

FIGURE 27.2   Major Vessels of the Venous System. 395

FIGURE 27.3   The Interior of the Heart. 396

FIGURE 27.4   Decision Tree for Coding Acute Type 1 Myocardial Infarction 401

FIGURE 27.5   Types of Cerebral Infarction. 411

FIGURE 27.6   Pacemaker Insertion 430

FIGURE 27.7   Angioplasty with Stent Insertion. 435

FIGURE 27.8   Coronary Artery Bypass Graft 437

FIGURE 27.9   Central Venous Catheter (CVC). 446

FIGURE 27.10   Peripherally Inserted Central Catheter (PICC). 446

FIGURE 27.11   Open Aneurysmectomy. 450

FIGURE 27.12   Open Surgical Aneurysm Repair via Tube Graft. 450

FIGURE 27.13   Endovascular Aneurysm Repair 451

FIGURE 27.14   Aorta and Lower Side Branches 453

TABLE 28.1   Section of the Neoplasm Table in the Alphabetic Index
of Diseases and Injuries 463

FIGURE 28.1   The Lymphatic System. 469

FIGURE 29.1   Examples of Open and Closed Fractures 498

FIGURE 29.2   Sample Tabular List Seventh-Character Values. 500

FIGURE 29.3   Gustilo Classification of Open Fractures 501

TABLE 29.1   Definitions of Terms Used for Qualifiers for "Detachment" Procedures 512

FIGURE 30.1   Skin Layers. 520

FIGURE 31.1   Decision Tree for Coding Adverse Effects of Drugs or Poisoning
Due to Drugs or Medicinal or Biological Substances 531

FIGURE 31.2   Excerpt from ICD-10-CM Table of Drugs and Chemicals 531

About the Author and Contributors

Nelly Leon-Chisen, RHIA, is the director of coding and classification at the American Hospital Association (AHA), where she heads the Central Office on ICD-10-CM and ICD-10-PCS and the Central Office on HCPCS. She represents the AHA as one of the Cooperating Parties responsible for the development of *AHA Coding Clinic® for ICD-10-CM and ICD-10-PCS,* the *ICD-10-CM Official Guidelines for Coding and Reporting,* and the *ICD-10-PCS Official Coding Guidelines.* She is the executive editor for the *AHA Coding Clinic®* publications.

Ms. Leon-Chisen's other ICD-10 activities include past membership in the ICD-10-PCS Technical Advisory Panel, past co-chair of the Workgroup for Electronic Data Interchange (WEDI) ICD-10 Implementation Workgroup, and numerous testimonies on ICD-10-CM and ICD-10-PCS before the ICD-9-CM Coordination and Maintenance Committee and the National Committee on Vital and Health Statistics. She was also the AHA lead project manager on the joint American Hospital Association–American Health Information Management Association (AHIMA) ICD-10-CM Field Study. She was a first-generation AHIMA-approved ICD-10 Trainer.

Ms. Leon-Chisen has lectured on ICD-9-CM, ICD-10, and POA coding, data quality, and DRGs throughout the United States, Europe, Asia, and Latin America. She has often served as a speaker for the popular *AHA Coding Clinic®* webinar series. She has broad health information management (HIM) experience in hospital inpatient and outpatient management, consulting, and teaching. She has been an instructor in the HIM and Health Information Technology programs for the University of Illinois and Truman Community College, both in Chicago. She is a past president of the Chicago Area Health Information Management Association and the recipient of its Distinguished Member Award. She is the recipient of the Professional Achievement Award from the Illinois Health Information Management Association. She was a member of the Advisory Board of the Health Information Technology Program of DeVry University in Chicago.

The Central Office on ICD-9-CM was first created through a written Memorandum of Understanding between the AHA and the National Center for Health Statistics in 1963 to do the following:

- Serve as the U.S. clearinghouse for issues related to the use of ICD-9-CM
- Work with the National Center for Health Statistics and the Centers for Medicare & Medicaid Services to maintain the integrity of the classification system
- Recommend revisions and modifications to the current and future revisions of the ICD
- Develop educational material and programs on ICD-9-CM

The Central Office on ICD-10-CM and ICD-10-PCS provides expert advice by serving as the clearinghouse for the dissemination of information on ICD-10-CM and ICD-10-PCS.

In 2014, the Central Office stopped providing ICD-9-CM advice and fully transitioned to ICD-10-CM/PCS advice while launching the stand-alone publication *AHA Coding Clinic® for ICD-10-CM and ICD-10-PCS.*

Acknowledgments

Nelly Leon-Chisen gratefully acknowledges the invaluable contributions of Anita Rapier, Gretchen Young-Charles, and Denene M. Harper, members of the American Hospital Association's Central Office on ICD-10-CM and ICD-10-PCS, who assisted in the revision and review of the manuscript for the handbook and the case summary exercises, as well as the preparation of instructors' ancillary materials.

Anita Rapier, RHIT, CCS, is a senior coding consultant at the AHA Central Office on ICD-10-CM and ICD-10-PCS. She is also the managing editor of *AHA Coding Clinic® for ICD-10-CM and ICD-10-PCS,* for which she is responsible for developing educational material. She has more than 25 years of experience in health information management and has held several positions in HIM, including education, quality, compliance, hospital-based outpatient and acute care, and long-term care. Ms. Rapier has presented numerous educational seminars and has authored articles on coding and compliance. She is also a speaker for the popular *AHA Coding Clinic®* webinar series.

Gretchen Young-Charles, RHIA, is a senior coding consultant at the AHA Central Office on ICD-10-CM and ICD-10-PCS. In this role, she develops educational articles on official coding advice for publication in *AHA Coding Clinic® for ICD-10-CM and ICD-10-PCS.* Ms. Young-Charles has more than 25 years of experience in the HIM field. She has worked in numerous HIM roles, including education, quality, and hospital-based outpatient and acute care. She also spent a number of years with the Peer Review Organization for the state of Illinois. She is also a speaker for the popular *AHA Coding Clinic®* webinar series.

Denene M. Harper, RHIA, is a senior coding consultant at the AHA Central Office on ICD-10-CM and ICD-10-PCS. She is responsible for writing articles on official coding advice for publication in *AHA Coding Clinic® for ICD-10-CM and ICD-10-PCS.* Ms. Harper has more than 25 years of experience in the HIM field, including hospital-based outpatient and acute care, utilization review, and quality improvement. She is also the moderator for the popular *AHA Coding Clinic®* webinar series.

In addition, Nelly Leon-Chisen gratefully acknowledges the significant contributions of Janatha R. Ashton, MS, RHIA, who authored the original case summary exercises in appendix C, and Therese M. (Teri) Jorwic, who revised those exercises and converted them from ICD-9 to ICD-10.

Therese M. (Teri) Jorwic, MPH, RHIA, CCS, CCS-P, FAHIMA, is a former assistant professor in Health Information Management at the University of Illinois at Chicago. She has presented numerous workshops and developed educational material for in-class and online courses on ICD-10-CM/PCS, ICD-9-CM, and HCPCS/CPT coding as well as on reimbursement systems for hospitals, physicians, and other health care providers. She also has presented workshops for associations and served as external faculty for the AHIMA ICD-10 Academy programs.

Thanks are due to Richard Hill, a senior editor at the American Hospital Association, who read the author's drafts and helped me to say in plain English what I wanted to say, even without being a coding professional himself. Additional thanks are due to Jennifer Gillespie, who has served as the production manager since the 2019 edition.

A sincere thanks to the representatives of the Cooperating Parties: Donna Pickett, RHIA, MPH; Mady Hue, RHIA; and Sue Bowman, RHIA, CCS—whose collaboration and friendship continue to make *Coding Clinic* advice and the Official Coding Guidelines a reality.

Thanks are also in order for the coding professionals and instructors who were early adopters of this handbook, and who provided many helpful suggestions (and, the author is a tad ashamed to say, corrections) to the early versions of the handbook. Their efforts made this work a better resource for students. Special thanks in this regard are due to Minnette Terlep, Linda Holtzman, Ann Zeisset, Lisa DeLiberto, Margaret Foley, Alicia Reinbolt, Noemi Staniszewski, Pat Poli, and Anne Pavlik.

Finally, Ms. Leon-Chisen wishes to acknowledge the tradition of excellence in coding education established by Faye Brown through the *ICD-9-CM Coding Handbook.* Ms. Brown's work served as the foundation on which the present handbook was built. The author humbly hopes this handbook can continue educating generations of coding professionals as the field implements ICD-10-CM and ICD-10-PCS.

How to Use This Handbook

This edition of the handbook is designed as a versatile resource:

- Textbook for academic programs in health information technology and administration
- Text for in-service training programs
- Self-instructional guide for individuals who would like to learn coding or refresh their skills outside a formal program
- Reference tool for general use in the workplace

The general and basic areas of information covered in chapters 1 through 10 are designed to meet the requirements of various basic courses on the use of ICD-10-CM and ICD-10-PCS. They may also be used as a foundation for moving on to the study of individual chapters of ICD-10-CM and ICD-10-PCS. Chapters 11 through 32 of the handbook include advanced material for both continuing education students and professionals in the field.

This handbook is designed to be used in conjunction with the ICD-10-CM and ICD-10-PCS coding manuals (either in book or PDF format) or comparable software. The ICD-10-CM and ICD-10-PCS classifications must be consulted throughout the learning process, and the material in this text cannot be mastered without using them. The official versions are available in PDF format from the Centers for Disease Control and Prevention (CDC) National Center for Health Statistics (ICD-10-CM) and the Centers for Medicare & Medicaid Services (ICD-10-PCS). Several publishers offer unofficial printed versions. There may be minor variations between the way material is displayed in this handbook and the way it is displayed in printed or digital versions.

The chapters in this handbook are not arranged in the same sequence as the chapters in ICD-10-CM or ICD-10-PCS. The first section of the handbook (chapters 1–11) provides discussions on the format and conventions followed in ICD-10-CM and ICD-10-PCS, as well as basic coding guidelines and introductory material on Z codes and External cause of morbidity codes. The next eight sections (chapters 12–32) progress from the less-complicated ICD-10-CM/PCS chapters to the more difficult. Faculty in academic and in-service programs can rearrange this sequence to suit their particular course outlines.

Appendix A, Coding and Reimbursement, contains basic information on the role of coding with reimbursement models for hospitals, physician practices, and other health care settings.

Appendix B, Reporting of the Present on Admission Indicator, contains information on the reporting of the Medicare requirement associated with the hospital inpatient reporting of all ICD-10-CM diagnosis codes.

Appendix C, Case Summary Exercises, is designed for students who have learned the basic coding principles and need additional practice applying the principles to actual cases. The exercises are geared for students with beginning to intermediate levels of knowledge. The case summaries are based on actual health records of both inpatients and outpatients. The patients described often have multiple conditions that may or may not relate to the current episode of care. Some exercises include several episodes of care for a patient in various settings.

Additional resources for educators are available for download on the AHA Central Office website: www.CodingClinicAdvisor.com. AHA offers materials designed to supplement classroom work and exercises in this handbook. Available materials include slide decks covering the key points of each chapter and exercise test banks. Please visit www.CodingClinicAdvisor.com and register as an educator to download these training materials.

Students using the handbook edition without answers will need to ask their instructors for the answers. After students have completed the exercises, they can check their answers against the instructor's edition, which lists the appropriate codes for each exercise, with the codes for the principal diagnosis and principal procedure sequenced first. Explanatory comments discuss why certain codes are appropriate and others are not and why some conditions listed in the case summaries are not coded at all. The comments also indicate how the principal diagnosis and procedure codes were designated, and which symptoms are inherent to certain conditions and so are not coded separately.

The *ICD-10-CM Official Guidelines for Coding and Reporting* and the *ICD-10-PCS Official Coding Guidelines*, referenced throughout this handbook, may be downloaded from the AHA Central Office website: www.CodingClinicAdvisor.com.

To use this handbook effectively, readers should work through the coding examples provided throughout the text until they fully understand the coding principles under discussion. Readers should be able to arrive at correct code assignments by following the instructions provided and reviewing the pertinent handbook material until it is fully understood. Exercises in the body of each chapter should be completed as they come up in the discussion, rather than at the end of the chapter or section. Most chapters provide a review exercise with additional material that covers the entire chapter. There is also a final review exercise, located before appendix A in this handbook, that offers additional coding practice. Answers to all of these exercises are provided in the edition with answers.

The handbook follows three conventions:

* In some examples, **a hyphen is used at the end of a code to indicate that additional characters are required but cannot be assigned in the example because certain information needed for assignment of these characters is not given.** This is done to emphasize concepts and specific guidelines without going too deeply into specific coding situations.

* **The underlining of codes in text examples indicates correct sequencing;** that is, the underlined code must be sequenced first in that particular combination of codes. When no code is underlined, there is no implicit reason why any of the codes in the series should be sequenced first. In actual coding, of course, other information in the health record may dictate a different sequence. This underlining convention is used in the handbook solely as a teaching device. It is not an element of the ICD-10-CM/PCS coding system.

* In the edition with answers, **the underlining of words in exercise questions indicates the appropriate term to be referenced in using the alphabetic indexes. The underlining of codes in the answer column of the exercises indicates correct code sequencing,** as it does in the examples in the main text.

Changes in Code Usage

Official coding guidelines approved by the four Cooperating Parties responsible for administering the ICD-10-CM and ICD-10-PCS systems in the United States (American Hospital Association, American Health Information Management Association, Centers for Medicare & Medicaid Services, and National Center for Health Statistics) are published on a yearly basis. The fiscal year 2021 (FY 2021) updates to the ICD-10-CM and ICD-10-PCS code sets have been incorporated into this edition of the handbook. The FY 2021 version of the ICD-10-CM and ICD-10-PCS guidelines have been incorporated into this edition as well.

AHA Coding Clinic® for ICD-10-CM and ICD-10-PCS advice published through Second Quarter 2020 has been included in this edition of the handbook.

Format AND Conventions AND Current Coding Practices FOR ICD-10-CM AND ICD-10-PCS

CHAPTER 1

Introduction to the ICD-10-CM Classification

CHAPTER OVERVIEW

- ICD-10-CM is a medical diagnosis classification system.
- The Tabular List of Diseases and Injuries displays codes in alphanumeric order. There are three-, four-, five-, six-, and seven-character codes.
- The Alphabetic Index of Diseases and Injuries uses a specific pattern to the indentions.
  - Main terms are flush to the left-hand margin.
  - Subterms are indented. The more specific the subterm, the farther the indent.
  - Carryover lines are two indents from the indent level of the preceding line.
  - There are also strict alphabetization rules.

LEARNING OUTCOMES

After studying this chapter, you should be able to:

Explain the basic principles of the medical classification system ICD-10-CM.

Demonstrate understanding of the three-, four-, five-, six-, and seven-character subdivisions.

Explain the alphabetization rules and indention patterns.

TERM TO KNOW

ICD-10-CM
International Classification of Diseases, Tenth Revision, Clinical Modification; a medical classification system used for the collection of information regarding disease and injury

INTRODUCTION

The International Classification of Disease, Tenth Revision, Clinical Modification (ICD-10-CM) is a clinical modification of the World Health Organization's (WHO) ICD-10. It expands ICD-10 codes to facilitate more precise coding of clinical diagnoses. ICD-10-CM is a closed classification system—it provides one and only one place to classify each condition. Despite the large number of different conditions to be classified, the system must limit its size to be usable. Certain conditions that occur infrequently or are of low importance are often grouped together in residual codes labeled "other" or "not elsewhere classified." A final residual category is provided for diagnoses not stated specifically enough to permit more precise classification. Occasionally, these two residual groups are combined in one code.

Medical coding professionals must understand the basic principles behind the classification system to use ICD-10-CM appropriately and effectively. This knowledge is also the basis for understanding and applying the official coding advice provided through the *AHA Coding Clinic*®, published by the Central Office of the American Hospital Association. It is important for medical coding professionals in all health care settings to keep current with *the ICD-10-CM Official Guidelines for Coding and Reporting*, as well as the *Coding Clinic*. This official advice is developed through the editorial board for the *Coding Clinic* and is approved by the four cooperating parties: the American Hospital Association (AHA), the American Health Information Management Association (AHIMA), the Centers for Medicare & Medicaid Services (CMS), and the Centers for Disease Control and Prevention's (CDC) National Center for Health Statistics (NCHS). In addition, representatives from several physician specialty groups provide the *Coding Clinic* editorial advisory board with clinical input.

DEVELOPMENT OF ICD-10-CM

ICD-10 was released by WHO in 1993 and contains only diagnosis codes. ICD-10-CM is the clinical modification developed under the leadership of the NCHS for use in the United States. ICD-10-CM was officially implemented in the United States in October 2015. All modifications to ICD-10 need to conform to the WHO conventions for ICD. ICD-10-CM is in the public domain. However, neither the codes nor the code titles may be changed except through the Coordination and Maintenance Process overseen jointly by the CDC and CMS. ICD-10-CM consists of more than 72,000 codes.

FORMAT

ICD-10-CM is divided into the Tabular List and the Alphabetic Index. The Tabular List is an alphanumeric list of codes divided into chapters based on body system or condition. The Index is an alphabetical list of terms and their corresponding codes.

TABULAR LIST OF DISEASES AND INJURIES

The main classification of diseases and injuries in the Tabular List of Diseases and Injuries consists of 22 chapters. (See the table of contents reproduced in figure 1.1.) Approximately half of the first 21 chapters are devoted to conditions that affect a specific body system; the rest classify conditions according to etiology. Chapter 2, for example, classifies neoplasms of all body systems, whereas chapter 10 addresses diseases of the respiratory system only. Chapter 22 is a newly created chapter containing codes for special purposes.

In addition, Z codes represent factors influencing health status and contact with health services that may be recorded as diagnoses. V, W, X, and Y codes are used to indicate the external circumstances responsible for injuries and certain other conditions. V, W, X, Y, and Z codes are

FIGURE 1.1   Table of Contents from ICD-10-CM

Preface

Introduction

ICD-10-CM Conventions

ICD-10-CM Official Guidelines for Coding and Reporting

ICD-10-CM Index to Diseases and Injuries

ICD-10-CM Neoplasm Table

Table of Drugs and Chemicals

ICD-10-CM Index to External Causes

ICD-10-CM Tabular List of Diseases and Injuries

CHAPTER 1—Certain infectious and parasitic diseases

CHAPTER 2—Neoplasms

CHAPTER 3—Diseases of the blood and blood-forming organs and certain
disorders involving the immune mechanism

CHAPTER 4—Endocrine, nutritional and metabolic diseases

CHAPTER 5—Mental, behavioral and neurodevelopmental disorders

CHAPTER 6—Diseases of the nervous system

CHAPTER 7—Diseases of the eye and adnexa

CHAPTER 8—Diseases of the ear and mastoid process

CHAPTER 9—Diseases of the circulatory system

CHAPTER 10—Diseases of the respiratory system

CHAPTER 11—Diseases of the digestive system

CHAPTER 12—Diseases of the skin and subcutaneous tissue

CHAPTER 13—Diseases of the musculoskeletal system and connective tissue

CHAPTER 14—Diseases of the genitourinary system

CHAPTER 15—Pregnancy, childbirth and the puerperium

CHAPTER 16—Certain conditions originating in the perinatal period

CHAPTER 17—Congenital malformations, deformations and chromosomal
abnormalities

CHAPTER 18—Symptoms, signs and abnormal clinical and laboratory findings
not elsewhere classified

CHAPTER 19—Injury, poisoning and certain other consequences of external causes

CHAPTER 20—External causes of morbidity

CHAPTER 21—Factors influencing health status and contact with health services

CHAPTER 22

reviewed briefly in chapter 12 of this handbook and in more detail in the chapters discussing the conditions to which they apply.

The variation in chapter titles in ICD-10-CM's table of contents represents the compromises made during the development of a statistical classification system based partially on etiology, partially on anatomical site, and partially on the circumstances of onset. The result is a classification system based on multiple axes. In contrast, a single-axis classification would be based entirely on the etiology of the disease, the anatomical site of the disease, or the nature of the disease process.

Codes in the Tabular List appear in alphanumeric order. References from the Alphabetic Index to the Tabular List are by code number, not by page number. Code numbers and titles appear in bold type in the Tabular List. Instructional notes that apply to the section, category, or subcategory are also included in the Tabular List.

Code Structure

All ICD-10-CM codes have an alphanumeric structure, with all codes starting with an alphabetical character. The basic code structure consists of three characters. A decimal point is used to separate the basic three-character category code from its subcategory and subclassifications (for example, L98.491). Most ICD-10-CM codes contain a maximum of six characters, with a few categories having a seventh-character code value.

Each chapter in the main classification is structured to provide the following subdivisions:

- Sections (groups of three-character categories), e.g., Infections of the skin and subcutaneous tissue (L00–L08)

- Categories (three-character code numbers), e.g., L02, Cutaneous abscess, furuncle and carbuncle

- Subcategories (four-character code numbers), e.g., L02.2, Cutaneous abscess, furuncle and carbuncle of trunk

- Fifth-, sixth-, or seventh-character subclassifications (five-, six-, or seven-character code numbers), e.g., L02.211, Cutaneous abscess of abdominal wall

The ICD-10-CM Tabular List contains categories, subcategories, and codes. The basic code used to classify a particular disease or injury consists of three characters and is called a category (e.g., K29, Gastritis and duodenitis). Characters for categories, subcategories, and codes may be either a letter or a number. All categories are three characters. A three-character category that has no further subdivision is equivalent to a code. Subcategories are either four or five characters. Codes may be three, four, five, six, or seven characters. That is, each level of subdivision after a category is a subcategory. The final level of subdivision is a code.

Codes that have applicable seventh characters are still referred to as codes, not subcategories. A code that has an applicable seventh character is considered invalid without the seventh character.

For example:

- K29   Gastritis and duodenitis   *(category)*
  - K29.0   Acute gastritis   *(subcategory)*
    - K29.00   Acute gastritis without bleeding   *(code)*

- R10   Abdominal and pelvic pain   *(category)*
  - R10.8   Other abdominal pain   *(subcategory)*
    - R10.81   Abdominal tenderness   *(subcategory)*
      - R10.811   Right upper quadrant abdominal tenderness   *(code)*

Placeholder Character

ICD-10-CM uses the letter "x" as a placeholder character at certain codes to allow for future expansion. An example of this may be seen at the poisoning, adverse effect, underdosing (T36–T50), and toxic effects (T51–T65) codes. For these categories, the sixth character represents the intent: accidental, intentional self-harm, assault, undetermined, adverse effect, or underdosing. Where a placeholder exists, the "x" must be used for the code to be considered valid.

For example, "x" is used as the fifth character in the following codes where the sixth character of "1" represents accidental, and "2" represents intentional self-harm:

T37.5x1   Poisoning by antiviral drugs, accidental (unintentional)
T37.5x2   Poisoning by antiviral drugs, intentional self-harm
T52.0x1   Toxic effect of petroleum products, accidental (unintentional)
T52.0x2   Toxic effect of petroleum products, intentional self-harm

Certain categories have an additional seventh-character value. The applicable seventh-character value is required for all codes within the category, or as the notes in the Tabular List instruct. The seventh-character value must always be the seventh character in the code. If a code is not a full six characters, a placeholder character "x" must be used to fill in the empty characters when a seventh-character value is required. Seventh-character values can be seen in chapter 15 of ICD-10-CM, Pregnancy, Childbirth and the Puerperium (O00–O9A), as well as in chapter 19 of ICD-10-CM, Injury, Poisoning and Certain Other Consequences of External Causes (S00–T88), and in chapter 20 of ICD-10-CM, External Causes of Morbidity (V00–V99).

An example of the use of the placeholder character "x" and the seventh-character value is shown here with an excerpt from the Tabular List:

T16   **Foreign body in ear**
Includes: foreign body in auditory canal

The appropriate 7th character values are to be added to each code from category T16:

       A   initial encounter
       D   subsequent encounter
       S   sequela

T16.1   **Foreign body in right ear**
T16.2   **Foreign body in left ear**
T16.9   **Foreign body in ear, unspecified ear**

A child presents to the emergency department with a bean in the right ear. The mother has brought the child because she was not able to remove the bean at home. This encounter would be assigned code T16.1xxA. The Tabular List shows subcategory T16.1 as the descriptor best fitting this scenario. Category T16 requires a seventh-character value. Because the code subcategory has only four characters (T16.1), the placeholder "x" is inserted twice to preserve the code structure before the seventh character "A" is added to report this as the initial encounter.

ALPHABETIC INDEX

The Alphabetic Index consists of the Index of Diseases and Injuries, the Index to External Causes, the Neoplasm Table, and the Table of Drugs and Chemicals.

The Alphabetic Index includes entries for main terms, subterms, and more specific subterms. An indented format is used for ease of reference.

Main terms identify disease conditions or injuries. Subterms indicate site, type, or etiology for conditions or injuries. For example, acute appendicitis is listed under **Appendicitis,** acute, and stress fracture is listed under **Fracture, traumatic,** stress. Occasionally, it is necessary to think of a synonym or another alternative term in order to locate the correct entry. There are, however, exceptions to this general rule, including the following:

- Congenital conditions are often indexed under the main term **Anomaly** rather than under the name of the condition.
- Conditions that complicate pregnancy, childbirth, or the puerperium are usually found under such terms as **Delivery, Pregnancy,** and **Puerperal.** They may also appear under the main term for the condition causing the complication by referencing the subterm "complicating childbirth (labor)," "complicating pregnancy," or "complicating puerperium." (Examples of these types of entries appear under the main term **Hypertension** in the Alphabetic Index.)
- Many of the complications of medical or surgical care are indexed under the term **Complications** rather than under the name of the condition.
- Late effects of an earlier condition can be found under **Sequelae,** or under the condition (as in the case of traumatic injuries).

A clear understanding of the format of the Alphabetic Index is a prerequisite for accurate coding. Understanding the indention pattern of the entries is a very important part of learning how to use the Index. A variety of vendors provide printed versions and others have computer programs for coding, but the format may not be consistent across versions. The PDF version of the Index from the NCHS represents each indention level by a hyphen. In general, however, the following pattern is used by several codebook publishers:

- Main terms are set flush with the left-hand margin. They are printed in bold type and begin with a capital letter.
- Subterms are indented one standard indention (equivalent to about two word-processing spaces) to the right under the main term. They are printed in regular type and begin with a lowercase letter.
- More specific subterms are indented farther and farther to the right as needed, always indented by one standard indention from the preceding subterm and listed in alphabetical order.
- A dash (-) at the end of an index entry indicates that additional characters are required.

Carryover lines are indented two standard indentions from the level of the preceding line. Carryover lines are used only when the complete entry cannot fit on a single line. They are indented farther to avoid confusion with subterm entries.

In printed versions, entries are presented in two, three, or four columns per page, dictionary style.

The subterms listed under the main term **Metrorrhagia** in the following entry provide an example:

Metrorrhagia N92.1	[main term]
climacteric N92.4	[subterm]
menopausal N92.4	[subterm]
postpartum NEC (atonic) (following delivery	[subterm]
of placenta) O72.1	[carryover line]
delayed or secondary O72.2	[more specific subterm]
preclimacteric or premenopausal N92.4	[subterm]
psychogenic F45.8	[subterm]

Each of the subterms (climacteric, menopausal, postpartum, preclimacteric, and psychogenic) is indented one standard indention from the level of the main term and is listed in alphabetical order. The fifth line is a carryover line set two standard indentions from the preceding line. The sixth line is a more specific entry ("delayed or secondary" under the subterm "postpartum").

EXERCISE 1.1

A reproduction of a page from the Alphabetic Index is shown below. Label the numbered lines as either main terms, subterms, or carryover lines. Each hyphen is meant to represent one level of indention.

---

1. **Railroad neurosis** F48.8

---

2. **Railway spine** F48.8

Raised—see also Elevated
3. --antibody titer R76.0

Rake teeth, tooth M26.39
Rales R09.89
4. **Ramifying renal pelvis** Q63.8

Ramsay-Hunt disease or syndrome—(see also
5. --Hunt's disease) B02.21

---

6. -meaning dyssynergia cerebellaris myoclonica G11.1
Ranula K11.6
-congenital Q38.4

---

7. **Rape**

---

8. -adult
--confirmed T74.21
--suspected T76.21
-alleged, observation or examination, ruled out

---

9. --adult Z04.41
--child Z04.42

---

10. -child
--confirmed T74.22
--suspected T76.22

Alphabetization Rules

To locate main terms and subterms quickly and efficiently, it is important to understand the alphabetization rules followed in the Alphabetic Index. Letter-by-letter alphabetization is used. The system of alphabetization ignores the following:

- Single spaces between words
- Single hyphens within words
- The final "s" in the possessive forms of words

The following list shows an example of letter-by-letter alphabetization with these modifications:

Beckwith-Wiedemann syndrome Q87.3	[ignores hyphen]
Beer drinker's heart (disease) I42.6	[ignores space between words]
Blood-forming organs, disease D75.9	[ignores hyphen]
Bloodgood's disease—see **Mastopathy**, cystic	[ignores possessive form]

Numerical Entries

Subterm entries that contain numerical characters or words indicating numbers are the first entries under the appropriate main term or subterm. Subterm entries are listed in alphabetical order when they include numbers written in their spelled-out form. For example, **Paralysis,** nerve, fourth, comes before, rather than after, **Paralysis,** nerve, third.

There are two different patterns for displaying numerical entries, depending on the book publisher or software used. One version arranges Roman numerals (such as "II") and Arabic numerals (such as "2") in numerical order (for example, I, II, III, IV, V, VI, VII, VIII, IX, X, and so forth). However, the official government version arranges Roman numerals as letters in alphabetical order, as shown in the following example (each hyphen below represents one level of indention):

Deficiency . . .

factor

--Hageman D68.2

--I (congenital) (hereditary) D68.2

--II (congenital) (hereditary) D68.2

--IX (congenital) (functional) (hereditary) (with functional defect) D67

--multiple (congenital) D68.8

---acquired D68.4

--V (congenital) (hereditary) D68.2

--VII (congenital) (hereditary) D68.2

--VIII (congenital) (functional) (hereditary) (with functional defect) D66

---with vascular defect D68.0

--X (congenital) (hereditary) D68.2

--XI (congenital) (hereditary) D68.1

--XII (congenital) (hereditary) D68.2

--XIII (congenital) (hereditary) D68.2

Connecting Words

Words such as "with," "in," "due to," and "associated with" are used to express the relationship between the main term and a subterm (or between the subterm and a sub-subterm); these words indicate an associated condition or etiology. Subterms preceded by "with" or "without" are not listed in alphabetical order in the version of the Index from NCHS. Such subterms appear immediately below the main term or any appropriate subterm entries. Coding professionals who fail to remember this feature of the alphabetization rules often make coding errors by overlooking the appropriate subterm. Please note that some publishers and encoder software vendors have deviated from this practice and listed the subterms "with" and "without" in alphabetical order. Review the following subterm entries under the main term **Bronchitis** using the instructions at the end of this example. Note that each hyphen represents one level of indention:

Bronchitis (diffuse) (fibrinous) (hypostatic) (infective) (membranous) J40

1 -with
--influenza, flu or grippe—see Influenza, with respiratory manifestations NEC

2 --obstruction (airway) (lung) J44.9

3 --tracheitis (15 years of age and above) J40
---acute or subacute J20.9
---chronic J42
---under 15 years of age J20.9

4 -acute or subacute (with bronchospasm or obstruction) J20.9

5 --with
---bronchiectasis J47.0
---chronic obstructive pulmonary disease J44.0

6 --chemical (due to gases, fumes or vapors) J68.0

7 --due to
---fumes or vapors J68.0
---*Haemophilus influenzae* J20.1
---*Mycoplasma pneumoniae* J20.0
---radiation J70.0
---specified organism NEC J20.8
---*Streptococcus* J20.2
---virus
----coxsackie J20.3
----echovirus J20.7
----parainfluenzae J20.4
----respiratory syncytial J20.5
----rhinovirus J20.6
--viral NEC J20.8

8 -allergic (acute) J45.909

9 --with
---exacerbation (acute) J45.901
---status asthmaticus J45.902

10 -arachidic T17.528

Refer to sections 1, 4, 8, and 10 as indicated in the example. Note that the subterms preceded by the connecting word "with" immediately follow the main term **Bronchitis** and precede the subterms beginning with the letter "a" (sections 4, 8, and 10).

Refer to sections 5, 6, and 7 as indicated in the example. Note that the more specific subterms preceded by the connecting word "with" immediately follow the subterm "acute or subacute." In this case, the subterms beginning with the word "with" precede the subterms beginning with the letters "c" and "d" (sections 6 and 7).

Also note that the subterms indented under the connecting word "with" are listed in alphabetical order. For example, sections 1, 2, and 3 indicated in the example are in alphabetical order.

Index Tables

The main body of the Alphabetic Index uses a table for the systematic arrangement of subterms under the main entry **Neoplasm.** This table simplifies access to complex combinations of subterms. The location of the Neoplasm Table will vary in printed editions of the codebook, depending on the publisher. It may be found following the Index entry **Neoplasm** or following the Alphabetic Index and before the Table for Drugs and Chemicals. The use of this table is discussed in chapter 29 of this handbook. The Table of Drugs and Chemicals is discussed in chapter 32 of this handbook.

The format and alphabetization rules used within the tables are the same as those followed in the rest of the Alphabetic Index. Although the uses of these two tables are discussed in detail later in this handbook, it is useful for the reader to become familiar with the location and format of the tables at this point in the discussion.

CHAPTER 2
ICD-10-CM Conventions

CHAPTER OVERVIEW

- A variety of notes appear in ICD-10-CM.

  — *General notes* commonly provide general information on usage in a specific section.

  — *Inclusion notes* and *exclusion notes* indicate when certain conditions are or are not included in a subdivision.

  — Additional instructional notes direct the coding professional to create a complete statement on the condition.

- Two main abbreviations (NEC and NOS) are used in ICD-10-CM.

- Cross-reference notes advise the coding professional to look elsewhere before assigning a code.

- Punctuation marks and relational terms have specialized meanings in ICD-10-CM.

LEARNING OUTCOMES

After studying this chapter, you should be able to:

List the different types of instructional notes.

Explain the importance of additional notes to the coding process.

Describe the difference between the abbreviations NEC and NOS.

Use your knowledge of cross-reference notes to navigate ICD-10-CM.

Define the specialized meanings of punctuation marks and relational terms in ICD-10-CM.

TERMS TO KNOW

NEC
not elsewhere classified; used in the Alphabetic Index to indicate that there is no separate code for the condition even though the diagnostic statement is specific

NOS
not otherwise specified; equivalent to the term "unspecified"

REMEMBER . . .

These conventions are not just helpful; they are necessary to successful coding.

INTRODUCTION

ICD-10-CM follows certain conventions to provide large amounts of information in a succinct and consistent manner. A thorough understanding of these conventions is fundamental to accurate coding. The conventions and instructions of the classification are applicable to all health care settings, unless otherwise indicated.

ICD-10-CM conventions include the following:

- Instructional notes
- Abbreviations
- Cross-reference notes
- Punctuation marks
- Relational terms ("and," "with," "without," "due to")

INSTRUCTIONAL NOTES

A variety of notes appear as instructions to the coding professional. These include general notes, inclusion and exclusion notes, "code first" notes, "use additional code" notes, and "code also" notes.

General Notes

General notes in the Tabular List of Diseases and Injuries provide general information on usage in a specific section, such as the note under chapter 15 of ICD-10-CM, Pregnancy, Childbirth and the Puerperium, that explains that codes from this chapter are for use only on maternal records, never on newborn records.

Inclusion and Exclusion Notes

Codes in a classification system must be mutually exclusive, with no overlapping of content. In ICD-10-CM, therefore, it is sometimes necessary to indicate when certain conditions are or are not included in a given subdivision. This is accomplished by means of inclusion and exclusion notes.

The location of inclusion and exclusion notes is extremely important. When this type of note is located at the beginning of a chapter or a section in ICD-10-CM, that advice applies to all codes within the chapter or section and is not repeated with individual categories or specific codes. Keep in mind that instructional notes affecting the code under consideration may be located on a previous page.

Inclusion Notes

Inclusion notes are introduced by the word "includes" when placed at the beginning of a chapter or section. Inclusion notes are used to further define, or give examples of, the content of the chapter, section, or category. Conditions listed in an inclusion note may be synonyms or conditions similar enough to be classified to the same code. Inclusion notes are not exhaustive; rather, they list certain conditions to reassure the coding professional, particularly when the title in the Tabular List may not seem to apply.

An example of an inclusion note can be found in the Tabular List, chapter 1, Certain Infectious and Parasitic Diseases (A00–B99). The inclusion note states that this chapter includes diseases generally recognized as communicable or transmissible. This note applies to all codes listed from A00 through B99.

Inclusion notes may also appear immediately under a three-character code title to further define, or give examples of, the content of the category. An example of this type of inclusion note can be found in the Tabular List at category D50, Iron deficiency anemia. The inclusion note states that codes in this category include asiderotic anemia and hypochromic anemia.

Inclusion Terms

Lists of terms are included under some codes. The terms are some of the conditions that may be reported with those codes. The terms may be synonyms for the code title. In the case of "other specified codes," the terms may be a list of the various conditions that are assigned to that code. As in the case of the inclusion notes, the list of inclusion terms is not meant to be exhaustive. The Index may also list additional terms classified to a code that are not repeated as inclusion terms.

Exclusion Notes

Exclusion notes are introduced by the word "excludes." Excluded conditions are listed in alphabetical order, with the code number or code range shown in parentheses. Exclusion notes are the opposite of inclusion notes; they indicate that a particular condition is not assigned to the code to which the note applies. The basic message of an excludes note is "code this condition elsewhere."

There are two types of exclusion notes in ICD-10-CM—each has a different use, but both indicate that codes excluded are independent of each other.

"Excludes1"

An "excludes1" note means "NOT CODED HERE!" An "excludes1" note instructs that the code excluded should never be used at the same time as the code above the "excludes1" note. This instruction is used when two conditions cannot occur together and therefore both codes cannot be used together. For example:

Q03   Congenital hydrocephalus
Excludes1: acquired hydrocephalus (G91.-)

In this example, the congenital form of the condition cannot be reported with the acquired form of the same condition.

There is an exception to the "excludes1" definition when the two conditions are unrelated to each other. For example, code **F45.8, Other somatoform disorders,** has an "excludes1" note for "sleep related teeth grinding" (G47.63) because "teeth grinding" is an inclusion term under F45.8. Only one of these two codes should be assigned for teeth grinding. However, psychogenic dysmenorrhea is also an inclusion term under F45.8, and a patient could have both this condition and sleep-related teeth grinding. In this case, the two conditions are clearly unrelated to each other, and so it would be appropriate to report F45.8 and G47.63 together. If it is not clear whether the two conditions involving an "excludes1" note are related or not, query the provider.

When applying the "excludes1" note instruction for two related conditions, assign only the code referenced in the "excludes1" note. For example, in the Tabular List, an "excludes1" note below code **I96, Gangrene, not elsewhere classified,** excludes "gangrene in other peripheral vascular diseases (I73.-)." This note should be interpreted to mean gangrene documented with another peripheral vascular disease is not coded here. Instead, code I73.- should be assigned for gangrene in other peripheral vascular disease.

"Excludes2"

An "excludes2" note means "NOT INCLUDED HERE!" An "excludes2" note instructs that the condition excluded is not part of the condition represented by the code. However, a patient may have both conditions at the same time. When an "excludes2" note appears under a code, it is acceptable to use both the code and the excluded code together. For example:

> **F90   Attention-deficit hyperactivity disorders**
> Excludes2: anxiety disorders (F40.-, F41.-)
> mood [affective] disorders (F30–F39)

In this example, the "excludes2" note serves as a warning that if a patient has an anxiety disorder, rather than attention-deficit hyperactivity disorder, the user should go to categories F40–F41 rather than remain in category F90. However, if a patient has both attention-deficit hyperactivity and an anxiety disorder, a code from category F90 could be used along with a code from categories F40–F41.

"Code First" and "Use Additional Code"

Certain conditions have both an underlying etiology and multiple body system manifestations due to the underlying etiology. In the Tabular List, "code first" and "use additional code" instructional notes indicate the proper sequencing order of these conditions—etiology (underlying condition) followed by manifestation. The "use additional code" note is found at the etiology code as a clue to identify the manifestations commonly associated with the disease. The "code first" note is found at the manifestation code to provide instructions that the underlying condition, if present, should be sequenced first.

The manifestation codes usually have the phrase "in diseases classified elsewhere" as part of the code title. Codes with this phrase are never used as a first-listed or principal diagnosis code. For such codes, a "use additional code" note appears at the etiology code, and a "code first" note appears at the manifestation code. An example of this convention is category F02, Dementia in other diseases classified elsewhere.

Other notes of this type provide a list introduced by the phrase "such as," meaning that any of the listed codes or any other appropriate code can be assigned first. Code **J99, Respiratory disorders in diseases classified elsewhere,** provides a list of conditions that may be the underlying disease.

It is not necessary to report the code identified in a "use additional code" note in the diagnosis field immediately following the primary code. There is no strict hierarchy inherent in the guidelines, nor in the ICD-10-CM classification, regarding the sequencing of secondary diagnosis codes.

"Code Also"

"Code also" notes in ICD-10-CM indicate that two codes may be required to fully describe a condition. This note does not provide sequencing direction. The sequencing order will depend on the circumstances of admission (i.e., reason for the encounter). An example of this note can be found under code **G47.01, Insomnia due to medical condition,** where the instructional note tells us to code also the associated medical condition.

ABBREVIATIONS

ICD-10-CM uses two main abbreviations:

- NEC, for "not elsewhere classified"
- NOS, for "not otherwise specified"

Although their meanings appear simple, these abbreviations are often misunderstood and misapplied. It is very important to understand not only their meanings but also their differences, because they provide guidance for correct code selection.

NEC

The abbreviation NEC is used in the Alphabetic Index and the Tabular List to indicate that there is no separate code for the condition, even though the diagnostic statement may be very specific. NEC is used when the information in the medical record provides detail for which a specific code does not exist. It represents "other specified." In the Tabular List, such conditions are ordinarily classified to a code with a fourth or sixth character 8 (or a fifth character 9) with a title that includes the words "other specified" or "not elsewhere classified," which permits the grouping of related conditions to conserve space and limit the size of the classification system. For example, a disease of the pleura specified as hydropneumothorax is included in code **J94.8, Other specified pleural conditions.**

NOS

The abbreviation NOS is the equivalent of "unspecified" and is used in the Alphabetic Index and the Tabular List. Codes so identified are to be used only when neither the diagnostic statement nor the medical record provides information that permits classification to a more specific code. The codes in these cases are ordinarily classified to codes with a fourth or sixth character 9 (or a fifth character 0). Conditions listed as both "not elsewhere classified" and "unspecified" are sometimes combined in one code.

Note that a main term followed by a list of subterms in the Alphabetic Index usually displays the unspecified code; the subterms must always be reviewed to determine whether a more specific code can be assigned. For example, in the Index, the main term **Cardiomyopathy** displays code I42.9. Subterms such as "alcoholic" or "congestive" are provided for more specific cardiomyopathies. Code I42.9 should be assigned only when there is no information in the medical record to identify one of these subterms.

CROSS-REFERENCE NOTES

Cross-reference notes are used in the Alphabetic Index to advise the coding professional to look elsewhere before assigning a code. The cross-reference instructions include "see," "see also," "see category," and "see condition."

"See"

The "see" cross-reference indicates that the user must refer to an alternative term. This instruction is mandatory; coding cannot be completed without following this advice. For example, the entry for **Hemarthrosis,** traumatic, uses a "see" cross-reference to advise the user to reference the entry for **Sprain,** by site.

"See Also"

The "see also" cross-reference advises the coding professional that there is another place in the Alphabetic Index that must be checked when the entries under consideration do not provide a code for the specific condition or procedure. It is not necessary to follow this cross-reference when the original entries provide all the information necessary.

For example, the cross-reference for the term **Psychoneurosis** advises the user to "see also Neurosis" when none of the specific subterms provides a code. To locate the code for neurasthenic psychoneurosis, it would not be necessary to follow this cross-reference because there is a subterm "neurasthenic" under the term **Psychoneurosis.** However, if the diagnosis were psychasthenic psychoneurosis, the code could be located only by following the "see also" reference to the term **Neurosis** and then looking for the subterm "psychasthenic."

"See Category"

The "see category" variation of the "see" cross-reference provides the three-character alphanumeric identifier for a category. The coding professional must refer to that category in the Tabular List and select a code from the options provided there. For example, a cross-reference under the Index entry for main term **Mononeuropathy,** subterm "in diseases classified elsewhere," refers the user to category G59.

"See Condition"

Occasionally, the Index advises the user to refer to the main term of a condition. For example, when a user looks up the main term **Arterial** to find the code for arterial thrombosis, the Index advice is to "see condition." Therefore, the user should then go to the main term **Thrombosis.** This cross-reference ordinarily appears when the adjective rather than the term (in noun form) has been referenced for the condition itself.

PUNCTUATION MARKS

Several punctuation marks are used in ICD-10-CM, most of which have a specialized meaning in addition to the usual English language usage.

Parentheses

Parentheses are used in ICD-10-CM to enclose supplementary words or explanatory information that may be either present or absent in the statement of diagnosis without affecting the code to which it is assigned. Such terms are considered to be "nonessential modifiers" and are used to suggest that the terms in parentheses are included in the code but need not be stated in the diagnosis. This is a significant factor in correct code assignment. Terms enclosed in parentheses in either the Tabular List or the Alphabetic Index do not affect the code assignment in any way; they serve only as reassurance that the correct code has been located.

For example, refer to the main term **Pneumonia,** which has several nonessential modifiers enclosed in parentheses. Unless a more specific subterm is located, this code will be assigned for pneumonia described by any of the terms in parentheses. Diagnoses of acute pneumonia and purulent pneumonia, for example, are both coded J18.9 because both terms appear in parentheses as nonessential modifiers. Pneumonia not otherwise specified is also assigned to code J18.9 because none of the terms in parentheses is required for this code assignment.

It is important to distinguish between the use of nonessential and essential modifiers. Essential modifiers are listed as subterms in the Alphabetic Index, not in parentheses, and they do affect code assignment. In contrast, words in parentheses are nonessential and do not affect the code assignment. For example, scoliosis described as acquired or postural is classified as M41.9, as the words "acquired" and "postural" are nonessential modifiers and do not affect the code; on the other hand, the term "congenital" is an essential modifier, and the code for this term is Q67.5.

The nonessential modifiers in the Index to Diseases apply to subterms following a main term, except when a nonessential modifier and a subentry are mutually exclusive, in which case the subentry takes precedence. For example, in ICD-10-CM's Alphabetic Index under the main term **Enteritis,** "acute" is a nonessential modifier, and "chronic" is a subentry. In this case, the nonessential modifier "acute" does not apply to the subentry "chronic."

EXERCISE 2.1

Referring only to the title and inclusion notes for code J40, mark an "X" next to each of the diagnostic statements listed below that is included in code J40.

1. Catarrhal bronchitis _____

2. Chronic bronchitis _____

3. Allergic bronchitis _____

4. Tracheobronchitis NOS _____

5. Asthmatic bronchitis _____

Square Brackets

Square brackets are often used in the Tabular List to enclose synonyms, alternative wordings, abbreviations, and explanatory phrases that provide additional information—for example, human immunodeficiency virus [HIV]. They are similar to parentheses in that the bracketed words are not required for the statement of diagnosis.

Square brackets are also used around codes. In this usage, the brackets indicate that the code inside the brackets can only be a manifestation code. Preceding the code in brackets will be another code, which must be assigned first for the underlying condition. The code in the brackets in this situation indicates that both conditions must be assigned, and the code in the brackets can never be assigned as the principal diagnosis. In the following example from the Alphabetic Index, the first code represents an underlying disease, and the second code enclosed in brackets represents a manifestation:

Nephropathy . . .
    sickle-cell D57.- [N08]

Colons

Colons are used in the Tabular List in both inclusion notes and exclusion notes after an incomplete term that needs one or more of the modifiers following the colon in order for the term to apply. The exclusion statement under code N92.6 in the Tabular List is an example of this usage. Here, the colon following the subterm "irregular menstruation with" indicates that if the condition is described as irregular menstruation with lengthened intervals or scanty bleeding, or irregular menstruation with shortened intervals or excessive bleeding, code N92.6 is excluded.

N92.6   Irregular menstruation, unspecified
    Irregular bleeding NOS
    Irregular periods NOS
    Excludes1: irregular menstruation with:
            lengthened intervals or scanty bleeding (N91.3–N91.5)
            shortened intervals or excessive bleeding (N92.1)

EXERCISE 2.2

Referring only to the title and inclusion notes provided for the four-character code D04.5, mark an "X" next to each diagnosis listed below that is included in code D04.5.

1. Carcinoma in situ of anal margin   _____

2. Carcinoma in situ of perianal skin   _____

3. Carcinoma in situ of skin of breast   _____

4. Carcinoma in situ of breast   _____

5. Carcinoma in situ of anal skin   _____

RELATIONAL TERMS

"And"

The word "and" should be interpreted to mean either "and" or "or" when it appears in a code title. For example, cases of "tuberculosis of bones," "tuberculosis of joints," and "tuberculosis of bones and joints" are classified to subcategory A18.0, Tuberculosis of bones and joints.

"With" and "In"

The words "with" and "in" should be interpreted to mean "associated with" or "due to" when they appear in a code title, the Alphabetic Index (either under a main term or subterm), or an instructional note in the Tabular List. The classification presumes a causal relationship between the two conditions linked by these terms in the Alphabetic Index or the Tabular List. These conditions should be coded as related even in the absence of provider documentation explicitly linking them, unless the documentation clearly states the conditions are unrelated, or unless another guideline exists that specifically requires a documented linkage between two conditions (for example, a sepsis guideline for "acute organ dysfunction that is not clearly associated with the sepsis"). If conditions are not specifically linked by these relational terms in the classification, or if a guideline requires that a linkage between two conditions be explicitly documented, provider documentation must link the conditions in order for them to be coded as related. The word "with" in the Alphabetic Index is sequenced immediately following the main term or subterm and is not in alphabetical order.

The following example from the Alphabetic Index for the main term **Diabetes** and the subterm "with" demonstrates the linkage between conditions:

Diabetes, diabetic (mellitus) (sugar) E11.9

-with

--amyotrophy E11.44

--arthropathy NEC E11.618

--autonomic (poly) neuropathy E11.43

--cataract E11.36

--Charcot's joints E11.610

--chronic kidney disease E11.22

The diagnoses of diabetes and chronic kidney disease are coded as **E11.22, Type 2 diabetes mellitus with diabetic chronic kidney disease.** This link can be assumed because chronic kidney disease is listed under the subterm "with."

The following example from the Alphabetic Index for the main term **Anemia** and the subterm "in" demonstrates the linkage between conditions:

> **Anemia** (essential) (general) (hemoglobin deficiency) (infantile) (primary) (profound) D64.9
>
> -in (due to) (with)
>
> --chronic kidney disease D63.1
>
> --end stage renal disease D63.1
>
> --failure, kidney (renal) D63.1
>
> --neoplastic disease (*see also* Neoplasm) D63.0

The diagnoses of anemia and chronic kidney disease are coded as **D63.1, Anemia in chronic kidney disease.** This linkage can be assumed because the chronic kidney disease is listed under the subterm "in (due to) (with)."

"Due To"

The words "due to" in either the Alphabetic Index or the Tabular List indicate that a causal relationship between two conditions is present. ICD-10-CM occasionally makes such an assumption when both conditions are present. For example, certain conditions affecting the mitral valve are assumed to be rheumatic in origin, regardless of whether or not the diagnostic statement specifies this causal relationship. However, for other combinations of conditions, a causal relationship should not be presumed if it is not indicated in the diagnostic statement. When the physician's statement indicates a causal relationship, the coding professional should locate the subterm "due to" under the relevant term in the Alphabetic Index to select the appropriate code to look up in the Tabular List.

CHAPTER 3

Uniform Hospital Discharge Data Set

CHAPTER OVERVIEW

- The Uniform Hospital Discharge Data Set (UHDDS) is used for reporting inpatient data.
- The following items are always found in the UHDDS:
  — General demographic information
  — Expected payer
  — Hospital identification
  — Principal diagnosis
  — Other diagnoses that have specific significance
  — All significant procedures
- The rules for identifying the first-listed diagnosis for an outpatient encounter differ from those for selecting the principal diagnosis for an inpatient encounter.
- Following all the coding guidelines will ensure accurate and ethical coding.

LEARNING OUTCOMES

After studying this chapter, you should be able to:

Correctly identify a principal diagnosis.

Understand the guidelines for assigning a principal diagnosis.

Understand when other diagnoses have significance and should be reported.

Explain the difference between a principal diagnosis and an admitting diagnosis.

Explain the importance of accurate and ethical coding.

TERMS TO KNOW

MS-DRG system
Medicare Severity Diagnosis-Related Group system; a patient classification system used in hospital inpatient reimbursement

Other reportable diagnoses
conditions that coexist with the principal diagnosis at the time of admission, develop subsequently, or affect patient care during the hospital stay

Principal diagnosis
the condition established after study that is chiefly responsible for admission of the patient to the hospital

UHDDS
Uniform Hospital Discharge Data Set; information used for reporting inpatient data

REMEMBER . . .

The admitting diagnosis is not an element of the UHDDS. Diagnoses that have no impact on patient care or that are related to an earlier episode are not reported on the UHDDS.

INTRODUCTION

The Uniform Hospital Discharge Data Set (UHDDS) is used for reporting inpatient data in acute care, short-term care, and long-term care hospitals. It uses a minimum set of items based on standard definitions that could provide consistent data for multiple users. Only those items that meet the following criteria have been included in the UHDDS:

- Easily identified
- Readily defined
- Uniformly recorded
- Easily abstracted from the medical record

Its use is required for claims reporting for Medicare and Medicaid patients. In addition, many other health care payers use most of the UHDDS as a uniform billing system.

DATA ITEMS

The UHDDS requires the following items:

- Principal diagnosis
- Other diagnoses that have significance for the specific hospital episode
- All significant procedures

The four cooperating parties responsible for developing and maintaining ICD-10-CM (the American Hospital Association, the American Health Information Management Association, the Centers for Medicare & Medicaid Services, and the Centers for Disease Control and Prevention's National Center for Health Statistics) have developed official guidelines for designating the principal diagnosis and for identifying other diagnoses that should be reported in certain situations. The UHDDS also contains a core of general information that pertains to the patient and to the specific episode of care, such as the age, sex, and race of the patient; the expected payer; and the hospital's identification.

The UHDDS definitions were originally developed in 1985 for hospital reporting of inpatient data elements. Since that time, the application of UHDDS definitions has been expanded to include all nonoutpatient settings. In addition to their application to acute care, short-term care, and long-term care hospitals, the definitions for principal diagnosis and other (secondary) diagnoses also apply to psychiatric hospitals, home health agencies, rehabilitation facilities, nursing homes, hospice, and other settings. Nearly all guidelines discussed below for selection of the principal diagnosis and other diagnoses apply to all these settings. Please note that one exception is the guideline regarding coding of an uncertain (unconfirmed) diagnosis (a diagnosis documented at the time of discharge as "probable," "suspected," "likely," "questionable," "possible," "compatible with," "consistent with," or "still to be ruled out," or another similar term indicating uncertainty) as if the condition existed or were established. The guideline regarding uncertain diagnosis applies only to inpatient admissions to acute care, short-term care, long-term care, and psychiatric hospitals. Coding of uncertain (unconfirmed) diagnoses is discussed in more detail in chapter 7 of this handbook.

Principal Diagnosis

The principal diagnosis is defined as the condition established after study to be chiefly responsible for admission of the patient to the hospital for care. It is important that the principal diagnosis be designated correctly because its establishment is significant in cost comparisons, in care analysis, and in utilization review. Accurate designation of the principal diagnosis is crucial for reimbursement because many third-party payers (including Medicare) base reimbursement primarily on the principal diagnosis. The principal diagnosis is ordinarily, but not always, listed first in the physician's diagnostic statement; the entire medical record must be reviewed to determine the condition that should be designated as the principal diagnosis.

The words "after study" in the definition of principal diagnosis are important, but their meaning is sometimes confusing. In many cases, it is not the admitting diagnosis but rather the diagnosis found after workup, or even after surgery, that proves to be the reason for admission. For example:

- A patient admitted with urinary retention may prove to have hypertrophy of the prostate, which is causing the urinary retention. In this case, the prostatic hypertrophy is the principal diagnosis unless treatment was directed only to the urinary retention.

- A patient is admitted because of chronic cough, difficulty with breathing, and malaise; a bronchoscopy with biopsy is performed for a lung mass. The mass is confirmed to be adenocarcinoma of the lung. In this case, the lung adenocarcinoma is the principal diagnosis because, after study, it is determined to be the underlying cause of the patient's malaise and respiratory symptoms as well as the reason for admission.

- A patient is admitted with severe abdominal pain. The white blood cell count is elevated to 16,000, with shift to the left. The patient is taken to surgery, where an acute ruptured appendix is removed. After study, the principal diagnosis is determined to be acute ruptured appendicitis.

- A patient is admitted with severe abdominal pain in the right lower quadrant, and an admitting diagnosis of probable acute appendicitis is given. The white blood cell count is slightly elevated. The patient is taken to surgery, where a normal appendix is found but an inflamed Meckel's diverticulum is removed. After study, the principal diagnosis is determined to be Meckel's diverticulum.

The circumstances of inpatient admission always govern the selection of the principal diagnosis, and the coding directives in the ICD-10-CM classification take precedence over all other guidelines. The importance of consistent, complete documentation in the medical record cannot be overemphasized. Without such documentation, the application of all coding guidelines is a difficult, if not impossible, task.

There are special instructions related to the selection of principal diagnosis when a patient is admitted as an inpatient from the hospital's observation unit or from outpatient surgery. The coding advice provided below applies if a single bill is submitted to a payer. If separate inpatient and outpatient bills are submitted, then the advice does not apply. Instead, hospitals should apply codes for the current encounter based on individual payer billing instructions.

For example:

- *Admission following medical observation:* A patient may be treated in a hospital's observation unit to determine whether the condition improves sufficiently for the patient to be discharged. If the condition either worsens or does not improve, the physician may decide to admit the patient as an inpatient of the same hospital for this same medical condition. The principal diagnosis reported is the medical condition that led to the hospital admission.

- *Admission following postoperative observation:* A patient undergoing outpatient surgery may require postoperative admission to an observation unit to monitor a condition (or complication) that develops postoperatively. If the patient subsequently requires inpatient admission to the same hospital, the UHDDS definition of principal diagnosis applies: "that condition established after study to be chiefly responsible for occasioning the admission of the patient to the hospital for care."

- *Admission from outpatient surgery:* A patient undergoing outpatient surgery may be subsequently admitted for continuing inpatient care at the same hospital. The following guidelines should be followed in selecting the principal diagnosis for the inpatient admission:

—If the reason for the inpatient admission is a complication, assign the complication as the principal diagnosis.

—If no complication or other condition is documented as the reason for the inpatient admission, assign the reason for the outpatient surgery as the principal diagnosis.

—If the reason for the inpatient admission is another condition unrelated to the surgery, assign the unrelated condition as the principal diagnosis.

- *Admissions/encounters for rehabilitation:* A patient may require inpatient or outpatient rehabilitation services. The following guidelines should be followed for the selection of the principal diagnosis or first-listed diagnosis when the purpose for the admission/ encounter is rehabilitation:

—Sequence first the code for the condition for which the service is being performed. For example, for an admission/encounter for rehabilitation for right-sided dominant hemiplegia following a cerebrovascular infarction, report code **I69.351, Hemiplegia and hemiparesis following cerebral infarction affecting right dominant side,** as the first-listed or principal diagnosis.

—If the condition for which the rehabilitation service was required is no longer present, report the appropriate aftercare code—or report the traumatic injury with the appropriate seventh character for subsequent encounter—as the first-listed or principal diagnosis.

Example 1: If a patient with severe degenerative osteoarthritis of the hip underwent hip replacement, and the current encounter/admission is required for rehabilitation, report code **Z47.1, Aftercare following joint replacement surgery,** as the first-listed or principal diagnosis.

Example 2: If the patient requires rehabilitation post hip replacement for right intertrochanteric femur fracture, report code **S72.141D, Displaced intertrochanteric fracture of right femur, subsequent encounter for closed fracture with routine healing,** as the first-listed or principal diagnosis.

Please note that the above guidelines regarding admissions/encounters for rehabilitation apply to coding for the billing form (UB-04), but they do not apply to coding for the etiologic diagnosis on the Inpatient Rehabilitation Facility Patient Assessment Instrument (IRF PAI). The IRF PAI has separate and distinct instructions, which are outside the scope of this handbook.

The following official guidelines for designating the principal diagnosis apply to all systems and etiologies. (Guidelines that apply only to specific body systems or etiologies are discussed in the relevant chapters of this handbook. To download the current version of the complete *ICD-10-CM Official Guidelines for Coding and Reporting,* please visitwww.codingclinicadvisor.com.)

1. *Two or more diagnoses that equally meet the definition for principal diagnosis:* In the unusual situation that two or more diagnoses equally meet the criteria for principal diagnosis as determined by the circumstances of the admission and the diagnostic workup and/or therapy provided, either may be sequenced first when neither the Alphabetic Index nor the Tabular List directs otherwise. However, it is not simply the fact that both conditions exist that makes this choice possible. When treatment is totally or primarily directed toward one condition, or when only one condition would have required inpatient care, that condition should be designated as the principal diagnosis. Also, if another coding guideline (general or disease specific) provides sequencing direction, that guideline must be followed.

Example 1: A patient is admitted with unstable angina and acute congestive heart failure. The unstable angina is treated with nitrates, and intravenous Lasix is given to manage the heart failure. Both diagnoses meet the definition of principal diagnosis equally, and either may be sequenced first.

Example 2: A patient is admitted with acute atrial fibrillation with rapid ventricular response and is also in heart failure with pulmonary edema. The patient is digitalized to reduce the ventricular rate and given intravenous Lasix to reduce the cardiogenic pulmonary edema. Both conditions meet the definition of principal diagnosis equally, and either may be sequenced first.

Example 3:   A patient is admitted with severe abdominal pain, nausea, and vomiting due to acute pyelonephritis and diverticulitis. Both underlying conditions are treated, and the physician believes both equally meet the criteria for principal diagnosis. In this instance, either condition may be listed as principal diagnosis.

2. *Two or more comparable or contrasting conditions:* In the rare instance that two or more comparable or contrasting conditions are documented as either/or (or similar terminology), both diagnoses are coded as though confirmed and the principal diagnosis is designated according to the circumstances of the admission and the diagnostic workup and/or therapy provided. When no further determination can be made as to which diagnosis more closely meets the criteria for principal diagnosis, either may be sequenced first. Note that this guideline does not apply for outpatient encounters.

Example 1:   A patient with the same complaints as those outlined in example 3 above is admitted with a final diagnosis of acute pyelonephritis versus diverticulum of the colon. The patient is treated symptomatically and discharged for further studies. In this case, both conditions meet the criteria for principal diagnosis equally, and either can be designated as the principal diagnosis.

Example 2:   The treatment of another patient with the same symptoms and the same final diagnoses is directed almost entirely toward the acute pyelonephritis, indicating that the physician considers this condition the more likely problem and that, after study, it is the condition that occasioned the admission. In this case, both conditions are coded, but the acute pyelonephritis is sequenced first because of the circumstances of the admission.

3. *Original treatment plan not carried out:* In a situation in which the original treatment plan cannot be carried out due to unforeseen circumstances, the criteria for designation of the principal diagnosis do not change. The condition that occasioned the admission is designated as the principal diagnosis even though the planned treatment was not carried out.

Example 1:   A patient with benign hypertrophy of the prostate is admitted for the purpose of a transurethral resection of the prostate (TURP). Shortly after admission, but before the patient is taken to the operating suite, the patient falls and sustains a fracture of the left femur. The TURP is canceled; hip pinning is carried out the following day. The principal diagnosis remains benign hypertrophy of the prostate even though that condition was not treated.

Example 2:   A patient with a diagnosis of carcinoma of the breast confirmed from an outpatient biopsy is admitted for the purpose of modified radical mastectomy. Before the preoperative medications are administered the next morning, the patient indicates that she has decided against having the procedure until she is able to consider possible alternative treatment more thoroughly. No treatment is given, and she is discharged. The carcinoma of the breast remains the principal diagnosis because it is the condition that occasioned the admission even though no treatment was rendered.

Other Diagnoses

Other reportable diagnoses are defined as those conditions that coexist with the principal diagnosis at the time of admission or develop subsequently or affect patient care for the current hospital episode. Diagnoses that have no impact on patient care during the hospital stay are not reported even when they are present. Diagnoses that relate to an earlier episode and have no bearing on the current hospital stay are not reported.

For UHDDS reporting purposes, the definition of "other diagnosis" includes only those conditions that affect the episode of hospital care in terms of any of the following:

- Clinical evaluation
- Therapeutic treatment
- Further evaluation by diagnostic studies, procedures, or consultation
- Extended length of hospital stay
- Increased nursing care and/or other monitoring

All these factors are self-explanatory except the first. Clinical evaluation means that the physician is aware of the problem and is evaluating it in terms of testing, consultations, or close clinical observation of the patient's condition. In most cases, a patient who is being evaluated clinically will also meet one of the other criteria. Note that a physical examination alone does not qualify as further evaluation or clinical evaluation; the physical examination is a routine part of every hospital admission. No particular order is mandated for sequencing other diagnoses. However, the more significant diagnoses should be sequenced early in the list when the number of diagnoses that may be reported is limited.

Reporting Guidelines for Other Diagnoses

The following guidelines and examples should be studied carefully because they provide the rationale for determining other diagnoses that should be reported:

1. *Previous conditions stated as diagnoses:* Physicians sometimes include in the diagnostic statement historical information or status post procedures performed on a previous admission that have no bearing on the current stay. Such conditions are not reported. However, history codes (categories Z80–Z87; subcategories Z91.4- and Z91.5-; and codes Z91.81, Z91.82, Z92.1–Z92.81, and Z92.83–Z92.89) may be used as secondary codes if the historical condition or family history has an impact on current care or influences treatment.

   Example: A patient is admitted with acute myocardial infarction; the physician notes in the history that the patient is status post cholecystectomy and had been hospitalized one year earlier for pneumonia. At discharge, the physician documents the final diagnoses as acute myocardial infarction, status post cholecystectomy, and history of pneumonia. Only the acute myocardial infarction is coded and reported; the other conditions included in the diagnostic statement have no bearing on the current episode of care.

2. *Other diagnosis with no documentation supporting reportability:* If the physician has included a diagnosis in the final diagnostic statement, it should ordinarily be coded. However, if there is no supporting documentation in the medical record, the physician should be consulted as to whether the diagnosis meets reporting criteria; if it does, the physician should be asked to add the necessary documentation. Reporting of conditions for which there is no supporting documentation is in conflict with UHDDS criteria.

   Example 1: A 10-year-old boy is admitted with open fracture of the tibia and fibula following a bicycle accident. On physical examination, the physician notes that there is a nevus on the leg and that the patient has a small, asymptomatic inguinal hernia. All these diagnoses are documented on the face sheet. The fracture is reduced with internal fixation, but neither the nevus nor the hernia is treated or further evaluated on this admission. The nevus and hernia are not reported because there is nothing to indicate that they had any effect on the episode of care.

Example 2:   A patient is admitted with an acute myocardial infarction. The physician also includes in the diagnostic statement a strabismus and a bunion noted on the physical examination. Review of the medical record reveals that no further reference to these conditions was made in terms of further evaluation or treatment; therefore, no codes for either the strabismus or the bunion are assigned.

3. *Chronic conditions that are not the thrust of treatment:* The criteria for selection of chronic conditions to be reported as "other diagnoses" include the severity of the condition, the use or consideration of alternative measures to treat the principal diagnosis due to the coexisting condition, the use of diagnostic or therapeutic services for the particular coexisting condition, the need for close monitoring of medications because of the coexisting condition, or modifications of nursing care plans because of the coexisting condition (for example, an increase in the nursing care required for the principal diagnosis due to the coexisting condition).

Chronic conditions such as (but not limited to) hypertension, Parkinson's disease, chronic obstructive pulmonary disease, and diabetes mellitus are systemic diseases that ordinarily should be coded even in the absence of documented intervention or further evaluation. Some chronic conditions affect the patient for the rest of his or her life; such conditions almost always require some form of continuous clinical evaluation or monitoring during hospitalization and therefore should be coded. This advice applies to inpatient coding.

For outpatient encounters/visits, chronic conditions that require or affect patient care treatment or management should be coded.

Example 1:   A patient is admitted following a hip fracture, and a diagnosis of Parkinson's disease is noted in the history and physical examination. Nursing notes indicate that the patient required additional care because of the Parkinson's disease. Both diagnoses are reported.

Example 2:   A patient is admitted with pneumonia, and the presence of diabetes mellitus is documented in the record. His blood sugar levels are monitored by laboratory studies, and nursing personnel also check his blood sugar before each meal. The patient is continued on his diabetic diet. Although no active diabetes treatment is provided, ongoing monitoring is required, and the condition is reported.

Example 3:   A patient is admitted with acute diverticulitis, and the physician documents in the admitting note a history of hypertension. Review of the medical record indicates that blood pressure medications were given throughout the stay. The hypertension is reportable, and the physician should be asked to add it to the diagnostic statement.

Example 4:   A patient is admitted in congestive heart failure. She has known hiatal hernia and degenerative arthritis. Neither condition is further evaluated or treated; by their nature, the conditions do not require continuing clinical evaluation. Only the code for the congestive heart failure is assigned; the other conditions are not reportable.

Example 5:   A 60-year-old diabetic patient is transferred from an extended care facility for treatment of a pressure ulcer. The physician notes in the history and physical exam that the patient is status post left below-the-knee amputation due to peripheral vascular disease. This condition, which requires additional nursing care, and the patient's diabetes are both reported.

4. *Conditions that are an integral part of a disease process should not be reported as additional diagnoses, unless otherwise instructed by the classification.*

Example 1:   A patient is admitted with nausea and vomiting due to infectious gastro-enteritis. Nausea and vomiting are common symptoms of infectious gastro-enteritis and are not reported.

Example 2:   A patient is admitted with severe joint pain and rheumatoid arthritis. Severe joint pain is a characteristic part of rheumatoid arthritis and is not reportable.

Example 3:   A patient is seen in the physician's office complaining of urinary frequency and is diagnosed with benign prostatic hypertrophy. Although urinary frequency is a common symptom of benign prostatic hypertrophy, both conditions are reported because of the instructional note in the Tabular List under code N40.1 to use additional codes to identify associated symptoms when specified.

5. *Conditions that are not an integral part of a disease process should be coded when present.*

Example 1:   A patient is admitted by ambulance following a cerebrovascular accident suffered at work. The patient was in a coma but gradually recovers consciousness. Diagnosis at discharge is reported as cerebrovascular thrombosis with coma. In this case, coma is coded as an additional diagnosis because it is not implicit in a cerebrovascular accident and is not always present.

Example 2:   A five-year-old boy is admitted with a 104-degree fever associated with acute pneumonia. During the first 24 hours, the patient also experiences convulsions due to the high fever. Both the pneumonia and the convulsions are reported because convulsions are not routinely associated with pneumonia. No code is assigned for fever, however, because it is commonly associated with pneumonia.

6. *Abnormal findings:* Codes from sections R70–R97 for nonspecific abnormal findings (laboratory, radiology, pathology, and other diagnostic results) should be assigned only when the physician has not been able to arrive at a related diagnosis but indicates that an abnormal finding is considered to be clinically significant by listing it in the diagnostic statement. This differs from the coding practices in the outpatient setting when one is coding encounters for diagnostic tests that have been interpreted by a physician.

A code should never be assigned on the basis of an abnormal finding alone. To make a diagnosis on the basis of a single lab value or abnormal diagnostic finding is risky and carries the possibility of error. A value reported as either lower or higher than the normal range does not necessarily indicate a disorder. Many factors influence the values in a lab sample; these include the collection device, the method used to transport the sample to the lab, the calibration of the machine that reads the values, and the condition of the patient. For example, a patient who is dehydrated may show an elevated hemoglobin due to increased viscosity of the blood. When findings are clearly outside the normal range and the physician has ordered other tests to evaluate the condition or has prescribed treatment without documenting an associated diagnosis, it is appropriate to ask the physician whether a diagnosis should be added or whether the abnormal finding should be listed in the diagnostic statement. Incidental findings on X-ray, such as asymptomatic hiatal hernia or a diverticulum, should not be reported unless further evaluation or treatment is carried out.

Example 1:   A low potassium level treated with intravenous or oral potassium is clinically significant and should be brought to the attention of the physician if no related diagnosis has been recorded.

Example 2:   A hematocrit of 28 percent, even though asymptomatic and not treated, is evaluated with serial hematocrits. Because the finding is outside the range of normal laboratory values and has been further evaluated, the physician should be asked whether an associated diagnosis should be documented.

Example 3: A routine preoperative chest X-ray on an elderly patient reveals collapse of a vertebral body. The patient is asymptomatic, and no further evaluation or treatment is carried out. Collapse of a vertebral body is a common finding in elderly patients and is insignificant for this episode.

Example 4: In the absence of a cardiac problem, an isolated electrocardiographic finding of bundle branch block is ordinarily not significant, whereas a finding of a Mobitz II block may have important implications for the patient's care and warrants asking the physician whether it should be reported for this admission.

Example 5: The physician lists an abnormal sedimentation rate as part of the diagnostic statement. The physician has been unable to make a definitive diagnosis during the hospitalization in spite of further evaluation and considers the abnormal finding a significant clinical problem. Code **R70.0, Elevated erythrocyte sedimentation rate,** should be assigned.

Admitting Diagnosis

Although the admitting diagnosis is not an element of the UHDDS, it must be reported for some payers and may also be useful in quality-of-care studies. Ordinarily, only one admitting diagnosis can be reported. The inpatient admitting diagnosis may be reported as one of the following:

- A significant finding (symptom or sign) representing patient distress or an abnormal finding on outpatient examination
- A possible diagnosis based on significant findings (working diagnosis)
- A diagnosis established on an ambulatory care basis or during a previous hospital admission
- An injury or a poisoning
- A reason or condition that is not actually an illness or injury, such as a follow-up examination or pregnancy in labor

If the admitting diagnosis is reported, the code should indicate the diagnosis provided by the physician at the time of admission. Although the admitting diagnosis may not agree with the principal diagnosis on discharge, the admitting diagnosis should not be changed to conform to the principal diagnosis. Examples of admitting diagnoses and subsequent principal diagnoses follow:

- *Admitting:* K92.2 Gastrointestinal bleeding
  Principal: K26.0 Acute duodenal ulcer with hemorrhage
- *Admitting:* N63.10 Lump in right breast
  Principal: C50.911 Carcinoma of right female breast
- *Admitting:* K81.0 Acute cholecystitis
  Principal: K80.00 Acute cholecystitis with cholelithiasis
- *Admitting:* I50.9 Congestive heart failure
  Principal: I21.09 Acute myocardial infarction, anterior wall
- *Admitting:* I21.9 Suspected acute myocardial infarction
  Principal: I71.01 Dissection of thoracic aorta

PROCEDURES

The UHDDS requires that all significant procedures be reported. The UHDDS definitions of significant procedures and other reporting guidelines are discussed in chapter 9 of this handbook, along with other information on coding operations and procedures.

RELATIONSHIP OF UHDDS TO OUTPATIENT REPORTING

The UHDDS definition of principal diagnosis does not apply to the coding of outpatient encounters. In contrast to inpatient coding, no "after study" element is involved in outpatient code assignment because ambulatory care visits do not permit the continued evaluation ordinarily needed to meet UHDDS criteria. If the physician does not identify a definite condition or problem at the conclusion of a visit or an encounter, the documented chief complaint should be reported as the reason for the encounter/visit.

RELATIONSHIP OF UHDDS TO LONG-TERM CARE REPORTING

The UHDDS definition of principal diagnosis has been expanded since its initial development so that it now applies to coding in all nonoutpatient settings (acute care, short-term care, long term care and psychiatric hospitals; home health agencies; rehabilitation facilities; nursing homes; hospice; and so forth). Other diagnoses documented by the physician (e.g., chronic conditions) that affect a resident's continued care should also be coded. However, in long term care (LTC) settings, such as skilled nursing facilities, intermediate care facilities, or nursing homes, there are some differences in the application of the principal and secondary diagnoses.

The diagnostic listing in LTC is dynamic and depends on many factors, including the point in time when codes are assigned. LTC has a longer time frame than an acute care stay: in LTC, ICD-10-CM codes are assigned upon admission; concurrently as diagnoses arise; and at the time of discharge, transfer, or expiration of a resident.

The first-listed diagnosis is the diagnosis chiefly responsible for the admission to, or continued residence in, a skilled nursing facility and should be sequenced first. For example, when an admission is coded, the first-listed diagnosis is the condition chiefly responsible for the admission to the facility. If the diagnosis codes are assigned during the resident's stay, the first-listed diagnosis is the condition chiefly responsible for the continued stay in the facility.

Example 1: A patient is admitted to a nursing home for convalescence following an acute illness. Code assignment is based on the condition being treated as documented in the medical record. It would also be appropriate to assign codes for any late effects, residual conditions, signs, or symptoms that are present. When the reason for the admission is strictly for convalescence and there is no other definitive diagnosis, assign code **Z51.89, Encounter for other specified aftercare,** as the first-listed diagnosis.

Example 2: A patient is admitted to LTC following hospital treatment of a fracture of the right femur. The reason for the LTC admission is to allow the patient to regain strength and the fracture to heal. Assign code **S72.90xD, Unspecified fracture of right femur, subsequent encounter for closed fracture with routine healing,** as the principal diagnosis. The seventh character "D" is used for encounters after the patient has received active treatment for the condition and is now receiving routine care during the healing or recovery phase. Code also any other coexistent conditions that require treatment.

Example 3: A nursing home resident is transferred to the hospital for treatment of pneumonia. She returns to the nursing home while still receiving antibiotics for the pneumonia. However, the main reason she is returning to the nursing home is because it has been her residence since she had a cerebrovascular accident (CVA) with residuals several years ago. The appropriate code from subcategory I69.3, Sequelae of cerebral infarction, is assigned as the principal diagnosis to identify the neurological deficits that resulted from the acute CVA. The appropriate code for the pneumonia is assigned as a secondary diagnosis for as long as the patient receives treatment for the condition.

ETHICAL CODING AND REPORTING

Although coded medical data are used for a variety of purposes, they have become increasingly important in determining payment for health care. Medicare reimbursement depends on the following:

- The correct designation of the principal diagnosis
- The presence or absence of additional codes that represent complications, comorbidities, or major complications or comorbidities as defined by the Medicare Severity Diagnosis-Related Group system
- Procedures performed

Other third-party payers may apply slightly different reimbursement methods, but the accuracy of ICD-10-CM and ICD-10-PCS coding is always vital.

Accurate and ethical ICD-10-CM and ICD-10-PCS coding depends on correctly following all instructions in the coding manuals as well as all official guidelines developed by the cooperating parties and coding advice published in the quarterly *AHA Coding Clinic®*. Accurate and ethical reporting requires the correct selection of those conditions that meet the criteria set by the UHDDS and the official guidelines mentioned above. Over-coding and over-reporting may result in higher payment, but those practices are unethical and may be considered fraudulent. On the other hand, it is important to be sure that all appropriate codes are reported, as failure to include all diagnoses or procedures that meet reporting criteria may result in financial loss for the health care provider.

It is important to abide by the American Health Information Management Association Standards of Ethical Coding, which are available for download at http://library.ahima.org/Coding Standards#.Xr8gqMV7kSk.

Occasionally, certain codes are identified by Medicare or another payer as being unacceptable as the principal diagnosis. This does not mean that the code should not be assigned when it is correct; it means that the third-party payer may question or deny payment. Coding professionals must code correctly and then make whatever adjustment is required for reporting, or they run the risk of developing incorrect coding practices that will distort data used for other purposes.

Hospitals sometimes identify a need to code nonreportable diagnoses or procedures for internal use. This is acceptable if the facility has a system for maintaining this information outside the reporting system.

There are a variety of payment policies that may have an impact on coding. Those policies may contradict each other or may be inconsistent with ICD-10-CM/PCS rules and conventions. Therefore, it is not possible to write coding guidelines that are consistent with all existing payer guidelines.

The following advice is shared to help providers resolve coding disputes with payers:

- First, determine whether the problem is really a coding dispute and not a coverage issue. Always contact the payer for clarification if the reason for the denial is unclear.

- If a payer really does have a policy that clearly conflicts with official coding rules or guidelines, every effort should be made to resolve the issue with the payer. Provide the applicable coding rule/guideline to the payer.

- If a payer refuses to change its policy, obtain the payer requirements in writing. If the payer refuses to provide its policy in writing, document all discussions with the payer, including dates and the names of individuals involved in the discussion. Confirm the existence of the policy with the payer's supervisory personnel.

- Keep a permanent file of the documentation obtained regarding payer coding policies. It may come in handy in the event of an audit.

CHAPTER 4

The Medical Record as a Source Document

CHAPTER OVERVIEW

- The medical record is the source document for coding.
- Medical records contain a variety of reports. These include the following:
  - Reason the patient came to the hospital
  - Tests performed and their findings
  - Therapies provided
  - Descriptions of surgical procedures
  - Daily records of patient progress
- The discharge summary provides a synopsis of the patient's stay.

LEARNING OUTCOMES

After studying this chapter, you should be able to:

Explain what is present in a medical record.

Understand when it is appropriate to query a physician about his or her documentation.

TERMS TO KNOW

POA indicator
present on admission indicator; a data element that applies to diagnosis codes for claims involving inpatient care

Provider
a physician or any qualified health care practitioner (such as a nurse practitioner or physician assistant) who is legally accountable for establishing the patient's diagnosis

REMEMBER . . .

Coding professionals must make sure that the medical record documentation supports the principal diagnosis.

. . . Refer to appendix B of this handbook for more information on the POA indicator.

INTRODUCTION

The source document for coding and reporting diagnoses and procedures is the medical record. Although discharge diagnoses are usually recorded on the face sheet, a final progress note, or the discharge summary, further review of the medical record is needed to ensure complete and accurate coding. Operations and procedures are frequently not listed on the face sheet or are not described in sufficient detail, making a review of operative reports, pathology reports, and other special reports imperative. The entire record should be reviewed to determine the specific reason for the encounter and the conditions treated.

In some institutions, midlevel providers, such as nurse practitioners and physician assistants, are involved in the care of the patient and can document diagnoses in the medical record. It is appropriate to base code assignments on the documentation of midlevel providers if they are considered legally accountable for establishing a diagnosis within the regulations governing the provider and the facility. The *ICD-10-CM Official Guidelines for Coding and Reporting* use the term "provider" to mean physician or any qualified health care practitioner who is legally accountable for establishing the patient's diagnosis. The term "provider" in the remaining text of this chapter is used in the same way.

Providers sometimes fail to list reportable conditions that developed during the stay but were resolved prior to discharge. Conditions such as urinary tract infection or dehydration, for example, are often not included in the diagnostic statement even though progress notes, providers' orders, and laboratory reports make it clear that such conditions were treated. It is inappropriate to assign a diagnosis based solely on a provider's orders for prescribed medications without the provider's documentation of the diagnosis being treated. If enough information is present to strongly suggest that an additional diagnosis should be reported, the provider should be consulted; no diagnosis should be added without the approval of the provider. Because diagnostic statements sometimes include diagnoses that represent past history or existing diagnoses that do not meet the Uniform Hospital Discharge Data Set (UHDDS) guidelines for reportable diagnoses, the coding professional must review the medical record to determine whether these diagnoses should be coded for this encounter.

It is customary to list the principal diagnosis first in the diagnostic statement. However, many providers are unaware of coding and reporting guidelines, and, consequently, this custom is not consistently followed. Because the correct designation of the principal diagnosis is of critical importance in reporting diagnostic information, the coding professional must make sure that medical record documentation supports the designation of principal diagnosis. If it appears that another diagnosis should be designated as the principal diagnosis, or if it seems that conditions not listed should be reported, follow the health care facility's procedures for obtaining a corrected diagnostic statement.

CONTENTS OF THE MEDICAL RECORD

Medical records contain a variety of reports that document the reason the patient came to the hospital, the tests performed and their findings, the therapies provided, descriptions of any surgical procedures, and daily records of the patient's progress. Each report contains important information needed for accurate coding and reporting of the principal diagnosis, other diagnoses, and the procedures performed.

A number of standard reports can be found in almost any medical record, but other reports will be included depending on the condition for which the patient is being treated, the extent of workup and therapy provided, and the provider's style of documentation. For example, a provider may list final diagnoses on the admission record (face sheet), on progress notes, or on the discharge summary. Consultants may record their consultation notes as progress notes or in separate reports.

Review of the inpatient medical record should begin with the discharge summary, when available, because it provides a synopsis of the patient's hospital stay, including the reason for admission, significant diagnostic findings, the treatment given, the patient's course in the hospital, the follow-up plan, and the final diagnostic statement. The history section usually indicates the reason for admission (principal diagnosis), which may require confirmation by review of the history and physical examination and admitting and emergency department records.

The section of the discharge summary that describes the patient's course in the hospital usually indicates treatment that has been given and any further workup that has been done. This section is particularly useful in determining whether all listed diagnoses meet the criteria for reporting and identifying other conditions that may merit reporting.

Conditions mentioned elsewhere in the body of the discharge summary do not necessarily warrant reporting, but they may provide clues for more specific review to make a final determination. The medical record should be reviewed further to determine whether such conditions meet the criteria for reportable diagnoses as defined in the UHDDS. The medication record is often helpful in indicating that therapeutic treatment may have been administered, but the coding professional should not assume a diagnosis solely on the basis of medication administration or abnormal findings in diagnostic reports. In addition, recorded diagnoses do not always contain sufficient information to provide the specificity required in coding. For example, a diagnosis of pneumonia may not indicate the organism responsible for the infection; a review of diagnostic studies of the sputum may provide this information. The provider should be asked to confirm that the organism discovered on the positive culture is the causative agent. Then, the provider should indicate his or her confirmation by documenting it in the medical record; this step must be taken before a code identifying the specific type of pneumonia can be assigned. A diagnosis of fracture may indicate which bone was fractured but not the particular part of the bone, information that is necessary for accurate code assignment. The X-ray or the operative report should supply these data. It is appropriate to utilize imaging reports to provide greater specificity of the anatomical site as documented by the provider. For example, coding professionals may need to review an X-ray report to identify the location of a fracture, or an imaging report, such as a magnetic resonance imaging (MRI) study, to determine the location of the infarction or stroke in a patient diagnosed with a cerebral infarction or hemorrhagic stroke.

Some facilities develop their own additional coding guidelines to provide assistance in determining when a provider query is appropriate. For example, if the test findings are outside the normal range and the provider has ordered other tests to evaluate the condition or prescribed treatment, internal guidelines could advise the coding professional to ask the provider whether a diagnosis should be added. However, a facility's internal guidelines must align with the Official Coding Guidelines. For example, internal guidelines should not direct the coding professional to use test results to interpret provider documentation or conclude that a provider query is unnecessary for code assignment.

The following examples illustrate diagnoses that are often recorded with less-than-complete information but can be coded more specifically by referring to diagnostic reports within the medical record and then obtaining the appropriate provider confirmation. Note the variation in code assignment when more information is available and is confirmed by the provider:

- *Diagnosis:*   C53.9   Cancer of cervix
  Pathology report: D06.9   Carcinoma, in situ, of cervix
- *Diagnosis:*   N39.0   Urinary tract infection
  Laboratory report: N39.0 + B96.20   *E. coli* in urine
- *Diagnosis:*   S72.90xA   Fracture of femur, initial encounter
  X-ray report: S72.21xB   Open fracture of subtrochanteric neck of the right femur, initial encounter

Diagnosing a patient's condition is solely the responsibility of the provider. Code assignment is generally based on the provider's documentation, not on clinical criteria used by the provider to establish the diagnosis. Coding professionals should not disregard provider documentation and decide on their own—based on clinical criteria, abnormal test results, and so forth—whether or not a condition should be coded. The provider's diagnostic statement that a patient has a particular condition is sufficient for coding assignment.

It is also appropriate to base code assignment on the documentation of other physicians (e.g., consultants, residents, anesthesiologists) involved in the care and treatment of the patient so long as there is no conflicting information from the attending physician. A physician query is not necessary if a physician involved in the care and treatment of the patient, including any of the consulting physicians, has documented a diagnosis and there is no conflicting documentation from another physician. If documentation from different physicians conflicts, the attending physician should be queried for clarification because he or she is ultimately responsible for the final diagnosis.

Code assignment is generally based on provider documentation. However, the *ICD-10-CM Official Guidelines for Coding and Reporting* outline a few exceptions where documentation by clinicians other than the patient's provider is acceptable. The exceptions are body mass index (BMI), depth of nonpressure chronic ulcers, pressure ulcer stage, coma scale, NIH stroke scale (NIHSS), and social determinants of health codes. Patient self-reported documentation may also be used to assign codes for social determinants of health, as long as either a clinician or provider accepts the patient self-reported information and incorporates it into the health record. The reason for these exceptions is that typically this information is documented by other clinicians involved in the care of the patient (e.g., a dietitian often documents BMI, a nurse often documents pressure ulcer stages, and an emergency medical technician often documents the coma scale). However, it is important to note that the associated diagnosis (such as overweight, obesity, pressure ulcer, or acute stroke) must be documented by the patient's provider. If there is conflicting medical record documentation, either from the same clinician or different clinicians, the patient's attending provider should be queried for clarification.

For inpatient coding, if the provider does not confirm pathological or radiological findings in the medical record, query him or her regarding the clinical significance of the findings and request that appropriate documentation be provided. Although the pathologist or radiologist provides a written interpretation of a tissue biopsy or an X-ray image, that is not equivalent to the attending physician's medical diagnosis, which is based on the patient's complete clinical picture. The attending physician is responsible for, and directly involved in, the care and treatment of the patient. For example, if the attending physician documented "breast mass" and the pathologist documented "carcinoma of the breast," that would be conflicting information requiring clarification from the attending physician.

The only exception to this guidance about querying the provider to document the clinical significance of findings is for the coding of 2019 novel coronavirus disease (COVID-19). The coding guidelines for inpatient encounters allow the reporting of this diagnosis on the basis of a positive COVID-19 test result alone.

When coding outpatient laboratory, pathology, and radiology encounters in hospital-based as well as stand-alone facilities, it is appropriate to assign codes on the basis of the written interpretation by a radiologist or pathologist.

Not all reportable services or procedures during an encounter or admission are performed or documented by physicians. It is appropriate to assign a procedure code based on documentation by the nonphysician professional who provided the service. This guidance applies only to procedure coding where there is documentation to substantiate the code. It does not apply to diagnosis coding. The documentation from the nonphysician professional who provided the service may be the only evidence that the service was provided. This is true of services such as infusions carried out by nurses and therapies provided by physical, respiratory, or occupational therapists.

Outpatient records generally contain less information than inpatient records do; nevertheless, all available reports for the encounter should be reviewed prior to code assignment. Code assignment depends on the information available at the time of code assignment. Documentation for the current encounter should clearly reflect those diagnoses that are current and relevant for that encounter. Conditions documented on previous encounters may not be clinically relevant for the current encounter. When a recurring condition is still reportable for the outpatient encounter or inpatient admission, that condition should be documented in the medical record for that encounter/admission. However, if the condition is not documented in the current medical record, it would be inappropriate to go back to previous encounters to retrieve a diagnosis without physician confirmation.

For ambulatory records, an additional data element called "patient's reason for visit" (PRV) is usually reported. The PRV is reported on unscheduled outpatient visits (e.g., emergency department or urgent care visits) to identify the main reason the patient sought treatment. The reason may differ from the physician's final diagnosis at the end of the encounter. If there are multiple conditions present, the code most likely to justify the patient encounter should be reported. This data element is found at Form Locator 70a–c on the UB-04 paper claim. Both the UB-04 paper claim and the electronic claim allow the reporting of three diagnosis codes for the patient's reason for visit.

The "present on admission" (POA) indicator is a data element approved by the National Uniform Billing Committee for inpatient reporting. The POA indicator applies to the diagnosis codes for claims involving inpatient admissions to general acute care hospitals or other facilities. Please refer to appendix B of this handbook for more detailed information on this topic.

CHAPTER 5

Basic ICD-10-CM Coding Steps

CHAPTER OVERVIEW

- There are three basic steps for locating codes to be assigned.
  - Locate the main term in the Alphabetic Index. Search for subterms, notes, or cross-references.
  - Verify the alphanumeric code in the Tabular List.
  - Assign the verified code or codes.
- It is important to understand basic coding techniques before moving on to the harder, system-based chapters of this handbook.

LEARNING OUTCOMES

After studying this chapter, you should be able to:

Locate code entries in the Alphabetic Index.

Determine the course of action when there are discrepancies between the Alphabetic Index and the Tabular List.

Perform basic coding techniques.

TERMS TO KNOW

Alphabetic Index of Diseases and Injuries and the **Index to External Causes**
include entries for main terms (diseases, conditions, or injuries) and subterms (site, type, or etiology), the Neoplasm Table, and the Table of Drugs and Chemicals

Tabular List
contains categories, subcategories, and valid codes

REMEMBER . . .

You cannot begin to code unless you have determined the principal diagnosis and other reportable diagnoses from the medical record.

INTRODUCTION

Once the medical record has been reviewed to determine the principal/first-listed diagnosis and other reportable diagnoses, the following steps to locate the codes to be assigned should be undertaken:

1. Locate the main term in the Alphabetic Index.
   - Review subterms and nonessential modifiers related to the main term.
   - Follow any cross-reference instructions.
   - Refer to any notes in the Alphabetic Index.
   - A dash (-) at the end of an Index entry indicates that additional characters are required.
2. Verify the alphanumeric code in the Tabular List.
   - Read the code title.
   - Read and follow any instructional notes. Refer to other codes as instructed.
   - Determine whether any additional characters must be added.
   - Determine laterality (right, left, or bilateral) and any applicable extensions.
3. Assign the verified code or codes.

It is imperative that these steps be followed without exception; the condition to be coded must first be located in the Alphabetic Index and then verified in the Tabular List. Relying on memory or using only the Index or Tabular List may lead to incorrect code assignment.

LOCATE THE CODE ENTRY IN THE ALPHABETIC INDEX

The first step in coding is to locate the main term in the Alphabetic Index. In the ICD-10-CM Alphabetic Index, the condition is listed as the main term, usually expressed as a noun. General terms such as "admission," "encounter," and "examination" are used to locate code entries for the Z code section. Some conditions are indexed under more than one main term. For example, anxiety reaction can be located in either of the following Index entries:

> **Anxiety . . .**
> -reaction F41.1
> **Reaction** . . .
> -anxiety F41.1

If a main term cannot be located, consider a synonym, an eponym, or another alternative term. Once the main term is located, search for subterms, notes, or cross-references. Subterms provide many types of more-specific information and must be checked carefully, following all the rules of alphabetization. The main term code entry should not be assigned until all subterm possibilities have been exhausted. During this process, it may be necessary to refer again to the medical record to determine whether any additional information is available to permit assignment of a more specific code. If a subterm cannot be located, the nonessential modifiers following the main term should be reviewed to see whether the subterm may be included there. If not, alternative terms should be considered.

EXERCISE 5.1

Without referring to the Alphabetic Index of Diseases and Injuries, underline the word that indicates the main term for each diagnosis.

1. Acute myocardial infarction

2. Chronic hypertrophy of tonsils and adenoids

3. Acute suppurative cholecystitis

4. Syphilitic aortic aneurysm

5. Normal, spontaneous delivery, full-term infant

6. Drug overdose due to barbiturates

7. Urinary tract infection due to *E. coli*

8. Hemorrhagic pneumonia

9. Admission for adjustment of artificial arm

10. Bilateral inguinal hernia

VERIFY THE ALPHANUMERIC CODE IN THE TABULAR LIST

Once an alphanumeric code entry has been located in the Alphabetic Index, refer to that code in the Tabular List; a code should not be assigned without such verification. In addition to the title for the code entry, it may be necessary to review the titles for the chapter, section, and category to be sure the correct code has been identified. Although the title for the code entry in the Tabular List does not always match exactly the Alphabetic Index entry, it is usually clear whether it applies. For example:

- Appendicitis (K37) has an additional modifier of "unspecified" in the Tabular List. This is an alert to look elsewhere when the type of appendicitis is stated in the medical record.

- Painful menstruation (N94.6) has the title **Dysmenorrhea, unspecified,** in the Tabular List. Although the title in the Tabular List is not identical to the term in the Alphabetic Index, it is clear that N94.6 is the right code for this condition.

Any significant discrepancy between the Index entry and the tabular listing should alert the coding professional to the need to review the Alphabetic Index for a more appropriate term.

All instructional terms and notes should be read and followed when they apply, with particular attention to exclusion notes. Ordinarily, the alphanumeric code listed with the main term entry in the Index is for an unspecified condition. It is important to review other codes in the related area to determine whether a more specific code can be assigned.

CODING DEMONSTRATIONS

Follow the steps outlined above to determine the correct code for each of the diagnostic statements listed below:

- **Hirsutism**

  Refer to the main term **Hirsutism** in the Alphabetic Index, which provides a code of L68.0. Note that there are no subterms. Verify this by referring to code L68.0 in the Tabular List. In this case, the Index entry and Tabular List title are identical and code L68.0 should be assigned.

- **Portal vein obstruction**

  Refer to the main term **Obstruction** in the Alphabetic Index and the subterm for portal (circulation) (vein), which provides a code of I81. In the Tabular List, the title for code 181 is "Portal (vein) thrombosis" but an inclusion term is "portal (vein) obstruction." If you are uncertain whether thrombosis and obstruction are the same condition for the purposes of coding, check the Index for the main term **Thrombosis.**

- **Abscess abdominal wall due to *Staphylococcus***

  Look up the main term **Abscess** in the Alphabetic Index and then the subterm "abdomen, abdominal"; and then the subterm "wall." The code entry is L02.211. Read the "use 'additional code' note" in the Tabular List that advises you to also assign a code to identify the organism involved (B95–B96). Hint: if you have trouble locating this note, check under the category title L02. Look up **Infection,** staphylococcal, and the subterm "as cause of disease classified elsewhere" in the Alphabetic Index and find code B95.8. In the Tabular List, the code title for B95.8 is "Unspecified staphylococcus as the cause of diseases classified elsewhere." Review the medical record for any mention of the specific type of *Staphylococcus*. If one is mentioned, consider assigning the code B95.61, B95.62, or B95.7; if not, assign code B95.8 as an additional code.

- **Aplasia of pulmonary artery**

  Refer to the main term **Aplasia** in the Alphabetic Index. Check the subterms, and note that there is no entry for pulmonary artery. However, there is a cross-reference note after **Aplasia** to "see also Agenesis." Follow the cross-reference advice and refer to the main term **Agenesis.** You immediately see a more specific subterm for "artery, pulmonary," with code entry Q25.79. The title for this code in the Tabular List is "Other congenital malformations of pulmonary artery," and it is clearly the correct code for this condition. As additional confirmation that this is the correct code, "agenesis of pulmonary artery" is listed as an inclusion term.

- **Acute bronchopneumonia due to aspiration of oil**

  Locate the main term **Bronchopneumonia** in the Alphabetic Index. Note the cross-reference instruction to "see Pneumonia, broncho." Follow the cross-reference by turning to the main term **Pneumonia** (acute) (double) (migratory). . . . Note that the term "acute" is a nonessential modifier enclosed in parentheses following the main term **Pneumonia.** This nonessential modifier applies also to the subterms, and so the term "acute" has now been accounted for but does not directly affect code assignment. Refer to the following subterms listed under the main term:

> **Pneumonia (acute) (double) (migratory) . . .**
> -broncho-, bronchial (confluent) (croupous)
>   (diffuse) (disseminated) (hemorrhagic) . . .
> --aspiration—see Pneumonia, aspiration

Note the cross-reference to "see Pneumonia, aspiration." Refer back to the subterm "aspiration" and locate the code J69.0. Search through the main term and subterms cited above and underline the component parts of the diagnostic statement that have been located so far. Note that all component parts of the diagnostic statement except "of oil" have been located. Refer back to "Pneumonia, aspiration," and you will see that there are additional subterms here under the connecting words "due to," with a subterm for "oils, essences," that takes you to code J69.1. Refer to code J69.1 in the Tabular List, and note that the title for this code is "Pneumonitis due to inhalation of oils and essences." Although the title is not worded exactly the same as the diagnosis, there is such a close correlation that it is clear that this is the code that should be assigned. Assign code J69.1 because it covers all elements of the diagnosis and no instructional notes contradict its use.

REVIEW EXERCISE 5.2

Using the Alphabetic Index and the Tabular List, code the following diagnoses

1. Chronic hypertrophy of tonsils and adenoids

2. Fibrocystic disease of breast (female)

3. Acute suppurative mastoiditis with subperiosteal abscess

4. Recurrent direct left inguinal hernia with gangrene

5. Acute upper respiratory infection with influenza

6. Benign cyst of right breast

7. Bunion, right great toe

8. Nondisplaced abduction fracture anterior acetabular column, subsequent encounter with routine healing

9. Bronchiectasis with acute bronchitis

10. Acute bleeding peptic ulcer

11. Dementia with aggressive behavior

12. Hereditary retinal degeneration

CHAPTER 6

Basic ICD-10-CM Coding Guidelines

CHAPTER OVERVIEW

- There are basic principles that all coding professionals must follow.
- It is important to use both the Alphabetic Index and the Tabular List during the coding process.
  - Follow all instructional notes.
  - Even if commonly used codes have been memorized, refer to the Alphabetic Index and Tabular List.
- Always assign codes to the highest level of detail.
  - All characters must be used.
  - None can be omitted or added.
- NEC and NOS codes should be assigned only when appropriate.
- Combination codes should be used if they are available.
  - Assign multiple codes as needed to fully describe a condition.
  - Avoid coding irrelevant information.

LEARNING OUTCOMES

After studying this chapter, you should be able to:

- Determine what level of detail to assign to a code.
- Understand how to use combination codes.
- Explain how to assign multiple codes to fully describe a condition.
- Identify what qualifications determine whether an unconfirmed diagnosis is coded as though it were an established diagnosis.
- Explain the difference between "rule out" and "ruled out."
- Code "borderline" diagnoses.
- Code acute and chronic conditions.
- Code a condition labeled "impending," "threatened," or "late effect."

TERMS TO KNOW

Combination code
a single code used to classify two diagnoses, a diagnosis with a secondary condition, or a diagnosis with an associated complication

NEC
not elsewhere classified

NOS
not otherwise specified

"Rule out"
indicates that a diagnosis is still possible

"Ruled out"
indicates that a diagnosis once considered likely is no longer possible

REMEMBER . . .

For the current version of the *ICD-10-CM Official Guidelines for Coding and Reporting,* visit www.codingclinicadvisor.com.

INTRODUCTION

The basic coding guidelines discussed in this chapter apply throughout the ICD-10-CM classification system. Following these principles is vital to accurate code selection and correct sequencing. Guidelines that apply to specific chapters of ICD-10-CM will be discussed in the relevant chapters of this handbook. To download a copy of the current version of the complete *ICD-10-CM Official Guidelines for Coding and Reporting,* please visit www.codingclinicadvisor.com. This handbook has been prepared using the 2021 version of the Official Coding Guidelines. Adherence to the guidelines when assigning ICD-10-CM diagnosis codes is required under the Health Insurance Portability and Accountability Act. The instructions and conventions of the classification take precedence over guidelines.

USE BOTH THE ALPHABETIC INDEX AND THE TABULAR LIST

Section I of the ICD-10-CM Official Coding Guidelines contains the conventions, general coding guidelines, and chapter-specific guidelines. The conventions for ICD-10-CM are the general rules for use of the classification independent of the guidelines. These conventions are incorporated within the Alphabetic Index and Tabular List of ICD-10-CM as instructional notes.

The first coding principle is that both the Alphabetic Index and the Tabular List must be used to locate and assign appropriate codes. The diagnosis, condition, or reason for visit to be coded must first be located in the Index, and the code provided there must then be verified in the Tabular List. The Index does not provide the full code. Selection of the full code, including laterality and any applicable seventh character, can only be done using the Tabular List. Follow all instructional notes to ensure that more specific subterms or other instructional notes are not overlooked. Experienced coding professionals should not rely on their memory for commonly used codes. Consistent reference to the Alphabetic Index and the Tabular List is imperative.

ASSIGN CODES TO THE HIGHEST LEVEL OF DETAIL

A second basic principle is that codes with the highest number of characters available must be used. This can be accomplished by following these steps:

1. Assign a three-character disease code only if it is not further divided (when there are no four-character codes within that category).

2. Assign a four-character code only when there are no five-character codes within that subcategory.

3. Assign a five-character code only when there are no six-character codes for that subcategory.

4. Assign a six-character code when a sixth-character subclassification is provided.

5. Assign a seventh-character value when provided.

All characters must be used. None can be omitted, and none can be added. The one exception to this rule is the placeholder character "x." For codes with less than six characters that require a seventh character, a placeholder "x" should be assigned for all characters less than six. The seventh-character value must always be the seventh character of a code. An example of this exception is at categories T36–T50 (poisoning, adverse effects, and underdosing codes).

The following examples demonstrate these basic coding principles:

- Refer to the Tabular List category J40, Bronchitis, not specified as acute or chronic. Code J40 has no fourth-character subdivisions; therefore, the three-character code is assigned.

- Refer to the Tabular List category K35, Acute appendicitis. This category includes fourth characters that indicate the presence of generalized or localized peritonitis. In addition, there are fifth characters and sixth characters that indicate whether there is an abscess, gangrene, or perforation of the appendix. Because fourth-character, fifth-character, and sixth-character subdivisions are provided, K35 cannot be assigned as a three-character code.

- Refer to the Tabular List category J45, Asthma. Category J45 has five fourth-character subdivisions (J45.2, J45.3, J45.4, J45.5, and J45.9). It also uses a final-character (fifth- or sixth-character) subclassification to specify whether there is any mention of status asthmaticus or acute exacerbation. Any code assignment from category J45 must have five characters (for subcategories J45.2–J45.5) or six characters (for subcategory J45.9) to ensure coding accuracy.

- Refer to the Tabular List category T27, Burn and corrosion of respiratory tract. Category T27 has eight four-character subdivisions to specify whether the condition is burn or corrosion and to provide detail about the part of the respiratory tract affected. The general note at category T27 also indicates that the appropriate seventh character is to be added to each code from this category. Because the codes from category T27 are only four characters long, the placeholder character "x" is used as a fifth- and sixth-character placeholder before the seventh character can be added. For example, an initial encounter for burn of the larynx and trachea would be coded to T27.0xxA.

ASSIGN RESIDUAL CODES (NEC AND NOS) AS APPROPRIATE

The main term entry in the Alphabetic Index is usually followed by the code number for the unspecified condition. This code should never be assigned without a careful review of subterms to determine whether a more specific code can be located. When the review does not identify a more specific code entry in the Index, the titles and inclusion notes in the subdivisions under the three-character, four-character, or five-character code in the Tabular List should be reviewed. The residual NOS (not otherwise specified) code should never be assigned when a more specific code is available. The following examples demonstrate this basic coding principle:

- Refer to the Alphabetic Index for nontraumatic hematoma of breast, which is classified as N64.89. In the Tabular List, this code is listed as "other" specified disorders of the breast. Even though the diagnosis is very specific, no separate code is provided for it.

- Refer to the Alphabetic Index for phlebitis. Note that phlebitis, not otherwise specified, is assigned to code **I80.9, Phlebitis and thrombophlebitis of unspecified site.** Now, suppose that review of the medical record provides even further specificity, that the diagnosis is phlebitis of not only the lower extremity but the right popliteal vein. The more specific code **I80.221, Phlebitis and thrombophlebitis of right popliteal vein,** should be assigned.

ASSIGN COMBINATION CODES WHEN AVAILABLE

A combination code is a single code used to classify any of the following: two diagnoses, a diagnosis with an associated secondary process (manifestation), or a diagnosis with an associated complication. Combination codes can be located in the Index by referring to subterm entries, with particular reference to subterms that follow connecting words such as "with," "due to," "in," and "associated with." Other combination codes can be identified by reading inclusion and exclusion notes in the Tabular List.

Only the combination code is assigned when that code fully identifies the diagnostic conditions involved or when the Alphabetic Index so directs. For example:

K80.00	Acute cholecystitis with cholelithiasis
J02.0	Acute pharyngitis due to streptococcal infection
K41.11	Bilateral recurrent femoral hernia with gangrene
H40.812	Glaucoma with increased episcleral venous pressure, left eye

---

EXERCISE 6.1

Code the following diagnoses.

1. Influenza with gastroenteritis

2. Acute cholecystitis with cholelithiasis and choledocholithiasis

3. Meningitis due to *Salmonella* infection

4. Atherosclerotic heart disease (native vessel)
    with unstable angina pectoris

Occasionally, a combination code lacks the necessary specificity to describe the manifestation or complication; in such cases, an additional code may be assigned. Directions in the Tabular List provide guidance regarding the use of an additional code or codes that may provide more specificity. For example, code O99.01- classifies anemia complicating pregnancy. Because it does not indicate the type of anemia, an additional code can be assigned for this purpose.

ASSIGN MULTIPLE CODES AS NEEDED

Multiple coding is the use of more than one code to fully identify the component elements of a complex diagnostic or procedural statement. A complex statement is one that involves connecting words or phrases such as "with," "due to," "incidental to," "secondary to," or similar terminology. Directions in the Tabular List provide guidance regarding the use of an additional code or codes that may provide more specificity. When no combination code is provided, multiple codes should be assigned as needed to fully describe the condition regardless of whether there is advice to that effect.

Mandatory Multiple Coding

The term "dual classification" is used to describe the required assignment of two codes to provide information about both a manifestation and the associated underlying disease or etiology. Mandatory multiple coding is identified in the Alphabetic Index by the use of a second code in brackets. The first code identifies the underlying condition, and the second identifies the manifestation. Both codes must be assigned and sequenced in the order listed.

In the Tabular List, the need for dual coding is indicated by the presence of a "use additional code" note with the code for the underlying condition, and a "code first underlying condition" note with the manifestation code. In printed versions of the manuals, the manifestation code is in italics. Manifestation codes cannot be designated as the principal diagnosis, and a code for the underlying condition (if present) must always be listed first, except in a few situations where other directions are provided. A code in brackets in the Alphabetic Index can be used only as a secondary code for the specific condition or procedure indexed in this way. For example:

G20 + F02.80   Dementia in Parkinson's disease
D66 + M36.2   Arthritis in hemophilia

EXERCISE 6.2

Code the following diagnoses according to the coding principles for correct sequencing of codes.

1. Amyloid heart

2. Chorioretinitis due to histoplasmosis

3. Combined spinal cord degeneration with anemia
   due to dietary vitamin B12 deficiency

4. Otomycosis, right ear

5. Cataract associated with hypoparathyroidism

Discretionary Multiple Coding

The "code first" notes appear in the Tabular List under certain codes that are not specifically manifestation codes, but codes in which the condition may be due to an underlying cause. When there is a "code first" note and an underlying condition is present, the underlying condition should be sequenced first, if applicable. For example, malignant ascites (R18.0) has a note to "code first" the malignancy, such as malignant neoplasm of ovary (C56.-). In this situation, code C56.- would be assigned first, followed by code R18.0.

The "code, if applicable, any causal condition first" note indicates that multiple codes should be assigned only if the causal condition is documented as being present. For example, "Other retention of urine" (R33.8) requires that the code to identify enlarged prostate (N40.1) be assigned as the first-listed code or principal diagnosis, but only if enlarged prostate is documented as being the cause of the urinary retention.

The instruction to "use additional code" indicates that multiple codes should be assigned only if the condition mentioned is documented as being present. Examples include the following:

- Malignant neoplasm of base of tongue (C01) requires an additional code to identify history of tobacco dependence (Z87.891), but only when history of tobacco dependence is documented in the medical record.

• Urinary tract infection (N39.0) requires an additional code to identify the organism if it is documented, such as positive culture of *E. coli* (B96.20).

EXERCISE 6.3

Code the following diagnoses.

1. Acute cystitis due to *E. coli* infection

2. Alcoholic gastritis due to chronic alcoholism

3. Diverticulitis of colon with intestinal hemorrhage

4. Diabetic neuralgia due to type 2 diabetes mellitus,

   patient on insulin

5. Erythema multiforme with arthritis

6. Fulminant hepatitis, type A, with hepatic coma

Avoid Indiscriminate Multiple Coding

Indiscriminate coding of irrelevant information should be avoided. For example, codes for symptoms or signs characteristic of the diagnosis and integral to it should not be assigned. Codes are never assigned solely on the basis of findings of diagnostic tests, such as laboratory, X-ray, or electrocardiographic tests, unless the diagnosis is confirmed by the physician. This guideline applies to inpatient admissions and differs from the coding practices in the outpatient setting when one is coding encounters for diagnostic tests that have been interpreted by a physician. Codes should not be assigned for conditions that do not meet Uniform Hospital Discharge Data Set criteria for reporting. For example, diagnostic reports often mention such conditions as hiatal hernia, atelectasis, and right bundle branch block with no further mention to indicate any relevance to the care given. Assigning a code is inappropriate for reporting purposes unless the physician provides documentation to support the condition's significance for the episode of care.

The only exception to this guidance about querying the provider to document the clinical significance of findings is for the coding of 2019 novel coronavirus disease (COVID-19). The coding guidelines for inpatient encounters allow the reporting of this diagnosis on the basis of a positive COVID-19 test result alone.

Codes designated as unspecified are never assigned when a more specific code for the same general condition is assigned. For example, diabetes mellitus with unspecified complication (E11.8) would never be assigned when a code for diabetes with renal complication (E11.29) is assigned for the same episode of care.

Laterality

Some ICD-10-CM codes indicate laterality, specifying whether the condition occurs on the left or right or whether the condition is bilateral. If the condition is bilateral but no bilateral code is provided, assign separate codes for the left side and the right side. If the side is not identified in the medical record, assign the code for unspecified side. For example:

Q70.10   Webbed fingers, unspecified hand

Q70.11   Webbed fingers, right hand

Q70.12   Webbed fingers, left hand

Q70.13   Webbed fingers, bilateral

When a patient has a bilateral condition (e.g., cataracts in both eyes), and each side is treated during separate encounters (e.g., cataract surgery is performed on each eye in separate encounters), assign a "bilateral" code for the encounter to treat the first side. (The code is "bilateral" for the first encounter because the condition exists on both sides at that time.) For the second encounter, assign the appropriate unilateral code for the side where the condition still exists. The bilateral code would not be assigned for the subsequent encounter because the patient no longer has the condition in the previously treated site. However, if the treatment on the first side did not completely resolve the condition, the bilateral code would still be appropriate for the encounter to re-treat the first side.

CODE UNCERTAIN DIAGNOSES AS IF ESTABLISHED

When a diagnosis for an inpatient admission to a short-term, acute care hospital, a long-term care hospital, or a psychiatric hospital is qualified as "possible," "probable," "suspected," "likely," "questionable," "?" or "rule out" at the time of discharge, the condition should be coded and reported as though the diagnosis were established. Other terms that fit the definition of a probable or suspected condition are "consistent with," "compatible with," "indicative of," "suggestive of," "appears to be," "concern for," and "comparable with." Note that exceptions to this guideline are made for the coding of HIV infection/illness and the coding of Zika, COVID-19, and influenza due to certain identified influenza viruses (e.g., avian influenza or other novel influenza A virus). In these exceptions, code only cases confirmed by physician documentation. The guideline regarding uncertain diagnoses does not apply to coding or reporting for outpatient services, home health services, hospice services, or physician services regardless of the setting. Instead, the coding professional should be guided by the Diagnostic Coding and Reporting Guidelines for Outpatient Services (Hospital-based and Physician Office). For these patients, code to the highest degree of certainty, such as symptoms, signs, or abnormalities. For example ("admitted" in the following examples refers to acute care inpatient hospital admissions):

- A patient is admitted with severe generalized abdominal pain.
  The physician's diagnostic statement on discharge is
  abdominal pain, probably due to acute gastritis.
  Only the code for gastritis is assigned as the pain is implicit in the diagnosis.   K29.00

- A patient is admitted and discharged with a final diagnosis of
  probable peptic ulcer with a recommendation for additional workup.   K27.9

- A patient is admitted as an inpatient and discharged with possible
  posttraumatic brain syndrome, nonpsychotic.   F07.81

- A patient is seen in the outpatient clinic with malaise. The
  physician's diagnostic statement is possible viral syndrome.
  Only the malaise is coded.   R53.81

Caution should be used in coding uncertain diagnoses of conditions such as epilepsy, HIV disease, and multiple sclerosis as if they were established. Incorrect reporting of such conditions can have serious personal consequences for the patient, such as the inability to obtain a driver's license and possible social and job discrimination. Physicians are often unaware that the Official Coding Guidelines require a diagnosis qualified as uncertain to be coded as if established; therefore, be sure to consult the physician before assigning codes for such uncertain conditions.

"Rule Out" versus "Ruled Out"

It is important to distinguish between the terms "rule out," which indicates that a diagnosis is still considered to be possible, and "ruled out," which indicates that a diagnosis originally considered as likely is no longer a possibility.

For inpatient episodes of care, diagnoses qualified by the term "rule out" are coded as if established in the same way that diagnoses described as possible or probable are coded. A diagnosis described as "ruled out" is never coded. If an alternative condition has been identified, that diagnosis should be coded; otherwise, a code for the presenting symptom or other precursor condition should be assigned. Here are some examples of codes assigned according to this coding principle:

- Rule out gastric ulcer . . .   K25.9 *[condition is coded]*
- Acute appendicitis, ruled out;
  Meckel's diverticulum found at surgery . . . Q43.0 *[code only the diverticulum]*
- Rule out angiodysplasia of the colon . . . K55.20 *[condition is coded]*

"Borderline" Diagnoses

Care should be exercised with diagnoses documented as "borderline." A borderline diagnosis is not the same as an uncertain diagnosis and is handled differently. Borderline diagnoses are coded as confirmed unless the classification provides a specific entry (e.g., borderline diabetes mellitus). If a borderline condition has a specific index entry in ICD-10-CM, it should be coded as such. Because borderline conditions are not uncertain diagnoses, this coding principle applies to all care settings (inpatient and outpatient). Query for clarification whenever the documentation is unclear regarding a borderline condition.

Use of Sign/Symptom and "Unspecified" Codes

Although every attempt should be made to report specific diagnosis codes when supported by the available medical record, the use of sign/symptom and "unspecified" codes is acceptable, and may even be necessary, in situations such as the following:

- If a definitive diagnosis has not been established by the end of the encounter
- If a more specific code cannot be assigned because of insufficient or unavailable clinical information about a particular health condition

An unspecified code should be reported when it is the code that most accurately reflects what is known about the patient's condition at the time of the encounter.

ACUTE AND CHRONIC CONDITIONS

When the same condition is described in the medical record as both acute (or subacute) and chronic, it should be coded according to the Alphabetic Index subentries for that condition. If separate subterms for acute (or subacute) and chronic are listed at the same indention level in the Alphabetic Index, both codes are assigned, with the code for the acute condition sequenced first. (Note that a condition described as subacute is coded as acute if there is no separate subterm entry for subacute.) For example, refer to the Alphabetic Index entry for acute and chronic bronchitis:

Bronchitis . . .
-acute or subacute . . . J20.9 . . .
-chronic . . . J42

Because both subterms appear at the same indention level, both codes are assigned if the provider documents acute and chronic bronchitis, with code J20.9 sequenced first.

When only one term is listed as a subterm, with the other in parentheses as a nonessential modifier, only the code listed for the subterm is assigned. For example, for a diagnosis of acute and chronic adenoiditis, the Alphabetic Index entry is as follows:

Adenoiditis (chronic) J35.02 . . .
-acute J03.90

The only code assigned in this situation is **J03.90, Acute tonsillitis, unspecified.**

In some cases, a combination code has been provided for use when the condition is described in the medical record as both acute and chronic. For example, code J96.20 includes both acute and chronic respiratory failure. When there are no subentries for acute (or subacute) or chronic, these modifiers are disregarded in coding the condition. For example, refer to the term **Mastopathy,** cystic. Neither acute nor chronic is listed as a subterm, and so code N60.1- is assigned.

EXERCISE 6.4

Code the following diagnoses.

1. Acute and chronic appendicitis

2. Subacute and chronic pyelonephritis

3. Acute and chronic cervicitis

4. Acute and chronic abscess of the broad ligament

5. Acute and chronic bilateral canaliculitis

IMPENDING OR THREATENED CONDITION

Selection of a code for a condition described at the time of discharge, or at the conclusion of an outpatient encounter, as impending or threatened depends first on whether the condition actually occurred. If so, the threatened/impending condition is coded as a confirmed diagnosis.

For example, a medical record shows a diagnosis of threatened premature labor at 28 weeks' gestation. Review of the medical record indicates that a stillborn was delivered during the hospital stay. This is coded as **O60.14x0, Preterm labor third trimester with preterm delivery third trimester, not applicable or unspecified,** because the threatened condition did occur.

However, if neither the threatened/impending condition nor a related condition occurred, refer to the Alphabetic Index to answer the following two questions: Is the condition indexed under the main term **Threatened** or **Impending**? Is there a subterm for impending or threatened under the main term for the condition? If such terms appear, assign the code provided. There are several subterms under each of the main terms **Impending** and **Threatened,** as well as several main terms with such subentries. For example, if a patient is admitted with threatened abortion but the abortion is averted, the code **O20.0, Threatened abortion,** is assigned because there is an Index entry for "threatened" under the main term **Abortion.**

When neither impending nor threatened is indexed for a condition, the precursor condition that actually existed is coded; a code is not assigned for the condition described as impending or threatened. For example, a patient is admitted with a diagnosis of impending gangrene of the lower extremities, but the gangrene is averted by prompt treatment. Because the gangrene does not occur and there is no index entry for impending gangrene, a code must be assigned for the presenting situation that suggested the possibility of gangrene, such as redness or swelling of the extremity.

REPORTING THE SAME DIAGNOSIS CODE MORE THAN ONCE

Each unique ICD-10-CM diagnosis code may be reported only once for an encounter. This applies both to bilateral conditions when there are no distinct codes identifying laterality and to two different conditions classified to the same ICD-10-CM diagnosis code.

LATE EFFECTS

A late effect is a residual condition that remains after the termination of the acute phase of an illness or injury. Such conditions may occur at any time after an acute injury or illness. There is no set period of time that must elapse before a condition is considered to be a late effect. Some late effects are apparent early; others may make an appearance long after the original injury or illness has been resolved. Certain conditions due to trauma, such as contractures and scarring, are inherent late effects no matter how early they occur.

Late effects include conditions reported as such or as sequela of a previous illness or injury. The fact that a condition is a late effect may be inferred when the diagnostic statement includes terms such as the following:

- Late
- Old
- Due to previous injury or illness
- Following previous injury or illness
- Traumatic, unless there is evidence of current injury

EXERCISE 6.5

Mark an "X" next to each diagnostic statement given below that identifies a late effect of an injury or illness. For each such statement, underline the residual condition once and the cause of the late effect twice.

1. Hemiplegia due to previous cerebrovascular accident   _____

2. Joint contracture of fracture, right index finger   _____

3. Scoliosis due to old infantile paralysis   _____

4. Laceration of tendon of finger two weeks ago; admitted now for tendon repair   _____

5. Keloid secondary to injury nine months ago   _____

6. Intellectual disability due to previous viral encephalitis   _____

Locating Late Effect Codes

Codes that indicate the cause of a late effect can be located by referring to the main term **Sequelae** in the Alphabetic Index of Diseases and Injuries (with the exception of late effects due to injury, poisoning, and certain other consequences of external causes). Note that ICD-10-CM provides only a limited number of codes to indicate the cause of a late effect:

B90.0–B90.9	Sequelae of tuberculosis
B91	Sequelae of poliomyelitis
B92	Sequelae of leprosy
B94.0–B94.9	Sequelae of other and unspecified infectious and parasitic diseases
E64.0–E64.9	Sequelae of malnutrition and other nutritional deficiencies
E68	Sequelae of hyperalimentation
G09	Sequelae of inflammatory diseases of central nervous system
G65.0–G65.2	Sequelae of inflammatory and toxic polyneuropathies
I69.0–I69.9	Sequelae of cerebrovascular disease
O94	Sequelae of complication of pregnancy, childbirth, and the puerperium

Two Codes Required

Complete coding of late effects requires two codes:

- The condition or nature of the late effect
- The late effect code

The condition or nature of the late effect is sequenced first, followed by the code for the cause of the late effect, except in a few instances where the Alphabetic Index or the Tabular List directs otherwise. If the late effect is due to injury, poisoning, or certain other consequences of external causes (S00–T88), a seventh-character value for "sequelae" should be assigned to the injury code as well as the external causes code (V01–Y95). For example:

M19.111 + S42.301S	Post-traumatic osteoarthritis of right shoulder due to old fracture of right humerus
G83.10 + B91	Paralysis of leg due to old poliomyelitis
N29 + B90.1	Tuberculous calcification of kidney

There are three exceptions to the coding principle that requires two codes for late effect:

• When the residual effect is not stated, the cause of the late effect code is used alone.

• When no late effect code is provided in ICD-10-CM but the condition is described as being a late effect, only the residual condition is coded. Note that conditions described as due to previous surgery are not coded as late effects; instead, they are classified as history of or complications of previous surgery, depending on the specific situation.

• When the late effect code has been expanded at the fourth-, fifth-, or sixth-character level(s) to include the manifestation condition, only the cause of the late effect code is assigned. For example, code **I69.010, Attention and concentration deficit following nontraumatic subarachnoid hemorrhage,** includes both the cause of the late effect (nontraumatic subarachnoid hemorrhage) and the manifestation (attention and concentration deficit).

LATE EFFECT VERSUS CURRENT ILLNESS OR INJURY

A late effect code is not used with a code for a current injury or illness of the same type, with one exception: Codes from category I69, Sequelae of cerebrovascular disease, may be assigned as an additional code with codes from I60–I67, if the patient has a current cerebrovascular disease and residual deficits from an old cerebrovascular disease. For example, a patient with residual aphasia due to subdural hemorrhage two years ago who is admitted because of acute cerebral thrombosis would have the following codes assigned: **I66.9, Occlusion and stenosis of unspecified cerebral artery,** and **I69.220, Aphasia following other nontraumatic intracranial hemorrhage.**

EXERCISE 6.6

Code the following diagnoses.

1. Residuals of poliomyelitis

2. Sequela of old crush injury to left foot

3. Stroke two years ago with residual hemiplegia of the right dominant side

4. Contracture of hip following partial hip replacement one year ago

REVIEW EXERCISE 6.7

Code the following diagnoses.

1. Traumatic arthritis, right ankle, following
   fracture, right ankle

2. Cicatricial contracture of left hand due to burn

3. Brain damage following cerebral abscess
   seven months ago

4. Flaccid hemiplegia due to old cerebral infarction

5. Bilateral neural deafness resulting from childhood
   measles 10 years ago

6. Mononeuritis, median nerve, resulting
   from previous crush injury to right arm

7. Posttraumatic, painful arthritis, left hand

8. Residuals of previous severe burn, left wrist

9. Locked-in state (paralytic syndrome) due to old
   cerebrovascular infarction

10. Borderline diabetes mellitus

11. Impending myocardial infarction

12. Borderline hypothyroidism

Introduction to the ICD-10-PCS Classification

CHAPTER OVERVIEW

- All ICD-10-PCS codes have an alphanumeric structure, no decimal points, and seven characters.
- ICD-10-PCS is divided into 17 sections relating to the general type of procedure.
- Codes in the Medical and Surgical Section specify the section, body system, root operation, body part, approach, device, and qualifier.
- ICD-10-PCS is divided into the Alphabetic Index and the Tables.

LEARNING OUTCOMES

After studying this chapter, you should be able to:

Explain the structure, format, and conventions of ICD-10-PCS.

TERMS TO KNOW

Approach
the fifth character in the code in the Medical and Surgical Section; the way the procedure site is reached (for example, open or percutaneous)

Character
an axis of classification that specifies information about the procedure performed

Qualifier
the seventh character in the code in the Medical and Surgical Section; it carries additional information for that particular procedure

Root operation
the third character in the code in the Medical and Surgical Section corresponding to the objective of the procedure; in this section alone, there are 31 possible objectives

Value
one of the 34 letters or numbers that can be selected to represent one of the characters in an ICD-10-PCS code

REMEMBER . . .

In the alphanumeric structure of ICD-10-PCS, do not confuse the letters "O" and "I" with the numbers 0 and 1.

INTRODUCTION

The *International Classification of Diseases, Tenth Revision, Procedure Coding System* (ICD-10-PCS) is a classification of operations and procedures developed for use in the United States; it is not part of the World Health Organization classification. ICD-10-PCS is used by hospitals to report inpatient procedures; it is not used in other health care settings. As with ICD-10-CM, ICD-10-PCS is a closed classification system providing one and only one place to classify each procedure. Similar to ICD-10-CM, hospital coding professionals must understand the basic principles behind the classification system to use ICD-10-PCS appropriately and effectively. This knowledge is also the basis for understanding and applying the official coding advice provided through the *AHA Coding Clinic*. It is important for medical coding professionals to keep current with the *ICD-10-PCS Official Guidelines for Coding and Reporting*, as well as with the *Coding Clinic*.

ICD-10-PCS uses standardized terminology to provide precise and stable definitions for all procedures performed. As such, ICD-10-PCS does not include eponyms, which are usually the name of the surgeon (or surgeons) who developed the procedure (e.g., Whipple procedure for pancreaticoduodenectomy). Instead, such procedures are coded to the operation that identifies the objective of the procedure. General information on ICD-10-PCS, including conventions and definitions of the components of a code, is provided in this chapter. Procedures specific to certain body systems will be covered in the relevant chapters of this handbook.

DEVELOPMENT OF ICD-10-PCS

ICD-10-PCS was developed by 3M under contract to the Centers for Medicare & Medicaid Services (CMS). Development of ICD-10-PCS was completed in 1998 and has been updated annually since then. ICD-10-PCS was officially implemented in the United States on October 1, 2015, for hospital reporting of inpatient procedures. Proposals for updating ICD-10-PCS are now handled through the Coordination and Maintenance Process overseen jointly by the National Center for Health Statistics and CMS. The goal of the revisions is to keep current with medical technology and coding needs.

The guiding principles that were followed in the development of ICD-10-PCS are these:

- Diagnostic information is not included in the procedure description.
- Explicit "not otherwise specified" (NOS) options are not provided.
- "Not elsewhere classified" (NEC) options are provided on a limited basis.
- All possible procedures are defined regardless of the frequency of occurrence. If a procedure could be performed, a code was created.

The 17 sections in ICD-10-PCs represent nearly 77,000 codes. ICD-10-PCS uses a table structure that permits the specification of a large number of codes on a single page in the tabular division.

FORMAT AND ORGANIZATION

Format

ICD-10-PCS is divided into the Alphabetic Index and the Tables. Codes can be located in alphabetical order within the Index. The Index will refer to a specific location within a Table, and the complete code can be obtained only by referring to the Tables. The complete list of ICD-10-PCS code titles is typically not included in published codebooks, but it is available for download from the CMS website (www.cms.gov/Medicare/Coding/ICD10).

Alphabetic Index

The Index is arranged in alphabetical order based on the type of procedure being performed. The ICD-10-PCS Index does not provide a complete code (with a few exceptions), but it points to a specific location in the Tables by specifying the first three or four characters of the code. The purpose of the Alphabetic Index is to locate the appropriate table in which you will find the information needed to complete the other characters of the code. Coding professionals are not required to consult the Index first before proceeding to the Tables to complete the code.

For example, "cholecystectomy" may be looked up by "Excision, gallbladder," or "Resection, gallbladder." The term **Cholecystectomy** has two reference notes as follows:

Cholecystectomy

—see Excision, Gallbladder 0FB4

—see Resection, Gallbladder 0FT4

The Index entries "0FB4" and "0FT4" are not complete codes, but rather they point the user to the appropriate Table identified by the first three values (for example, 0FT, which is shown in figure 7.1).

Tables

The ICD-10-PCS Tables are composed of grids specifying the valid combinations of characters that make up a procedure code. Within a Table, valid codes include all combinations of choices in characters 4 through 7 contained in the same row of the Table.

FIGURE 7.1   Sample Excerpt of ICD-10-PCS Table

Section	0	Medical and Surgical
Body System	F	Hepatobiliary System and Pancreas
Operation	T	Resection: Cutting out or off, without replacement, all of a body part

Body Part	Approach	Device	Qualifier
0 Liver 1 Liver, Right Lobe 2 Liver, Left Lobe 4 Gallbladder G Pancreas	0 Open 4 Percutaneous Endoscopic	Z No Device	Z No Qualifier
5 Hepatic Duct, Right 6 Hepatic Duct, Left 7 Hepatic Duct, Common 8 Cystic Duct 9 Common Bile Duct C Ampulla of Vater D Pancreatic Duct F Pancreatic Duct, Accessory	0 Open 4 Percutaneous Endoscopic 7 Via Natural or Artificial Opening 8 Via Natural or Artificial Opening Endoscopic	Z No Device	Z No Qualifier

FIGURE 7.2 Structure of Codes in the Medical and Surgical Section

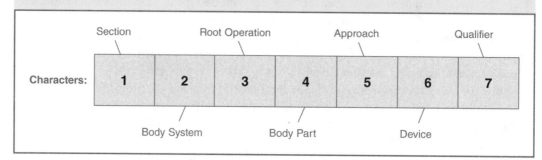

Code Structure

All ICD-10-PCS codes have an alphanumeric structure, with all codes made up of seven characters and no decimal points. It is important to distinguish between "character" and "value" before we go any further. Each **character** in a code is an axis of classification that represents an aspect of the procedure. A **value** is one of the 34 letters or numbers that can be selected to represent one of the characters in an ICD-10-PCS code. These values are made up of digits 0–9, or the letters A–H, J–N, and P–Z. The letters "O" and "I" are not used so as not to be confused with the digits "0" and "1."

Refer to figure 7.2 for the structure and meaning of each character for codes within the Medical and Surgical Section.

Within a defined code range, each of the second through seventh characters has a standard meaning—but these characters may have different meanings across sections. Within a defined code range, a character specifies the same type of information in that axis of classification, as follows: The first character represents the axis for section, the second for body system, the third for root operation, the fourth for body part, the fifth for approach, the sixth for device, and the seventh for qualifier. These specific components of a code and their definitions will be covered in more detail later.

The number of unique values used in an axis of classification differs as needed. This means that within different axes of the classification, there may be different unique values. For example, the body part axis will have many more unique values than the approach axis, because there are many more body parts than surgical approaches.

As with words in their context, the meaning of any single value is a combination of its axis of classification and any preceding values on which it may be dependent. For example, the meaning of a body part value in the Medical and Surgical Section is always dependent on the body system value. The body part value "0" in the "central nervous system and cranial nerves" body system specifies "brain," and the body part value "0" in the "peripheral nervous system" body system specifies "cervical plexus." (Refer to figure 7.3 for a graphic representation of this example).

Relational Terms

The term "and," when used in a code description, usually means "and/or." For example, the description "lower arm and wrist muscle" means lower arm and/or wrist muscle. The exception is when "and" is used to describe a combination of multiple body parts and separate values exist for each body part in the description (e.g., there is a code description "skin and subcutaneous tissue" that, when used as a qualifier, includes separate body part values for skin and subcutaneous tissue).

FIGURE 7.3 Examples of Body Part Values

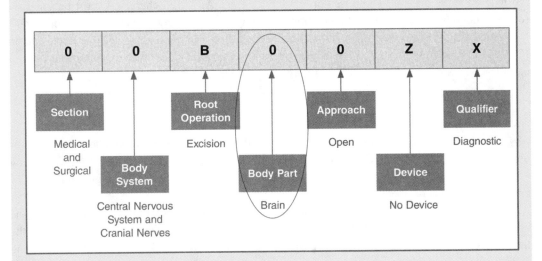

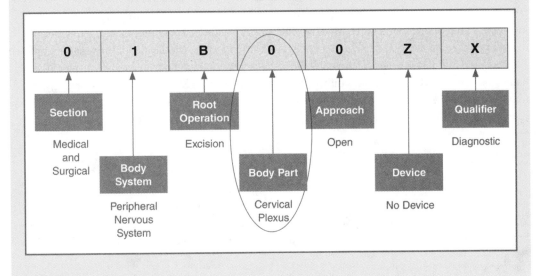

EXERCISE 7.1

Without referring to the handbook material or ICD-10-PCS, mark the following statements either true or false.

1. The ICD-10-PCS Index includes eponyms to identify procedures. _____

2. All ICD-10-PCS codes have an alphanumeric structure, _____
    with all codes made up of seven characters.

3. All complete ICD-10-PCS codes can be located within the Index. _____

4. The ICD-10-PCS Tables specify the valid combinations of characters _____
    that make up a procedure code.

5. The letters "O" and "I" are not used as ICD-10-PCS values _____
    so as not to be confused with the digits "0" and "1."

CODE CHARACTERS AND THEIR DEFINITIONS

All ICD-10-PCS codes are composed of seven characters. All seven characters must be specified for the code to be valid. If the documentation is incomplete for coding purposes, the provider must be queried for the necessary information. This section discusses each character that makes up an ICD-10-PCS code, and the definition of each, as well as the main values that are applicable to build an ICD-10-PCS code in the Medical and Surgical Section.

Character 1: Section

The first character in the code always refers to the section. A section refers to a broad procedure category or section where the code is found. ICD-10-PCS is divided into 17 sections relating to the general type of procedure. Table 7.1 displays the ICD-10-PCS sections along with the first character of each code specifying the section.

As shown in table 7.1, the number 0 represents the Medical and Surgical Section, while the other sections each have their own numeric or alphabetical values. For example, Obstetrics has the first character 1. There are also some limited ancillary diagnostic codes, such as "B" for Imaging and "C" for Nuclear Medicine. There is no section for laboratory tests, as most facilities do not code lab tests for inpatient records. The majority of the procedures that would normally be reported in an inpatient setting can be found in the Medical and Surgical Section. Therefore, the following discussion regarding the component characters of a code refers strictly to the Medical and Surgical Section. The Medical- and Surgical-Related Section and the Ancillary Section are both covered in chapter 10 of this handbook. Chapter 10 also includes information about codes from Section X, New Technology, which may be used in the inpatient setting. The Obstetrics Section, which covers procedures performed on products of conception, is discussed in chapters 23 and 24 of this handbook.

Character 2: Body System

The second character in an ICD-10-PCS code represents the body system. This character indicates the general physiological system or anatomical region involved (e.g., gastrointestinal). Within the Medical and Surgical Section, these characters will retain the same value in all codes. For example, a central nervous system procedure in this section will always have the value "0" for

TABLE 7.1 ICD-10-PCS Sections and Their Corresponding Character Values

Value	Section	Value	Section
0	Medical and Surgical	9	Chiropractic
1	Obstetrics	B	Imaging
2	Placement	C	Nuclear Medicine
3	Administration	D	Radiation Therapy
4	Measurement and Monitoring	F	Physical Rehabilitation and Diagnostic Audiology
5	Extracorporeal or Systemic Assistance and Performance	G	Mental Health
6	Extracorporeal or Systemic Therapies	H	Substance Abuse Treatment
7	Osteopathic	X	New Technology
8	Other Procedures		

the second character, while a respiratory system procedure will have the value "B" for the second character.

For additional detail, some traditional body systems have been assigned multiple values. For example, the circulatory system has been subdivided into heart and great vessels, upper arteries, lower arteries, upper veins, and lower veins. Within the conventions of ICD-10-PCS, each of these areas is considered a separate body system with its own unique value. Refer to table 7.2 for the body systems in the Medical and Surgical Section, along with their corresponding character values.

The diaphragm is used as the frame of reference for body part values classified as upper or lower in the "upper arteries," "lower arteries," "upper veins," "lower veins," and "muscles and tendons" body systems. For example, veins located above the diaphragm are found in the "upper veins" body system, and veins located below the diaphragm are found in the "lower veins" body system.

Three body systems refer to anatomical regions, as follows:

- Anatomical regions, general
- Anatomical regions, upper extremities
- Anatomical regions, lower extremities

The "general anatomical regions" body system codes should only be used when a procedure is performed on an anatomical region (e.g., drainage of a body cavity), rather than on a specific body part. "General anatomical regions" body systems can also be used on the rare occasions when no information is available to support assignment of a code to a more specific body part within a body system.

TABLE 7.2 Medical and Surgical Section Body Systems and Values

Value	Body System	Value	Body System
0	Central nervous and cranial nerves	J	Subcutaneous tissue and fascia
1	Peripheral nervous	K	Muscles
2	Heart and great vessels	L	Tendons—includes synovial membrane
3	Upper arteries	M	Bursae and ligaments—includes synovial membrane
4	Lower arteries		
5	Upper veins	N	Head and facial bones
6	Lower veins	P	Upper bones
7	Lymphatic and hemic—includes lymph vessels and lymph nodes	Q	Lower bones
		R	Upper joints—includes synovial membrane
8	Eye	S	Lower joints—includes synovial membrane
9	Ear, nose, sinus—includes sinus ducts	T	Urinary
B	Respiratory	U	Female reproductive
C	Mouth and throat	V	Male reproductive
D	Gastrointestinal	W	Anatomical regions, general
F	Hepatobiliary and pancreas	X	Anatomical regions, upper extremities
G	Endocrine	Y	Anatomical regions, lower extremities
H	Skin and breast—includes skin and breast glands and ducts		

EXERCISE 7.2

Referring to table 7.2, mark an "X" next to each term or phrase identifying a body system as classified by a unique value within ICD-10-PCS.

1. Respiratory   _____

2. Heart and great vessels   _____

3. Circulatory   _____

4. Musculoskeletal   _____

5. Upper bones   _____

Character 3: Root Operation

The third character refers to the root operation. Root operation is one of the most important concepts that the user needs to understand to identify and select the correct ICD-10-PCS code. Mastering the definitions of these root operations is the key to "building" a code in ICD-10-PCS. Root operation refers to the objective of the procedure. Different root operations are distinguished by their objectives—namely, what is the procedure trying to accomplish?

In the Medical and Surgical Section, there are 31 different root operations. Each root operation is precisely defined in the classification. The definitions are easily found in the Table. For example, in the excerpts of the Tables shown in figure 7.1 (page 63) and figure 7.4 (page 70), the root operation "Resection" is defined on the third line of the first row as "cutting out or off, without replacement, all of a body part."

Root operations include terms such as "Alteration," "Bypass," "Change," "Creation," "Dilation," "Excision," "Resection," "Fusion," "Insertion," "Occlusion," and "Repair." The complete list of root operations in the Medical and Surgical Section, along with their corresponding values, is included in table 7.3.

Some of the root operations used in ICD-10-PCS may not necessarily coincide with terminology used by physicians in their documentation. However, because many of the terms used to construct ICD-10-PCS codes are defined within the system, the physician is not expected to use the

TABLE 7.3   ICD-10-PCS Root Operations and Their Corresponding Values

Value	Root Operation	Value	Root Operation	Value	Root Operation	Value	Root Operation
0	Alteration	8	Division	J	Inspection	S	Reposition
1	Bypass	9	Drainage	K	Map	T	Resection
2	Change	B	Excision	L	Occlusion	V	Restriction
3	Control	C	Extirpation	M	Reattachment	W	Revision
4	Creation	D	Extraction	N	Release	U	Supplement
5	Destruction	F	Fragmentation	P	Removal	X	Transfer
6	Detachment	G	Fusion	Q	Repair	Y	Transplantation
7	Dilation	H	Insertion	R	Replacement		

exact terms used in ICD-10-PCS code descriptions. Instead, it is the coding professional's responsibility to determine the correlation between the documentation of procedures in the medical record and the ICD-10-PCS definitions.

It is not necessary to query the physician when the correlation between the documentation and the defined ICD-10-PCS terms is clear. For example, if the physician documents "partial resection," the coding professional can independently correlate "partial resection" to the root operation "Excision" without querying the physician for clarification because partial resection meets the definition of excision within ICD-10-PCS, namely, "cutting out or off, without replacement, a portion of a body part."

Because of the large number of root operations and their importance in assigning ICD-10-PCS codes, specific root operations are covered in more detail in chapter 9 of this handbook.

Character 4: Body Part

The fourth character indicates the specific part of the body system or anatomical site where the procedure was performed (for example, appendix). Within ICD-10-PCS, body part values may refer to an entire organ (e.g., liver) or to specific portions of an organ (e.g., liver, right lobe). The ICD-10-PCS Body Part Key is a helpful alphabetical listing of specific alternative names for muscles, veins, nerves, and other anatomical sites, along with the corresponding ICD-10-PCS body part that should be used for code selection. For example, the key indicates that procedures that refer to the term "abdominal aortic plexus" should be coded using the body part "abdominal sympathetic nerve."

If a procedure is performed on a portion of a body part that does not have a separate body part value, the value corresponding to the whole body part value should be selected. For example, a procedure that is done on the alveolar process of the mandible would get coded to the "mandible" body part, right or left.

If procedures performed on body parts are identified with the prefix "peri" (meaning "around" or "near") and the site of the procedure is not further defined, then the procedure should be coded to the body part named. For example, a procedure identified as "perirenal" is coded to the body part "kidney." However, care must be exercised in applying this guideline because it only applies when a more specific body part value is not available. For example, a procedure documented as "repair of periurethral laceration," in which the tissue torn was vulvar rather than urethral, is coded to the body part "vulva" because a specific body part exists in ICD-10-PCS for the vulva. If the body part "vulva" were not available in ICD-10-PCS, then the "peri" guideline would apply, and "periurethral" would be coded to the body part "urethra."

A procedure site documented as involving the periosteum is coded to the corresponding bone body part. For example, excisional debridement of the right heel down to and including the periosteum of the calcaneus is coded **0QBL0ZZ Excision of right tarsal, open approach.**

If a procedure is performed on a continuous section of a tubular body part, code the body part value corresponding to the furthest anatomical site from the point of entry. For example, a procedure performed on a continuous section of artery from the femoral artery to the external iliac artery, with the point of entry at the femoral artery, is coded to the "external iliac" body part, right or left.

Occasionally, surgeries are performed in which organs are reconfigured to create new organs. If additional surgery on the new organ is required in the future, the ICD-10-PCS body part value would be selected on the basis of the current function of the organ. For example, a patient undergoes a urinary diversion, in which a new bladder is created from part of the small intestine, as a treatment for bladder cancer; at a later date, when that patient has a polyp removed from the artificial neobladder made up of small intestine, the ICD-10-PCS procedure code for the removal is assigned to the body part "bladder" rather than to "small intestine."

Branches of body parts. Where ICD-10-PCS does not provide a body part value to a specific branch of a body part, the body part is typically coded to the closest proximal branch that has a specific body part value. For example, a procedure performed on the mandibular branch of the trigeminal nerve is coded to the "trigeminal nerve" body part value. In the cardiovascular body systems, if a general body part is available in the correct root operation table, and coding to a proximal branch would require assigning a code in a different body system, the procedure is coded using the general body part value. For example, occlusion of the bronchial artery is coded to the body part value "upper artery" in the body system "upper arteries," and not to the body part value "thoracic aorta, descending" in the body system "heart and great vessels."

Bilateral body part values. ICD-10-PCS provides values for some bilateral body parts. However, not every paired organ or body part has a "bilateral" value. If the identical procedure is performed on both sides, and a bilateral body part value exists for that body part, the procedure code is assigned once using the bilateral body part value. For example, refer to figure 7.4 to code bilateral oophorectomy. The identical procedure was performed on both ovaries, and there is a body part value that includes bilateral ovaries. Because there is a value for "bilateral," we would report a single code.

If no bilateral body part value exists, each procedure should be coded separately using the appropriate body part value. For example, consider bilateral hip replacement. There are body part values for "right hip" and for "left hip," but not for bilateral hips. If the exact same procedure were performed on both hips, two separate codes should be reported to identify that both hips were replaced.

Skin, subcutaneous tissue, and fascia overlying a joint. If a procedure is performed on the skin, subcutaneous tissue, or fascia overlying a joint, the procedure is coded to the following body part:

- Shoulder is coded to upper arm.
- Elbow is coded to lower arm.
- Wrist is coded to lower arm.
- Hip is coded to upper leg.
- Knee is coded to lower leg.
- Ankle is coded to foot.

FIGURE 7.4   Excerpt from Table Showing Bilateral Body Part

Section	0	Medical and Surgical
Body System	U	Female Reproductive System
Operation	T	Resection: Cutting out or off, without replacement, all of a body part

Body Part	Approach	Device	Qualifier
0 Ovary, Right 1 Ovary, Left 2 Ovaries, Bilateral 5 Fallopian Tube, Right 6 Fallopian Tube, Left 7 Fallopian Tubes, Bilateral 9 Uterus	0 Open 4 Percutaneous Endoscopic 7 Via Natural or Artificial Opening 8 Via Natural or Artificial Opening Endoscopic F Via Natural or Artificial Opening With Percutaneous Endoscopic Assistance	Z No Device	Z No Qualifier
4 Uterine Supporting Structure C Cervix F Cul-de-sac G Vagina	0 Open 4 Percutaneous Endoscopic 7 Via Natural or Artificial Opening 8 Via Natural or Artificial Opening Endoscopic	Z No Device	Z No Qualifier
J Clitoris L Vestibular Gland M Vulva	0 Open X External	Z No Device	Z No Qualifier
K Hymen	0 Open 4 Percutaneous Endoscopic 7 Via Natural or Artificial Opening 8 Via Natural or Artificial Opening Endoscopic X External	Z No Device	Z No Qualifier

CHAPTER 7

*Introduction
to the
ICD-10-PCS
Classification*

Fingers and toes. If a body system does not contain a separate body part value for fingers, procedures performed on the fingers are coded to the body part value for the hand. If a body system does not contain a separate body part value for toes, procedures performed on the toes are coded to the body part value for the foot. For example, excision of a finger tendon is coded to one of the hand tendon body part values in the "tendons" body system.

We have now covered most of the body part guidelines, except for a few that are reserved for the body system. Procedures on the following body parts are covered in more detail in later chapters of this handbook:

- Upper intestinal tract and lower intestinal tract are addressed in chapter 19, Diseases of the Digestive System.

- Tendons, ligaments, bursae, and fascia near a joint are addressed in chapter 22, Diseases of the Musculoskeletal System and Connective Tissue.

- Coronary arteries are addressed in chapter 27, Diseases of the Circulatory System.

Character 5: Approach

The fifth character refers to the technique or approach used to reach the procedure site (e.g., open). Seven approaches are listed in the Medical and Surgical Section. Approaches can be external, through the skin or mucous membrane, or through an orifice. The following list breaks down the approaches.

- External
- Through the skin or mucous membrane
  —Open
  —Percutaneous
  —Percutaneous endoscopic
- Through an orifice
  —Via natural or artificial opening
  —Via natural or artificial opening endoscopic
  —Via natural or artificial opening with percutaneous endoscopic assistance

As with root operations, each approach is precisely defined in the classification. Refer to table 7.4 for the approaches shown in the Medical and Surgical Section, along with their corresponding values and definitions, and to figure 7.5 for illustrations of surgical approaches.

In addition to the approach definitions listed in table 7.4, there are a handful of guidelines related to the selection of the approach, as follows:

- *Open approach with percutaneous endoscopic assistance*: code to "open" approach. Example: laparoscopic-assisted sigmoidectomy is coded to "open."

- *Percutaneous endoscopic approach with extension of incision.* Procedures performed using the percutaneous endoscopic approach, with incision or extension of an incision to assist in the removal of all or a portion of a body part or to anastomose a tubular body part to complete the procedure, are coded to the approach value Percutaneous Endoscopic. *Examples*: Laparoscopic sigmoid colectomy with extension of stapling port for removal of specimen and direct anastomosis is coded to the approach value percutaneous endoscopic.

- *External approach.* The following procedures should be coded to "external":
  —Procedures performed within an orifice on structures that are visible without the aid of any instrumentation. Example: resection of tonsils.
  —Procedures performed indirectly by the application of external force through the intervening body layers. Example: closed reduction of fracture.

- *Percutaneous procedure via device*: Code to "percutaneous." Example: fragmentation of kidney stone via percutaneous nephrostomy.

TABLE 7.4 Medical and Surgical Section Approaches

Value	Approach	Definition
X	External	Procedures performed directly on the skin or mucous membrane and procedures performed indirectly by the application of external force through the skin or mucous membrane
0	Open	Cutting through the skin or mucous membrane and any other body layers necessary to expose the site of the procedure
3	Percutaneous	Entry, by puncture or minor incision, of instrumentation through the skin or mucous membrane and/or any other body layers necessary to reach the site of the procedure
4	Percutaneous endoscopic	Entry, by puncture or minor incision, of instrumentation through the skin or mucous membrane and/or any other body layers necessary to reach and visualize the site of the procedure
7	Via natural or artificial opening	Entry of instrumentation through a natural or artificial external opening to reach the site of the procedure
8	Via natural or artificial opening endoscopic	Entry of instrumentation through a natural or artificial external opening to reach and visualize the site of the procedure
F	Via natural or artificial opening with percutaneous endoscopic assistance	Entry of instrumentation through a natural or artificial external opening, and entry, by puncture or minor incision, of instrumentation through the skin or mucous membrane and any other body layers necessary to aid in the performance of the procedure

EXERCISE 7.3

Identify the ICD-10-PCS approach value used for each of the procedures below:

Procedure	Approach Value
1. Appendectomy via abdominal incision	_____
2. Arthroscopic knee chondroplasty	_____
3. Adenoidectomy	_____
4. Bronchoscopy	_____
5. Laparoscopic-assisted hysterectomy	_____
6. Vaginal endometrial ablation	_____
7. Insertion of intravenous pacemaker lead	_____
8. Endoscopic carpal tunnel release	_____
9. Chest tube removal	_____
10. EGD and biopsy of stomach	_____

Character 6: Device

The sixth character is used to identify whether a device was used in a procedure. Only devices that remain in or on the patient's body after the procedure is completed are coded. If no device remains after the procedure is completed, the device value "Z," representing "no device," is used as the sixth character to complete the code structure. In limited root operations, the classification allows the reporting of temporary devices, or devices used intraoperatively, for specific procedures involving clinically significant devices—in which the purpose of the device is to be used for a brief duration during the procedure or the current inpatient stay. For further details, refer to the discussion regarding the seventh character, qualifier, later in this chapter.

Device values fall into four basic categories:

- Grafts and prostheses

- Implants

- Simple or mechanical appliances

- Electronic appliances

Occasionally, a device that is intended to remain after the procedure is completed must be removed before the end of the operative episode in which it was inserted (for example, the device is too small or a complication occurs). In this situation, both the insertion and removal of the device should be coded.

Materials that are integral to a procedure are not coded as devices. Examples of integral materials are sutures, ligatures, clips, radiological markers, and temporary postoperative wound drains. Drains placed in the operative wound site at the close of the procedure to prevent reaccumulation of fluids are not coded separately. A drain placed at the end of an open surgical drainage procedure is considered the same as any other temporary postsurgical wound drain used to prevent buildup of fluid and is not coded separately.

The ICD-10-PCS Index contains entries to provide guidance on the selection of codes related to devices. In addition, two resources have been created to assist with identification of devices:

- Device Key

- Device Aggregation Table

The Device Key lists devices by their common names, as well as their brand names, with the corresponding ICD-10-PCS terms to assist in selecting the appropriate device value. For example, the key indicates that both the common device name "Total artificial (replacement) heart" and the brand name "AbioCor® Total Replacement Heart" should be coded to the ICD-10-PCS value for "synthetic substitute" device.

The Device Aggregation Table provides a mechanism for directing coding professionals and secondary data users to correlate a specific device value, used in the original root operation where the device was placed, with its more general device value used in other root operations. The Device Aggregation Table provides all the entries that refer to a particular device value, and this table may be used to get a better sense of how these devices are classified. The table provides general and specific information about devices, the applicable operation(s), and the body system(s).

Often, in root operations such as "Removal" and "Revision," the device value is the aggregate general device of an entire family of specific device values. For example, in figure 7.6, the Device Aggregation Table indicates that, for the root operation "Insertion," there are two specific cardiac lead devices available—one for defibrillators and one for pacemakers. However, when coding a less-specific root operation such as "Removal" or "Revision," the device value is less specific. In these cases, only the general device "cardiac lead" is available and the type of cardiac device for the lead (i.e., defibrillator or pacemaker) is not specified.

Within ICD-10-PCS, "intraluminal device" is the most generic value for any device that resides in the lumen of a tubular or hollow body part. It is used when the device does not have a more specific device value. When a more specific type of intraluminal device value is available, the more specific value should be used. For example, an intravenous cardiac lead is a device that resides

FIGURE 7.5   Illustrations of Medical and Surgical Section Approaches

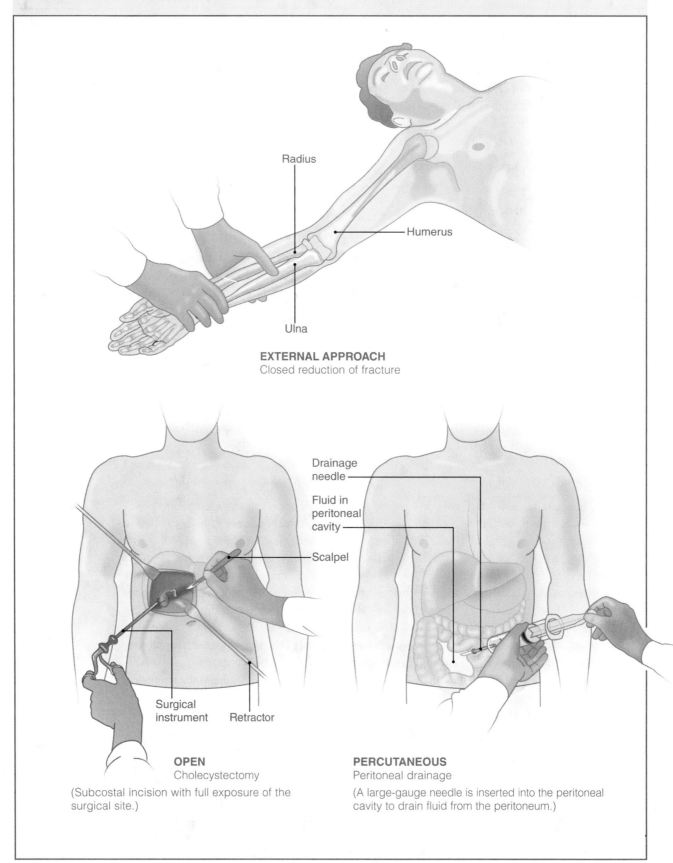

Radius

Humerus

Ulna

EXTERNAL APPROACH
Closed reduction of fracture

Drainage needle

Fluid in peritoneal cavity

Scalpel

Surgical instrument   Retractor

OPEN
Cholecystectomy

(Subcostal incision with full exposure of the surgical site.)

PERCUTANEOUS
Peritoneal drainage

(A large-gauge needle is inserted into the peritoneal cavity to drain fluid from the peritoneum.)

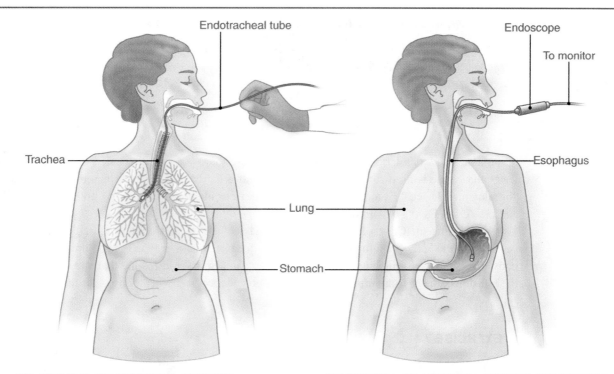

VIA NATURAL OR ARTIFICIAL OPENING
Insertion of endotracheal tube

(The tube is inserted through the mouth into the trachea.)

VIA NATURAL OR ARTIFICIAL OPENING ENDOSCOPIC
Gastroscopy

(The endoscope is inserted through the mouth into the stomach.)

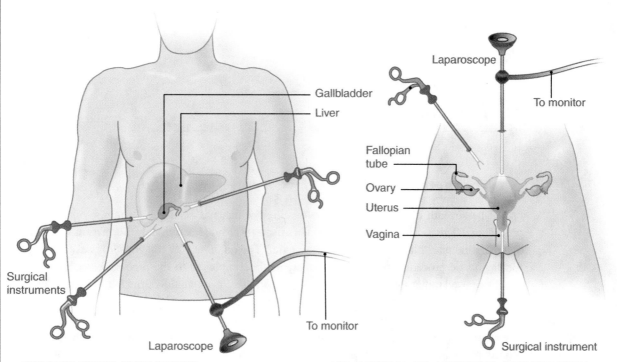

PERCUTANEOUS ENDOSCOPIC
Laparoscopic cholecystectomy

(Several small incisions are made in the abdomen, through which surgical instruments and a laparoscope with a video camera are placed into the abdominal cavity.)

VIA NATURAL OR ARTIFICIAL OPENING WITH PERCUTANEOUS ENDOSCOPIC ASSISTANCE
Laparoscopic-assisted vaginal hysterectomy

(A vaginal hysterectomy is done with laparoscopic assistance; ovaries and fallopian tubes may be detached using a laparoscope, and the uterus is detached and all of the organs are removed through the vagina.)

FIGURE 7.6   Excerpt from the Device Aggregation Table

Specific Device	For Operation	In Body System	General Device
Cardiac Lead, Defibrillator	Insertion	Heart and Great Vessels	Cardiac Lead
Cardiac Lead, Pacemaker	Insertion	Heart and Great Vessels	Cardiac Lead

in the lumen of a tubular body part; however, because there is a specific device value for "cardiac lead," that value is used for insertion or removal of a cardiac lead, rather than the more general "intraluminal device." Examples of intraluminal devices include biliary stents, embolization coils, and the Zenith Flex® AAA Endovascular Graft.

According to ICD-10-PCS, an "infusion device" is any device that is used to infuse substances into the body. An infusion catheter can be a device that is inserted in the lumen of a tubular body part, such as a vein, but an infusion catheter can also be inserted in other sites. The fact that the infusion catheter is an infusion device takes precedence over whether it is intraluminal or not.

EXERCISE 7.4

Mark an "X" next to each term or phrase that can be considered a codeable device within ICD-10-PCS.

1. Joint prosthesis   _____

2. Cardiac pacemaker   _____

3. Prolene sutures   _____

4. Neurostimulator   _____

5. Mesh graft   _____

Character 7: Qualifier

The seventh character indicates a qualifier, which has a unique meaning within individual procedures. This position within the code is used to provide additional information. Examples of qualifiers include "diagnostic" and "stereotactic." The qualifier "X" (diagnostic) is exclusively used for diagnostic procedures. If there is a therapeutic component to the procedure, the qualifier "Z" should be used rather than the qualifier "X." When there is no qualifier, the letter "Z" is used as the seventh-character value to complete the code structure.

If a patient undergoes two separate procedures, one diagnostic and the other therapeutic, both procedures are coded separately. For example, suppose a patient undergoes a diagnostic drainage procedure (biopsy) and a therapeutic drainage procedure; if the biopsy uses a different approach or samples a different site than the therapeutic drainage procedure, separate codes are required to capture the two procedures.

As noted earlier, in limited root operations, the classification allows the reporting of temporary devices and devices used intraoperatively. These devices are identified with the qualifier values "temporary" and "intraoperative." For example, Table 04L, "Occlusion—Lower Arteries," provides a code for the occlusion of the abdominal aorta with a temporary intraluminal device.

CHAPTER 8

Basic ICD-10-PCS Coding Steps

CHAPTER OVERVIEW

- The Uniform Hospital Discharge Data Set (UHDDS) requires all significant procedures to be reported. Significant procedures meet any one of the following conditions:
  - The procedure is surgical in nature.
  - It carries an anesthetic risk.
  - It carries a procedural risk.
  - It requires specialized training.
- ICD-10-PCS contains the Alphabetic Index and the Tables.

LEARNING OUTCOMES

After studying this chapter, you should be able to:

Identify main terms in the Alphabetic Index.

Navigate the Tables to find the appropriate Table.

TERM TO KNOW

Principal procedure
procedure performed for definitive treatment (rather than for diagnostic or exploratory purposes)

INTRODUCTION

This chapter covers the steps to take in locating ICD-10-PCS codes. In addition, it discusses general information on reporting procedures as well as selection of the principal procedure.

The following steps should be undertaken to locate the procedure codes using ICD-10-PCS:

1. Locate the main term in the Alphabetic Index

   • Follow any cross-reference instructions.

   • Obtain the first three or four characters for the procedure.

   • In a few instances, the Index provides complete seven-character codes.

2. Find the applicable Table.

   • Review the section, body system, and root operation definition, and verify that the first three characters referenced by the Index are correct.

3. Continue building the ICD-10-PCS code by selecting a value from each column for the remaining four characters, as follows:

   • Select a value from the body part column for the fourth character.

   • Select a value from the approach column for the fifth character.

   • Select a value from the device column for the sixth character.

   • Select a value from the qualifier column for the seventh character.

It is important to note that valid codes can be built using all combinations of choices in characters 4 through 7 that are in the same row of the Table. Because all ICD-10-PCS codes are seven characters long, the code must specify all seven characters to be valid.

LOCATE THE MAIN TERM IN THE ALPHABETIC INDEX

The first step in coding is to locate the main term in the Alphabetic Index. The Index can be used to access the Tables. Main terms may be common procedure terms (e.g., **Appendectomy, Cholecystectomy**), root operation values (e.g., Resection, Excision), or body parts. Subterms provide more specific information. Each indention level of the Index is represented below by a hyphen. Please note that some publishers have adopted the convention used in the ICD-10-CM Index of adding a dash (-) at the end of an Index entry to indicate that additional characters are required.

The following examples demonstrate the different main terms and subterms used in ICD-10-PCS.

• When the main term is a root operation value (e.g., Excision), the subterms will be body parts where the operation was performed, as shown below:

Excision

-Abdominal Wall 0WBF

-Acetabulum

--Left 0QB5

--Right 0QB4

-Adenoids 0CBQ

- When the main term is a common procedure, references are provided to the corresponding ICD-10-PCS root operation and body part, as shown below:

Claviculectomy

—see Excision, Upper Bones 0PB

—see Resection, Upper Bones 0PT

Condylectomy

—see Excision, Head and Facial Bones 0NB

—see Excision, Upper Bones 0PB

—see Excision, Lower Bones 0QB

- When the main term is an anatomical term, helpful references are provided to identify specific ICD-10-PCS body parts, as shown below:

Adductor hallucis muscle

—*use* Foot Muscle, Right

—*use* Foot Muscle, Left

It is not necessary to start with the Alphabetic Index before proceeding to the Tables to complete a code. A valid code may be chosen directly from the Tables, but looking up the code will require a thorough familiarity with the body systems and root operations.

EXERCISE 8.1

Without referring to the Alphabetic Index, underline the word(s) in each item that indicates the main term(s) for each procedure.

1. Laparoscopic cholecystectomy

2. Resection of pancreas

3. Bilateral oophorectomy

4. Incision and drainage of abscess, neck

5. Bowel resection with transverse colostomy

6. Fusion of L5-S1 vertebral joints

7. Lysis of intestinal adhesions

FIND THE APPLICABLE TABLE

Once the first three or more characters of a code have been located in the Alphabetic Index, refer to the appropriate Table. There is no need to follow the reference notes to see other terms if the Index provides the first three or four characters of a code. For example, the main term **Cholecystectomy** refers us to "0FT4" for "Resection, gallbladder." Looking up the main term **Resection** with the subterm "gallbladder" will not yield the complete seven-character code. Instead, it will reference the same Table: 0FT4.

To find the appropriate Table:

- If using the PDF version of ICD-10-PCS available for download from the Centers for Medicare & Medicaid Services website, the appropriate Table can be accessed directly by clicking the hyperlinked character values provided in the Index entry (e.g., 0FT4).

- If using a published ICD-10-PCS book, it will be necessary to manually locate the appropriate Table. The Tables are arranged in a series, beginning with section 0, Medical and Surgical, and body system 0, Central Nervous System and Cranial Nerves, and proceeding in numerical order. Sections 0 through 9 are followed by sections B through D, F through H, and X. The same convention is followed within each Table for the second through seventh characters—numeric values in order first, followed by alphabetical values in order.

EXERCISE 8.2

Without referring to ICD-10-PCS, identify the order in which the following Tables (represented by the first three characters) can be located.

1. 0JQ _____

2. 0J9 _____

3. B31 _____

4. 09B _____

5. 09W _____

CODING DEMONSTRATIONS

Follow the steps outlined above to determine the correct code for each of the procedural statements listed below.

Total Laparoscopic Cholecystectomy

Refer to main term **Cholecystectomy.** Note that there are two references: "see Excision, Gallbladder [0FB4]" and "see Resection, Gallbladder [0FT4]." There is no need to find the Index entry for the main term **Excision,** subterm "gallbladder," or main term **Resection,** subterm "gallbladder," as they will both refer to the same Tables. If you are unfamiliar with the differences between these two root operations, you can review the definitions of "Excision" and "Resection" in appendix A of ICD-10-PCS, or you can locate both Tables (0FB and 0FT) and read the definitions of the root operations there.

FIGURE 8.1 Excerpt of 0FT Table from ICD-10-PCS

Section	0	Medical and Surgical
Body System	F	Hepatobiliary System and Pancreas
Operation	T	Resection: Cutting out or off, without replacement, all of a body part

Body Part	Approach	Device	Qualifier
0 Liver 1 Liver, Right Lobe 2 Liver, Left Lobe 4 Gallbladder G Pancreas	0 Open 4 Percutaneous Endoscopic	Z No Device	Z No Qualifier
5 Hepatic Duct, Right 6 Hepatic Duct, Left 7 Hepatic Duct, Common 8 Cystic Duct 9 Common Bile Duct C Ampulla of Vater D Pancreatic Duct F Pancreatic Duct, Accessory	0 Open 4 Percutaneous Endoscopic 7 Via Natural or Artificial Opening 8 Via Natural or Artificial Opening Endoscopic	Z No Device	Z No Qualifier

Review Table 0FB. Reading across the first row of the Table, the first character, "0," refers to Medical and Surgical Section; the second character, "F," refers to the body system "hepatobiliary system and pancreas"; and the third character, "B," refers to the root operation "Excision." Excision is defined on the 0FB Table as "cutting out or off, without replacement, a portion of a body part." Because the procedure is total cholecystectomy, "Excision" is not the correct root operation.

Review Table 0FT. The third character, "T," refers to the root operation "Resection." Resection is defined on the 0FT Table as "cutting out or off, without replacement, all of a body part." Based on this review, it becomes clear that "Excision, gallbladder" is the root operation for a partial cholecystectomy, and "Resection" is the root operation for a total cholecystectomy; therefore, 0FT is the correct Table.

Continue building the remainder of the code by selecting the remaining values among the appropriate characters from the four columns shown in figure 8.1. In the first column—body part—select the value of "4" for gallbladder. From the second column—approach—because this was a laparoscopic procedure, select the value "4" for percutaneous endoscopic. Moving across the Table, select as the sixth character "Z" for device, because no device was used for this procedure, and select as the last character "Z," representing no qualifier. The ICD-10-PCS procedure code, then, is 0FT44ZZ. Figure 8.1 shows the 0FT Table used for this demonstration, with the appropriate value circled for each character of the code.

Note that within an ICD-10-PCS Table, valid codes include all combinations of choices in characters 4 through 7 contained in the same row of the Table. For example, using the Table in figure 8.1 to assign the code for total cholecystectomy, the value "8" is not valid as the fifth character for approach because it is not on the same row as the body part "4" for gallbladder.

Below Knee Amputation, Distal Portion, Right Leg

Look up the main term **Amputation** in the Alphabetic Index. Note the cross-reference instruction to "see Detachment." Follow the cross-reference by turning to the main term **Detachment,** and then the subterm "leg." Note that additional subterms specify "lower" and then "left" and "right." In this instance, the Index provides code 0Y6H0Z for the right lower leg—it is almost complete, except that it only has six characters.

FIGURE 8.2 Excerpt of 0Y6 Table from ICD-10-PCS

Section	**0** Medical and Surgical
Body System	**Y** Anatomical Regions, Lower Extremities
Operation	**6** Detachment: Cutting off all or a portion of the upper or lower extremities

Body Part	Approach	Device	Qualifier
2 Hindquarter, Right **3** Hindquarter, Left **4** Hindquarter, Bilateral **7** Femoral Region, Right **8** Femoral Region, Left **F** Knee Region, Right **G** Knee Region, Left	**0** Open	**Z** No Device	**Z** No Qualifier
C Upper Leg, Right **D** Upper Leg, Left **H** Lower Leg, Right **J** Lower Leg, Left	**0** Open	**Z** No Device	**1** High **2** Mid **3** Low

Refer to Table 0Y6 (shown as figure 8.2) and locate the appropriate row for the body part character "H" for lower leg, right. Because the only acceptable values for approach and device for this body part are "0" and "Z," they have already been provided in the Index. Review the values available for the qualifier. As this particular case refers to a "below the knee, distal portion" amputation, select the value "3" for "low." The ICD-10-PCS procedure code, then, is 0Y6H0Z3.

UNIFORM HOSPITAL DISCHARGE DATA SET FOR REPORTING PROCEDURES

The Uniform Hospital Discharge Data Set (UHDDS) requires all significant procedures to be reported. In addition, Medicare requires the reporting of any procedure that affects payment, whether or not it meets the definition of a significant procedure. Other procedures may be reported at the hospital's discretion. Most hospitals do not code ancillary or diagnostic procedures in the inpatient setting.

A significant procedure is defined as one that meets any of the following conditions:

- Is surgical in nature
- Carries an anesthetic risk
- Carries a procedural risk
- Requires specialized training

Surgery includes incision, excision, destruction, amputation, introduction, insertion, endoscopy, repair, suturing, and manipulation. Any procedure performed under anesthesia other than topical carries an anesthetic risk. Procedural risk is more difficult to define, but any procedure that has a recognized risk of inducing functional impairment, physiological disturbance, or possible trauma during an invasive procedure is included in this group. Procedures requiring specialized training are those that are performed by specialized professionals, qualified technicians, or clinical teams specifically trained to perform certain procedures or whose services are directed primarily to carrying them out. This definition implies training over and above that which is ordinarily provided in the education of physicians, nurses, or technicians.

Meeting Various Reporting Requirements

Under the Health Insurance Portability and Accountability Act of 1996, for administrative simplification purposes, standard code sets have been designated for electronic claims transactions. ICD-10-PCS is the standard for hospitals when reporting surgery and procedures for inpatients, whereas the American Medical Association's Current Procedural Terminology and the Health Care Procedure Coding System level II codes are the standards for hospital reporting of outpatient procedures and physician reporting.

A hospital may also code outpatient procedures using the ICD-10-PCS system for internal or non-claim-related purposes, if desired. In addition, hospitals may report ICD-10-PCS codes for outpatient services, for specific payers under contractual agreements, or as required by their state data-reporting requirements.

Designating the Principal Procedure

The principal procedure as described by the UHDDS is one performed for definitive treatment (rather than for diagnostic or exploratory purposes) or one that is necessary to care for a complication. If two or more procedures appear to meet this definition, the one most related to the principal diagnosis is designated the principal procedure. If both are equally related to the principal diagnosis, the most resource-intensive or complex procedure is usually designated as principal. When more than one procedure is reported, the principal procedure should be identified as that which relates to the principal diagnosis. Coding professionals are advised to follow UHDDS definitions for reporting unless a particular payer has substantially different reporting requirements.

The following additional guidance is provided for selecting principal procedures in relation to the principal diagnosis when more than one procedure is performed:

- A procedure was performed for definitive treatment of the principal diagnosis, and another procedure for a secondary diagnosis was also performed.

  Sequence as principal procedure the procedure performed for definitive treatment most related to the principal diagnosis.

- A procedure was performed for definitive treatment, and diagnostic procedures were performed for both the principal diagnosis and a secondary diagnosis.

  Sequence as principal procedure the procedure performed for definitive treatment most related to the principal diagnosis.

- A diagnostic procedure was performed for the principal diagnosis, and a procedure was performed for definitive treatment of a secondary diagnosis.

  Sequence the diagnostic procedure as the principal procedure because the procedure most related to the principal diagnosis takes precedence.

- No procedures related to the principal diagnosis were performed; however, procedures were performed to diagnose and definitively treat a secondary diagnosis.

  Sequence as principal procedure the procedure performed for definitive treatment of the secondary diagnosis because there were no procedures (definitive or nondefinitive treatment) related to the principal diagnosis.

It is important to follow UHDDS definitions because principal procedures are significant in the reporting of surgical quality indicators.

CHAPTER 9

ICD-10-PCS
Root Operations in the
Medical and Surgical Section

CHAPTER OVERVIEW

The 31 Medical and Surgical root operations can be divided into nine groups that share similar attributes:

- Root operations to take out some or all of a body part
- Root operations to take out solids, fluids, or gases from a body part
- Root operations that involve cutting or separation only
- Root operations to put in or put back or move some or all of a body part
- Root operations to alter the diameter or route of a tubular body part
- Root operations that always involve a device
- Root operations that involve examination only
- Root operations that include other repairs
- Root operations that include other objectives

LEARNING OUTCOMES

After studying this chapter, you should be able to:

Identify the objectives of each root operation.

Distinguish among the different root operations in the Medical and Surgical Section.

Discuss the general guidelines applicable to root operations.

TERM TO KNOW

Root operation
the third character in an ICD-10-PCS code, which refers to the objective of the procedure

CHAPTER 9

*ICD-10-PCS
Root Operations
in the Medical
and Surgical
Section*

INTRODUCTION

The previous chapters introduce the structure of ICD-10-PCS codes and discuss the basic steps to select ICD-10-PCS codes. Character 3 in the built code, root operations, is one of the most important concepts the user needs to understand to identify and select the correct ICD-10-PCS code. The root operation refers to the objective of the procedure. This chapter covers in detail the 31 root operations in the Medical and Surgical Section and their corresponding definitions. In addition, applicable guidelines from the *ICD-10-PCS Official Coding Guidelines* (2021 edition) are introduced.

ROOT OPERATION GUIDELINES

The majority of the *ICD-10-PCS Official Coding Guidelines* relate to the third character in a code, which represents the root operation. In this section, we start with the general guidelines applicable to all root operations and then move on to overarching concepts such as coding multiple procedures and discontinued procedures. Guidelines related to specific root operations are covered under the applicable root operation.

To determine the appropriate root operation, the full definition of the root operation must be applied. The definitions for the root operations (within the ICD-10-PCS classification) are included in the classification in appendix A of ICD-10-PCS as well as within each ICD-10-PCS Table (see figure 9.1).

Components of a procedure specified in the root operation definition or explanation as integral to that root operation are not coded separately. The full definition of each root operation provided in the Table must be carefully considered, as that definition will guide whether or not a procedure gets coded separately. For example, resection of a joint as part of a joint replacement procedure is included in the definition for "Replacement" and is not coded separately. Also not coded separately are procedural steps necessary to reach the operative site (such as incision or approach) or to close the operative site (such as suturing), including anastomosis of a tubular body part. For example, in a resection of sigmoid colon with anastomosis of descending colon to rectum, the anastomosis is not coded separately.

FIGURE 9.1   Table Excerpt Demonstrating Location of Root Operation Definition

Section	0	Medical and Surgical	Root operation definition
Body System	F	Hepatobiliary System and Pancreas	
Operation	T	Resection: Cutting out or off, without replacement, all of a body part	

Body Part	Approach	Device	Qualifier
0 Liver 1 Liver, Right Lobe 2 Liver, Left Lobe 4 Gallbladder G Pancreas	0 Open 4 Percutaneous Endoscopic	Z No Device	Z No Qualifier
5 Hepatic Duct, Right 6 Hepatic Duct, Left 7 Hepatic Duct, Common 8 Cystic Duct 9 Common Bile Duct C Ampulla of Vater D Pancreatic Duct F Pancreatic Duct, Accessory	0 Open 4 Percutaneous Endoscopic 7 Via Natural or Artificial Opening 8 Via Natural or Artificial Opening Endoscopic	Z No Device	Z No Qualifier

Excision/Resection followed by replacement. If an excision or resection of a body part is followed by a replacement procedure, code both procedures to identify each distinct objective, except when the excision or resection is considered integral and preparatory for the replacement procedure. For example, for mastectomy followed by reconstruction, both resection and replacement of the breast are coded to fully capture the distinct objectives of the procedures performed. Another example is resection of a joint as part of a joint replacement procedure. Since the resection of the joint is considered integral and preparatory for the replacement of the joint, the resection is not coded separately.

CHAPTER 9

ICD-10-PCS
Root Operations
in the Medical
and Surgical
Section

Coding Multiple Procedures

Multiple procedures performed during the same operative episode are coded separately if they meet one of the following four conditions:

1. *The same root operation is performed on different body parts as defined by distinct values of the body part character.* One example is the diagnostic excision of the liver and pancreas. This guideline is straightforward, except that it requires knowing how "body part" is used in the context of ICD-10-PCS. Refer to the excerpt of the Table in figure 9.1. Note that liver is an individual body part, but "liver, right lobe" and "liver, left lobe" are listed separately because each of these body parts has a distinct value. Therefore, separate biopsies of the right and left lobes of the liver are coded separately because the right and left lobes have different values in the fourth character for "body part."

2. *The same root operation is repeated in multiple body parts, and those body parts are separate and distinct body parts classified to a single ICD-10-PCS body part value.* For example, suppose a surgeon performs excision of the sartorius muscle and excision of the gracilis muscle during the same encounter. These muscles are distinct body parts that are both included in the upper leg muscle body part value. The two procedures done during the surgical encounter should be coded separately to make it apparent that two excisions were performed. Another example is extraction of multiple toenails; the toes are separate and distinct body parts, so each extraction would be coded separately. The same root operation repeated in different locations within the same body part should be coded only once. For example, excision of several fibroid tumors from the uterus is not coded multiple times because the excisions are not being performed on separate body parts. This example differs from the previous example of excision of the sartorius muscle and excision of the gracilis muscle, which are separate and distinct body parts—not different locations within the same body part.

3. *Multiple root operations with distinct objectives are performed on the same body part.* An example is destruction of sigmoid lesion and bypass of sigmoid colon.

4. *The intended root operation is attempted using one approach but is converted to a different approach.* For example, laparoscopic cholecystectomy converted to an open cholecystectomy is coded as percutaneous endoscopic "Inspection" and open "Resection." The following four ICD-10-CM diagnosis codes are available to identify procedures converted to open procedures. They may only be used as additional diagnosis codes.

   Z53.31 Laparoscopic surgical procedure converted to open procedure
   Z53.32 Thoracoscopic surgical procedure converted to open procedure
   Z53.33 Arthroscopic surgical procedure converted to open procedure
   Z53.39 Other specified procedure converted to open procedure

Coding Discontinued or Incomplete Procedures

When a planned procedure is begun but cannot be completed, it is coded to the extent to which it was actually performed according to the following principles:

88

CHAPTER 9

ICD-10-PCS
Root Operations
in the Medical
and Surgical
Section

- If the intended procedure is discontinued or otherwise not completed, code the procedure to the root operation performed.

- If a procedure is discontinued before any other root operation is performed, code the root operation "Inspection" of the body part or anatomical region inspected.

The following examples show how to code discontinued procedures:

- A patient is admitted for transurethral removal of ureteral stone. The scope is passed as far as the bladder, but the surgeon is unable to pass it into the ureter. Code only "Inspection" of the bladder.

- A patient is admitted for cholecystectomy with exploration of common duct. When the abdominal cavity is entered, extensive metastatic malignancy involving the stomach and duodenum with probable primary neoplasm in the pancreas is found. The procedure is discontinued and the operative wound closed. Code only the exploratory laparotomy as "Inspection" of the peritoneal cavity.

- A planned aortic valve replacement procedure is discontinued after the initial thoracotomy and before any incision is made in the heart muscle when the patient becomes hemodynamically unstable. This procedure is coded as an open "Inspection" of the mediastinum.

When a procedure is considered to have "failed" in that it did not achieve the hoped-for result or because every objective of the procedure could not be accomplished, the procedure is coded as performed. For example, an almost immediate reocclusion of the coronary artery occasionally occurs after the completion of a percutaneous coronary angioplasty, which makes it necessary to return to the operating room to perform a coronary artery bypass to correct the problem. The angioplasty might be described as a failed procedure, but, in fact, the procedure was performed and should be coded. Note that failure to achieve the therapeutic objective is not classified as a complication of the procedure.

It is important to distinguish a failed procedure from an attempted but unsuccessful procedure. In the example of the percutaneous coronary angioplasty, the procedure was performed, so the "Dilation" is coded. On the other hand, if a procedure is attempted but is not successful, the procedure would not be coded. For example, if a patient had an attempted foreign body removal from the right cornea with an eye spud and the procedure was unsuccessful, the attempted removal would not be considered an "Extirpation"; only "Inspection" would be coded.

Coding Biopsies

A biopsy is defined as the taking of tissue from a living person for the purpose of microscopic study. A biopsy code is not assigned when a lesion removed for therapeutic purposes is sent to the laboratory for examination, even though the term "biopsy" may be used in describing the procedure. Surgical specimens are routinely sent to the pathology laboratory for study; this procedure is not considered a biopsy, and assigning a biopsy code is inappropriate. Biopsies may be coded with several different root operations depending on how the biopsy was performed, keeping in mind the definitions for the different root operations. For example, biopsies may be reported with the root operations "Excision" (e.g., lymph node sampling), "Extraction" (e.g., bone marrow biopsy), or "Drainage" (e.g., fine needle aspiration [FNA] of lung fluid) with the qualifier "diagnostic."

When FNA of tissue, such as lymph tissue, is done, report "Extraction" of the body part for the tissue aspirated if that body part is available in the appropriate ICD-10-PCS Table. If the appropriate body part value is not available under "Extraction," the root operation "Excision" should be reported for FNA of tissue. FNA of gas or fluid should be reported to the root operation "Drainage."

Biopsy followed by more definitive treatment. If a diagnostic "Excision," "Extraction," or "Drainage" procedure (biopsy) is followed by a more definitive procedure, such as "Destruction," "Excision," or "Resection" at the same procedure site, both the biopsy and the more definitive treatment are coded. For example, a biopsy of the breast is followed by partial mastectomy at the same procedure site; both the biopsy and the partial mastectomy procedure are coded.

89

CHAPTER 9

*ICD-10-PCS
Root Operations
in the Medical
and Surgical
Section*

Coding Procedures on Overlapping Body Layers

Occasionally, a procedure may involve overlapping body layers. In those instances, the following guideline applies: *If a root operation such as "Excision," "Extraction," "Repair," or "Inspection" is performed on overlapping layers of the musculoskeletal system, the body part specifying the deepest layer is coded.* For example, an excisional debridement that includes skin and subcutaneous tissue as well as muscle is coded to the body part "muscle."

MEDICAL AND SURGICAL ROOT OPERATIONS

The 31 Medical and Surgical root operations can be divided into nine groups that share similar attributes:

- Root operations to take out some or all of a body part
- Root operations to take out solids, fluids, or gases from a body part
- Root operations that involve cutting or separation only
- Root operations that put in or put back or move some or all of a body part
- Root operations that alter the diameter or route of a tubular body part
- Root operations that always involve a device
- Root operations that involve examination only
- Root operations that include other repairs
- Root operations that include other objectives

Root Operations to Take Out Some or All of a Body Part

This group of root operations includes "Excision," "Resection," "Detachment," "Destruction," and "Extraction." Table 9.1 provides an overview of these root operations, including the objective of the procedure, the site of the procedure, and an example of each root operation.

"Excision," "Resection," and "Detachment" are similar in that they all cut out or off without replacement. The difference between these three root operations is based on the site and extent of the procedure—some ("Excision") or all ("Resection") of a body part or an extremity ("Detachment").

TABLE 9.1 Root Operations to Take Out Some or All of a Body Part

Root Operation	Objective of Procedure	Site of Procedure	Example
Excision	Cutting out/off without replacement	Some of a body part	Breast lumpectomy
Resection	Cutting out/off without replacement	All of a body part	Total mastectomy
Detachment	Cutting off without replacement	Some/all of an upper or lower extremity	Amputation above elbow
Destruction	Eradicating without replacement	Some/all of a body part	Fulguration of endometrium
Extraction	Pulling out or off without replacement	Some/all of a body part	Suction dilation and curettage

CHAPTER 9

*ICD-10-PCS
Root Operations
in the Medical
and Surgical
Section*

Excision versus Resection

"Excision" is defined as cutting out or off, without replacement, "a portion" of a body part, while "Resection" is cutting out or off, without replacement, "all" of a body part. This distinction is a key concept within ICD-10-PCS; "all" of a body part is uniquely defined in ICD-10-PCS, and it can vary for different organs. For example, a breast lumpectomy is "Excision," while a total mastectomy is "Resection." When the excision is a biopsy, the qualifier "diagnostic" is used.

ICD-10-PCS contains values for anatomical subdivisions of a body part, such as lobes of the lungs or liver and regions of the intestine. Resection of the specific body part is coded whenever all of the body part is cut out or off; excision of a less-specific body part is not coded. It is important to review the body part values within the Table to confirm whether the procedure should be coded as "Resection" or "Excision." For example, refer back to the "Resection" Table in figure 9.1 on page 86. The body part column shows unique values for "liver"; "liver, right lobe"; and "liver, left lobe." Removal of the entire right lobe of the liver is therefore a "Resection" (cutting out all of a body part) because each lobe of the liver is listed as a body part in this Table.

Adjunct information about the anastomotic technique used to complete a procedure (e.g., end-to-end or side-to-end anastomosis after a colectomy) is not specified in ICD-10-PCS. Only the specific excision or resection code is assigned.

Surgeons may use terms such as "radical resection" or "radical excision." Care should be exercised when coding such procedures, as the term "radical" can have different meanings depending on the procedure, and the term is not always reliable information for coding the procedure. The coding professional should instead be guided by the information in the operative report.

Each organ or structure that was resected or excised and for which there is a distinctly defined body part should be coded separately. ICD-10-PCS guideline B3.2a states that if, during the same operative session, the same root operation is repeated at different body parts that are defined by distinct values of the body part character, multiple procedures should be coded.

Excision for Graft

For procedures involving harvesting of graft tissue, the following guideline applies: *If an autograft is obtained from a different procedure site in order to complete the objective of the procedure, a separate procedure is coded except when the seventh-character qualifier value in the ICD-10-PCS Table fully specifies the site from which the autograft was obtained.* For example, for a coronary bypass with excision of saphenous vein graft, the excision of the saphenous vein is coded separately because there is no seventh-character qualifier to specify the saphenous vein as the site of the autograft harvest. However, for a replacement of breast with autologous deep inferior epigastric artery perforator (DIEP) flap, there is a seventh-character qualifier value for "deep inferior epigastric artery perforator flap" in the "Replacement" Table; therefore, excision of the DIEP flap is not coded separately.

Detachment, Destruction, and Extraction

The root operation "Detachment" is used exclusively for extremity amputation procedures at any level. For "Detachment," the body part value is the site of the detachment, with a qualifier, if applicable, to further specify the level where the extremity was amputated.

"Destruction" and "Extraction" share the site of procedure—some or all of a body part. "Destruction" is defined as physical eradication of all or a portion of a body part by the direct use of energy, force, or a destructive agent. With "Destruction," none of the body part is physically taken out. Examples of the root operation "Destruction" are fulguration, ablation, cauterization, and cryoablation. "Extraction" is defined as pulling or stripping out or off all or a portion of a body part by use of force. When the extraction procedure is a biopsy, the qualifier "diagnostic" is used. Examples of the root operation "Extraction" are dilation and curettage, vein stripping, nonexcisional biopsy, and dermabrasion.

91

CHAPTER 9

ICD-10-PCS
Root Operations
in the Medical
and Surgical
Section

EXERCISE 9.1

Code these procedures.

1. Laparoscopic excision of right ovarian cyst

2. Diagnostic dilatation and curettage

3. Below-the-knee amputation, distal portion, right leg

4. Laparoscopic total right oophorectomy

5. Rectal polyp fulguration via sigmoidoscope

6. Wedge biopsy of right breast

7. Surgical removal of entire sigmoid colon via abdominal incision

Root Operations to Take Out Solids, Fluids, or Gases from a Body Part

The next group of root operations includes "Drainage," "Extirpation," and "Fragmentation." These root operations share the same site of procedure, namely "within a body part." Table 9.2 provides an overview of these root operations, including the objective of the procedure, the site of the procedure, and an example of each root operation.

The differences between these three root operations are that "Drainage" takes or lets out fluids or gases, "Extirpation" takes or cuts out solid matter from a body part, and "Fragmentation" breaks solid matter into pieces. The root operation "Drainage" is applicable to both diagnostic

TABLE 9.2 Root Operations to Take Out Solids/Fluids/Gases from a Body Part

Root Operation	Objective of Procedure	Site of Procedure	Example
Drainage	Taking/letting out fluids/gases	Within a body part	Incision and drainage
Extirpation	Taking/cutting out solid matter	Within a body part	Thrombectomy
Fragmentation	Breaking solid matter into pieces	Within a body part	Lithotripsy

CHAPTER 9

ICD-10-PCS
Root Operations
in the Medical
and Surgical
Section

and therapeutic drainage procedures. The qualifier "diagnostic" is used to identify "Extraction" or "Drainage" root operations that are biopsies. Note that a separate procedure to put in a drainage device is coded to the root operation "Drainage" with the device value "drainage device."

For "Extirpation," the solid matter may be an abnormal by-product of a biological function or a foreign body; it may be embedded in a body part or in the lumen of a tubular body part. The solid matter may or may not have been previously broken into pieces. For "Fragmentation," a physical force (e.g., manual, ultrasonic) applied directly or indirectly is used to break the solid matter into pieces. The solid matter may be an abnormal by-product of a biological function or a foreign body. While the root operations "Extirpation" and "Fragmentation" may seem to be closely related, the key difference is that for "Fragmentation" the pieces of solid matter are not taken out.

EXERCISE 9.2

Code these procedures.

1. Incision and drainage of external perianal abscess

2. Percutaneous mechanical thrombectomy,
   left brachial artery

3. Hysteroscopy with intraluminal lithotripsy
   of left fallopian tube calcification

Root Operations Involving Cutting or Separation Only

This group of root operations is made up of two root operations: "Division" and "Release." Table 9.3 provides an overview of these root operations, including the objective and site of the procedure and an example of each root operation.

"Division" is cutting into/separating a body part. This procedure is performed *within* a body part. With "Division," all or a portion of the body part is separated into two or more portions. Examples of "Division" include neurotomy, spinal cordotomy, and osteotomy.

"Release" is freeing a body part from an abnormal physical constraint. The site of procedure is *around* a body part. With "Release," some of the restraining tissue may be taken out, but none of the body part is taken out. The body part value coded is the body part being freed, not the tissue being manipulated or cut to free the body part. An example is lysis of intestinal adhesions; the value selected should be the specific intestine body part value.

Release versus Division: If the sole objective of the procedure is to free a body part without cutting the body part, that procedure should be identified as root operation "Release." An example

---

TABLE 9.3   Root Operations Involving Cutting or Separation Only

Root Operation	Objective of Procedure	Site of Procedure	Example
Division	Cutting into/separating a body part	Within a body part	Neurotomy
Release	Freeing a body part from constraint	Around a body part	Adhesiolysis

93

CHAPTER 9

ICD-10-PCS
Root Operations
in the Medical
and Surgical
Section

is freeing a nerve root from surrounding scar tissue without cutting the nerve. However, if the sole objective of the procedure is separating, or transecting, a body part (e.g., severing the nerve root to relieve pain), that procedure should be identified as root operation "Division."

Root Operations to Put In, Put Back, or Move Some or All of a Body Part

The next grouping of root operations includes "Transplantation," "Reattachment," "Transfer," and "Reposition." Table 9.4 provides an overview of these root operations, including the objective of the procedure, the site of the procedure, and an example of each root operation.

The root operation "Transplantation" refers to putting in a living body part taken from another individual or animal to physically take the place and/or function of all or a portion of a similar body part. The native body part may or may not be removed, and the transplanted body part may take over all or a portion of the native body part's function. Examples include organ transplants such as liver or kidney transplants. Please note that a procedure in which autologous or nonautologous cells are put in is coded to the Administration Section (rather than the Medical and Surgical Section), even though the procedure may be referred to as a transplantation—for example, stem cell transplantation.

Another root operation in this group is "Reattachment." This root operation involves putting back in, or on, all or a portion of a separated (detached) body part to its normal location or other suitable location. Vascular circulation and nervous system pathways may or may not be reestablished. Examples of this root operation are reattachment of fingers or hand.

The root operation "Transfer" is moving, without taking out, all or a portion of a body part to another location to take over the function of all or a portion of a body part. The body part transferred remains connected to its vascular and nervous supply. Examples include tendon transfer and skin pedicle flap transfer.

The root operation "Transfer" contains qualifiers that can be used to specify when a transfer flap is composed of more than one tissue layer, such as a musculocutaneous flap. For procedures involving transfer of multiple tissue layers including skin, subcutaneous tissue, fascia, or muscle, the procedure is coded to the body part value that describes the deepest tissue layer in the flap, and the qualifier can be used to describe the other tissue layer(s) in the transfer flap. For example, a musculocutaneous flap transfer is coded to the appropriate body part value in the body system "muscles," and the qualifier is used to describe the additional tissue layer(s) in the transfer flap.

The root operation "Reposition" refers to moving a body part to normal or other suitable location. Although both "Transfer" and "Reposition" involve moving a body part, a transfer is performed with the objective that the body part will take over or replace the function of a body part. Reposition, on the other hand, is moving a body part to where it should normally be or to another

TABLE 9.4 Root Operations to Put In/Put Back or Move Some/All of a Body Part

Root Operation	Objective of Procedure	Site of Procedure	Example
Transplantation	Putting in a living body part from a person/animal	Some/all of a body part	Kidney transplant
Reattachment	Putting back a detached body part	Some/all of a body part	Reattach finger
Transfer	Moving a body part to function for a similar body part	Some/all of a body part	Skin transfer flap
Reposition	Moving a body part to normal or other suitable location	Some/all of a body part	Move undescended testicle

CHAPTER 9

ICD-10-PCS
Root Operations
in the Medical
and Surgical
Section

appropriate position. Examples of "Reposition" procedures are the reposition of undescended testicle and reduction of displaced fracture.

EXERCISE 9.3

Code these procedures.

1. Percutaneous right foot tenotomy

2. Laparotomy with lysis of large intestine adhesions

3. Reattachment of severed left index finger

4. Liver transplant with donor matched liver

5. Closed reduction of dislocation of the right shoulder joint

---

Root Operations to Alter the Diameter or Route of a Tubular Body Part

Four root operations are performed to alter the diameter or route of a tubular body part: "Restriction," "Occlusion," "Dilation," and "Bypass." Tubular body parts are defined in ICD-10-PCS as the hollow body parts that provide a route of passage for solids, liquids, or gases. They include the cardiovascular system and body parts in the gastrointestinal, genitourinary, biliary, and respiratory tracts. Table 9.5 provides an overview of these root operations.

The objective of the root operation "Restriction" is to *partially* close, or narrow, the diameter of an orifice or a lumen, whereas the objective of the root operation "Occlusion" is to *completely* close an orifice or a lumen. The orifice may be a natural orifice or an artificially created orifice. Both "Restriction" and "Occlusion" include intraluminal and extraluminal methods.

TABLE 9.5 Root Operations to Alter the Diameter or Route of a Tubular Body Part

Root Operation	Objective of Procedure	Site of Procedure	Example
Restriction	Partially closing orifice/lumen	Tubular body part	Gastroesophageal fundoplication
Occlusion	Completely closing orifice/lumen	Tubular body part	Fallopian tube ligation
Dilation	Expanding orifice/lumen	Tubular body part	Percutaneous transluminal coronary angioplasty (PTCA)
Bypass	Altering route of passage	Tubular body part	Coronary artery bypass graft (CABG)

CHAPTER 9

*ICD-10-PCS
Root Operations
in the Medical
and Surgical
Section*

- An example of "Restriction" is gastroesophageal fundoplication. In this procedure, the upper part of the stomach is wrapped around the lower esophageal sphincter to strengthen the sphincter, prevent acid reflux, and repair a hiatal hernia. Essentially, the procedure partially closes the valve between the esophagus and stomach (lower esophageal sphincter), which stops acid from backing up into the esophagus easily.

- An example of "Occlusion" is fallopian tube ligation where the tubes are clipped or blocked, which is performed to completely close the fallopian tube to prevent pregnancy.

The objective of the root operation "Dilation" is to expand, or enlarge, the diameter of the orifice or lumen of a tubular body part. As with "Restriction" and "Occlusion," the orifice may be a natural orifice or an artificially created orifice, and "Dilation" may include intraluminal or extraluminal methods. For example, percutaneous transluminal angioplasty is performed to expand the lumen of narrow coronary vessels to improve blood circulation.

The objective of the root operation "Bypass" is to alter the route of passage of the contents of a tubular body part. "Bypass" may include rerouting contents of a body part to a downstream area of the normal route, to a similar route and body part, or to an abnormal route and dissimilar body part. "Bypass" includes one or more anastomoses, with or without the use of a device. "Bypass" procedures are coded by identifying the body part bypassed "from" and the body part bypassed "to." Other specific guidelines for bypass procedures are covered in this handbook in chapter 19, Diseases of the Digestive System, and chapter 27, Diseases of the Circulatory System. An example of a "Bypass" root operation is a coronary artery bypass graft procedure whereby blood flow is rerouted through a new artery or vein that is grafted around diseased sections of the coronary arteries to increase blood flow to the heart muscle.

Root Operations That Always Involve a Device

The next grouping involves six root operations that always involve a device: "Insertion," "Replacement," "Supplement," "Change," "Removal," and "Revision." Table 9.6 provides an overview of these root operations.

The objective of the root operation "Insertion" is to put in a nonbiological device that monitors, assists, performs, or prevents a physiological function but does not physically take the place of a body part. This root operation represents those procedures whose sole objective is to put in a device without doing anything else to the body part. Examples include insertion of radioactive implant and insertion of central venous catheter.

TABLE 9.6   Root Operations That Always Involve a Device

Root Operation	Objective of Procedure	Site of Procedure	Example
Insertion	Putting in nonbiological device	In/on a body part	Central line insertion
Replacement	Putting in device that replaces a body part	Some/all of a body part	Total hip replacement
Supplement	Putting in device that reinforces or augments a body part	In/on a body part	Abdominal wall herniorrhaphy using mesh
Change	Exchanging device without cutting/puncturing	In/on a body part	Drainage tube change
Removal	Taking out device	In/on a body part	Central line removal
Revision	Correcting a malfunctioning displaced device	In/on a body part	Revision of pacemaker insertion

CHAPTER 9

*ICD-10-PCS
Root Operations
in the Medical
and Surgical
Section*

The objective of the root operation "Replacement" is to put in a device (biological or synthetic material) that takes the place of some, or all, of a body part. The body part may have previously been taken out or replaced, or it may be taken out, physically eradicated, or rendered nonfunctional during the "Replacement" procedure. Examples include hip replacement, bone graft, and free skin graft. Remember that excision or resection is considered integral and preparatory for the replacement procedure. For example, resection of a hip joint as part of a joint replacement procedure is preparatory to the insertion of the joint prosthesis and the resection is not coded separately.

The objective of the root operation "Supplement" is to put in a device (biological or synthetic material) that physically reinforces and/or augments the function of a body part. The biological material may be nonliving or living, and may be derived from the patient, another person, or an animal. The body part may have been previously replaced, and the "Supplement" procedure is performed to physically reinforce and/or augment the function of the replaced body part. Common examples include hernia repair using mesh and mitral valve ring annuloplasty.

The root operation "Change" involves procedures whereby similar devices are exchanged without cutting or puncturing the skin or mucous membrane. All procedures with the root operation "Change" are reported with an external approach. Examples of "Change" root operations include urinary catheter change and changing of gastrostomy tube.

The root operation "Removal" involves procedures for taking out, or off, a device from a body part. This root operation should be coded only when it is not an integral part of another root operation. For example, if a device is taken out and a similar device is put in without cutting or puncturing the skin or mucous membrane, the root operation is "Change," and "Removal" is not coded separately. Examples of "Removal" include drainage tube removal and removal of external fixation device.

The root operation "Revision" applies to procedures whose objective is to correct, to the extent possible, the position or function of a previously placed device without taking the entire device out and putting a whole new device in its place. This root operation may include taking out and/or putting in part of the device; in such cases, "Removal" of the old device would not be coded separately. It is important to understand that a complete redo of a procedure is coded to the root operation performed, rather than "Revision." Examples of "Revision" include adjustment of pacemaker leads and adjustment of hip prosthesis.

Note that for the root operations "Change," "Removal," and "Revision," general body part values are used when the specific body part value is not in the Table.

Some procedures are performed on the device only, and not on a body part. Examples include irrigation of gastrostomy tube and replacement of pulse generator. In such instances, these procedures are reported with the root operations "Change," "Irrigation," "Removal," and "Revision."

EXERCISE 9.4

Code these procedures.

1. Cystoscopy with intraluminal dilation of bladder neck stricture

2. Total right knee arthroplasty with insertion of
   total knee prosthesis

97

CHAPTER 9

ICD-10-PCS
Root Operations
in the Medical
and Surgical
Section

3. Laparoscopic bilateral fallopian tube ligation using clips

_____

4. Left ventral hernia repair (open) with Marlex mesh

_____

5. Open revision of right knee replacement, with removal
   and exchange of the polyethylene unicondylar lateral component

_____

Root Operations That Involve Examination Only

Two root operations involve examination of a body part: "Inspection" and "Map." Refer to table 9.7 for an overview of these root operations.

If the examination's objective is visual or manual exploration of some or all of a body part, the root operation is "Inspection." The visual exploration may be accomplished with or without optical instrumentation. Manual exploration may be performed directly or through intervening body layers. Examples of "Inspection" root operations include diagnostic arthroscopy and exploratory laparotomy.

Three important guidelines apply to the root operation "Inspection":

• *Inspection of a body part(s) performed in order to achieve the objective of a procedure is not coded separately.* For example, a fiberoptic bronchoscopy (which is the procedure to inspect the lung) is performed to irrigate the bronchus. The root operation "Inspection" is not coded because the objective of the procedure is not to visually explore the bronchus but to perform the irrigation.

• *If multiple tubular body parts are inspected, the most distal body part (the body part farthest from the starting point of the inspection) is coded. If multiple nontubular body parts in a region are inspected, the body part that specifies the entire area inspected is coded.* For example, in a cystourethroscopy, both the bladder and the ureters are examined using a cystoscope inserted through the urethra. The most distal (or farthest away) body part in this situation is the ureter, so the body part value for the ureter is selected. An example of "Inspection" of multiple nontubular body parts in a region is an exploratory laparotomy whereby the abdominal contents are inspected. In this instance, the body part value would be "peritoneal cavity" because this body part specifies the entire area inspected.

TABLE 9.7   Root Operations That Involve Examination Only

Root Operation	Objective of Procedure	Site of Procedure	Example
Inspection	Visual/manual exploration	Some/all of a body part	Diagnostic cystoscopy
Map	Location of electrical impulses/ functional areas	Brain/cardiac conduction mechanism	Cardiac electrophysiological study

CHAPTER 9

*ICD-10-PCS
Root Operations
in the Medical
and Surgical
Section*

• *When both an "Inspection" procedure and another procedure are performed on the same body part during the same episode, if the "Inspection" procedure is performed using a different approach than the other procedure, the "Inspection" procedure is coded separately.* For example, if an endoscopic inspection of the duodenum and an open excision of the duodenum are performed during the same procedural episode, the two procedures would be coded separately. The different approaches are endoscopic for the "Inspection" and open for the "Excision."

The root operation "Map" should be used if the examination's objective is to locate the route of passage of electrical impulses or functional areas in a body part. The applicability of the root operation "Map" is limited to the cardiac conduction mechanism and the central nervous system. Examples include cardiac electrophysiological study, heart catheterization with cardiac mapping, percutaneous mapping of basal ganglia, or intraoperative whole brain mapping via craniotomy.

Root Operations That Include Other Repairs

This grouping includes two root operations: "Control" and "Repair." Refer to table 9.8 for an overview of these root operations.

The root operation "Control" describes stopping or attempting to stop postprocedural bleeding or other acute bleeding. It includes irrigation or evacuation of hematoma at the operative site. The bleeding site is coded to the general anatomical region's body system and not to a specific body part. Examples of this root operation are control of post-prostatectomy hemorrhage and control of post-tonsillectomy hemorrhage. It is important to note that the root operation "Control" should not be coded if an attempt to stop the postprocedural bleeding or other acute bleeding is unsuccessful. If stopping the bleeding requires performing a more definitive root operation such as "Bypass," "Detachment," "Excision," "Extraction," "Reposition," "Replacement," or "Resection," the more definitive root operation is coded instead of "Control."

Physicians may refer to interventions to control bleeding in other situations, and coding professionals will need to review the procedure performed in order to select the appropriate code. For example, a procedure to control bleeding from duodenal ulcers by using clips on vessels in the duodenum is coded to "Control" of the duodenum rather than to a vascular system body part. In a similar example, control of epistaxis with silver nitrate or sutures placed to surround a small ruptured arterial bleeding vessel of the external right naris is coded **093K7ZZ, Control bleeding in nasal mucosa and soft tissue, via natural or artificial opening.**

The root operation "Repair" represents a broad range of procedures for restoring, to the extent possible, a body part to its normal anatomical structure and function. This root operation is only used when the procedure performed does not meet the definition of one of the other root operations. Examples of "Repair" include herniorrhaphy and suturing of laceration. Most of the body's organs and tissues are vascular and, as such, bleed when they are cut or eroded. Repair of a cut or eroded body part is coded to that body part, rather than to a vascular system body part.

TABLE 9.8   Root Operations That Include Other Repairs

Root Operation	Objective of Procedure	Site of Procedure	Example
Control	Stopping, or attempting to stop, postprocedural or other acute bleeding	Anatomical region	Post-prostatectomy bleeding control
Repair	Restoring body part to its normal structure	Some/all of a body part	Suture laceration

Root Operations That Include Other Objectives

The last group of root operations is made up of those procedures that include other objectives not included in the previous groups. This group includes the root operations "Fusion," "Alteration," and "Creation." Table 9.9 provides an overview of these root operations.

The root operation "Fusion" refers to joining together portions of an articular body part, rendering the articular body part immobile. The procedure may be accomplished by a fixation device, a bone graft, or other means. The most common example of this root operation is spinal fusion. Specific guidelines related to coding of spinal fusion are covered in detail in chapter 22 of this handbook, Diseases of the Musculoskeletal System and Connective Tissue.

The root operation "Alteration" is coded for all procedures performed solely to improve appearance. This root operation refers to modifying a body part for cosmetic purposes without affecting the function of the body part. All methods, approaches, and devices used for the objective of improving appearance are coded here. Note that coding of the root operation "Alteration" requires diagnostic confirmation that the procedure was performed to improve appearance. Examples include face lift and breast augmentation.

The last root operation, "Creation," is defined as putting in or on biological or synthetic material to form a new body part that to the extent possible replicates the anatomic structure or function of an absent body part. Examples include creation of a vagina in a male patient, creation of a penis in a female patient, and creation of an aortic valve from a truncal valve using zooplastic tissue in a child with truncus arteriosus (a condition in which the aorta and the pulmonary trunk are fused into the single great vessel).

In summary, ICD-10-PCS requires mastering the 31 root operations in the Medical and Surgical Section as the key to selecting the appropriate codes. These concepts are applied in future chapters in this handbook as the more common procedures for each body system are discussed.

CHAPTER 9

ICD-10-PCS
Root Operations
in the Medical
and Surgical
Section

TABLE 9.9   Root Operations That Include Other Objectives

Root Operation	Objective of Procedure	Site of Procedure	Example
Fusion	Rendering joint immobile	Joint	Spinal fusion
Alteration	Modifying body part for cosmetic purposes without affecting function	Some/all of a body part	Face lift
Creation	Putting in or on biological or synthetic material to form a new body part that to the extent possible replicates the anatomic structure or function of an absent body part	Perineum	Artificial vagina/penis

100

CHAPTER 9

ICD-10-PCS
Root Operations
in the Medical
and Surgical
Section

EXERCISE 9.5

Code these procedures.

1. Thoracotomy with exploration of right pleural cavity

2. Reopening of thoracotomy site with drainage and control
    of postoperative hemopericardium

3. Open cosmetic plastic repair of deformed left ear lobe

4. Exploratory laparotomy peritoneal cavity

5. Arthroscopic left subtalar arthrodesis with
    internal fixation device

6. Partial removal of right ovary

7. Endometrial ablation using hysteroscope

8. Percutaneous excisional biopsy of the liver

9. Total left hip replacement with cemented
    ceramic on ceramic bearing prosthesis

10. Total nephrectomy, left kidney

ICD-10-PCS
Medical- and Surgical-Related, Ancillary, and New Technology Procedure Sections

CHAPTER OVERVIEW

- ICD-10-PCS provides codes for Medical- and Surgical-Related, Ancillary, and New Technology Procedures in addition to the Medical and Surgical Section.

- There are nine sections in the Medical- and Surgical-Related Procedures. These sections include obstetric procedures, placement, administration of substances, measurement and monitoring of body functions, extracorporeal or systemic assistance and performance, extracorporeal or systemic therapies, osteopathic procedures, other procedures, and chiropractic procedures.

- There are six sections in the Ancillary Procedures. These sections include imaging, nuclear medicine, radiation therapy, physical rehabilitation and diagnostic audiology, mental health, and substance abuse treatment.

- The New Technology Section codes uniquely identify new technology procedures not currently classified elsewhere in ICD-10-PCS. This section may include codes for medical and surgical procedures, medical- and surgical-related procedures, ancillary procedures, or infusions of new technology drugs.

LEARNING OUTCOMES

After studying this chapter, you should be able to:

Identify the objectives of each root operation.

Distinguish between the different root operations in the Medical- and Surgical-Related Section.

Discuss the general guidelines applicable to root operations.

Correctly assign codes for ancillary services.

Understand the structure of codes for new technologies.

TERM TO KNOW

Root operation
the third character in an ICD-10-PCS code, which refers to the objective of the procedure

CHAPTER 10

ICD-10-PCS
Medical- and
Surgical-
Related,
Ancillary,
and New
Technology
Procedure
Sections

INTRODUCTION

The previous chapter introduces the Medical and Surgical Section of ICD-10-PCS, where the majority of the hospital inpatient procedures are classified. In addition to the Medical and Surgical Section, ICD-10-PCS has sections for Medical- and Surgical-Related Procedures, Ancillary Procedures, and New Technology, which are covered in this chapter.

Many hospitals do not code minor ancillary procedures for inpatient stays. However, for the sake of completeness, ICD-10-PCS includes codes for these minor procedures, which a hospital may use to collect data on these services. Codes in the New Technology Section may affect hospital inpatient Medicare payments, so it is important to understand their application.

MEDICAL- AND SURGICAL-RELATED PROCEDURES

There are nine sections in the Medical- and Surgical-Related Procedures. These sections include obstetric procedures, placement, administration of substances, measurement and monitoring of body functions, extracorporeal or systemic assistance and performance, extracorporeal or systemic therapies, osteopathic procedures, other procedures, and chiropractic procedures, as shown in table 10.1. The obstetric procedures (section 1) are covered in detail in chapter 23 of this handbook, Complications of Pregnancy, Childbirth, and the Puerperium.

TABLE 10.1 Medical- and Surgical-Related Sections

Section Value	Description
1	Obstetrics
2	Placement
3	Administration
4	Measurement and Monitoring
5	Extracorporeal or Systemic Assistance and Performance
6	Extracorporeal or Systemic Therapies
7	Osteopathic
8	Other Procedures
9	Chiropractic

Placement Section

Codes in the Placement Section follow the same conventions used in the Medical and Surgical Section. All seven characters retain the same meaning in both sections, as shown in figure 10.1.

The root operations in the Placement Section are different from those in the Medical and Surgical Section covered in chapter 9 of this handbook. The Placement Section root operations include only those procedures that are performed without making an incision or a puncture. There are two body system (character 2) values in this section: "anatomical regions" (W) and "anatomical

FIGURE 10.1 Structure of Codes in the Placement Section

Character 1	Character 2	Character 3	Character 4	Character 5	Character 6	Character 7
Section	Body System	Root Operation	Body Region	Approach	Device	Qualifier

orifices" (Y). In addition, there are two body region (character 4) values: external body regions (e.g., abdominal wall) and natural orifices (e.g., ear). With a few exceptions, most hospitals do not assign codes from the Placement Section for inpatient stays.

Table 10.2 provides an overview of the root operations (third character) in the Placement Section with their corresponding values and definitions. The root operations "Change" and "Removal" are common to other sections. The remaining five root operations, unique to the Placement Section, are:

- Compression
- Dressing
- Immobilization
- Packing
- Traction

CHAPTER 10

ICD-10-PCS
Medical- and
Surgical-
Related,
Ancillary,
and New
Technology
Procedure
Sections

TABLE 10.2 Placement Section Root Operation Values and Definitions

Value	Description	Definition
0	Change	Taking out or off a device from a body region and putting back an identical or similar device in or on the same body region without cutting or puncturing the skin or a mucous membrane
1	Compression	Putting pressure on a body region
2	Dressing	Putting material on a body region for protection
3	Immobilization	Limiting or preventing motion of a body region
4	Packing	Putting material in a body region
5	Removal	Taking out or off a device from a body region
6	Traction	Exerting a pulling force on a body region in a distal direction

Devices in this section specify the material or device (e.g., splint, traction apparatus, bandage) and include casts for fractures and dislocations. When the placement of devices requires extensive design, fabrication, or fitting, ICD-10-PCS classifies these procedures to the Rehabilitation Section. The devices classified to the Placement Section are off-the-shelf devices.

Examples of procedures in the Placement Section are the following:

Cast change, lower right arm

Character 1 Section	Character 2 Body System	Character 3 Root Operation	Character 4 Body Region	Character 5 Approach	Character 6 Device	Character 7 Qualifier
2	W	0	C	X	2	Z
Placement	Anatomical regions	Change	Lower arm, right	External	Cast	No qualifier

Application of compression dressing to abdominal wound

Character 1 Section	Character 2 Body System	Character 3 Root Operation	Character 4 Body Region	Character 5 Approach	Character 6 Device	Character 7 Qualifier
2	W	3	0	X	6	Z
Placement	Anatomical regions	Compression	Abdominal wall	External	Pressure dressing	No qualifier

104

CHAPTER 10

ICD-10-PCS
Medical- and
Surgical-
Related,
Ancillary,
and New
Technology
Procedure
Sections

Application of dressing to right hand

Character 1 Section	Character 2 Body System	Character 3 Root Operation	Character 4 Body Region	Character 5 Approach	Character 6 Device	Character 7 Qualifier
2	W	2	E	X	4	Z
Placement	Anatomical regions	Dressing	Hand, right	External	Bandage	No qualifier

Placement of stereotactic head frame

Character 1 Section	Character 2 Body System	Character 3 Root Operation	Character 4 Body Region	Character 5 Approach	Character 6 Device	Character 7 Qualifier
2	W	3	0	X	Y	Z
Placement	Anatomical regions	Immobilization	Head	External	Other device	No qualifier

Caution should be exercised with the root operation "Immobilization" because ICD-10-PCS classifies several similar-sounding procedures to different sections based on the setting where the procedure is performed. When the splint and braces are placed in inpatient settings (except for the rehabilitation setting), they are coded to "Immobilization," Table 2W3 in the Placement Section. However, for the rehabilitation setting, these procedures are coded to F0DZ6EZ and F0DZ7EZ in the Physical Rehabilitation and Diagnostic Audiology Section.

Removal of stereotactic head frame

Character 1 Section	Character 2 Body System	Character 3 Root Operation	Character 4 Body Region	Character 5 Approach	Character 6 Device	Character 7 Qualifier
2	W	5	0	X	Y	Z
Placement	Anatomical regions	Removal	Head	External	Other device	No qualifier

Cervical traction using a traction apparatus

Character 1 Section	Character 2 Body System	Character 3 Root Operation	Character 4 Body Region	Character 5 Approach	Character 6 Device	Character 7 Qualifier
2	W	6	2	X	0	Z
Placement	Anatomical region	Traction	Neck	External	Traction apparatus	No qualifier

Note that "traction" in this section includes only traction performed using a mechanical traction apparatus. When manual traction is performed by a physical therapist, it should be classified to the Manual Therapy Techniques in section F, Physical Rehabilitation and Diagnostic Audiology.

Administration Section

The Administration Section includes services such as injections, infusions, and transfusions, along with related procedures such as irrigation and tattooing. The structure of codes in this section is shown in figure 10.2.

FIGURE 10.2 Structure of Codes in the Administration Section

Character 1	Character 2	Character 3	Character 4	Character 5	Character 6	Character 7
Section	Body System	Root Operation	Body System/Region	Approach	Substance	Qualifier

There are three body system (character 2) values in this section:

0   Circulatory
C   Indwelling device
E   Physiological systems and anatomical regions

There are three root operations in the Administration Section, and they are classified according to the broad category of substance administered. Blood products are classified to the root operation "Transfusion," and cleansing substances are classified to "Irrigation." All other therapeutic, diagnostic, nutritional, physiological, or prophylactic substances administered are classified to "Introduction."

Character 5 (approach) uses values defined in the Medical and Surgical Section. The percutaneous approach is used for intradermal, subcutaneous, and intramuscular injections. Catheter utilization to introduce substances into the circulatory system is also classified to the percutaneous approach.

Examples of procedures for each root operation in the Administration Section are as follows:

Infusion of chemotherapy, central vein insertion

Character 1 Section	Character 2 Body System	Character 3 Root Operation	Character 4 Body System/ Region	Character 5 Approach	Character 6 Substance	Character 7 Qualifier
3	E	0	4	3	0	5
Administration	Physiological systems and anatomical regions	Introduction	Central vein	Percutaneous	Antineoplastic	Other antineoplastic

Peritoneal dialysis via indwelling catheter

Character 1 Section	Character 2 Body System	Character 3 Root Operation	Character 4 Body System/ Region	Character 5 Approach	Character 6 Substance	Character 7 Qualifier
3	E	1	M	3	9	Z
Administration	Physiological systems and anatomical regions	Irrigation	Peritoneal cavity	Percutaneous	Dialysate	No qualifier

106

CHAPTER 10

ICD-10-PCS
Medical- and
Surgical-
Related,
Ancillary,
and New
Technology
Procedure
Sections

Transfusion of embryonic stem cells into central vein

Character 1 Section	Character 2 Body System	Character 3 Root Operation	Character 4 Body System/ Region	Character 5 Approach	Character 6 Substance	Character 7 Qualifier
3	0	2	4	3	A	Z
Administration	Circulatory	Transfusion	Central vein	Percutaneous	Stem cells, embryonic	No qualifier

Measurement and Monitoring Section

The Measurement and Monitoring Section classifies procedures that determine the level of a physiological or physical function. Two body system values are used for character 2: "physiological systems" and "physiological devices." The two root operations (character 3) in this section differ in only one respect: "Measurement" describes a single level taken, at a point in time; "Monitoring" describes a series of tests performed repetitively over a period of time. In this section, the sixth character defines the physiological or physical function being tested (e.g., pressure, temperature). The structure of codes in this section is shown in figure 10.3.

FIGURE 10.3   Structure of Codes in the Measurement and Monitoring Section

Character 1	Character 2	Character 3	Character 4	Character 5	Character 6	Character 7
Section	Body System	Root Operation	Body System	Approach	Function/Device	Qualifier

Examples of procedures in the Measurement and Monitoring Section are the following:

Single external EKG (electrocardiogram) reading

Character 1 Section	Character 2 Body System	Character 3 Root Operation	Character 4 Body System	Character 5 Approach	Character 6 Function/Device	Character 7 Qualifier
4	A	0	2	X	4	Z
Measurement and monitoring	Physiological systems	Measurement	Cardiac	External	Electrical activity	No qualifier

Holter monitoring

Character 1 Section	Character 2 Body System	Character 3 Root Operation	Character 4 Body System	Character 5 Approach	Character 6 Function/Device	Character 7 Qualifier
4	A	1	2	X	4	5
Measurement and monitoring	Physiological systems	Monitoring	Cardiac	External	Electrical activity	Ambulatory

CHAPTER 10

*ICD-10-PCS
Medical- and
Surgical-
Related,
Ancillary,
and New
Technology
Procedure
Sections*

EXERCISE 10.1

Code the following procedures.

1. Percutaneous irrigation of pleural cavity using irrigating substance

2. Transplant of autologous bone marrow via central vein

3. Placement of cast on right lower arm

4. Insertion of nasal packing

5. Cardiac pacemaker rate check (external)

6. Application of compression dressing to the back

Extracorporeal or Systemic Assistance and Performance Section

The Extracorporeal or Systemic Assistance and Performance Section includes procedures that use equipment to support a physiological function, such as breathing (e.g., mechanical ventilation), circulating the blood (e.g., hemodialysis), or restoring the natural rhythm of the heart (e.g., cardioversion). These procedures are typically performed in a critical care setting.

The structure of codes in this section is shown in figure 10.4.

FIGURE 10.4   Structure of Codes in the Extracorporeal or Systemic Assistance and Performance Section

Character 1	Character 2	Character 3	Character 4	Character 5	Character 6	Character 7
Section	Body System	Root Operation	Body System	Duration	Function	Qualifier

There is a single body system (character 2) value, "physiological systems" (A). This section contains three root operations: "Assistance," "Performance," and "Restoration." "Assistance" and "Performance" vary only in the degree of control exercised over the physiological function. Assistance takes over a portion of a physiological function, whereas performance takes over the function completely—both by extracorporeal means. The root operation "Restoration" is defined as returning, or attempting to return, a physiological function to its original state by extracorporeal means. "Restoration" defines only external cardioversion and defibrillation procedures. Cardioversion procedures are classified to the root operation "Restoration" whether the procedure is successful or fails.

CHAPTER 10

*ICD-10-PCS
Medical- and
Surgical-
Related,
Ancillary,
and New
Technology
Procedure
Sections*

Character 5 differs from other sections in that it describes the duration of the procedure, rather than the approach. In the case of the respiratory body system, character 5 specifies whether the procedure's duration was less than 24 consecutive hours, 24 to 96 consecutive hours, or greater than 96 consecutive hours. In other body systems, character 5 specifies whether the procedure was a single occurrence, multiple occurrences, intermittent, or continuous. In ICD-10-PCS, the duration value ("single" versus "multiple") is assigned based on documentation of a single (continuous) treatment or multiple (separate) treatments. Character 6 describes the body function being acted upon (e.g., respiration assisted by ventilation).

Examples of codes representing the three root operations from this section are the following:

Continuous positive airway pressure for sleep apnea—eight hours

Character 1 Section	Character 2 Body System	Character 3 Root Operation	Character 4 Body System	Character 5 Duration	Character 6 Function	Character 7 Qualifier
5	A	0	9	3	5	7
Extracorporeal or systemic assistance and performance	Physiological systems	Assistance	Respiratory	Less than 24 consecutive hours	Ventilation	Continuous positive airway pressure

Continuous mechanical ventilation for six consecutive days

Character 1 Section	Character 2 Body System	Character 3 Root Operation	Character 4 Body System	Character 5 Duration	Character 6 Function	Character 7 Qualifier
5	A	1	9	5	5	Z
Extracorporeal or systemic assistance and performance	Physiological systems	Performance	Respiratory	Greater than 96 consecutive hours	Ventilation	No qualifier

External cardioversion

Character 1 Section	Character 2 Body System	Character 3 Root Operation	Character 4 Body System	Character 5 Duration	Character 6 Function	Character 7 Qualifier
5	A	2	2	0	4	Z
Extracorporeal or systemic assistance and performance	Physiological systems	Restoration	Cardiac	Single	Rhythm	No qualifier

Extracorporeal or Systemic Therapies Section

The Extracorporeal or Systemic Therapies Section describes other systemic procedures not defined by the root operations "Assistance" and "Performance" in section 5, Extracorporeal or Systemic Assistance and Performance. The structure of codes in this section is shown in figure 10.5.

FIGURE 10.5   Structure of Codes in the Extracorporeal or Systemic Therapies Section

Character 1	Character 2	Character 3	Character 4	Character 5	Character 6	Character 7
Section	Body System	Root Operation	Body System	Duration	Qualifier	Qualifier

109

CHAPTER 10

*ICD-10-PCS
Medical- and
Surgical-
Related,
Ancillary,
and New
Technology
Procedure
Sections*

This section contains a single body system value, "physiological systems." There are 10 root operations in the Systemic Therapies Section. The meaning of each root operation as used in ICD-10-PCS is consistent with the terminology used in the medical community, except for "Decompression" and "Hyperthermia," as follows:

- *Atmospheric control:* Extracorporeal control of atmospheric pressure and composition.

- *Decompression:* Extracorporeal elimination of undissolved gas from body fluids. "Decompression" describes a single type of procedure: treatment for decompression sickness (the bends) in a hyperbaric chamber.

- *Electromagnetic therapy:* Extracorporeal treatment by electromagnetic rays.

- *Hyperthermia:* Extracorporeal raising of body temperature. It is important to distinguish the objective of the hyperthermia procedure for proper code assignment. Hyperthermia may be used to treat temperature imbalance, in which case it is coded to the Extracorporeal or Systemic Therapies Section. However, hyperthermia is also used as an adjunct radiation treatment for cancer, in which case ICD-10-PCS classifies it to the Radiation Therapy Section.

- *Hypothermia:* Extracorporeal lowering of body temperature.

- *Pheresis:* Extracorporeal separation of blood products. This procedure is used in medical practice for two main purposes: to treat diseases in which too much of a blood component is produced, such as leukemia, or to remove a blood product, such as platelets, from a donor for transfusion into a patient who needs it.

- *Phototherapy:* Extracorporeal treatment by light rays. Phototherapy to the circulatory system refers to exposing the blood to light rays outside the body using a machine that recirculates the blood and returns it to the body after phototherapy.

- *Shock wave therapy:* Extracorporeal treatment by shock waves.

- *Ultrasound therapy:* Extracorporeal treatment by ultrasound.

- *Ultraviolet light therapy:* Extracorporeal treatment by ultraviolet light.

Character 5, duration, specifies whether the procedure was single or multiple. This section is different from others in that two characters, 6 and 7, are qualifiers, but no qualifier is used for character 6 (i.e., the sixth-character value is always "Z"). This is to comply with the overall structure of all ICD-10-PCS codes to be seven characters long. The seventh-character qualifier identifies various blood components separated out in pheresis procedures, such as red blood cells, white blood cells, platelets, plasma, stem cells from cord blood, and hematopoietic stem cells.

Examples are the following:

Donor peripheral lymphocyte apheresis procedure, multiple

Character 1 Section	Character 2 Body System	Character 3 Root Operation	Character 4 Body System	Character 5 Duration	Character 6 Qualifier	Character 7 Qualifier
6	A	5	5	1	Z	1
Extracorporeal or systemic therapies	Physiological systems	Pheresis	Circulatory	Multiple	No qualifier	Leukocytes

Shock wave therapy for heel pain, single treatment

Character 1 Section	Character 2 Body System	Character 3 Root Operation	Character 4 Body System	Character 5 Duration	Character 6 Qualifier	Character 7 Qualifier
6	A	9	3	0	Z	Z
Extracorporeal or systemic therapies	Physiological systems	Shock wave therapy	Musculoskeletal	Single	No qualifier	No qualifier

CHAPTER 10

*ICD-10-PCS
Medical- and
Surgical-
Related,
Ancillary,
and New
Technology
Procedure
Sections*

EXERCISE 10.2

Code the following procedures.

1. Continuous hyperbaric oxygenation

2. Ultrasound therapy of peripheral vascular vessels, single treatment

3. Hemodialysis, prolonged intermittent treatment for 8 hours

4. Failed cardioversion

5. Pheresis of hematopoietic stem cells, single episode

Osteopathic Section

The Osteopathic Section is one of the smallest sections in ICD-10-PCS. There is a single body system ("anatomical regions") and a single root operation ("Treatment"). The structure of codes in this section is shown in figure 10.6.

FIGURE 10.6   Structure of Codes in the Osteopathic Section

Character 1	Character 2	Character 3	Character 4	Character 5	Character 6	Character 7
Section	Body System	Root Operation	Body Region	Approach	Method	Qualifier

Character 6, method, in this section defines the osteopathic method of the procedure. The following osteopathic methods are specified: articulatory raising, fascial release, general mobilization, high velocity–low amplitude, indirect, low velocity–high amplitude, lymphatic pump, muscle energy–isometric, muscle energy–isotonic, and other method.

One example is muscle energy–isotonic osteopathic treatment of neck.

Character 1 Section	Character 2 Body System	Character 3 Root Operation	Character 4 Body Region	Character 5 Approach	Character 6 Method	Character 7 Qualifier
7	W	0	1	X	8	Z
Osteopathic	Anatomical regions	Treatment	Cervical	External	Muscle energy isotonic	None

Other Procedures Section

The Other Procedures Section contains codes for medical- and surgical-related procedures not included in the other medical- and surgical-related sections. The structure of codes in this section is shown in figure 10.7. There is a single root operation, "Other procedures." This root operation is defined as methodologies that attempt to remediate or cure a disorder or disease. There are relatively few codes in this section, including some nontraditional, whole body therapies such as acupuncture, meditation, and yoga therapy. Character 6, method, defines the method of the procedure, such as computer assisted procedure, robotic assisted procedure, or acupuncture. Note that the procedure codes for robotic assisted and computer assisted procedures are coded in addition to the primary procedure (e.g., cholecystectomy). Another procedure included in this section is the fertilization portion of an in-vitro fertilization procedure.

FIGURE 10.7   Structure of Codes in the Other Procedures Section

Character 1	Character 2	Character 3	Character 4	Character 5	Character 6	Character 7
Section	Body System	Root Operation	Body Region	Approach	Method	Qualifier

Here are two examples:

Robotic assisted laparoscopic cholecystectomy (the robotic assistance only)

Character 1 Section	Character 2 Body System	Character 3 Root Operation	Character 4 Body Region	Character 5 Approach	Character 6 Method	Character 7 Qualifier
8	E	0	W	4	C	Z
Other procedures	Physiological systems and anatomical regions	Other procedures	Trunk region	Percutaneous endoscopic	Robotic assisted procedure	No qualifier

Suture removal of left arm

Character 1 Section	Character 2 Body System	Character 3 Root Operation	Character 4 Body Region	Character 5 Approach	Character 6 Method	Character 7 Qualifier
8	E	0	X	X	Y	8
Other procedures	Physiological systems and anatomical regions	Other procedures	Upper extremity	External	Other method	Suture removal

Chiropractic Section

The last section in the Medical- and Surgical-Related Procedures is the Chiropractic Section. This section consists of a single body system, "anatomical regions," and a single root operation, "Manipulation." "Manipulation" is defined in ICD-10-PCS as a manual procedure that involves a directed thrust to move a joint past the physiological range of motion without exceeding the anatomical limit. The structure of codes in this section is similar to the structure of codes in the Other Procedures Section (see figure 10.7). An example for this section is the following:

Chiropractic mechanically assisted manipulation of right wrist

Character 1 Section	Character 2 Body System	Character 3 Root Operation	Character 4 Body Region	Character 5 Approach	Character 6 Method	Character 7 Qualifier
9	W	B	7	X	K	Z
Chiropractic	Anatomical regions	Manipulation	Upper extremity	External	Mechanically assisted	None

112

CHAPTER 10

ICD-10-PCS
Medical- and
Surgical-
Related,
Ancillary,
and New
Technology
Procedure
Sections

EXERCISE 10.3

Code the following procedures.

1. Acupuncture to the back using anesthesia

2. Blood collection from indwelling vascular access device

3. Osteopathic manipulation of lower back using high velocity– low amplitude

4. Open excision of acoustic neuroma with computer assisted magnetic resonance imaging

5. Chiropractic manipulation of low back with high-velocity, short-lever arm thrust contact

ANCILLARY PROCEDURES

There are six sections in ICD-10-PCS for ancillary procedures, as follows:

B   Imaging
C   Nuclear Medicine
D   Radiation Therapy
F   Physical Rehabilitation and Diagnostic Audiology
G   Mental Health
H   Substance Abuse Treatment

The ancillary sections do not include root operations. Instead, character 3 in these sections represents the root type of the procedure.

Codes in these sections include characters not previously defined, such as contrast, modality qualifier, and equipment. Section G, Mental Health, and section H, Substance Abuse Treatment, are covered in chapter 15 of this handbook, Mental Disorders.

Imaging Section

The Imaging Section follows the same conventions established in the Medical and Surgical Section, except that the third and fifth characters introduce definitions not used in previous sections. The third character defines root type, rather than root operation, and the fifth character defines contrast, if used. In addition, contrast is differentiated by whether it is low or high osmolar contrast. The sixth-character qualifier in this section can be used to specify that an image is taken without contrast and is followed by one with contrast (unenhanced and enhanced).

The structure of codes in this section is shown in figure 10.8.

CHAPTER 10

*ICD-10-PCS
Medical- and
Surgical-
Related,
Ancillary,
and New
Technology
Procedure
Sections*

FIGURE 10.8 Structure of Codes in the Imaging Section

Character 1	Character 2	Character 3	Character 4	Character 5	Character 6	Character 7
Section	Body System	Root Type	Body Part	Contrast	Qualifier	Qualifier

The Imaging Section utilizes the following five root types:

- *Value 0—Plain radiography:* Planar display of an image developed from the capture of external ionizing radiation on photographic or photoconductive plate.

- *Value 1—Fluoroscopy:* Single-plane or biplane real-time display of an image developed from the capture of external ionizing radiation on a fluorescent screen. The image may also be stored by either digital or analog means.

- *Value 2—Computerized tomography (CT scan):* Computer-reformatted digital display of multiplanar images developed from the capture of multiple exposures of external ionizing radiation.

- *Value 3—Magnetic resonance imaging (MRI):* Computer-reformatted digital display of multiplanar images developed from the capture of radio-frequency signals emitted by nuclei in a body site excited within a magnetic field.

- *Value 4—Ultrasonography:* Real-time display of images of anatomy or flow information developed from the capture of reflected and attenuated high-frequency sound waves.

Examples include the following:

X-ray of right upper arm

Character 1 Section	Character 2 Body System	Character 3 Root Type	Character 4 Body Part	Character 5 Contrast	Character 6 Qualifier	Character 7 Qualifier
B	P	0	E	Z	Z	Z
Imaging	Non-axial upper bones	Plain radiography	Upper arm, right	None	None	None

Retrograde pyelogram (kidneys, ureters, bladder) with low osmolar contrast

Character 1 Section	Character 2 Body System	Character 3 Root Type	Character 4 Body Part	Character 5 Contrast	Character 6 Qualifier	Character 7 Qualifier
B	T	1	4	1	Z	Z
Imaging	Urinary system	Fluoroscopy	Kidneys, ureters and bladder	Low osmolar	None	None

CT scan of brain without contrast, followed by high osmolar contrast

Character 1 Section	Character 2 Body System	Character 3 Root Type	Character 4 Body Part	Character 5 Contrast	Character 6 Qualifier	Character 7 Qualifier
B	0	2	0	0	0	Z
Imaging	Central nervous system and cranial nerves	Computerized tomography	Brain	High osmolar	Unenhanced and enhanced	None

CHAPTER 10

*ICD-10-PCS
Medical- and
Surgical-
Related,
Ancillary,
and New
Technology
Procedure
Sections*

MRI of liver and spleen with contrast

Character 1 Section	Character 2 Body System	Character 3 Root Type	Character 4 Body Part	Character 5 Contrast	Character 6 Qualifier	Character 7 Qualifier
B	F	3	6	Y	Z	Z
Imaging	Hepatobiliary system and pancreas	Magnetic resonance imaging	Liver and spleen	Other contrast	None	None

Bilateral ovarian ultrasound

Character 1 Section	Character 2 Body System	Character 3 Root Type	Character 4 Body Part	Character 5 Contrast	Character 6 Qualifier	Character 7 Qualifier
B	U	4	5	Z	Z	Z
Imaging	Female reproductive system	Ultrasonography	Ovaries, bilateral	None	None	None

Nuclear Medicine Section

The Nuclear Medicine Section is organized like the Imaging Section, with the only significant difference being that the fifth character in the Nuclear Medicine Section is used to define the radionuclide (radiation source) instead of the contrast material used in the procedure. Similar to the Imaging Section, the third character classifies the procedure by root type, rather than root operation. The sixth and seventh characters are qualifiers and are not used in this section.

The structure of the codes in this section is shown in figure 10.9.

FIGURE 10.9   Structure of Codes in the Nuclear Medicine Section

Character 1	Character 2	Character 3	Character 4	Character 5	Character 6	Character 7
Section	Body System	Root Type	Body Part	Radionuclide	Qualifier	Qualifier

The following seven root types are used in the Nuclear Medicine Section:

- *Value 1—Planar nuclear medicine imaging:* Introduction of radioactive materials into the body for single-plane display of images developed from the capture of radioactive emissions.

- *Value 2—Tomographic (tomo) nuclear medicine imaging:* Introduction of radioactive materials into the body for three-dimensional displays of images developed from the capture of radioactive emissions.

- *Value 3—Positron emission tomographic (PET) imaging:* Introduction of radioactive materials into the body for three-dimensional displays of images developed from the simultaneous capture, 180 degrees apart, of radioactive emissions.

- *Value 4—Nonimaging nuclear medicine uptake:* Introduction of radioactive materials into the body for measurements of organ function, from the detection of radioactive emissions.

- *Value 5—Nonimaging nuclear medicine probe:* Introduction of radioactive materials into the body for the study of distribution and fate of certain substances by the detection of radioactive emissions from an external source.

- *Value 6—Nonimaging nuclear medicine assay:* Introduction of radioactive materials into the body for the study of body fluids and blood elements by the detection of radioactive emissions.
- *Value 7—Systemic nuclear medicine therapy:* Introduction of unsealed radioactive materials into the body for treatment.

Examples include the following:

Brain PET scan with C-11

Character 1 Section	Character 2 Body System	Character 3 Root Type	Character 4 Body Part	Character 5 Radionuclide	Character 6 Qualifier	Character 7 Qualifier
C	0	3	0	B	Z	Z
Nuclear medicine	Central nervous system and cranial nerves	Positron emission tomographic (PET) imaging	Brain	Carbon 11	None	None

I-131 thyroid uptake study

Character 1 Section	Character 2 Body System	Character 3 Root Type	Character 4 Body Part	Character 5 Radionuclide	Character 6 Qualifier	Character 7 Qualifier
C	G	4	2	G	Z	Z
Nuclear medicine	Endocrine system	Nonimaging nuclear medicine uptake	Thyroid gland	Iodine 131	None	None

Radiation Therapy Section

The ICD-10-PCS Radiation Therapy Section contains the radiation procedures used for cancer treatment. The structure of the codes in this section is shown in figure 10.10.

FIGURE 10.10   Structure of Codes in the Radiation Therapy Section

Character 1	Character 2	Character 3	Character 4	Character 5	Character 6	Character 7
Section	Body System	Root Type	Body Part	Modality Qualifier	Isotope	Qualifier

The differences in character meanings for this section are as follows:

- Character 3 defines root type, which is the basic radiation delivery modality used (beam radiation, brachytherapy, stereotactic radiosurgery, or other radiation).
- Character 5 specifies further the treatment modality used (e.g., photons, electrons, heavy particles, contact radiation).
- Character 6 defines the radioactive isotope used, if applicable.
- Character 7 is a qualifier and is not specified in this section.

CHAPTER 10

ICD-10-PCS
Medical- and
Surgical-
Related,
Ancillary,
and New
Technology
Procedure
Sections

Examples include the following:

External beam radiation to left breast (photons 1.33 MeV)

Character 1 Section	Character 2 Body System	Character 3 Root Type	Character 4 Body Part	Character 5 Modality Qualifier	Character 6 Isotope	Character 7 Qualifier
D	M	0	0	1	Z	Z
Radiation therapy	Breast	Beam radiation	Breast, left	Photons 1–10 MeV	None	None

Endobronchial brachytherapy, HDR, Ir-192

Character 1 Section	Character 2 Body System	Character 3 Root Type	Character 4 Body Part	Character 5 Modality Qualifier	Character 6 Isotope	Character 7 Qualifier
D	B	1	1	9	8	Z
Radiation therapy	Respiratory system	Brachytherapy	Bronchus	High dose rate (HDR)	Iridium-192 (Ir-192)	None

Brachytherapy (also referred to as internal radiation) involves placing a radioactive implant inside the body in or near a tumor. Brachytherapy is coded to the modality "Brachytherapy" in the Radiation Therapy Section. When a radioactive brachytherapy source is left in the body at the end of the procedure, the implantation of the brachytherapy source is also coded, using the device value "radioactive element" in the appropriate "Insertion" table of the Medical and Surgical Section. The Radiation Therapy Section code identifies the specific modality and isotope of the brachytherapy, and the Medical and Surgical Section "Insertion" code identifies the implantation of the brachytherapy source that remains in the body at the end of the procedure.

For example, right breast brachytherapy with implantation via percutaneous catheters of a low dose rate iridium 192 brachytherapy source left in the body at the end of the procedure is coded to **DM11B8Z, Low dose rate (LDR) brachytherapy of right breast using iridium 192 (Ir-192)** and **0HHT31Z, Insertion of radioactive element into right breast, percutaneous approach.**

After resection of a brain tumor, cesium-131 brachytherapy seeds embedded in a collagen matrix may be implanted at the treatment site. The cesium-131 implantation is coded to the central nervous system and cranial nerves body system, body part "brain," root operation "Insertion," with the device value "radioactive element, cesium-131 collagen implant" (code 00H004Z). A code from the Radiation Therapy Section is not assigned because the device value for the "Insertion" procedure identifies both the implantation of the radioactive element and a specific brachytherapy isotope that is not included in the Radiation Therapy Section tables.

When a patient undergoes a separate procedure to place a temporary applicator for delivering brachytherapy, the placement of the applicator is coded to the root operation "Insertion" and the device value "other device." The brachytherapy is coded separately using the modality "Brachytherapy" in the Radiation Therapy Section.

For example, a tandem and ovoid applicator may be inserted vaginally into the uterus to deliver intrauterine brachytherapy to treat cervical cancer. When this is done as a separate procedure, assign code **0WHR7YZ, Insertion of other device into genitourinary tract, via natural or artificial opening,** for the placement of the tandem and ovoid applicator. Also assign a code for the brachytherapy, such as **DU11B7Z, Low dose rate (LDR) brachytherapy of cervix using cesium 137 (Cs-137),** when the radioactive implant is delivered via the applicator.

However, when the intrauterine brachytherapy applicator is placed concomitantly with delivery of the brachytherapy dose, the procedure is coded with a single code using the modality "Brachytherapy" in the Radiation Therapy Section.

CHAPTER 10

ICD-10-PCS
Medical- and
Surgical-
Related,
Ancillary,
and New
Technology
Procedure
Sections

EXERCISE 10.4

Code the following procedures.

1. Intravascular ultrasound bilateral internal carotid arteries

2. MRI of the brain with contrast

3. PET scan of the lungs with F-18

4. Right breast brachytherapy, via percutaneous needles, LDR, Palladium 103 left at the end of procedure

5. CT scan of the lungs without contrast

Physical Rehabilitation and Diagnostic Audiology Section

The structure of the codes in the Physical Rehabilitation and Diagnostic Audiology Section is shown in figure 10.11.

FIGURE 10.11 Structure of Codes in the Physical Rehabilitation and Diagnostic Audiology Section

Character 1	Character 2	Character 3	Character 4	Character 5	Character 6	Character 7
Section	Section Qualifier	Root Type	Body System and Region	Type Qualifier	Equipment	Qualifier

This section contains character definitions unlike the other sections in ICD-10-PCS, as follows:

- Character 2 is a section qualifier that specifies whether the procedure is a rehabilitation or diagnostic audiology procedure.
- Character 3 defines the general procedure root type.
- Character 4 defines the body system and body region combined, where applicable.
- Character 5 specifies further the procedure type.
- Character 6 specifies any equipment used.

This section contains 14 root types, which are defined in table 10.3.
The following important coding notes apply to this section:

- Treatment procedures include swallowing dysfunction exercises, bathing and showering techniques, wound management, gait training, and a host of activities typically associated with rehabilitation.
- Assessments are further classified into more than 100 different tests or methods. The majority of these assessments focus on the faculties of hearing and speech; others focus

CHAPTER 10

*ICD-10-PCS
Medical- and
Surgical-
Related,
Ancillary,
and New
Technology
Procedure
Sections*

Table 10.3 Physical Rehabilitation and Diagnostic Audiology Root Types

Value	Description	Definition
0	Speech assessment	Measurement of speech and related functions
1	Motor and/or nerve function assessment	Measurement of motor, nerve, and related functions
2	Activities of daily living assessment	Measurement of functional level for activities of daily living
3	Hearing assessment	Measurement of hearing and related functions
4	Hearing aid assessment	Measurement of the appropriateness and/or effectiveness of a hearing device
5	Vestibular assessment	Measurement of the vestibular system and related functions
6	Speech treatment	Application of techniques to improve, augment, or compensate for speech and related functional impairment
7	Motor treatment	Exercise or activities to increase or facilitate motor function
8	Activities of daily living treatment	Exercise or activities to facilitate functional competence for activities of daily living
9	Hearing treatment	Application of techniques to improve, augment, or compensate for hearing and related functional impairment
B	Hearing aid treatment	Application of techniques to improve the communication abilities of individuals with cochlear implant
C	Vestibular treatment	Application of techniques to improve, augment, or compensate for vestibular and related functional impairment
D	Device fitting	Fitting of a device designed to facilitate or support achievement of a higher level of function
F	Caregiver training	Training in activities to support patient's optimal level of function

on various aspects of body function and on the patient's quality of life, such as muscle performance, neuromotor development, and reintegration skills.

- The fifth character used in "Device Fitting" describes the device being fitted rather than the method used to fit the device.

- "Caregiver Training" is divided into 18 different broad subjects taught to help a caregiver provide proper patient care. Examples include bathing, dressing, feeding, and eating.

Examples of codes from this section include the following:

Hydrotherapy whirlpool treatment of skin ulcer of right heel

Character 1 Section	Character 2 Section Qualifier	Character 3 Root Type	Character 4 Body System and Region	Character 5 Type Qualifier	Character 6 Equipment	Character 7 Qualifier
F	0	8	G	5	B	Z
Physical rehabilitation and diagnostic audiology	Rehabilitation	Activities of daily living treatment	Integumentary lower extremity	Wound management	Physical agents	None

119

CHAPTER 10

ICD-10-PCS
Medical- and
Surgical-
Related,
Ancillary,
and New
Technology
Procedure
Sections

Bedside swallowing assessment of stroke patient

Character 1 Section	Character 2 Section Qualifier	Character 3 Root Type	Character 4 Body System and Region	Character 5 Type Qualifier	Character 6 Equipment	Character 7 Qualifier
F	0	0	Z	H	Z	Z
Physical rehabilitation and diagnostic audiology	Rehabilitation	Speech assessment	None	Bedside swallowing and oral function	None	None

EXERCISE 10.5

Code the following procedures.

1. Aphasia assessment by speech therapist

2. Prosthetic device fitting, below knee leg prosthetic

3. Caregiver training in keeping wound clean and dressing change

NEW TECHNOLOGY SECTION

The New Technology Section was introduced with the FY 2016 revisions to the ICD-10-PCS classification. Codes in this section have the value "X" in the first-character position and may therefore be referred to as Section X codes. Codes in this section uniquely identify new technology procedures not currently classified elsewhere in ICD-10-PCS. The New Technology Section may include codes for medical and surgical procedures, medical- and surgical-related procedures, ancillary procedures, or infusions of new technology drugs. The codes are requested via the Centers for Medicare & Medicaid Services' New Technology Application Process. Unlike many of the codes in the Medical- and Surgical-Related and Ancillary Sections that hospitals may choose not to report for inpatients, procedures from the New Technology Section may significantly affect the Medicare reimbursement that hospitals receive. It is important to note, however, that inclusion of a code in the New Technology Section does not automatically confer approval of a Medicare New Technology add-on payment.

Figure 10.12 shows the structure of the codes in the New Technology Section. These codes have many similarities to those in other sections in ICD-10-PCS, the main difference being use of the seventh character. In other sections, the seventh character is referred to as the "qualifier," and the information specified varies depending on the section. In the New Technology Section, the seventh character is used exclusively to identify the new technology group.

FIGURE 10.12   Structure of Codes in the New Technology Section

Character 1	Character 2	Character 3	Character 4	Character 5	Character 6	Character 7
Section	Body System	Root Operation	Body Part	Approach	Device/ Substance/ Technology	New Technology Group

CHAPTER 10

ICD-10-PCS
Medical- and
Surgical-
Related,
Ancillary,
and New
Technology
Procedure
Sections

As with other sections in ICD-10-PCS, character 2 (body system) is a fixed set of values that combines the uses of body system, body region, and physiological system. The values for characters 3 (root operation), 4 (body part), and 5 (approach) are also the same as their counterparts in other sections of ICD-10-PCS (for example, root operation and approach have the same definitions presented in chapter 7 of this handbook). Character 6 (device/substance/technology) in the New Technology Section contains a general description of the key feature of the new technology.

The new technology group (character 7) is a number or letter that identifies the year a new technology code is added to the classification. For example, because FY 2016 was the first year for this section, the seventh-character value "1" (new technology group 1) identifies the New Technology Section codes added in FY 2016. Codes added in FY 2017 have the seventh-character value "2" (new technology group 2), and so on.

For example:

Introduction of Isavuconazole anti-infective into peripheral vein, percutaneous approach

Character 1 Section	Character 2 Body System	Character 3 Root Operation	Character 4 Body Part	Character 5 Approach	Character 6 Device/ Substance/ Technology	Character 7 New Technology Group
X	W	0	3	3	4	1
New technology	Anatomical regions	Introduction	Peripheral vein	Percutaneous	Isavuconazole anti-infective	New technology group 1

Section X codes fully represent the specific procedure described in the code title and do not require additional codes from other ICD-10-PCS sections. When section X contains a code title that fully describes a specific new technology procedure, and it is the only procedure performed, only the section X code is reported for the procedure. There is no need to report an additional code from another section of ICD-10-PCS. For example, code **XW03341, Introduction of Isavuconazole anti-infective into peripheral vein, percutaneous approach, new technology group 1,** does not require an additional code from Table 3E0, Administration.

When multiple procedures are performed, New Technology section X codes are coded following the multiple procedures guideline. For example, for a dual filter cerebral embolic filtration used during transcatheter aortic valve replacement (TAVR), **X2A5312, Cerebral Embolic Filtration, Dual Filter in Innominate Artery and Left Common Carotid Artery, Percutaneous Approach, New Technology Group 2,** is assigned along with an ICD-10-PCS code for the TAVR procedure.

CHAPTER 11

Z Codes and External Cause of Morbidity Codes

CHAPTER OVERVIEW

- Z codes and External cause of morbidity codes follow the same format and conventions as the main ICD-10-CM classification.

- Certain Z codes are used as principal diagnosis codes in specific situations.

- Aftercare management Z codes are generally listed first to explain the reason for continued care after the initial treatment of an injury or disease.

- Z codes are also useful for coding admission for observation and evaluation and admission for palliative care.

- Z codes are also used for special investigative examinations when no problem, diagnosis, or condition is identified and for screening examinations.

- Z codes indicate personal history, family history, and genetic susceptibility to disease.

LEARNING OUTCOMES

After studying this chapter, you should be able to:

Locate Z codes and External cause of morbidity codes.

Explain how and when Z codes and External cause of morbidity codes are used.

TERMS TO KNOW

Aftercare management
continued care during the healing phase or long-term care due to the consequences of a disease

External cause of morbidity codes
codes for external causes to provide information for injury research and evaluation of injury prevention strategies

Palliative care
care focused on the management of pain and other symptoms of patients who are in the terminal phase of an illness

Z codes
codes for factors influencing health status and contact with health services

REMEMBER . . .

Z codes and External cause of morbidity codes are used throughout the classification.

INTRODUCTION

In addition to the main classification (A00.0 through T88.9), two special groups of codes are provided in ICD-10-CM:

- External causes of morbidity (V00–Y99)
- Factors influencing health status and contact with health services (Z codes: Z00–Z99)

USING Z CODES AND EXTERNAL CAUSE OF MORBIDITY CODES

Certain Z codes are designated as the principal (or first-listed) diagnosis in specific situations; others are assigned as additional codes when it is important to indicate a history, status, or problem that may affect health care. Some Z codes can be used as either the principal (or first-listed) diagnosis or as an additional code.

External cause codes are assigned as additional codes to indicate how the injury or health condition happened (cause), the intent (unintentional or accidental; intentional, such as suicide or assault), the place where the event occurred, the activity of the patient at the time of the event, and the person's status (e.g., civilian, military). External cause of morbidity codes are not used to report the intent for poisonings, toxic effects, adverse effects, or underdosing of drugs. ICD-10-CM classifies these conditions using codes in categories T36 through T65, which combine the substances involved with the external cause. These situations are discussed in chapter 31 of this handbook, Poisoning, Toxic Effects, Adverse Effects, and Underdosing of Drugs.

There is no national requirement for mandatory ICD-10-CM External cause code reporting. Unless a provider is subject to a state-based External cause code reporting mandate, or unless these codes are required by a particular payer, reporting of ICD-10-CM codes in chapter 20, External Causes of Morbidity, is not required. In the absence of a mandatory reporting requirement, providers are encouraged to report External cause codes voluntarily, as they provide valuable data for injury research and evaluation of injury prevention strategies.

Because Z codes and External cause codes are used throughout the classification, this chapter provides a general introduction before they are discussed in other chapters in the handbook.

LOCATING Z CODES AND EXTERNAL CAUSE OF MORBIDITY CODES

The format and conventions used throughout the main classification are also used in the Indexes and Tabular Lists for these supplementary classifications. Index entries for Z codes are included in the main Alphabetic Index. These are the key main terms:

- Admission
- Examination
- History
- Observation
- Aftercare
- Problem
- Status

The Tabular List for Z codes follows immediately after the External Causes of Morbidity (V00–Y99) section in the Tabular List.

Z CODES

Z codes are used as the principal (or first-listed) diagnosis in the following situations:

- To indicate that a person with a resolving disease or a chronic condition is being seen for specific aftercare, such as the removal of postoperative sutures
- To indicate that the patient is being seen for the sole purpose of special therapy, such as radiotherapy or chemotherapy
- To indicate that a person not currently ill is encountering the health service for a specific reason, such as to act as an organ donor, to receive prophylactic care, or to receive counseling
- To indicate the birth status of newborns

Z codes are assigned as additional diagnosis codes in the following situations:

- To indicate that a patient has a history, a health status, or another problem that is not in itself an illness or injury but may influence patient care. Note that the following Z codes can be listed first if the fact of the history itself is the reason for admission or encounter:

  Z85.-   Personal history of malignant neoplasm

  Z86.-   Personal history of certain other diseases

  Z80–Z84   Family history

- To indicate the outcome of delivery for obstetric patients

Admission or Encounter for Aftercare Management

Aftercare visit codes (Z42–Z51) are used when the initial treatment of a disease has been completed but the patient requires continued care during the healing or recovery phase or for long-term consequences of the disease. The aftercare code is not assigned when treatment is directed at a current acute disease. The diagnosis code is to be used in these cases. The exceptions to this rule are encounters for antineoplastic chemotherapy and immunotherapy (Z51.1-) or external beam radiotherapy (Z51.0). When the encounter is for the purpose of more than one type of antineoplastic therapy (e.g., radiation and chemotherapy), both codes are assigned and either can be sequenced first. (Chapter 28 of this handbook, Neoplasms, discusses the use of radiation and chemotherapy codes.)

Admission for aftercare management ordinarily involves planned care, such as the fitting and adjustment of an external prosthetic device (Z44.-), attention to an artificial opening (Z43.-), breast reconstruction following mastectomy (Z42.1), or removal of an internal fixation device not related to an injury (Z47.2).

There are codes for encounters for attention to dressings, sutures, and drains (Z48.0-). There are also codes to report aftercare following surgery for neoplasms (Z48.3), following organ transplant (Z48.2-), and following surgery on specific body systems (Z48.810–Z48.817). These codes should be reported along with any other aftercare codes or other diagnosis codes to provide more detail regarding an aftercare visit.

Palliative care is an alternative to aggressive treatment for patients who are in the terminal phase of an illness. Care is focused on the management of pain and other symptoms of the disease, which is often more appropriate than aggressive care when a patient is dying of an incurable illness. Code **Z51.5, Encounter for palliative care,** is used to classify admissions or encounters for comfort care, end-of-life care, hospice care, and terminal care for terminally ill patients. It may be used in any health care setting.

The aftercare Z codes should not be used for aftercare of injuries. For aftercare of an injury, assign the acute injury code with the appropriate seventh character for subsequent encounter (e.g., "D," "G," "K," or "P" for fractures). These codes are covered in more detail in chapter 29 of this handbook.

Aftercare codes are generally listed first to explain the specific reason for the encounter. They can be used occasionally as additional codes when aftercare is provided during an encounter for treatment of an unrelated condition but no applicable diagnosis code is available (e.g., the closure of a colostomy during an admission to treat an injury sustained in an automobile accident). After-care codes should be used in conjunction with any other aftercare or diagnosis code(s) to provide better detail on the specifics of an aftercare visit, unless otherwise directed by the classification. The sequencing of multiple aftercare codes depends on the circumstances of the encounter. Certain aftercare Z codes need a secondary diagnosis code to describe the resolving condition or sequelae. For others, the condition is included in the code title.

When the patient is admitted because of a complication of previous care, the appropriate code from the main classification is assigned rather than the aftercare Z code. (See chapter 32 of this handbook.)

Admission for Follow-Up Examination

When a patient is admitted for the purpose of surveillance after the initial treatment of a disease or injury has been completed, a code from category Z08, Z09, or Z39 is assigned as the principal diagnosis or reason for the encounter. Examples include:

Z09   Encounter for follow-up examination after completed treatment for conditions other than malignant neoplasm

Z08   Encounter for follow-up examination after completed treatment for malignant neo-plasm

Z39.2   Encounter for routine postpartum follow-up

If a recurrence, an extension, or a related condition is identified, the code for that condition is assigned as the principal diagnosis rather than a code from categories Z08, Z09, or Z39. Examples include the following:

- An asymptomatic patient who had a resection of the descending colon a year earlier is admitted for colonoscopy to evaluate the anastomosis and determine whether there is any recurrence of malignancy. Colonoscopy proved the anastomosis to be normal, and there was no evidence of cancer recurrence. In this case, code **Z08, Encounter for follow-up examination after completed treatment for malignant neoplasm,** is coded as the principal diagnosis, with the additional code **Z85.038, Personal history of other malignant neoplasm of large intestine,** and a code for the colonoscopy.

- An asymptomatic patient who had a resection of the descending colon a year earlier is admitted for colonoscopy to evaluate the anastomosis and determine whether there is any recurrence of malignancy. Colonoscopy showed the anastomosis to be normal, and there was no evidence of cancer recurrence. However, a polyp of the transverse colon was found, and it was removed; pathology examination showed it to be an adenomatous polyp. Code **D12.3, Benign neoplasm of transverse colon,** is assigned as the principal diagnosis, with code **Z85.038, Personal history of other malignant neoplasm of large intestine,** assigned as an additional code. In this case, code Z08 is not assigned because a related condition was identified.

- A patient who had a colon resection for removal of carcinoma of the descending colon one year ago is now seen for follow-up examination to evaluate the anastomosis and determine whether there is any recurrence of disease. Colonoscopy showed normal anastomosis but revealed a recurrence of cancer at the primary site. Code **C18.6, Malignant neoplasm of descending colon,** is assigned as the principal diagnosis. Code Z08 is not assigned.

- A patient who had surgical excision of a malignant neoplasm of the ovary one year ago, followed by chemotherapy, is admitted for follow-up examination. There is no evidence

125

CHAPTER 11

Z Codes and
External Cause
of Morbidity
Codes

of recurrence or metastasis, and no other pathologic condition is identified. Code **Z08, Encounter for follow-up examination after completed treatment for malignant neoplasm,** is assigned along with the additional code Z85.43 to indicate the history of ovarian cancer as the reason for the examination.

- A patient who had benign polyps of the colon removed one year ago is now admitted with complaints of pain in the left lower abdomen. A colonoscopy is performed to determine whether there is any recurrence of colon polyps, and the results are entirely normal. In this case, code **R10.32, Left lower quadrant pain,** is assigned rather than code Z09 because the abdominal pain was the reason for the admission.

Code **Z09, Encounter for follow-up examination after completed treatment for conditions other than malignant neoplasm,** may be assigned as the reason for encounter only when the patient is no longer receiving treatment.

Admission for Observation and Evaluation

A code from category Z03, Encounter for medical observation for suspected diseases and conditions ruled out, or category Z04, Encounter for examination and observation for other reasons, is assigned when a person without a diagnosis is suspected of having an abnormal condition, without signs or symptoms, that requires study but is ruled out after examination and observation. Categories Z03 and Z04 can also be used for administrative and legal observation status. Outpatient referral for surveillance or for further diagnostic studies does not contradict the use of a code from these categories. The observation codes are not used if an injury or illness, or any sign or symptom related to the suspected condition, is present. In those cases, the diagnosis or symptom code is used. When a related diagnosis is established, the code for that condition is assigned instead of a code from category Z03 or Z04. Codes from category Z05 are used for observation and evaluation of a newborn within the neonatal period for suspected disease or condition, ruled out (see chapter 26 of this handbook). For persons with a feared health complaint in whom no diagnosis is made, assign code Z71.1.

Codes from categories Z03 and Z04 are primarily used as the principal/first-listed diagnosis or reason for encounter. However, an observation code from category Z03 or Z04 may be assigned as a secondary diagnosis code. This may be appropriate when the patient is being observed for a condition that is ruled out and is unrelated to the principal/first-listed diagnosis (e.g., patient presents for treatment following injuries sustained in a motor vehicle accident and is also observed for suspected COVID-19 infection that is subsequently ruled out).

A code from category Z03 or Z04 is ordinarily assigned as a solo code, with two exceptions:

- When a chronic condition requires care or monitoring during the stay, a code for that condition can be assigned as an additional code. Codes for chronic conditions that do not affect the stay are not assigned.

- When admission is for the purpose of ruling out a serious injury, such as concussion, codes for minor injuries such as abrasions or contusions may be assigned as additional codes. This exception is based on the fact that such minor injuries in themselves would not require hospitalization.

The following examples may help coding professionals to better understand the use of categories Z03 and Z04:

- A law enforcement representative refers the patient for evaluation of a suspected mental disorder. None is found, and no other condition is identified. Code **Z04.6, Encounter for general psychiatric examination, requested by authority,** is assigned.

- An adult patient is seen in the emergency department because of alleged rape. Observation and examination reveal no physical findings, such as hemorrhage or laceration. Code **Z04.41, Encounter for examination and observation following alleged adult**

126

CHAPTER 11

*Z Codes and
External Cause
of Morbidity
Codes*

rape, is assigned as the principal diagnosis. Code Z04.41 covers the collection of specimens, advice given for prophylaxis of pregnancy, and any other provision of counseling services. When physical findings suggest that a rape has occurred, code Z04.41 is not assigned; rather, the condition identified is coded and designated as the principal diagnosis. Rape is not a medical diagnosis but a matter of jurisprudence. Confirmed adult rape is coded to **T74.21-, Adult sexual abuse, confirmed.** Suspected adult rape is coded to **T76.21-, Adult sexual abuse, suspected.**

• A patient presents with generalized complaints involving nonspecific abdominal pain, minimal weight loss, and change of bowel habits. Because of a strong family history of colon cancer, the patient is admitted for evaluation for suspected malignancy. The presence of a neoplasm is ruled out, and no alternative diagnosis is made; it seems obvious that the symptoms reported are largely subjective. Code **Z03.89, Encounter for observation for other suspected diseases and conditions ruled out,** is assigned with an additional code of **Z80.0, Family history of malignant neoplasm of digestive organs.**

Note that a code from categories Z03 through Z05 is not assigned when a patient is admitted to the observation unit of the hospital immediately following same-day (outpatient) surgery, even though the medical record may suggest that the admission is for observation. Hospitals are advised to contact their individual payers to obtain billing instructions on whether a single claim should be submitted or whether separate claims should be submitted. If a single bill is submitted to a payer, code the reason for the surgery as the first-listed diagnosis (reason for the encounter). If the patient develops complications during the outpatient encounter, including during the observation stay, code these complications as secondary diagnoses while reporting the reason for the surgery as the reason for the overall encounter. Additional codes are assigned for the procedures performed. However, if separate bills are submitted, this advice would not apply. Hospitals should apply codes for the current encounter based on the individual payer's billing instructions.

Consider the following examples:

• A patient is admitted following outpatient surgery for a right direct inguinal hernia repair for "continued observation." Review of the medical record indicates that the patient was admitted to observation because he was experiencing severe nausea and vomiting.

• If a single claim is submitted: Code **K40.90, Unilateral inguinal hernia, without obstruction or gangrene, not specified as recurrent,** is assigned as the first-listed diagnosis, rather than a code from category Z03 or Z04. In addition, code **R11.2, Nausea with vomiting, unspecified,** is assigned as the secondary diagnosis, and code **0YQ50ZZ, Repair right inguinal region, open approach,** is assigned for the procedure.

• If separate bills are submitted: For the outpatient surgery bill, assign code **K40.90, Unilateral inguinal hernia, without obstruction or gangrene, not specified as recurrent,** as the first-listed diagnosis, along with the appropriate Healthcare Common Procedural Coding System code for the surgical procedure. For the observation bill, code **R11.2, Nausea with vomiting, unspecified,** is assigned as the first-listed diagnosis, rather than a code from category Z03 or Z04.

Codes from subcategory Z03.7, Encounter for suspected maternal and fetal conditions ruled out, may either be used as a first-listed code or assigned as an additional code depending on the case. Generally, this subcategory may only be reported as the principal or first-listed diagnosis, except when there are multiple encounters on the same day and the medical records for the encounters are combined. These codes should be used in very limited circumstances on a maternal record when an encounter is for a suspected maternal or fetal condition that is ruled out during that encounter. For example, if a maternal or fetal condition is suspected due to an abnormal test result but the condition is not confirmed, assign a code from subcategory Z03.7. However, if the condition is confirmed, code the condition instead. Codes from subcategory Z03.7 are not for use if an illness or any sign or symptom related to the suspected condition or problem is present. In such cases, the

127

CHAPTER 11

Z Codes and
External Cause
of Morbidity
Codes

diagnosis/symptom code is used. Other codes may be used in addition to the code from subcategory Z03.7, but only if they are unrelated to the suspected condition being evaluated.

If a patient is admitted after a period in the outpatient observation unit for further evaluation unrelated to surgery, the principal diagnosis is the condition that provided the original reason for the outpatient observation. If a patient is admitted to an observation unit for a medical condition, and the medical condition worsens or does not improve, it may be necessary for the patient to be admitted to the hospital as an inpatient. In this case, the medical condition that led to the hospital admission would be the principal diagnosis.

Special Investigations and Examinations

When a patient receives only diagnostic services during an episode of care, a code for the condition or problem that was chiefly responsible for the encounter is assigned first. A code from category Z01, Encounter for other special examination without complaint, suspected or reported diagnosis, is assigned as the reason for the encounter only when no problem, diagnosis, or condition is identified as the reason for the examination. Additionally, the examinations or procedures performed are assigned procedure codes. Codes from category Z01 are rarely appropriate for inpatient coding and are never assigned as additional codes. For example:

- A patient is examined for a cough and fever and referred to the radiology department for a chest X-ray, which may rule out pneumonia. The radiologist's report indicates that the X-ray is normal. The code for the cough (R05) or the fever (R50.9) is listed as the reason for the encounter. A code for pneumonia is not assigned; neither is a code assigned from category Z01.

- A patient is examined for a cough and fever and referred to the radiology department for a chest X-ray, which may rule out pneumonia. The radiologist's report confirms a diagnosis of bronchopneumonia. Code **J18.0, Bronchopneumonia, unspecified organism,** is listed as the reason for the visit. Codes are not assigned for the cough or fever because these symptoms are implicit in the diagnosis of bronchopneumonia. No code from category Z01 is assigned.

- A patient examined for vertigo is referred to the clinical laboratory for blood work to rule out hypothyroidism. Code **R42, Dizziness and giddiness,** is assigned as the reason for the visit. A code for hypothyroidism is not assigned because hypothyroidism is not an established diagnosis. Code **Z01.89, Encounter for other specified special examination,** is not assigned.

- A patient is referred to the radiology department for a chest X-ray as part of a routine physical examination. Code **Z00.00, Encounter for general adult medical examination,** is listed as the reason for the encounter because there are no presenting symptoms and the X-ray was not performed to rule out any suspected disease.

Patients are often referred to hospital ancillary services for preoperative evaluations that involve a variety of tests performed in various departments. Patients may also be referred for preoperative blood typing. Preoperative and preprocedural laboratory examination Z codes are for use only in those situations when a patient is being cleared for a procedure or surgery and no treatment is given. In this situation, one of the following codes is assigned, with additional codes for the condition for which surgery is planned and for any findings related to the preoperative evaluation:

Z01.810	Encounter for preprocedural cardiovascular examination
Z01.811	Encounter for preprocedural respiratory examination
Z01.812	Encounter for preprocedural laboratory examination
Z01.818	Encounter for other preprocedural examination
Z01.83	Encounter for blood typing

128

CHAPTER 11

Z Codes and

External Cause

of Morbidity

Codes

For example:

- A patient with the diagnosis of cholelithiasis is referred to the radiology department for a preoperative chest X-ray. Code **Z01.818, Encounter for other preprocedural examination,** should be listed as the reason for the encounter, with an additional code for the cholelithiasis.

Some of the codes for routine health examinations distinguish between "with" and "without" abnormal findings (for example, code Z00.00 versus code Z00.01). Code assignment depends on the information that is known at the time the encounter is being coded. For example, if no abnormal findings were identified during the examination but the encounter is being coded before test results are back, it is acceptable to assign the code for "without abnormal findings." An examination with abnormal findings refers to a condition/diagnosis that is newly found, or a change in severity of a chronic condition, during a routine physical exam. When assigning a code for "with abnormal findings," an additional code(s) should be assigned to identify the specific abnormal finding(s).

For example:

- An adult patient diagnosed with hypertension presents for an annual physical examination. During the visit, the patient's blood pressure is noted to be elevated, and the physician adjusts the antihypertensive meds for better control. Code **Z00.01, Encounter for general adult medical examination with abnormal findings,** should be the first-listed diagnosis. This case is assigned the code "with abnormal findings" because the physician discovered the elevated and uncontrolled hypertension during the visit. Code **I10, Essential (primary) hypertension,** is assigned as an additional code to describe the abnormal finding (uncontrolled hypertension).

- A patient is seen for a well-child exam. He also has viral bronchitis, which was diagnosed during a previous visit, and is still under treatment. Code **Z00.129, Encounter for routine child health examination without abnormal findings,** is the first-listed diagnosis. This case is assigned "without abnormal findings" because the bronchitis is not newly diagnosed during the routine exam and a change in severity is not documented. Code **J20.8, Acute bronchitis due to other specified organisms,** is assigned for the viral bronchitis.

Screening Examinations

Codes from categories Z11 through Z13, Encounter for screening, are assigned to encounters for tests performed to identify a disease or disease precursors for the purpose of early detection and treatment for patients who test positive. Screening is performed on apparently well individuals who present no signs or symptoms relative to the disease. A screening mammogram is an example of such a test. If a screening examination identifies pathology, the code for the reason for the test (namely, the screening code from categories Z11–Z13) is assigned as the principal diagnosis or first-listed code, followed by a code for the pathology or condition found during the screening exam. For example:

- A patient undergoes routine mammography, which reveals no pathology. Code **Z12.31, Encounter for screening mammogram for malignant neoplasm of breast,** is assigned.

- An asymptomatic patient undergoes a screening mammography. The radiologist reports the presence of microcalcifications. Assign code **Z12.31, Encounter for screening mammogram for malignant neoplasm of breast,** followed by code **R92.0, Mammographic microcalcification found on diagnostic imaging of breast.**

- A patient with a family history of breast cancer in her mother, aunt, and older sister presents for a screening mammogram because she is considered at high risk for the disease. Assign code **Z12.31, Encounter for screening mammogram for malignant neoplasm of breast,** followed by code **Z80.3, Family history of malignant neoplasm of breast.**

Contact/Exposure

Category Z20 indicates contact with, and suspected exposure to, communicable diseases. These codes are for patients who are suspected to have been exposed to a disease by close personal contact with an infected individual or are located in an area where a disease is epidemic. Examples include contact with or exposure to an intestinal infectious disease, tuberculosis, HIV, Zika virus, or COVID-19.

Category Z77 indicates contact with and suspected exposures hazardous to health. Examples of contact/exposures covered in category Z77 include contact/exposure to hazardous nonmedicinal chemicals (such as lead or uranium), environmental pollution, or mold.

Codes Representing Patient History, Status, or Problems

Categories Z80 through Z84 indicate a family history. They may be assigned when the family history is the reason for examination or treatment.

Codes from categories Z85 through Z92 are used to indicate a personal history of a previous condition. When the condition mentioned is still present or still under treatment, or if a complication is present, a code from categories Z85 through Z92 is not assigned.

Status codes indicate that a patient is a carrier of a disease, has the sequelae or residual of a past disease or condition, or has another factor influencing his or her health status. Categories Z88 through Z99 indicate that the patient has a continuing condition or health status that may influence care, such as the fact that a tracheostomy (Z93.0), a colostomy (Z93.3), a cardiac pacemaker (Z95.0), or an aortocoronary bypass graft (Z95.1) is in place. Z codes indicating status are redundant when the diagnosis code itself indicates that the status exists. For example, in the case of an acute rejection crisis of a transplanted kidney, code **T86.11, Kidney transplant rejection,** is used. Because the patient's transplant status is implicit in that diagnosis, the additional code Z94.0, indicating kidney transplant status, is not meaningful and should not be assigned.

A diagnostic statement expressed as "status post" typically refers to an earlier surgery, injury, or illness and usually has no significance for the episode of care. No code for the condition is assigned in this case. A personal history code can be assigned if desired. Note the important distinction between history and status codes. History codes indicate that the problem no longer exists, while status codes indicate that the condition is present.

Codes from category Z79 are assigned to indicate a patient's continuous use of a prescribed drug for an extended period. For example, codes from category Z79 are assigned for long-term use of medication:

- As a prophylactic measure (e.g., to prevent deep vein thrombosis)
- As treatment of a chronic condition (e.g., arthritis)
- For a disease requiring a lengthy course of treatment (e.g., cancer)

A code from category Z79 is appropriately assigned when the patient is currently receiving long-term anticoagulant therapy (Z79.01), antithrombotics/antiplatelets (Z79.02), nonsteroidal anti-inflammatories (Z79.1), antibiotic therapy (Z79.2), hormonal contraceptives (Z79.3), insulin (Z79.4), steroids (Z79.51–Z79.52), or other long-term drug therapy (Z79.81–Z79.899). Subcategory Z79.8 includes long-term use of selective estrogen receptor modulators (Z79.810), aromatase inhibitors (Z79.811), other agents affecting estrogen receptors and estrogen levels (Z79.818), aspirin (Z79.82), bisphosphonates (Z79.83), hormone replacement therapy (Z79.890), opiate analgesic (Z79.891), and other long-term drug therapy (Z79.899). An additional code is assigned for the condition for which the medication is prescribed.

Note that coding guidelines do not provide a definition or time frame for long-term drug therapy. If a patient receives a drug on a regular basis and has multiple refills available for a prescription, it is appropriate to document long-term drug use. Documentation of long-term drug use is at the discretion of the health care provider.

130

CHAPTER 11

Z Codes and
External Cause
of Morbidity
Codes

Do not assign a code from category Z79 when the medication is prescribed to treat an acute illness or injury and is being given for a brief period of time (e.g., antibiotics to treat bronchitis). Codes from category Z79 are also not used when medications are given for detoxification or maintenance programs used to prevent withdrawal symptoms in patients with drug dependence. For example, long-term use of methadone for pain management is coded with **Z79.891, Long term (current) use of opiate analgesic,** but the use of methadone in a maintenance program to prevent withdrawal symptoms is coded using the drug dependence code (F11.2-).

Code Z51.81 is used to report encounters for therapeutic drug monitoring. If the drug being monitored is one that the patient has been receiving on a long-term basis, a code from category Z79 should be added.

Codes from categories Z55 through Z65, Persons with potential health hazards related to socioeconomic and psychosocial circumstances, are used to indicate certain problems that may affect the patient's care or prevent satisfactory compliance with the recommended regimen. Because codes from categories Z55 through Z65 represent information about social determinants of health, rather than medical diagnoses, they do not need to be derived from physician documentation; it is also acceptable to report them based on information documented by other clinicians involved in the care of the patient. Patient self-reported documentation may also be used to assign codes for social determinants of health, as long as a clinician or provider accepts the patient self-reported information and incorporates it into the health record. There is a growing interest in the social determinants of health as key influencers in health outcomes. Social determinants include societal and environmental conditions such as income, education level, language fluency, cultural differences, employment status, and level of health care access. Hospitals, payers, and others are interested in collecting data on the social determinants of health, with the understanding that this information will be critical for the population health efforts of health plans, hospitals, and health centers nationwide.

History, status, and problem codes ordinarily cannot be used as the principal diagnosis or reason for encounter, with the following exceptions:

- Family history codes from categories Z80 through Z84
- Personal status codes from categories Z85 through Z87 (except subcategory Z87.7, Personal history of [corrected] congenital malformations)
- Code **Z91.81, History of falling**

These codes can be used as the principal diagnosis or reason for encounter when the history is the reason for admission or encounter.

History, status, and problem codes can be used as additional codes for any patient regardless of the reason for the encounter, but they are ordinarily assigned only when the history, status, or problem has some significance for the episode of care. For example, a history of previously treated carcinoma or a family history of malignant neoplasm may be useful in explaining why certain tests are performed. Status subcategory Z96.6- indicates that the patient has had an orthopedic joint replacement, but this fact would probably be significant only if it limits the patient's movement to the extent that additional nursing care is required or when it prevents the patient's full participation in a rehabilitation program.

Genetic Susceptibility to Disease

Codes from category Z15 are used to report genetic susceptibility to disease. Genetic susceptibility refers to a genetic predisposition for contracting a disease. Patients with a genetic susceptibility to certain diseases may request prophylactic removal of an organ to prevent the disease from occurring.

It is important to distinguish genetic susceptibility from carrier state. An individual who is a carrier of a disease can pass it on to an offspring.

Subcategory Z15.0, Genetic susceptibility to malignant neoplasm, is further subdivided to identify the potential body site, such as breast (Z15.01), ovary (Z15.02), prostate (Z15.03), endometrium (Z15.04), and other (Z15.09).

131

CHAPTER 11

*Z Codes and
External Cause
of Morbidity
Codes*

Codes from category Z15 should not be used as principal or first-listed codes. Sequencing of category Z15 codes would depend on the circumstances of the encounter, as follows:

- If the patient has the condition to which he or she is susceptible, and that condition is the reason for the encounter, the code for the current condition is sequenced first, followed by the Z15.- code.

- If the patient is being seen for follow-up after completed treatment for this condition, and the condition no longer exists, a follow-up code should be sequenced first, followed by the appropriate personal history (Z85.- to Z87.-) and genetic susceptibility (Z15.-) codes.

- If the purpose of the encounter is genetic counseling associated with procreative management, assign first code **Z31.5, Encounter for procreative genetic counseling,** followed by a code from category Z15. Additional codes should be assigned for any applicable family or personal history.

Z Codes as Principal/First-Listed Diagnosis

Z codes may be assigned as the principal or first-listed diagnosis or as secondary diagnoses. The *ICD-10-CM Official Guidelines for Coding and Reporting* contain a list of Z codes that may only be a principal/first-listed diagnosis. In most situations, Z codes on that list may only be reported as the principal/first-listed diagnosis; exceptions are made for cases in which there are multiple encounters on the same day and the medical records for the encounters are combined, or when there is more than one Z code that meets the definition of principal diagnosis (e.g., a patient is admitted to home health care for aftercare and rehabilitation, and both diagnoses equally meet the definition of principal diagnosis). These codes should not be reported if they do not meet the definition of principal or first-listed diagnosis.

REVIEW EXERCISE 11.1

Code the following diagnoses.

1. Visit to change surgical dressing

2. Family history of polyps of the colon

3. Status post aortocoronary bypass procedure

4. Encounter for gastrostomy tube irrigation

5. Adjustment of cardiac pacemaker pulse generator

6. Long-term use of anticoagulant therapy

7. Dependence on respirator

8. Aftercare for end-of-life care

9. Encounter for screening mammogram

10. Encounter for radiation therapy

_____

11. Noncompliance with medication, unintentional,

    due to patient's advanced age

_____

12. Encounter for removal of sutures

_____

Coding OF Signs AND Symptoms

CHAPTER 12

Symptoms, Signs, and Ill-Defined Conditions

CHAPTER OVERVIEW

- Many symptoms and signs are classified to chapter 18 of ICD-10-CM if they point to multiple diseases or systems or if they are of an unexplained etiology.

- There are few situations in which a symptom code from chapter 18 is used as a principal diagnosis.

- Conversely, for outpatients, the symptom code is often used as the reason for the encounter.

- Codes from chapter 18 are assigned as secondary diagnoses only when the sign or symptom is not integral to a condition.

- The codes for nonspecific abnormal findings are rarely appropriate for use in an inpatient setting.

LEARNING OUTCOMES

After studying this chapter, you should be able to:

Explain the difference between a sign and a symptom.

Determine when to properly use a code from chapter 18 of ICD-10-CM for a principal diagnosis.

Determine when to properly use a code from chapter 18 for an additional diagnosis.

TERMS TO KNOW

Sign
objective evidence of disease observed by the examining physician

Symptom
subjective observation reported by the patient

REMEMBER . . .

In an inpatient situation, there are often more appropriate options than the codes found in chapter 18 of ICD-10-CM.

. . . For inpatients, a diagnosis described as possible, probable, and so on is considered to be an established diagnosis.

INTRODUCTION

A sign is defined as objective evidence of disease that can be observed by the examining physician. A symptom, on the other hand, is a subjective observation reported by the patient but not confirmed objectively by the physician.

Symptoms and signs are classified in two ways in ICD-10-CM: Signs and symptoms that point to a specific diagnosis have been assigned to a category in other chapters of ICD-10-CM. Those that can point to more than one disease or system, or that are of unexplained etiology, are classified to chapter 18 of ICD-10-CM. For example, irritable bowel syndrome with diarrhea is classified to code K58.0, in ICD-10-CM chapter 11, Diseases of the digestive system, whereas unspecified diarrhea is classified to code R19.7 in ICD-10-CM chapter 18.

SIGNS AND SYMPTOMS AS PRINCIPAL DIAGNOSES

Codes for symptoms, signs, and ill-defined conditions from chapter 18 of ICD-10-CM cannot be used as principal diagnoses or reasons for outpatient encounters when related diagnoses have been established, but they may be assigned as additional diagnoses. Examples include:

T40.1x1A + R40.20   Coma due to poisoning by heroin, initial encounter
I44.2 + R55   Syncope due to third-degree atrioventricular block

If the patient is an inpatient, a diagnosis described as possible, probable, and so on at the time of discharge is considered to be an established diagnosis. For example, a patient is admitted with severe generalized abdominal pain. The physician's diagnostic statement is abdominal pain, probably due to acute gastritis (K29.00). Only the code for the gastritis is assigned, as the abdominal pain is integral to the probable gastritis. Refer to chapter 6 of this handbook for more details on uncertain diagnoses.

There are only a few inpatient situations in which a symptom code from chapter 18 can be correctly designated the principal diagnosis, as follows:

1. When no related condition is identified and the symptom is the reason for the encounter, a code from chapter 18 of ICD-10-CM is assigned as the principal diagnosis even though other unrelated diagnoses may be listed. For example, a patient is admitted with tachycardia. An electrocardiogram (EKG) does not provide any conclusive evidence of the type of tachycardia or of any underlying cardiac condition. The patient also has insulin-dependent diabetes; blood sugars are monitored daily during the hospital stay. The reason for admission is tachycardia; therefore, code **R00.0, Tachycardia, unspecified,** is the principal diagnosis. Because the diabetes was treated during the hospital stay, an additional code is assigned for the diabetes mellitus.

2. Other situations in which codes from chapter 18 of the ICD-10-CM manual can be appropriately used as the principal diagnosis for an inpatient admission include the following:

   • Presenting signs or symptoms are transient, and no definitive diagnosis can be made.

   • The patient is referred elsewhere for further study or treatment before a diagnosis is made.

   • A more precise diagnosis cannot be made for any other reason.

   • The symptom is treated in an outpatient setting without the additional workup required to arrive at a more definitive diagnosis.

   • Provisional diagnosis of a sign or symptom is made for a patient who fails to return for further investigation or care.

   • A residual late effect is the reason for admission, and the Alphabetic Index directs the coding professional to an alternative sequencing.

137

CHAPTER 12

Symptoms,
Signs, and
Ill-Defined
Conditions

Generally speaking, symptom codes classified to other chapters of ICD-10-CM are not designated as principal diagnoses when a related condition has been identified. The symptom can be designated as principal diagnosis, however, when the patient is admitted for the sole purpose of treating the symptom and no treatment or further evaluation of the underlying disease takes place. For example, patients with dehydration secondary to gastroenteritis are sometimes admitted for the purpose of rehydration when the gastroenteritis itself could be managed on an outpatient basis. In this case, the code for dehydration can be designated as the principal diagnosis even though the cause of the dehydration is stated.

Note that these guidelines do not apply when coding and reporting hospital outpatient care or physician services. Outpatient encounters do not ordinarily permit the type of study that results in an established diagnosis, and treatment is often directed at relieving symptoms rather than treating the underlying condition. Words such as "possible" and "probable" are not considered to be established diagnoses for outpatient visits or encounters. The highest level of certainty is reported as the reason for encounter for outpatients. Therefore, if a diagnosis is not established, a symptom code is assigned as the reason for the encounter.

SIGNS AND SYMPTOMS AS ADDITIONAL DIAGNOSES

Unless otherwise instructed by the classification, codes from chapter 18 are assigned as secondary codes only when the symptom or sign is not integral to the underlying condition, and when the presence of the sign or symptom makes a difference in the severity of the patient's condition and/or the care given. For example, many but not all patients with cirrhosis of the liver have ascites. When ascites is present, it makes a difference in the care given, and so the chapter 18 code for ascites (R18.8) should be assigned as an additional code.

However, please note that for ascites in alcoholic cirrhosis, code R18.8 is not assigned as an additional diagnosis. Category R18, Ascites, excludes ascites in alcoholic cirrhosis, which is assigned instead to code **K70.31, Alcoholic cirrhosis of liver with ascites.**

Codes from chapter 18 are not assigned when the sign or symptom is implicit in the diagnosis or when the sign or symptom is included in the condition code. Care should be exercised to review instructional notes because ICD-10-CM contains a number of combination codes that identify both the definitive diagnosis and the common signs or symptoms of that diagnosis. When using one of these combination codes, an additional code should not be assigned for the sign or symptom. Such redundant coding is inappropriate. Additional examples include:

- Abdominal pain due to gastric ulcer—no symptom code is assigned to the abdominal pain because it is integral to the ulcer.

- Coma due to diabetes mellitus—the coma is not assigned a separate code because combination codes are provided for diabetes with associated coma.

- Patient admitted with chest pain, initially thought to be angina—diagnostic studies do not support this diagnosis, and the physician's diagnosis is chest pain, probable costochondritis (M94.0). The chest pain is not coded because it is implicit in the costochondritis.

ABNORMAL FINDINGS

Although categories R70 through R97 in chapter 18 are provided for coding nonspecific abnormal findings, it is rarely appropriate to assign one of these codes for acute inpatient hospital care. They are assigned only when (1) the physician has not been able to arrive at a definitive related diagnosis and lists the abnormal finding itself as a diagnosis and (2) the condition meets the Uniform Hospital Discharge Data Set criteria for reporting of other diagnoses.

For example, if the physician lists a diagnosis of abnormal electrocardiographic findings without any mention of associated disease, assigning code **R94.31, Abnormal electrocardiogram**

[ECG] [EKG], would be appropriate if there were evidence of further evaluation for a possible cardiac condition. On the other hand, if an elevated blood pressure reading is documented in the medical record, but the physician has not listed it as a diagnosis and there is no evidence of any follow-up or treatment, assigning a code for this abnormal finding would be inappropriate.

If the coding professional notes clinical findings outside of the normal range but no related diagnosis is stated, the medical record must be reviewed to determine whether additional tests and/or consultations were carried out related to these findings or whether specific related care was given. If such documentation is present, it is appropriate to ask the physician whether a code should be assigned.

For example, a patient with a low potassium level treated with oral or intravenous potassium has a clinically significant condition that probably should be reported; the physician should be asked whether a diagnosis should be added. On the other hand, a finding of degenerative arthritis on a routine postoperative chest X-ray of an elderly patient when no treatment or further diagnostic evaluation of the arthritis has been carried out does not warrant a code assignment.

GLASGOW COMA SCALE

The Glasgow coma scale is a scale for assessing the degree of consciousness, especially after a head injury. The scoring is determined by three factors: amount of eye opening, verbal responsiveness, and motor responsiveness. The test score can function as an indicator for certain diagnostic tests or treatments and for predicting the duration and ultimate outcome of coma.

The Glasgow coma scale was developed for adult patients; the pediatric version is used to assess the mental state of child patients. Like the adult version, the pediatric Glasgow coma scale is composed of three tests (eye, verbal, and motor responses), but the individual verbal and motor responses differ from the adult scale to accommodate children. Inclusion terms in subcategories R40.22 (Coma scale, best verbal response) and R40.23 (Coma scale, best motor response) clarify the usage for pediatric patients two to five years of age and for those under two years of age.

The coma scale codes in subcategory R40.2, Coma, can be used in combination with traumatic brain injury codes. These codes are primarily for use by trauma registries. Coma scale codes should be sequenced after the diagnosis code(s). One code from each subcategory (amount of eye opening, verbal responsiveness, and motor responsiveness) is needed to complete the scale. The seventh character indicates when the scale was recorded (e.g., in the field, at arrival to emergency department, at hospital admission, 24 hours or more after hospital admission, or unspecified time). The seventh character should match for all three codes.

At a minimum, the initial score documented upon presentation at the facility should be recorded. This may be a score from the emergency medicine technician or documented in the emergency department. A facility may choose to capture multiple Glasgow coma scale scores, if desired. Assign a code from R40.24-, Glasgow coma scale, total score, when only the total score is documented in the medical record. When individual score(s) are documented, one code from each subcategory R40.21- through R40.23- is assigned to complete the coma scale. Code R40.244- is used to report other coma, without a documented Glasgow coma scale score, or when there is only a partial score reported. Similar to the codes for Glasgow coma scale individual scores (subcategories R40.21-, R40.22-, and R40.23-), codes for the total score (subcategory R40.24-) require a seventh character to indicate when the scale was recorded.

Code assignment for the coma scale may be based on medical record documentation from clinicians who are not the patient's provider (i.e., the physician or other qualified health care practitioner legally accountable for establishing the patient's diagnosis), because this information is typically documented by other clinicians involved in the care of the patient. For example, an emergency medical technician often documents the coma scale. However, the associated diagnosis must be documented by the patient's provider. If there is conflicting medical record documentation—either from the same clinician or from different clinicians—the patient's attending provider should be queried for clarification.

139

CHAPTER 12

*Symptoms,
Signs, and
Ill-Defined
Conditions*

Occasionally, a patient is put in a medically induced coma. This type of reversible coma is induced with drugs to help protect the brain from swelling by decreasing blood flow as well as the metabolic rate of brain tissue. Do not report codes for individual or total Glasgow coma scale scores for a medically sedated patient or a patient with a medically induced coma.

NATIONAL INSTITUTES OF HEALTH STROKE SCALE

Codes in subcategory R29.7- are used to report the National Institutes of Health Stroke Scale (NIHSS) scores. The NIHSS is a clinical assessment tool to evaluate and document neurological status in acute stroke patients. It uses 15 items to evaluate the effect of acute cerebral infarction on the levels of consciousness, language, neglect, visual-field loss, extraocular movement, motor strength, ataxia, dysarthria, and sensory loss. The NIHSS identifies the patient's neurological status and the severity of the stroke.

Codes from R29.7- are intended to be used as secondary codes; the acute cerebral infarction (I63-) should be coded as the first-listed diagnosis. The R29.7- codes discretely identify NIHSS scores from 0 to 42. For example, a patient admitted with acute stroke and an NIHSS score of 30 should be coded with the principal diagnosis of **I63.9, Cerebral infarction, unspecified,** and the secondary diagnosis of **R29.730, NIHSS score 30.** If desired, a facility may choose to capture multiple stroke scale scores. At a minimum, the coding professional should report the initial score documented.

Similar to code assignment for the coma scale, code assignment from subcategory R29.7 may be based on medical record documentation from clinicians who are not the patient's provider because this information is typically documented by other clinicians involved in the care of the patient.

ILL-DEFINED CONDITIONS

Code **R99, Ill-defined and unknown cause of mortality,** is only for use in the very limited circumstances when a patient who has already died is brought into an emergency department or other health care facility and pronounced dead on arrival. This code should not be used to represent the discharge disposition of death.

EXERCISE 12.1

Code the following diagnoses and procedures as statements given at the time of discharge. Do not assign External cause of morbidity codes.

---

1. Dysuria

   Transurethral biopsy of bladder (via cystoscope)

---

2. Acute chest pain due to influenzal pleurisy

---

3. Gross, painless hematuria, cause undetermined

   Cystoscopy with control of bladder hemorrhage by cauterization

---

140

CHAPTER 12

Symptoms,
Signs, and
Ill-Defined
Conditions

4. Pyuria, intermittent, cause undetermined

5. Enlarged lymph node, left axilla

   Open biopsy, axillary lymph node

6. Elevated glucose tolerance test

7. Severe vertigo, left temporal headache, and nausea

8. Syncope, cause undetermined

9. Chest pain, probably angina pectoris (inpatient discharge)

10. Psychogenic dysuria

11. Arteriosclerotic gangrene, left foot

12. Chronic epistaxis, severe, recurrent

    Silver nitrate cauterization bleeding nasal mucosa

13. Severe epistaxis due to hypertension

    Nasal packing

14. Hereditary epistaxis

15. Generalized abdominal pain due to possible pancreatitis

    or cholecystitis (inpatient discharge)

16. Chronic fatigue syndrome

17. Fever and malaise due to viral syndrome

18. Fever of unknown etiology, headache

19. Prediabetes

Coding OF Infectious AND Parasitic Diseases, Endocrine Diseases AND Metabolic Disorders, AND Mental Disorders

CHAPTER 13

Infectious and Parasitic Diseases

CHAPTER OVERVIEW

- Chapter 1 of ICD-10-CM includes information on how to code infectious and parasitic diseases.
  - The primary axis of chapter 1 is the organism responsible for the disease.
  - When the main term for the condition is located, specific subterms always take precedence over general subterms.
- This chapter has information on coding specific infectious and parasitic diseases, including tuberculosis, Zika virus, West Nile virus, bacteremia, septicemia, systemic inflammatory response syndrome (SIRS), sepsis, toxic shock syndrome, and gram-negative bacterial infections.
- Also included in chapter 1 of ICD-10-CM is detailed information on all aspects of HIV/AIDS coding procedures.
- Chapter 22 of ICD-10-CM contains codes for special purposes, including coronavirus disease 2019 (COVID-19).

LEARNING OUTCOMES

After studying this chapter, you should be able to:

- Code infectious and parasitic diseases.
- Explain the differences between bacteremia, septicemia, SIRS, sepsis, and septic shock, and how to code these conditions.
- Explain how to code for HIV testing, diagnosis, and treatment.
- Explain how to code for COVID-19.

TERMS TO KNOW

Bacteremia
presence of bacteria in the bloodstream after a trauma or an infection

COVID-19
an infectious disease caused by the 2019 novel coronavirus SARS-CoV-2 that became a worldwide pandemic in 2020

Sepsis
SIRS due to infection; a severe case indicates organ dysfunction

Septicemia
a systemic disease associated with pathological microorganisms or toxins in the bloodstream

Septic shock
circulatory failure associated with severe sepsis

SIRS
systemic inflammatory response syndrome; a systemic response to infection or trauma with such symptoms as fever and tachycardia

REMEMBER . . .

Codes from chapter 1 of ICD-10-CM take precedence over codes from other chapters for the same condition.

. . . Coding for HIV/AIDS is not allowed unless the diagnostic statement reports the diagnosis with absolute certainty.

INTRODUCTION

Chapter 1 of ICD-10-CM classifies infectious and parasitic diseases that are easily transmissible (communicable). The primary axis for this chapter is the organism responsible for the condition. Infectious and parasitic conditions are classified in one of several ways, making careful use of the Alphabetic Index imperative. Some examples follow.

- A single code from chapter 1 is assigned to indicate the organism. For example, code B26.- is assigned for mumps. Some codes of this type use a fourth character to indicate a site or an associated condition. For example, code B37.1 is assigned for candidiasis of the lung.
- Combination codes frequently identify both the condition and the organism. For example:

J15.212   Pneumonia due to Methicillin resistant *Staphylococcus aureus*
B26.0   Orchitis due to mumps

Dual classification is also used extensively for chapter 1. For example:

B49 + J99   Bronchomycosis
B39.9 + H32   Chorioretinitis in histoplasmosis

Codes from chapter 1 take precedence over codes from other chapters for the same condition. For example, urinary tract infection due to candidiasis is classified to code **B37.49, Other urogenital candidiasis,** rather than to code **N39.0, Urinary tract infection, site not specified.**

Conditions that are not considered to be easily transmissible or communicable are classified in the appropriate body system chapter, with an additional code from category B95–B97 to indicate the responsible organism. For example, codes **N41.00, Acute prostatitis without hematuria,** and **B95.0, *Streptococcus*, group A, as the cause of diseases classified elsewhere,** are assigned for acute prostatitis due to group A *Streptococcus*.

Chapter 22 of ICD-10-CM contains codes for special purposes and has a new section for provisional assignment of codes for new diseases of uncertain etiology or for emergency use. Code **U07.1, COVID-19,** was created for infections due to SARS-CoV-2. This condition is discussed in more detail later in this chapter.

ORGANISM VERSUS SITE OR OTHER SUBTERM

A thorough search of the Alphabetic Index is required when coding infection. Once the main term for the condition has been located, a subterm for the organism always takes precedence over a more general subterm (such as "acute" or "chronic") when both subterms occur at the same indention level in the Alphabetic Index. For example, for a diagnosis of chronic cystitis due to gonococcus, the Alphabetic Index provides subterms for both chronic and gonococcal:

Cystitis (exudative) . . .
   chronic N30.20 . . .
   gonococcal A54.01

In this case, only code A54.01 is assigned because the subterm for the organism takes precedence over the subterm "chronic."

When the organism is specified but is not indexed under the main term for the condition, refer to the main term **Infection** or to the main term for the organism. For example, consider a diagnosis of candidal cystitis. No subterm for candidal is located under the main term **Cystitis,** but there is a main term entry **Infection,** followed by a subterm for *Candida,* which points the user to see the main term **Candidiasis, candidal;** listed there is the subterm "urogenital site, NEC." Code B37.49 is therefore assigned for this diagnosis rather than the code for cystitis.

WEST NILE VIRUS FEVER

Subcategory A92.3 is used to report West Nile virus infection. The virus is transmitted to humans by the bite of a mosquito that has bitten an infected bird. Most healthy people infected by the virus have few symptoms or have a mild illness consisting of fever, headache, and body aches prior to recovering. In elderly patients or those with a weakened immune system, the virus may cause encephalitis, meningitis, or permanent neurologic damage and may be life threatening. Subcategory A92.3 is further subdivided to distinguish between West Nile virus infection unspecified (A92.30), with encephalitis (A92.31), with other neurologic manifestation (A92.32), and with other complications (A92.39). With this expansion, milder cases of the disease are differentiated from those with more serious complications and neurologic manifestations.

ZIKA VIRUS

Code A92.5 is used to report Zika virus disease (Zika). Zika virus disease is a disease caused by the Zika virus, which is spread to people primarily through the bite of an infected mosquito. The most common symptoms are fever, rash, joint pain, and conjunctivitis. The illness is usually mild with symptoms lasting for several days to a week after being bitten by an infected mosquito. According to the Centers for Disease Control and Prevention, Zika virus infection during pregnancy can cause a serious birth defect called microcephaly (a condition in which a baby's head is much smaller than expected), as well as other severe fetal brain defects, such as intracranial calcifications, ventriculomegaly, and/or cerebral atrophy.

Code only a confirmed diagnosis of Zika virus (**A92.5, Zika virus disease**) as documented by the provider. This is an exception to the hospital inpatient guideline Section II, H. In this context, "confirmation" does not require documentation of the type of test performed; the physician's diagnostic statement that the condition is confirmed is sufficient. This code should be assigned regardless of the stated mode of transmission. If the provider documents "suspected," "possible," or "probable" Zika, do not assign code A92.5. Instead, assign a code or codes explaining the reason for the encounter (such as fever, rash, or joint pain), or assign code **Z20.821, Contact with and (suspected) exposure to Zika virus.** Assign code **Z86.1, Personal history of infectious and parasitic diseases,** if documentation in the medical record indicates that the patient has a past history of Zika virus infection.

TUBERCULOSIS

Tuberculosis (TB) is a bacterial disease caused by *Mycobacterium tuberculosis* and *Mycobacterium bovis*. People with weakened immune systems are at increased risk for contracting TB. It is spread through the air when a person with untreated pulmonary TB coughs or sneezes. Prolonged exposure to a person with untreated TB is usually necessary for infection to occur.

Tuberculosis is classified to categories A15 through A19 based on the general site (e.g., respiratory system) or type of tuberculosis (e.g., miliary), as follows:

A15   Respiratory tuberculosis
A17   Tuberculosis of nervous system
A18   Tuberculosis of other organs
A19   Miliary tuberculosis

Categories A15, A17, and A18 are subdivided further to specify the site. Tuberculosis usually affects the lungs (code A15.0), although other parts of the body can also be affected, such as intrathoracic lymph nodes (code A15.4), kidneys (code A18.11), and bones and joints (subcategory A18.0). Miliary tuberculosis (category A19) is the form of TB in which the bacillus spreads through all body tissues and organs, producing many thousands of tiny tubercular lesions.

Care should be taken to differentiate between a diagnosis of tuberculosis and a positive tuberculin skin test without a diagnosis of active tuberculosis. Code R76.11 classifies the following:

- Nonspecific reaction to tuberculin skin test without active tuberculosis

- Positive tuberculin skin test without active tuberculosis

- Positive PPD (skin test)

- Abnormal result of Mantoux test

- Tuberculin (skin test) positive

- Tuberculin (skin test) reactor

"Latent tuberculosis" refers to infection with *Mycobacterium tuberculosis*, but without active TB disease. The only sign of TB infection is a positive reaction to the tuberculin skin test or TB blood test. Persons with latent TB infection do not have any symptoms, are not infectious, and cannot spread TB infection to others. However, in persons with a weak immune system, the bacteria can become active, multiply, and cause tuberculosis disease. Latent tuberculosis is coded as **Z22.7, Latent tuberculosis.**

SEPSIS, SEVERE SEPSIS, AND SEPTIC SHOCK

For a diagnosis of sepsis, the appropriate code for the underlying systemic infection should be assigned. If the type of infection or causal organism is not further specified, assign code **A41.9, Sepsis, unspecified organism.**

Streptococcal sepsis is classified to category A40 with the third character specifying sepsis due to different streptococci strains, such as group A (A40.0), group B (A40.1), *Streptococcus pneumoniae* (A40.3), other (A40.8), or unspecified (A40.9). However, sepsis documented as "due to *Streptococcus* group D" is assigned to code **A41.81, Sepsis due to *Enterococcus*.**

Although sepsis is most commonly caused by bacterial infection, it may also be caused by viruses, fungi, and/or parasites. Sepsis caused by the *Candida* fungus is assigned code B37.7, and sepsis due to disseminated herpesviral disease is assigned code B00.7.

Assign code **A41.89, Other specified sepsis,** for a diagnosis of viral sepsis. Although codes in categories A30–A49 classify bacterial illnesses, ICD-10-CM does not provide a specific viral sepsis code, and A41.89 is the best available option. When the specific type of viral infection is not documented, code **B97.89, Other viral agents as the cause of diseases classified elsewhere,** should be assigned as an additional code to provide further specificity, and to convey that the sepsis is due to a viral infection.

Organisms that cause sepsis are sometimes transferred to other tissue, where they may seed infection in another site and lead to such conditions as arteritis, meningitis, and pyelonephritis. Additional codes are assigned for these manifestations when they are present.

A diagnosis of sepsis can neither be assumed nor ruled out on the basis of laboratory values alone. Negative or inconclusive blood cultures do not preclude a diagnosis of sepsis in patients with clinical evidence of the condition; however, the provider should be queried. A code for sepsis should never be assigned based on clinical definition or criteria, nor on clinical signs alone. A code for sepsis is assigned only when the physician makes such a diagnosis, regardless of the clinical criteria used to arrive at that diagnosis.

Bacteremia (R78.81) refers to the presence of bacteria in the bloodstream after trauma or mild infection. This condition is usually transient and ordinarily clears promptly through the action of the body's own immune system. Bacteriuria (R82.71) refers to the presence of bacteria in a microscopic examination of the urine, but it should not be confused with urinary tract infection (N39.0).

The unusual or imprecise diagnostic reference to a site-specific or organ-specific sepsis, such as urosepsis, may require further clarification for coding purposes. For example, the term "urosepsis" refers to pyuria or bacteria in the urine, not the blood. Unfortunately, urosepsis is sometimes stated as the diagnosis even though the condition has progressed from a localized urinary tract infection and has become a generalized sepsis. The term "urosepsis" is a nonspecific term and should not be considered synonymous with sepsis. It has no default code in the Alphabetic Index. When this term is documented, consult the provider for clarification.

Systemic inflammatory response syndrome (SIRS) generally refers to the systemic response to infection, trauma/burns, or other insult (such as cancer), with symptoms including fever, tachycardia, tachypnea, and leukocytosis. SIRS of noninfectious origin is coded to subcategory R65.1, with the code assignment depending on whether acute organ dysfunction is present (R65.11) or not (R65.10). Care must be exercised for code assignment, as ICD-10-CM does not provide a separate code or index entry for SIRS due to an infectious process, and the condition does not automatically equate to sepsis. For example, for a patient documented as SIRS secondary to pneumonia, assign only code **J18.9, Pneumonia, unspecified organism.** When sepsis is not present, no other code is required. If the medical record documentation appears to meet the criteria for sepsis, the provider should be queried for clarification.

Severe sepsis (subcategory R65.2) generally refers to sepsis with associated acute or multiple organ dysfunction. Subcategory R65.2 is further subdivided to identify whether the severe sepsis is associated with septic shock (R65.21) or without septic shock (R65.20). Septic shock generally refers to circulatory failure associated with severe sepsis and therefore represents a type of acute organ dysfunction. The physician must specifically record "septic shock" in the diagnostic statement in order for it to be coded as such. Septic shock indicates the presence of severe sepsis, and code **R65.21, Severe sepsis with septic shock,** must be assigned, even if the term "severe sepsis" is not documented.

A code from subcategory R65.2, Severe sepsis, should not be assigned unless severe sepsis or an associated acute organ dysfunction is documented. When a patient has sepsis and an acute organ dysfunction, but the documentation indicates that the acute organ dysfunction is related to a medical condition other than sepsis, codes from subcategory R65.2 should not be used. If the documentation is not clear as to whether an acute organ dysfunction is related to the sepsis or another medical condition, the provider should be queried. Because of the complex nature of severe sepsis, some cases may require querying the provider prior to code assignment.

Coding and Sequencing

Coding professionals should be guided by the following instructions when coding sepsis or severe sepsis. The coding of these conditions is dependent on the documentation available.

Severe Sepsis

The coding of severe sepsis requires a minimum of two codes:

- Sequence first a code for the underlying infection followed by a code from subcategory R65.2, Severe sepsis.
- If the causal organism is not documented, assign code **A41.9, Sepsis, unspecified organism,** for the infection.
- Also assign additional code(s) for the associated acute organ dysfunction.

If severe sepsis is present on admission and meets the Uniform Hospital Discharge Data Set definition of principal diagnosis—that is, the condition after study that necessitated the admission—assign first the code for the underlying systemic infection (e.g., A40.-, A41.-, or B37.7) followed by the appropriate code from subcategory R65.2 as required by the sequencing rules in the Tabular List. A code from subcategory R65.2 can never be assigned as a principal diagnosis.

When severe sepsis develops during an encounter (it was not present on admission), the underlying systemic infection code should be assigned first, and a code from subcategory R65.2 should be assigned as secondary diagnosis. In some cases, severe sepsis may be present on admission, but the diagnosis is not confirmed until sometime after admission. When the documentation is not clear as to whether severe sepsis was present on admission, the provider must be queried for clarification.

Sepsis and Severe Sepsis with a Localized Infection

When the reason for admission is both sepsis, or severe sepsis, and a localized infection (e.g., pneumonia or cellulitis), the code(s) for the underlying systemic infection should be assigned first and the code for the localized infection should be assigned as a secondary diagnosis. If the patient has severe sepsis, a code from subcategory R65.2 should also be assigned as a secondary diagnosis. On the other hand, if the patient is admitted with a localized infection, such as pneumonia, and the sepsis/severe sepsis does not develop until after admission, the code for the localized infection should be assigned first, followed by the appropriate sepsis/severe sepsis codes.

When the code for sepsis identifies the organism and the patient also has a localized infection due to the same organism, it is not necessary to separately assign a code for the organism responsible for the localized infection because the sepsis code clearly identifies the causal organism. For example, for a diagnosis of sepsis due to *Escherichia coli* urinary tract infection, assign code **A41.51, Sepsis due to** *Escherichia coli [E. coli],* and code **N39.0, Urinary tract infection, site not specified.** Code A41.51 clearly identifies the causal bacterium for both the sepsis and the urinary tract infection. Although there is a "Use additional code (B95–B97), to identify infectious agent" instructional note at code N39.0, assigning B96.20 as an additional code is redundant in this case.

Sepsis due to a Postprocedural Infection

As with all postprocedural complications, code assignment for sepsis due to a postprocedural infection is based on the provider's documentation of the relationship between the infection and the procedure. For such cases, the postprocedural infection code that identifies the site of the infection—such as a code for infection following a procedure (T81.40- through T81.43-) or infection of an obstetric surgical wound (O86.00–O86.03)—should be coded first, if known. Assign an additional code for sepsis following a procedure (T81.44) or sepsis following an obstetrical procedure (O86.04). Use an additional code to identify the infectious agent. For infections following infusion, transfusion, therapeutic injection, or immunization, a code from subcategory T80.2, Infections following infusion, transfusion, and therapeutic injection, or code **T88.0-, Infection following immunization,** should be assigned first, followed by the code to specify the infectious agent. In addition, for severe sepsis, the appropriate code from subcategory R65.2 should also be assigned along with the code(s) for any acute organ dysfunction.

Postprocedural infections can result in severe sepsis and postprocedural septic shock. In such cases, the code for the precipitating complication—such as codes **T81.4-, Infection following a procedure,** or **O86.0-, Infection of obstetric surgical wound**—should be coded first. The assignment of additional codes will differ based on whether septic shock is also present:

- If there is no septic shock, code **R65.20, Severe sepsis without septic shock,** and a code for the systemic infection are assigned.

- If there is septic shock, code **T81.12-, Postprocedural septic shock,** and a code for the systemic infection are assigned.

Sepsis and Severe Sepsis Associated with a Noninfectious Process (Condition)

In some cases, a noninfectious process (condition), such as trauma, may lead to an infection that can result in sepsis or severe sepsis. If sepsis or severe sepsis is documented as associated with a noninfectious condition, such as a burn or serious injury, and this condition meets the definition for principal diagnosis, the code for the noninfectious condition should be sequenced first, followed by the code for the resulting infection. If severe sepsis is present, a code from subcategory

R65.2 should also be assigned with any associated organ dysfunction(s) codes. It is not necessary to assign a code from subcategory R65.1, Systemic inflammatory response syndrome (SIRS) of non-infectious origin, for these cases.

If the infection meets the definition of principal diagnosis, it should be sequenced before the noninfectious condition. When both the associated noninfectious condition and the infection meet the definition of principal diagnosis, either condition may be assigned as principal diagnosis. Only one code from category R65, Symptoms and signs specifically associated with systemic inflammation and infection, should be assigned. Therefore, when a noninfectious condition leads to an infection resulting in severe sepsis, assign the appropriate code from subcategory R65.2, Severe sepsis. Do not additionally assign a code from subcategory R65.1, Systemic inflammatory response syndrome (SIRS) of non-infectious origin.

Sepsis and septic shock complicating abortion, pregnancy, childbirth, and the puerperium are discussed in chapter 23 of this handbook, Complications of Pregnancy, Childbirth, and the Puerperium. Newborn sepsis is discussed in chapter 26, Perinatal Conditions.

Note carefully in the following cases the different codes that would be assigned based on the information available:

1. Streptococcal sepsis: Assign code **A40.9, Streptococcal sepsis, unspecified.**

2. Severe sepsis: Assign first the code for the systemic infection (e.g., A40.-, A41.-, or B37.7) followed by the appropriate code from subcategory R65.2 as required by the sequencing rules in the Tabular List. Additional codes are also assigned to identify the specific acute organ dysfunction (e.g., renal, respiratory, or hepatic).

3. Septic shock: Assign first the code for the initiating systemic infection (e.g., A40.-, A41.-, or B37.7) followed by code **R65.21, Severe sepsis with septic shock,** or code **T81.12-, Postprocedural septic shock,** and codes for any associated acute organ dysfunction. Note that the sequencing instructions in the Tabular List preclude the assignment of the code for septic shock as a principal diagnosis.

4. Patient admitted due to both pneumonia and sepsis: Assign codes A41.9+J18.9.

5. Patient admitted with pneumonia, develops sepsis after admission: Assign codes J18.9+A41.9.

6. Sepsis due to a postprocedural infection: Assign a code from T81.40- to **T81.43-, Infection following a procedure,** or a code from O86.00 to **O86.03, Infection of obstetric surgical wound,** that identifies the site of the infection, followed by the code for the specific infection (e.g., A40.-, A41.-, or B37.7). Additionally, assign code **T81.44-, Sepsis following a procedure,** or O86.04, **Sepsis following an obstetrical procedure.**

7. For infections following infusion, transfusion, therapeutic injection, or immunization, a code from subcategory T80.2, Infections following infusion, transfusion, and therapeutic injection, or code **T88.0-, Infection following immunization,** should be assigned first, followed by the code to specify the infectious agent.

8. Bacteremia: Assign code R78.81.

9. Patient admitted with SIRS due to pneumonia, but patient is not septic: Assign code J18.9.

10. Patient admitted with sepsis due to aspiration pneumonia: Assign code **A41.9, Sepsis, unspecified organism,** as the principal diagnosis. Codes **J18.9, Pneumonia, unspecified organism,** and **J69.0, Pneumonitis due to inhalation of food and vomit,** are assigned as additional diagnoses.

TOXIC SHOCK SYNDROME

Toxic shock syndrome (A48.3) is caused by a bacterial infection. The symptoms include high fever of sudden onset, vomiting, watery diarrhea, and myalgia, followed by hypotension and sometimes shock. It was originally reported almost exclusively in menstruating women using high-absorbency tampons. The organism isolated was *Staphylococcus aureus.* A similar syndrome has been identi-fied in children and males infected with group A *Streptococcus.* An additional code from category B95 or B96 is reported to identify the responsible organism.

GRAM-NEGATIVE BACTERIAL INFECTION

Gram-negative bacteria are a specific group of organisms with particular staining characteristics. They are clinically similar, as is the case with *Klebsiella* and *Pseudomonas,* and are thought of as a group even when the specific organism cannot be determined. Occasionally, several gram-negative organ-isms may be seen, but no single organism is identified as the causative agent, resulting in a diagnosis of gram-negative infection. Gram-negative infections are ordinarily more severe and require more intensive care than gram-positive infections. Note that a code is never assigned solely on the basis of gram-stain results; the assignment is based on the physician's clinical evaluation of the condition.

When the infectious organism has been identified, a specific code is often provided, such as **J15.0, Pneumonia due to** *Klebsiella pneumoniae.* However, for certain infections classified in chapters other than chapter 1, no organism is identified as part of the infection code (e.g., **N39.0, Urinary tract infection, site not specified**). In these instances, an additional code from categories B95–B97 is assigned to indicate the responsible infectious agent. An instructional note will be found at the infection code advising users to assign an additional code to identify the organism. Two examples of codes for gram-negative bacterial infections follow:

J15.8	Pneumonia due to anaerobic gram-negative bacteria
N11.8 + B96.89	Chronic pyelonephritis due to gram-negative bacteria

Table 13.1 provides a sampling of gram-negative and gram-positive organisms. A more com-plete list can be obtained from the health care organization's clinical laboratory director.

TABLE 13.1   Gram-Negative and Gram-Positive Bacteria

Gram-Negative Bacteria		Gram-Positive Bacteria
Bacteroides (anaerobic)	Hemophilus	Actinomyces
Bordetella	Klebsiella	Clostridioides
Brucella	Legionella	Corynebacterium
Campylobacter	Moraxella	Enterococcus
Citrobacter	Morganella	Lactobacillus
Enterobacter	Neisseria	Listeria
Escherichia coli	Proteus	Mycobacterium
Francisella	Pseudomonas	Nocardia
Fusobacterium (anaerobic)	Salmonella	Peptococcus
Gardnerella	Shigella	Peptostreptococcus
Helicobacter	Trichinella vaginalis	Staphylococcus
	Veillonella (anaerobic)	Streptococcus
	Yersinia	

NOSOCOMIAL INFECTIONS

Nosocomial infections are secondary infections that are contracted as a result of medical treatment or develop during hospitalization. They are also known as "hospital-acquired infections." ICD-10-CM provides code **Y95, Nosocomial condition,** as an additional External cause of morbidity code to identify these infections.

DRUG-RESISTANT INFECTIONS

ICD-10-CM provides unique codes to classify methicillin-susceptible and methicillin-resistant *Staphylococcus aureus* (MRSA) infections. Such codes are available for sepsis (A41.01 and A41.02), infection (A49.01 and A49.02), infection in diseases classified elsewhere (B95.61 and B95.62), and pneumonia (J15.211 and J15.212).

When a patient is diagnosed with MRSA infection, and that infection has a combination code that includes the causal organism (e.g., sepsis, pneumonia), assign the appropriate combination code for the condition (e.g., code **A41.02, Sepsis due to Methicillin resistant *Staphylococcus aureus,*** or code **J15.212, Pneumonia due to Methicillin resistant *Staphylococcus aureus***). Do not assign code **B95.62, Methicillin resistant *Staphylococcus aureus* infection as the cause of diseases classified elsewhere,** as an additional code, because the combination code includes the type of infection and the MRSA organism.

Not every infection has a combination code that includes the causal organism. When there is documentation of a current infection (e.g., wound infection, stitch abscess, urinary tract infection) due to MRSA, and that infection does not have a combination code that includes the causal organism, assign the appropriate code to identify the condition, along with code **B95.62, Methicillin resistant *Staphylococcus aureus* infection as the cause of diseases classified elsewhere,** for the MRSA infection.

Many bacterial infections are resistant to current antibiotics. It is necessary to identify all infections documented as antibiotic resistant. Assign a code from category Z16, Resistance to antimicrobial drugs, following the infection code only if the infection code does not identify drug resistance. For example, for MRSA cases, do not assign a code from subcategory Z16.11, Resistance to penicillins, as an additional diagnosis. Drug resistance codes may be located in the Alphabetic Index by referring to the main term **Resistance, Organism(s), to Drug.** Codes from category Z16, Resistance to antimicrobial drugs, are assigned only as an additional code when the physician specifically documents an infection that has become drug resistant to identify the resistance and nonresponsiveness of a condition to antimicrobial drugs. Such statements as "multi-drug resistant" or "(specified drug) resistant condition" or similar terminology indicate this condition. The code for the infection should be assigned first, followed by the code from category Z16. For example:

J15.20 + Z16.24   Staphylococcal pneumonia resistant to penicillin and other antibiotics

It is important to distinguish colonization from infection. A patient may be referred to as being colonized or a carrier—meaning that an infectious organism (e.g., MRSA) is present on or in the body without necessarily causing illness. Colonization is not necessarily indicative of a disease process, and it may not be considered the cause of a patient's specific condition unless documented as such by the provider. A positive colonization test might be documented as "MRSA screen positive" or "MRSA nasal swab positive." ICD-10-CM provides codes under category Z22 for carrier or suspected carrier of infectious diseases and colonization status for several common infections, such as *Staphylococcus* (Z22.321 or Z22.322) and group B *Streptococcus* (Z22.330).

If a patient is documented as having both MRSA infection and MRSA colonization during a hospital admission, a code for the MRSA infection and code **Z22.322, Carrier or suspected carrier of Methicillin resistant *Staphylococcus aureus,*** may both be assigned.

EXERCISE 13.1

Code the following diagnoses.

1. Acute viral hepatitis (Australian antigen) with hepatitis delta and hepatic coma

2. Chronic gonococcal cystitis

3. Infectious gammaherpesviral mononucleosis with hepatomegaly

4. Postmeasles otitis media

5. Acute scarlet fever

6. Anaerobic gram-negative sepsis

7. Sepsis due to methicillin-resistant *Staphylococcus aureus* (MRSA)

8. Chronic moniliasis of vulva

9. Pulmonary tuberculosis, infiltrative

10. Late, latent syphilis

11. Herpes zoster of conjunctiva

12. Pneumonia due to schistosomiasis

13. Acute empyema due to group B streptococcal infection

14. Encephalitis due to typhus

15. Acute respiratory distress due to sin nombre virus

16. Adenoviral pneumonia

17. Chronic gonococcal urethritis

18. Chronic vulvitis due to monilia with microorganisms resistant to cephalosporin

19. Amebic abscess of brain and lung Long-term use of antibiotic

_____

20. Enterococcal septic shock due to acute postoperative
peritonitis (surgery performed during same admission)

AIDS AND OTHER HIV INFECTIONS

Because human immunodeficiency virus (HIV) infection is a major health care concern, the collection of accurate and complete data on conditions associated with HIV infection is important for health care resource planning. Code B20 is assigned for all types of HIV infections, which are described by a variety of terms, such as the following:

- AIDS
- Acquired immune deficiency syndrome
- Acquired immunodeficiency syndrome
- AIDS-related complex (ARC)
- AIDS-related conditions
- HIV infection, symptomatic

Unconfirmed Diagnosis of HIV Infection

Code **B20, Human immunodeficiency virus [HIV] disease,** is assigned only if provider documentation specifically indicates an AIDS diagnosis or that the patient has an HIV-related illness. Code B20 is not assigned when the diagnostic statement indicates that the infection is "suspected," "possible," "likely," or "?". This is an exception to the general guideline that directs the coding professional to assign a code for a diagnosis qualified as "suspected" or "possible" as if it were established. Confirmation in this case does not require documentation of a positive serology or culture for HIV; the provider's diagnostic statement that the patient is HIV-positive or has an HIV-related illness is sufficient. If documentation is unclear, the provider should be asked to state the diagnosis in positive terms.

Coding professionals should not assume that patients being treated with antiretroviral drugs have AIDS or HIV disease. The fact that a patient is receiving medication does not indicate AIDS or HIV disease. The protocol is to treat asymptomatic patients prophylactically with antiretroviral drugs to suppress the virus and prevent progression of the illness.

Serologic Testing for HIV Infection

When an asymptomatic patient with no prior diagnosis of HIV infection or positive-HIV status requests testing to determine his or her HIV status, use code **Z11.4, Encounter for screening for human immunodeficiency virus [HIV].** When the patient being tested for HIV shows signs or symptoms of illness or has been diagnosed with a condition related to HIV infection, assign code(s) for the signs and symptoms or the diagnosis rather than the screening code.

When the patient makes a return visit to learn the result of the serology test, code **Z71.7, Human immunodeficiency virus [HIV] counseling,** as the reason for the encounter when the test result is negative or inconclusive; code R75 is also assigned to indicate the test results.

When a patient is known to be in a high-risk group for HIV infection, code **Z72.89, Other problems related to lifestyle,** can be assigned as an additional code.

When the test result is positive but the patient displays no symptoms and has no related complications and no established diagnosis of HIV infection, code **Z21, Asymptomatic human immunodeficiency virus [HIV] infection status,** is assigned. Code Z21 is not assigned when the term "AIDS" is used, when the patient is under treatment for an HIV-related illness, or when the patient is described as having any active HIV-related condition; code B20 is assigned instead. Code **Z71.7, Human immunodeficiency virus [HIV] counseling,** can also be assigned as an additional code when counseling is provided for a patient who tests HIV-positive.

When a patient has had contact with, or has been exposed to, the HIV virus but shows no signs or symptoms of illness and has not been diagnosed with a condition related to HIV, assign code **Z20.6, Contact with and (suspected) exposure to human immunodeficiency virus [HIV].**

Newborns with HIV-positive mothers often test positive on ELISA (enzyme-linked immuno-sorbent assay) and/or Western blot HIV tests. This finding usually indicates the antibody status of the mother rather than the status of the newborn; antibodies can cross the placenta and remain for as long as 18 months after birth without the child being infected. Such inconclusive test results are also coded R75. (See chapter 26 of this handbook for further information on coding HIV infection in the newborn.)

Sequencing of HIV-Related Diagnoses

When a patient is admitted for treatment of an HIV infection or any related complications, code **B20, Human immunodeficiency virus (HIV) disease,** is sequenced as the principal diagnosis, with additional codes for the HIV-related conditions. When a patient with an HIV infection is admitted for treatment of an entirely unrelated condition, such as an injury, that unrelated condition is designated as the principal diagnosis, with code B20 and codes for any associated conditions assigned as additional codes.

When an obstetric patient is identified as having any HIV infection, a code from subcategory O98.7, Human immunodeficiency virus [HIV] disease complicating pregnancy, childbirth and the puerperium, is assigned, with code B20 assigned as an additional code. If an obstetric patient tests positive for HIV but has no symptoms and no history of an HIV infection, codes O98.7- and **Z21, Asymptomatic human immunodeficiency virus [HIV] infection status,** are assigned rather than B20.

EXERCISE 13.2

Code the following diagnoses and procedures.

1. Candidiasis, of esophagus, opportunistic, secondary to AIDS

2. *Pneumocystis carinii*
   AIDS

3. Positive HIV test in patient who is asymptomatic, presents
   no related symptoms, and has no history of HIV infection

4. Acute lymphadenitis due to HIV infection

5. Acute appendicitis (admitted for appendectomy)

   Kaposi's sarcoma of skin of chest, due to HIV infection

   Total laparoscopic appendectomy

   _____

6. Kaposi's sarcoma of oral cavity

   AIDS

   Excisional biopsy of oral cavity mucosa

   _____

7. Agranulocytosis due to HIV infection

   _____

8. Burkitt's tumor of inguinal region associated with AIDS

   _____

9. Background retinopathy due to AIDS

   _____

10. Inconclusive HIV test

   _____

COVID-19

Coronavirus disease 2019 (COVID-19) is a respiratory disease caused by the severe acute respiratory syndrome coronavirus 2 (SARS-CoV-2). In the name COVID-19, "CO" stands for "corona," "VI" for "virus," and "D" for "disease." Formerly, this disease was referred to as "2019 novel coronavirus" or "2019-nCoV." Common symptoms can include fever, cough, shortness of breath or difficulty breathing, chills, muscle pain, sore throat, headache, and new loss of taste or smell. Less common symptoms are gastrointestinal symptoms like diarrhea, nausea, or vomiting. Symptoms may appear from 2 to 14 days after exposure to the virus.

Effective April 1, 2020, code **U07.1, COVID-19,** was implemented in response to the global pandemic. This was an off-cycle, unprecedented update to the ICD-10-CM as an exception to the code set updating process established under the Health Insurance Portability and Accountability Act. The exception was made due to the critical need to uniquely identify COVID-19 in claims and surveillance data.

Unconfirmed Diagnosis of COVID-19

Code **U07.1, COVID-19,** is assigned only if the provider documentation either specifically documents a confirmed diagnosis of the COVID-19 or there is documentation of a positive COVID-19 test result. This is an exception to the *ICD-10-CM Official Guidelines for Coding and Reporting* hospital inpatient guideline Section II, part H. In this context, "confirmation" does not require documentation of a positive test result for COVID-19; the provider's documentation that the individual has COVID-19 is sufficient. In addition, the provider does not need to explicitly link the COVID-19 test result to the respiratory condition, the positive test results can be coded as a confirmed COVID-19 case as long as the test result itself is part of the medical record. Please note that the advice allowing coding from positive test results is limited to test results for COVID-19 and not the coding of other laboratory tests.

If a definitive diagnosis has not been established or if the provider documents "suspected," "possible," "probable, " or "inconclusive" COVID-19, do not assign code U07.1; instead, assign codes for any presenting signs or symptoms (such as fever).

Sequencing of COVID-19

Code **U07.1, COVID-19,** is sequenced first followed by the appropriate codes for associated manifestations when COVID-19 meets the definition of principal or first-listed diagnosis. For example, when the reason for the encounter/admission is a respiratory manifestation of COVID-19, assign code U07.1 as the principal/first-listed diagnosis and assign code(s) for the respiratory manifestation(s) as additional diagnoses. When the reason for the encounter/admission is a non-respiratory manifestation (e.g., viral enteritis) of COVID-19, assign code U07.1 as the principal/first-listed diagnosis and assign code(s) for the manifestation(s) as additional diagnoses. The exception to this sequencing rule is when another guideline requires that certain codes be sequenced first, such as in the case of obstetrics patients or patients with sepsis or transplant complications.

When COVID-19 is the reason for admission/encounter during pregnancy, childbirth or the puerperium, the appropriate code from subcategory O98.5-, Other viral diseases complicating pregnancy, childbirth and the puerperium, should be sequenced as the principal/first-listed diagnosis. Code U07.1 and the codes for associated manifestation(s) should be assigned as additional diagnoses. If the reason for admission/encounter is unrelated to COVID-19 but the patient tests positive for COVID-19 during the admission/encounter, the code for the reason for admission/encounter should be sequenced as the principal/first-listed diagnosis. The appropriate code from subcategory O98.5- , code U07.1, along with codes for associated COVID-19 manifestations, should be assigned as additional diagnoses. Codes from ICD-10-CM Chapter 15, Pregnancy, Childbirth and the Puerperium, take precedence over codes from other chapters, including code U07.1.

COVID-19 may present with respiratory symptoms of different degrees of severity, and it may progress to sepsis or severe sepsis. Whether a code for sepsis or code U07.1 is assigned as the principal diagnosis depends on the circumstances of admission and whether the sepsis meets the definition of principal diagnosis.

Note the different codes that would be assigned in the following cases based on a confirmed COVID-19 diagnosis along with available documentation of various acute respiratory illnesses:

* Pneumonia due to COVID-19: Assign codes U07.1 and **J12.89, Other viral pneumonia.**

* Acute bronchitis due to COVID-19: Assign codes U07.1 and **J20.8, Acute bronchitis due to other specified organisms.**

* Bronchitis not otherwise specified (NOS) due to COVID-19: Assign codes U07.1 and **J40, Bronchitis, not specified as acute or chronic.**

* COVID-19 with a lower respiratory infection, not otherwise specified (NOS), or an acute respiratory infection, NOS: Assign codes U07.1 and **J22, Unspecified acute lower respiratory infection.**

* COVID-19 associated with a respiratory infection, NOS: Assign codes U07.1 and **J98.8, Other specified respiratory disorders.**

* Acute respiratory distress syndrome (ARDS) due to COVID-19: Assign codes U07.1 and **J80, Acute respiratory distress syndrome.**

* Patient is admitted with pneumonia due to COVID-19, which then progresses to viral sepsis (not present on admission): Assign code U07.1 as the principal diagnosis, followed by the codes for the viral sepsis (A41.89) and viral pneumonia (J12.89).

- Patient is admitted with sepsis due to COVID-19 pneumonia, and the sepsis meets the definition of principal diagnosis: Assign the code for viral sepsis (A41.89) as the principal diagnosis followed by codes U07.1 and J12.89 as secondary diagnoses.

- Asymptomatic patient tests positive for COVID-19: Assign code U07.1. Although the individual is asymptomatic, the individual has tested positive and is considered to have COVID-19.

- Pregnant patient admitted with mild COVID-19 and acute bronchitis: Assign the appropriate code from subcategory O98.51, Other viral diseases complicating pregnancy, as the first-listed diagnosis, followed by codes U07.1 and J20.8 and an additional code for the number of weeks of gestation.

- Newborn tests positive for COVID-19 during the birth admission without documentation specifying the type of transmission: Assign first the appropriate code from category Z38, Liveborn infants according to place of birth and type of delivery, as the principal diagnosis, followed by code U07.1.

- Patient is admitted with viral enteritis due to COVID-19: Assign code U07.1 as the principal diagnosis, followed by the code for the viral enteritis (A08.39).

- Patient status post lung transplant contracts COVID-19: Assign code **T86.812, Lung transplant infection,** followed by code U07.1.

Contact/Exposure, Screening, Testing, or History of COVID-19

The following guidance applies to encounters related to contact/exposure to COVID-19, antibody testing, history of COVID-19, and follow-up visits post COVID-19.

- *Contact/exposure:*
    - If the exposed individual, whether symptomatic or asymptomatic, tests positive for the COVID-19 virus, assign code U07.1. Although the individual is asymptomatic, the individual has tested positive and is considered to have COVID-19 infection.
    - For asymptomatic individuals with actual or suspected exposure, assign code **Z20.828, Contact with and (suspected) exposure to other viral communicable diseases.**
    - For symptomatic individuals where there is an actual or suspected exposure to COVID-19, and infection has been ruled out, or the test results are inconclusive or unknown, assign code **Z20.828, Contact with and (suspected) exposure to other viral communicable diseases.**

- *Screening.* During the COVID-19 pandemic, a screening code is generally not appropriate. For encounters for COVID-19 testing, including preoperative testing, code as exposure to COVID-19 with code **Z20.828, Contact with and (suspected) exposure to other viral communicable diseases.**

- *Antibody Testing.* For an encounter for COVID-19 antibody testing that is not being performed to confirm a current COVID-19 infection nor is a follow-up test after resolution of COVID-19, assign code **Z01.84, Encounter for antibody response examination.** Antibody testing is a blood test performed to determine whether an individual has developed antibodies to a disease.

- *Personal History.* If a patient has a history of COVID-19, assign code **Z86.19, Personal history of other infectious and parasitic diseases.**

- *Follow-up Visits.* If a patient previously had COVID-19 and is being seen for a follow-up exam (and COVID-19 test results are negative), assign codes **Z09, Encounter for** follow-up examination after completed treatment for conditions other than malignant neoplasm, and **Z86.19**, Personal history of other infectious and parasitic diseases.

LATE EFFECTS

Chapter 1 provides four sequelae categories for use when there is a residual condition due to previous infection or parasitic infestation:

B90   Sequelae of tuberculosis
B91   Sequelae of poliomyelitis
B92   Sequelae of leprosy
B94   Sequelae of other and unspecified infectious and parasitic diseases

As discussed the code for the residual effect is sequenced first, followed by the appropriate sequelae code, except in a few instances where the Alphabetic Index instructs otherwise. A code for the infection itself is not assigned because it is no longer present. For example:

G93.9 + B94.1   Brain damage resulting from previous viral encephalitis (three years ago)
N29 + B90.1   Tuberculous calcification of kidney

CHAPTER 14

Endocrine, Nutritional, and Metabolic Diseases

CHAPTER OVERVIEW

- Diabetes mellitus is the condition coding professionals encounter most when working with chapter 4 of ICD-10-CM.
- Diabetes mellitus has two classification axes.
  - The first axis is the type of diabetes.
  - The fourth character identifies any associated complication.
- Diabetes causes many concurrent complications.
  - These complications may be either acute or chronic.
  - Assign as many codes as necessary to identify all the conditions.
- Codes from categories E08, E09, and E13 are used for classification of secondary diabetes.
- Nutritional disorders classified by ICD-10-CM include deficiencies of specific vitamins and minerals and obesity.
- Specific codes for cystic fibrosis identify site of manifestation involvement.
  - There may be pulmonary, gastrointestinal, or other site involvement.
  - Use codes together if different sites are involved.
- Fluid overload is a component of congestive heart failure.

LEARNING OUTCOMES

After studying this chapter, you should be able to:

Code diabetes mellitus properly.

Identify the differences when coding for diabetes during pregnancy and gestational diabetes.

Code fluid overload due to congestive heart failure.

Code nutritional disorders such as obesity.

TERMS TO KNOW

Diabetes mellitus
a chronic disorder of impaired carbohydrate, protein, and fat metabolism

Type 1 diabetes
also known as juvenile type; characterized by the body's failure to produce insulin

Type 2 diabetes
characterized by the body's production of insulin in an insufficient quantity or the body's inability to utilize such insulin

REMEMBER . . .

Coding professionals may use as many codes as necessary to identify all the conditions related to diabetes that a patient is experiencing.

INTRODUCTION

Chapter 4 of ICD-10-CM covers a variety of conditions that are related in a general way. Because diabetes mellitus is a common medical problem, it is the condition coding professionals encounter most often when working with this chapter.

DIABETES MELLITUS

Diabetes mellitus, classified in categories E08 through E13, is a chronic disorder of impaired carbohydrate, protein, and fat metabolism. The disorder is caused by either an absolute decrease in the amount of insulin secreted by the pancreas or a reduction in the biologic effectiveness of the insulin secreted. Other conditions include the term "diabetes," such as bronze diabetes and diabetes insipidus, but a diagnosis of diabetes without further qualification should be interpreted as diabetes mellitus.

FIGURE 14.1   Major Organs of the Endocrine System

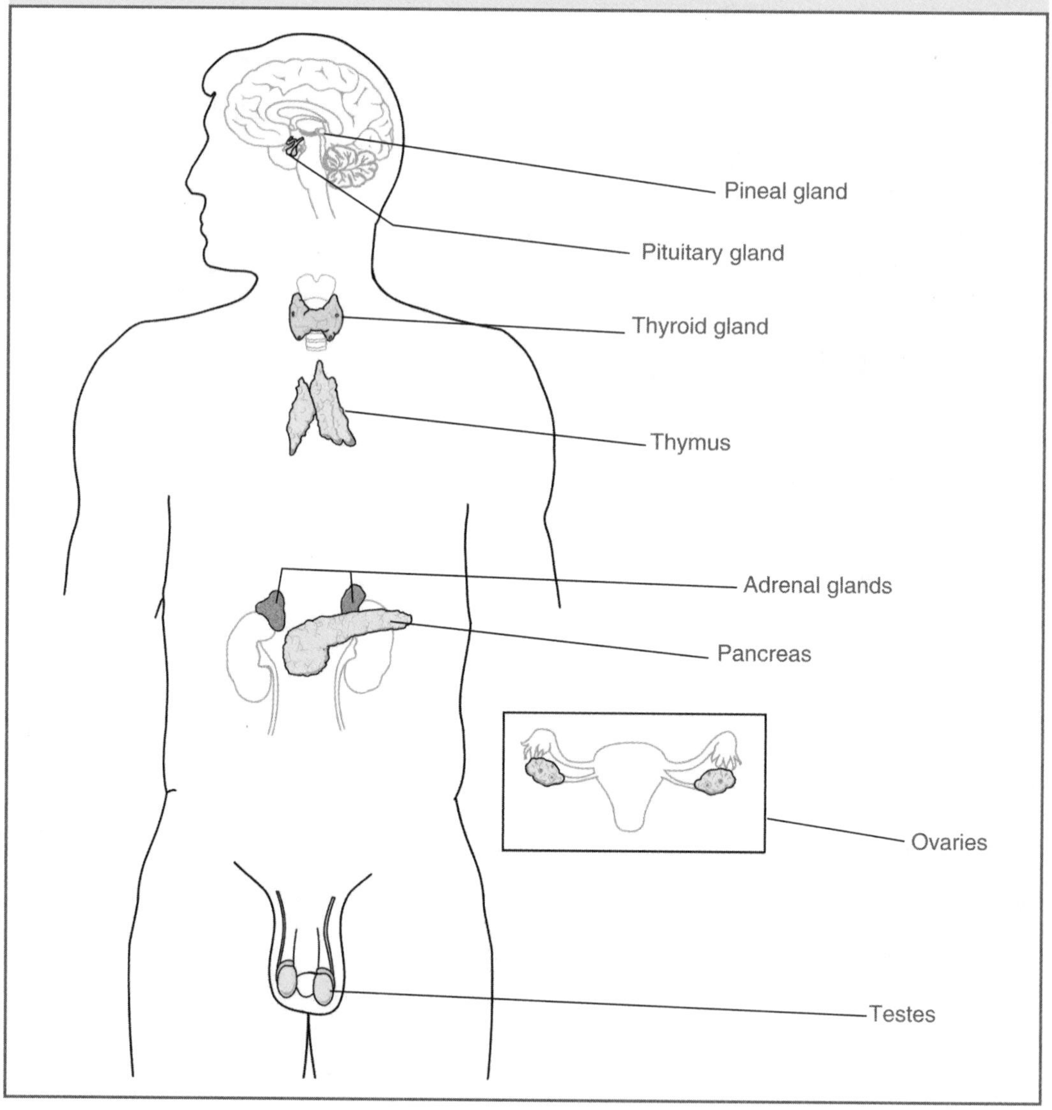

161

: **CHAPTER 14**
: *Endocrine,*
: *Nutritional,*
: *and Metabolic*
: *Diseases*

The diabetes mellitus codes are combination codes that include the type of diabetes mellitus, the body system affected, and the complications affecting that body system. The type of diabetes (e.g., secondary, type 1, type 2) is identified at the category level, while the fourth character identifies the presence of any associated complication and the fifth-character, sixth-character, and seventh-character subclassifications provide further specificity regarding the complication. As many codes within a particular category as are necessary to describe all of the complications of the diabetes mellitus may be used. It is not required that the diabetes mellitus and the associated conditions be listed together in the medical record.

The ICD-10-CM classification presumes a causal relationship between diabetes and several acute and chronic conditions. The term "with" means "associated with" or "due to" when it appears in a code title, the Alphabetic Index, or an instructional note in the Tabular List. For example, under the Alphabetic Index main term **Diabetes,** the subterm "with" indicates a range of conditions in which the classification assumes a linkage between the condition—such as dermatitis, foot ulcer, or gangrene—and the diabetes. However, if the physician documentation specifies that diabetes mellitus is not the underlying cause of the other condition, the condition should not be coded as a diabetic complication.

The "with" guideline does not apply to "not elsewhere classified" (NEC) Index entries that cover broad categories of conditions. Coding professionals should not assume a causal relationship when the diabetic complication is classified as "NEC." Specific conditions must be linked in the patient's medical documentation by the terms "with," "due to," or "associated with." An example is the Index main term **Diabetes,** subterm "with," sub-subterm "skin complication NEC." To link diabetes and a specific skin complication NEC, such as cellulitis or acne vulgaris, the provider would need to document the condition as a diabetic skin complication.

When the coding professional is unable to determine whether a condition is related to diabetes mellitus, or the ICD-10-CM classification does not provide coding instruction, it is appropriate to query the physician for clarification so that the appropriate codes may be reported.

If the provider has confirmed a diagnosis of diabetes mellitus, the appropriate code from categories E08–E13, Diabetes mellitus, should be assigned. Otherwise, a diagnosis of "borderline diabetes," "prediabetes," or "latent diabetes" should be assigned to code **R73.03, Prediabetes.** Abnormal glucose or abnormal glucose tolerance without further provider confirmation of the disease should be assigned to code **R73.09, Other abnormal glucose.**

Types of Diabetes Mellitus

There are three major types of diabetes mellitus: type 1 (or type I); type 2 (or type II); and secondary (e.g., due to an underlying condition or induced by a drug or chemical). The essential element in the selection of the codes in categories E08–E13 is the type of diabetes, not whether the patient is on insulin; the types are classified as follows:

E08 Diabetes mellitus due to underlying condition
E09 Drug or chemical induced diabetes mellitus
E10 Type 1 diabetes mellitus
E11 Type 2 diabetes mellitus
E13 Other specified diabetes mellitus

If the medical record documentation is not clear with regard to the type of diabetes, the default is category E11, Type 2 diabetes mellitus. When the type of diabetes is not documented but the record does indicate that the patient uses insulin, the default is still type 2. The fact that a patient is receiving insulin does not indicate that the diabetes is type 1.

Type 1 diabetes mellitus (category E10) may also be described as ketosis prone, juvenile type, juvenile onset, or juvenile diabetes. The age of a patient is not the sole determining factor, although most individuals with type 1 diabetes develop the condition before reaching puberty. Type 1 diabetes is characterized by the body's failure to produce insulin at all or by an absolute decrease in such production. These patients require regular insulin injections to sustain life, and they experience significant health problems when they do not follow the prescribed regimen for medication and diet. Careful monitoring is required to avoid serious complications. Code **Z79.4, Long term (current) use of insulin,** may be assigned for patients with type 1 diabetes because these patients require insulin.

Type 2 diabetes mellitus (category E11) may also be described as ketosis resistant. Insulin is produced, but either it is produced in insufficient quantity or the body is unable to utilize it adequately. Individuals with type 2 diabetes usually do not require insulin; the diabetes is ordinarily managed with oral hypoglycemic agents, diet, and exercise. Code **Z79.84, Long term (current) use of oral hypoglycemic drugs,** is assigned when the patient requires oral hypoglycemic medication. For some patients, however, ordinary diabetes management measures are not effective, and insulin therapy may be required to control persistent hyperglycemia.

When a patient with type 2 diabetes routinely uses insulin, assign code **Z79.4, Long term (current) use of insulin.** If the patient is treated with both oral medications and insulin, only the code for insulin use should be assigned. If the patient is treated with both insulin and an injectable non-insulin antidiabetic drug, assign codes Z79.4 and **Z79.899, Other long term (current) drug therapy.** If the patient is treated with both oral hypoglycemic drugs and an injectable non-insulin antidiabetic drug, assign codes Z79.84 and Z79.899.

Secondary diabetes is always caused by another condition or event. Secondary diabetes may be due to an underlying condition (E08), drug or chemically induced (E09), due to an infection, or the result of therapy (such as the surgical removal of the pancreas); or it may be some other specified type of diabetes (E13). It can also be the result of an adverse effect of correctly administered medications, the result of poisoning, or a late effect of using certain medications. Secondary diabetes is coded as follows:

- Secondary diabetes that is due to an underlying condition is coded to category E08, Diabetes mellitus due to underlying condition, with the underlying condition coded first. Underlying conditions include congenital rubella (P35.0), Cushing's syndrome (E24.-), cystic fibrosis (E84.-), malignant neoplasm (C00–C96), malnutrition (E40–E46), and pancreatitis and other diseases of the pancreas (K85.- and K86.-)

- Secondary diabetes that is induced by a drug or chemical is coded to category E09. For example, steroid-induced diabetes mellitus due to the prolonged use of prednisone for an unrelated condition is coded as **E09.9, Drug or chemical induced diabetes mellitus without complications,** followed by code **T38.0x5-, Adverse effect of glucocorticoids and synthetic analogues.**

- Codes from categories E10 and E11 are not assigned for secondary diabetes.

- The sequencing of the secondary diabetes codes is based on the Tabular List instructions for categories E08, E09, and E13. For category E08, the underlying condition should be coded first. For category E09, the responsible drug or chemical is coded first for poisoning. For cases of adverse effect, an additional code (T36–T50) is assigned with fifth or sixth character 5.

- Secondary diabetes mellitus that is due to pancreatectomy is coded to **E89.1, Postprocedural hypoinsulinemia.** Assign a code from category E13 and either code **Z90.410, Acquired total absence of pancreas,** or code **Z90.411, Acquired partial absence of pancreas,** as additional diagnoses. For example, postpancreatectomy diabetes mellitus due to surgical removal of part of the pancreas is coded to E89.1, E13.9, and Z90.411.

- For patients with secondary diabetes who routinely use insulin, code **Z79.4, Long term (current) use of insulin,** should be assigned. However, code Z79.4 should not be used if insulin is given temporarily to bring the patient's blood sugar under control during the encounter.

- Code **Z79.84, Long term (current) use of oral hypoglycemic drugs,** is assigned for the routine use of oral antidiabetic medication.

- Only the code for insulin use is assigned when the patient is treated with both oral medications and insulin.
- If the patient is treated with both insulin and an injectable non-insulin antidiabetic drug, assign codes **Z79.4, Long term (current) use of insulin,** and **Z79.899, Other long term (current) drug therapy.**
- If the patient is treated with both oral hypoglycemic drugs and an injectable non-insulin antidiabetic drug, assign codes **Z79.84, Long term (current) use of oral hypoglycemic drugs,** and **Z79.899, Other long term (current) drug therapy.**

Category E13, Other specified diabetes mellitus, includes diabetes mellitus due to genetic defects of beta-cell function and diabetes mellitus due to genetic defects in insulin action.

Diabetes type 1.5 is also assigned to category E13. This form of diabetes is described as latent autoimmune diabetes of adults (LADA), slow-progressing type 1 diabetes, and double diabetes. Individuals with type 1.5 diabetes have autoantibodies that gradually destroy beta cells that produce insulin. Within 5 to 10 years of diagnosis, they will require insulin.

Complications and Manifestations of Diabetes Mellitus

Type 1 and type 2 diabetes mellitus, as well as secondary diabetes mellitus, can lead to a variety of complications that involve either acute metabolic derangements (E08–E13 with .0- or .1-) or long-term complications (E08–E13 with .2- to .6-). Sequencing of the diabetes mellitus and the complication or manifestation is based on the reason for a particular encounter. Assign as many codes from categories E08–E13 as needed to identify all of the patient's associated conditions.

Acute Metabolic Complications

Hyperosmolarity, ketoacidosis, and hypoglycemia are acute metabolic complications. The subclassification for acute metabolic complications is as follows:

E08, E09, and E11–E13 with .01	Diabetic hyperosmolarity with coma
E08–E13 with .00	Diabetic hyperosmolarity without nonketotic hyperglycemic-hyperosmolar coma
E08–E13 with .11	Diabetic ketoacidosis with coma
E08–E13 with .10	Diabetic ketoacidosis without coma
E08–E13 with .641	Diabetic hypoglycemia with coma
E08–E13 with .649	Diabetic hypoglycemia without coma

Diabetes with hyperosmolarity (E08–E13 with .01 or .00) is a condition in which there is hyperosmolarity and dehydration without significant ketosis. This condition most often occurs in patients with type 2 diabetes. Coma may or may not be present.

Typical findings for patients with diabetic ketoacidosis (DKA) are glycosuria, strong ketonuria, hyperglycemia, ketonemia (blood ketone), acidosis (low arterial blood pH), and low plasma bicarbonate. Ketoacidosis is an acute, life-threatening complication of diabetes that occurs most commonly in patients with type 1 diabetes, but it can occur in patients with type 2 diabetes. When there is not enough insulin in the body for muscle and fat cells to absorb glucose to use for energy, fat is broken down and ketones are released into the bloodstream. In a person with diabetes, ketones build up in the bloodstream. The patient may experience excess thirst, frequent urination, nausea, vomiting, abdominal pain, weakness, and decrease in alertness. ICD-10-CM Index to Diseases and Injuries advises users to code "diabetes, by type, with ketoacidosis" when referencing ketoacidosis. For example, if the documentation reflects type 2 diabetes with ketoacidosis, assign a code from subcategory E11.1, Type 2 diabetes mellitus with ketoacidosis.

Diabetes with hypoglycemia may occur when an excessive amount of insulin is given, when the patient misses a meal, or when the patient is under stress. The condition may progress to coma.

164

CHAPTER 14 :

Endocrine,
Nutritional,
and Metabolic
Diseases

ICD-10-CM provides codes for diabetic hypoglycemia with coma (E08–E13 with .641) or without coma (E08–E13 with .649).

Chronic Complications

Patients with diabetes mellitus are susceptible to various chronic conditions that affect the renal, nervous, and peripheral vascular systems, particularly in the feet and the eyes. Onset may occur early or late in the course of the diabetes and may occur in both insulin-dependent and non-insulin-dependent patients.

Patients with diabetes often have several complications concurrently, in which case multiple codes from categories E08–E13 are assigned to identify all the associated diabetic conditions.

Diabetic Renal Complications

Patients with diabetes are particularly prone to developing complications that affect the kidneys, such as nephritis, nephrosis, or chronic kidney disease. Nephritis is an inflammation of the kidney that develops slowly, over a long period of time. Nephrosis is an advanced stage of renal disease characterized by massive edema and marked proteinuria. Chronic kidney disease is often the ultimate progression of such conditions.

Diabetic kidney complications are coded to E08–E13 with .21 for diabetic nephropathy, .22 for chronic kidney disease, and .29 for other kidney complication. When the renal condition has progressed to chronic kidney disease, the diagnosis is sometimes stated in a way that appears to require three codes, one for the diabetes with chronic kidney disease (E08–E13 with .22), one for an interim manifestation (N08), and one for the final or current problem (N18.1–N18.6, Chronic kidney disease). It is not necessary to code the intermediate condition, but all three codes may be assigned if the hospital prefers.

Patients who have both diabetes and hypertension may develop chronic kidney disease as a result. In this case, three codes are required: one code for the diabetes with renal manifestation, E08–E13 with .22; a second code from category I12 (or I13) with a fourth character 0 with chronic kidney disease stage 5 or end-stage renal disease or a fourth character 9 with chronic kidney disease stage 1 through stage 4, or unspecified; and a third code from category N18 to indicate the specific stage of the chronic kidney disease. No other manifestation code is assigned. An example follows:

E10.22 + I12.0 + N18.5   Progressive type 1 diabetic nephropathy with hypertensive renal disease and chronic kidney disease stage 5

However, when the patient has diabetes, hypertension, and chronic kidney disease and the provider documents a causal relationship between the diabetes and the chronic kidney disease in terms such as "diabetic CKD" or "diabetic nephropathy," the chronic kidney disease is not coded as hypertensive chronic kidney disease. A code from category I12 or I13 is not assigned; the hypertension is reported separately.

Diabetic Eye Disease

Retinopathy is a common complication of diabetes. Any disease of the retina said to be due to diabetes requires a code of E08–E13 with .3-. Diabetes with unspecified diabetic retinopathy is coded to E08–E13 with .31-. Nonproliferative diabetic retinopathy may be classified as mild (E08–E13 with .32-), moderate (E08–E13 with .33-), or severe (E08–E13 with .34-). Proliferative diabetic retinopathy is coded to E08–E13 with .35-. The sixth character provides additional information to identify the presence or absence of macular edema. The seventh character designates the laterality of the condition (e.g., right eye, left eye, bilateral, or unspecified eye).

ICD-10-CM presumes a causal relationship between diabetes and cataracts. Cataracts are considered a major cause of visual impairment in diabetic patients, as the incidence and progression of cataract is elevated in patients with diabetes mellitus. Diabetes and cataracts should be coded as related even in the absence of provider documentation explicitly linking them. For example:

165

. . . . **CHAPTER 14**

Endocrine,

Nutritional,

and Metabolic

Diseases

E11.36 — Type 2 diabetes mellitus with diabetic cataract

K86.1 + E08.36 + H25.9 — Secondary diabetes mellitus due to chronic pancreatitis with mature senile cataract

Diabetic Neurological Complications

Peripheral, cranial, and autonomic neuropathy are chronic manifestations of diabetes mellitus. The subclassification for diabetic neurological complications is as follows:

E08–E13 with .40 — Unspecified diabetic neuropathy

E08–E13 with .41 — Diabetic mononeuropathy

E08–E13 with .42 — Diabetic polyneuropathy

E08–E13 with .43 — Diabetic autonomic (poly)neuropathy

E08–E13 with .44 — Diabetic amyotrophy

E08–E13 with .49 — Other diabetic neurological complication

Do not use the code for autonomic neuropathy unless the diagnosis is stated as such by the physician. Examples of code assignments for diabetic neurological complications include the following:

E11.41 + H49.01 — Diabetic third (cranial) nerve palsy, right eye

E11.41 + G57.90 — Mononeuropathy of the lower limb due to type 2 diabetes

E10.40 — Diabetes type 1 with neuropathy

E10.43 + K31.84 — Type 1 diabetes with diabetic gastroparesis

Diabetic Circulatory Complications

Peripheral vascular disease is a frequent complication of diabetes mellitus. Diabetic peripheral vascular disease without gangrene is coded as E08–E13 with .51; diabetic peripheral vascular disease with gangrene is coded as E08–E13 with .52. Code **A48.0, Gas gangrene,** is assigned as an additional code for a diagnosis of gas gangrene.

Arteriosclerosis occurs earlier and more extensively in patients with diabetes. Like peripheral vascular disease, arteriosclerotic peripheral artery disease in patients with diabetes is coded to E08–E13 with .51 or .52. An additional code from subcategory I70.2, Arteriosclerosis of native arteries of extremities, is also assigned.

Diabetes with other circulatory complications is coded to E08–E13 with .59. However, coronary artery disease, cardiomyopathy, and cerebrovascular disease are not complications of diabetes and are not included in subcategories E08–E13 with .5-. These conditions are coded separately unless the physician documents a causal relationship with the diabetes.

Other Manifestations of Diabetes Mellitus

Common chronic complications of diabetes mellitus, besides renal, ophthalmic, neurological, or circulatory, are classified to E08–E13 with .6- as follows:

E08–E13 with .61- — Diabetic arthropathy

E08–E13 with .62- — Diabetic skin complications

E08–E13 with .63- — Diabetic oral complications

Ulcers of the lower extremities, particularly the feet, are common complications of diabetes. When a patient with diabetes mellitus has a skin ulcer, the classification presumes a causal relationship between the conditions unless the documentation clearly states the conditions are unrelated. For a diabetic foot ulcer, a code from E08 through E13 with .621 is assigned first, and an additional code of L97.4- or L97.5- is used to indicate the specific site of the ulcer. Other diabetic skin ulcers are coded to E08–E13 with .622, with an additional code to identify the site of the ulcer (L97.1–L97.9, L98.41–L98.49). If gangrene is present with the ulcer, assign .52 with the E08–E13 code.

166

CHAPTER 14

Endocrine,
Nutritional,
and Metabolic
Diseases

Organic impotence is often the result of either diabetic peripheral neuropathy or diabetic peripheral vascular disease. It is coded first to either E08–E13 with .40 or E08–E13 with .51, with an additional code of **N52.1, Erectile dysfunction due to diseases classified elsewhere.**

When either skin ulcer or organic impotence is specified as diabetic but without an indication as to whether the condition is due to neuropathy or peripheral vascular disease, code the condition as E08–E13 with .69 (with other specified complication), with an additional code for the complication. Codes E08–E13 with .69 are used for any other specified chronic manifestation that cannot be captured with the other codes in categories E08–E13. For example:

E10.69 + M75.01   Adhesive capsulitis of right shoulder due to type 1 diabetes mellitus

Complications due to Insulin Pump Malfunction

Some patients with diabetes use an insulin pump to receive insulin therapy. An insulin pump is a small, computerized device attached to the body that delivers insulin via a catheter. The pump may provide a continuous drip of insulin all day long, or it may allow the patient to self-administer an insulin bolus by pushing a button. Failure or malfunction of the pump may result in underdosing or overdosing of insulin. Both of these situations are considered mechanical complications and are assigned a code from subcategory T85.6, Mechanical complication of other specified internal and external prosthetic devices, implants and grafts, as the principal diagnosis or first-listed code. The appropriate T85.6- code is selected depending on the type of malfunction, as follows:

T85.614-   Breakdown (mechanical) of insulin pump
T85.624-   Displacement of insulin pump
T85.633-   Leakage of insulin pump

In addition, codes are assigned to specify underdose (T38.3x6-) or overdose (T38.3x1-), as well as the code for the type of diabetes mellitus and any associated complications.

DIABETES MELLITUS COMPLICATING PREGNANCY

Diabetes mellitus complicating pregnancy, delivery, or the puerperium is classified in chapter 15 of ICD-10-CM. Diabetes mellitus is a significant complicating factor in pregnancy. Pregnant women who have diabetes mellitus should first be assigned a code from category O24, Diabetes mellitus in pregnancy, childbirth and puerperium, followed by the appropriate diabetes code(s) (E08–E13) from chapter 4 of ICD-10-CM to indicate the type of diabetes involved.

Because diabetes mellitus inevitably complicates the pregnant state, is aggravated by the pregnancy, or is a main reason for obstetric care, it is appropriate to assign E08–E13 codes for a pregnant patient with diabetes mellitus. Assign also code **Z79.4, Long term (current) use of insulin,** if the diabetes mellitus is routinely treated with insulin.

Gestational Diabetes

A diagnosis of gestational diabetes refers to abnormal glucose tolerance that appears during pregnancy in a woman who was not previously diabetic. Gestational diabetes mellitus is not a true diabetes mellitus. It can occur during the second and third trimesters of pregnancy. It is thought to be due to metabolic or hormonal changes that occur during pregnancy. Patients with gestational diabetes are usually placed on a diabetic diet and sometimes require insulin therapy to maintain normal blood glucose levels during pregnancy, but the condition usually resolves during the postpartum period. Gestational diabetes can cause complications in the pregnancy similar to those of pre-existing diabetes mellitus. It also places the woman at greater risk of developing diabetes after the pregnancy. Subcategory O24.4, Gestational diabetes mellitus, is assigned for this condition. No other code from category O24 should be used with a code from O24.4.

167

CHAPTER 14

Endocrine,
Nutritional,
and Metabolic
Diseases

Subcategory O24.4 is further subdivided on the basis of whether the gestational diabetes occurs in pregnancy, childbirth, or puerperium as well as whether it is controlled by diet or medication (oral medication or insulin). If a patient with gestational diabetes is treated with both diet and medication, only the code for medication-controlled gestational diabetes mellitus is required. Neither code **Z79.4, Long-term (current) use of insulin,** nor code **Z79.84, Long term (current) use of oral hypoglycemic drugs,** should be assigned with codes from subcategory O24.4.

An abnormal glucose tolerance in pregnancy, without a diagnosis of gestational diabetes, is assigned a code from subcategory O99.81, Abnormal glucose complicating pregnancy, childbirth and the puerperium. Codes O24.4- (gestational diabetes) and O99.81- (abnormal glucose tolerance complicating pregnancy) should never be used together on the same record.

Neonatal Conditions Associated with Maternal Diabetes

Newborns with diabetic mothers sometimes experience either a transient decrease in blood sugar (**P70.0, Syndrome of infant of mother with gestational diabetes; P70.1, Syndrome of infant of a diabetic mother; P70.3, Iatrogenic neonatal hypoglycemia;** or **P70.4, Other neonatal hypoglycemia**) or a transient hyperglycemia (**P70.2, Neonatal diabetes mellitus**). The latter condition is sometimes referred to as pseudodiabetes and occasionally requires a short course of insulin therapy. Note, however, that these codes are assigned only when the maternal condition has actually had such an effect; the fact that the mother has diabetes in itself does not warrant the assignment of one of these codes for the newborn. When laboratory reports seem to indicate either a transient decrease in blood sugar or transient hyperglycemia, it is appropriate to check with the attending physician.

When an infant is born to a diabetic mother, and the infant presents no manifestations of infant of a diabetic mother syndrome, assign the appropriate Z38 code as the principal diagnosis. Code **Z83.3, Family history of diabetes mellitus,** should be assigned as an additional diagnosis. In addition, assign code **Z05.42, Observation and evaluation of newborn for suspected metabolic condition ruled out,** as an additional diagnosis for a newborn infant who requires special surveillance after being born to a diabetic mother but who lacks manifestations of infant of a diabetic mother syndrome.

EXERCISE 14.1

Code the following diagnoses. Do not assign External cause of morbidity codes.

1. Diabetes mellitus, type 1
   Diabetic nephrosis

2. Secondary diabetes mellitus due to pancreatic malignancy
   Diabetic cataract

3. Type 2 diabetes with ketoacidosis

4. Diabetes mellitus, type 2, with
   hyperosmolar, nonketotic coma

5. Diabetic Kimmelstiel-Wilson disease

6. Chronic kidney disease, stage IV due to type 1
   diabetes

_____

7. Impotence due to diabetic neuropathy

_____

HYPOGLYCEMIC AND INSULIN REACTIONS

Hypoglycemic reactions can occur in both diabetic and nondiabetic patients. In a diabetic patient, hypoglycemia with coma is coded as E08–E13 with .641, and codes E08–E13 with .649 are assigned for hypoglycemia when there is no mention of coma. Diabetes-related hypoglycemic reactions may occur when there is an imbalance between eating or exercise patterns and the dosage of insulin or oral hypoglycemic drugs. Hypoglycemia due to insulin may also occur in a patient newly diagnosed with type 1 diabetes during the initial phase of therapy while the dosage is being adjusted.

In a patient who does not have diabetes, code **E15, Nondiabetic hypoglycemic coma,** is assigned for hypoglycemic coma not otherwise specified. Code E15 also includes drug-induced insulin coma in a nondiabetic patient. Code **E16.2, Hypoglycemia, unspecified,** is assigned for hypoglycemia not otherwise specified.

Hypoglycemia without coma, due to a drug used as prescribed in a nondiabetic patient, requires code **E16.0, Drug-induced hypoglycemia without coma,** followed by a code from categories T36–T50 with a sixth character 5 to indicate adverse effect and the responsible drug. Hypoglycemic coma or shock in a nondiabetic patient resulting from the incorrect use of insulin or another antidiabetic agent is coded as poisoning (T38.3x- with a sixth character 1–4) with the poisoning code first, followed by code **E15, Nondiabetic hypoglycemic coma.**

EXERCISE 14.2

Code the following diagnoses. Do not assign External cause of morbidity codes.

_____

1. Neonatal hypoglycemia

_____

2. Hypoglycemic coma in patient without diabetes

_____

3. Patient with type 2 diabetes mellitus participated in a
   strenuous game of racquetball without adjusting his
   insulin dosage; he is admitted with blood sugar of 35
   and is diagnosed as being hypoglycemic

_____

4. Type 1 diabetic developed hypoglycemia even
   though she had taken only the prescribed dose of insulin
   and did not alter her exercise or eating regimen

_____

HISTORY OF DIABETES MELLITUS

Obesity is a risk factor for a patient developing diabetes mellitus and hypertension. If these conditions develop, and the patient undergoes bariatric surgery, a significant loss of weight may result in remission of the diabetes and/or hypertension. If the provider documents the patient has "resolved" or "history of" diabetes or hypertension and the patient has no existing manifestations related to diabetes or hypertension, assign codes **Z86.39, Personal history of other endocrine, nutritional and metabolic disease,** or **Z86.79, Personal history of other diseases of circulatory system.**

CODES FOR NUTRITIONAL DISORDERS

Nutritional disorders, such as deficiencies of specific vitamins and minerals, are classified in categories E40 through E64, with the exception of nutritional anemias, which are classified in categories D50 through D53.

Several codes are used to identify overweight and obesity, including the following:

E66.01   Morbid (severe) obesity due to excess calories

E66.09   Other obesity due to excess calories

E66.1   Drug-induced obesity

E66.2   Morbid (severe) obesity with alveolar hypoventilation

E66.3   Overweight

E66.8   Other obesity

E66.9   Obesity, unspecified

These codes are assigned only on the basis of the physician's diagnostic statement. Category E66, Overweight and obesity, requires the assignment of an additional code (Z68.-) for the body mass index (BMI), if known. BMI is a measure of weight for height used as a tool for indicating weight status in adults. Coding BMI is an exception to the guideline that requires that code assignment be based on the documentation by the provider. The BMI code assignment should be based on medical record documentation, which may be found in the notes of other clinicians involved in the care of the patient (i.e., physician or other qualified health care practitioner legally accountable for establishing the patient's diagnosis). BMI is typically documented by the dietitian or the nurse. Although BMI may be reported on the basis of another clinician's documentation, the codes for the associated diagnosis (such as overweight and obesity) must be based on the provider's documentation.

Being overweight may place a patient at increased risk for certain medical conditions. However, overweight may only be reported when it meets the definition of a reportable diagnosis per Section III, Reporting Additional Diagnoses, of the *ICD-10-CM Official Guidelines for Coding and Reporting*. Neither the code for overweight nor the BMI code is assigned when there is no documentation that the diagnosis "overweight" meets the definition of a reportable secondary diagnosis. Obesity and morbid obesity are always clinically significant and should be coded and reported when documented by the provider. The BMI code may be reported with these conditions when BMI is documented. BMI codes should not be assigned during pregnancy.

Occasionally, a patient's BMI may fluctuate during a hospital stay. If the BMI fluctuation is linked to a clinically significant condition, such as malnutrition or anorexia nervosa, code the most severe BMI value recorded during the admission. However, the BMI codes are not intended to report changes in BMI caused by fluid overload/retention. BMI fluctuation caused by weight gain due to excess fluid is not the same as that caused by loss or gain of body mass; weight from excess fluid can lead to an overestimate of the BMI, making it an inaccurate indicator of the patient's actual weight status.

Code **E66.2, Morbid (severe) obesity with alveolar hypoventilation,** also known as Pickwickian syndrome, involves sleep-disordered breathing that causes a person to stop breathing for short periods of time while sleeping. It may be related to both obesity and neurological conditions.

METABOLIC DISORDERS

Metabolic disorders other than diabetes are classified to categories E70–E88. A metabolic disorder occurs when abnormal reactions in the body disrupt the metabolism. These disorders involve an alteration in the normal metabolism of carbohydrates, lipids, proteins, water, and nucleic acids.

Fluid Overload

Fluid overload (E87.7-) is the excessive accumulation of fluid in the body. It may be caused by excessive parenteral infusion or deficiencies in cardiovascular or renal fluid volume regulation. However, when fluid overload is a component of congestive heart failure, it is not coded separately (per the guideline of not coding separately conditions that are an integral part of a disease process). If the fluid overload is noncardiogenic in nature (e.g., fluid overload due to dialysis noncompliance in a patient with congestive heart failure and end-stage renal disease), the "excludes2" note at code I50.9 allows the separate coding of both the congestive heart failure and fluid overload.

Cystic Fibrosis

Cystic fibrosis (E84.-), also known as mucoviscidosis or cystic fibrosis of the pancreas, is a disorder of the exocrine glands that causes the accumulation of thick, tenacious mucus. It is the primary cause of pancreatic deficiency and chronic malabsorption in children. Although cystic fibrosis affects the body in a number of ways, progressive respiratory insufficiency is the major cause of illness in patients with this disease. The symptoms primarily affect the digestive and respiratory systems. In some glands involved in digestion, like the pancreas, the thick mucus may become an obstruction, preventing digestive enzymes from reaching the intestines. The pulmonary manifestation results in mucus secretions that clog the airways and allow bacteria to multiply. Sometimes, this state progresses to complications such as acute and chronic bronchitis, bronchiectasis, pneumonia, atelectasis, peribronchial and parenchyma scarring, pneumothorax, and hemoptysis. Intra-abdominal complications such as meconium ileus, rectal prolapse, inguinal hernia, gallstones, ileocolic intussusception, and gastroesophageal reflux also occur.

Specific codes identify the site of manifestation involvement, such as pulmonary involvement (E84.0), meconium ileus (E84.11), other intestinal manifestations (E84.19), or other site involvement (E84.8). These manifestation codes may be used together if different sites are involved. Code E84.9, Cystic fibrosis, unspecified, should be used if the manifestation is not specified. If an infectious organism is involved with cystic fibrosis with pulmonary involvement, assign an additional code for the organism present.

Because there is no known cure for cystic fibrosis, therapy is directed toward the complications of the disease, with the major focus on the maintenance of adequate nutritional and respiratory status. Admissions due to the cystic fibrosis itself most often occur when the patient is brought in for workup to confirm the diagnosis.

Tumor Lysis Syndrome

Tumor lysis syndrome (TLS) refers to a group of serious, potentially life-threatening metabolic disturbances that can occur after antineoplastic therapy. TLS can develop spontaneously as a result of radiation therapy or corticosteroid therapy. However, it usually occurs following the administration of anticancer drugs and is often associated with leukemias and lymphomas. It is also seen in other hematological malignancies and solid tumors. When cancer cells are destroyed, they can release intracellular ions and metabolic by-products into the circulation, leading to TLS. Code E88.3, Tumor lysis syndrome, is used to report spontaneous TLS as well as TLS following antineoplastic drug therapy. Use an additional code (T45.1x5-) to identify an adverse effect of drug when TLS is drug induced.

EXERCISE 14.3

Code the following diagnoses and procedures. Do not assign External cause of morbidity codes.

1. Hypercholesterolemia and endogenous hyperglyceridemia

2. Cystic fibrosis with mild mental intellectual disabilities

3. Congenital myxedema
    Inappropriate antidiuretic hormone secretion syndrome

4. Hypokalemia

5. Uninodular toxic nodular goiter with thyrotoxicosis
    Open left thyroid lobectomy

6. Adenomatous goiter with thyrotoxicosis
    Percutaneous endoscopic substernal thyroidectomy, complete

7. Toxic diffuse goiter with thyrotoxic crisis

8. Hypothyroidism, ablative, following total thyroidectomy
    performed three years ago

9. Morbidly obese patient with a BMI of 39
    Laparoscopic gastroplasty with gastric banding
    restriction

10. Flushing and sleeplessness due to premature menopause

11. Fluid overload following blood transfusion due to
    transfusion associated circulatory overload (TACO)

12. Nutritional anemia with moderate protein-calorie malnutrition
    and BMI of 18

CHAPTER 15

Mental Disorders

CHAPTER OVERVIEW

- Mental disorders are classified in chapter 5 of the ICD-10-CM.

- Organic anxiety disorder is a psychosis and the direct effect of a medical condition. The medical condition should be coded first.

- Schizophrenia is classified in category F20, with a fourth character indicating the type of schizophrenia.

- Affective disorders are common mental diseases with multiple aspects, including biologic, behavioral, social, and psychological factors. The most common affective disorders are the following:

  — Major depressive disorder

  — Bipolar disorders

  — Anxiety disorders

- Nonpsychotic mental disorders are also classified. These include the following:

  — Reactions to stress (both acute and chronic)

  — Psychophysiologic disorders

- Substance abuse and dependence are classified as mental disorders in ICD-10-CM.

  — Use, abuse, and dependence are different conditions and should be coded differently.

  — Alcohol dependence syndrome, drug dependence, and nondependent abuse of drugs are classified to three different categories.

LEARNING OUTCOMES

After studying this chapter, you should be able to:

Code a variety of mental disorders.

Determine the differences among types of affective disorders.

Explain the difference between substance abuse and dependence, and code the conditions and therapies surrounding these two distinct conditions.

TERMS TO KNOW

Abuse
problematic use of drugs or alcohol but without dependence

Dependence
increased tolerance to drugs or alcohol with a compulsion to continue taking the substance despite the cost; withdrawal symptoms often occur upon cessation

REMEMBER . . .

Although coding assignments for mental disorders are made according to ICD-10-CM, psychiatrists often state diagnoses using the different terminology found in the *Diagnostic and Statistical Manual of Mental Disorders, Fifth Edition.*

INTRODUCTION

Mental disorders of all types are classified in chapter 5 of ICD-10-CM.

Psychiatrists ordinarily state diagnoses in accordance with the nomenclature used in the *Diagnostic and Statistical Manual of Mental Disorders, Fifth Edition* (DSM-5®), published by the American Psychiatric Association (APA). According to the APA, DSM-5 and the International Classification of Diseases (ICD) should be thought of as companion publications. Whereas the primary purpose of DSM-5 is to extensively describe the criteria used by psychiatrists to diagnose mental disorders, the objective of ICD is to provide codes for psychiatry and all other areas of medicine that can be used for insurance reimbursement and the monitoring of morbidity and mortality statistics. DSM-5 lists ICD-10-CM codes for specific mental disorders.

The disorder names used in DSM-5 and ICD do not always match. Coding professionals working with mental health records may find it useful to become familiar with DSM-5, but actual coding assignment is made according to the classifications in ICD-10-CM.

MENTAL DISORDERS DUE TO KNOWN PHYSIOLOGICAL CONDITIONS

Categories F01 through F09, Mental disorders due to known physiological conditions, include a range of mental disorders grouped together on the basis of having a demonstrable etiology in cerebral disease, brain injury, or other insult leading to cerebral dysfunction. The cerebral dysfunction may be primary or secondary. Primary cerebral dysfunction includes diseases, injuries, and insults affecting the brain directly and selectively. Secondary cerebral dysfunction includes systemic

FIGURE 15.1   Side View of the Brain

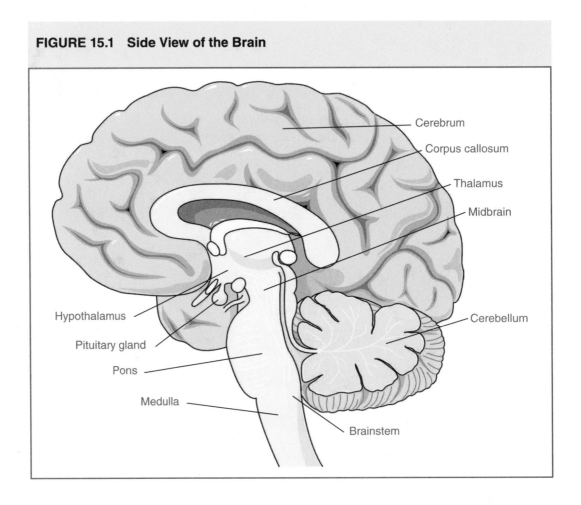

diseases and disorders that attack the brain as only one of the multiple organs or body systems involved.

This section includes the following categories:

F01 Vascular dementia
F02 Dementia in other diseases classified elsewhere
F03 Unspecified dementia
F04 Amnestic disorder due to known physiological condition
F05 Delirium due to known physiological condition
F06 Other mental disorders due to known physiological condition
F07 Personality and behavioral disorders due to known physiological condition
F09 Unspecified mental disorder due to known physiological condition

Instructional notes to code first the underlying physiological condition are provided for categories F02 through F09, except category F03, Unspecified dementia. Category F01, Vascular dementia, has an instructional note to code first the underlying physiological condition or sequelae of cerebrovascular disease.

Organic Brain Syndrome

Organic brain syndrome is an older general term used to describe decreased mental function due to a medical disease other than a psychiatric illness. In general, organic brain syndromes cause agitation; confusion; long-term loss of brain function (dementia); and severe, short-term loss of brain function (delirium). Organic brain syndrome is common in the elderly but is not part of the normal aging process. Organic brain syndrome, not otherwise specified, is coded to **F09, Unspecified mental disorder due to known physiological condition.** The underlying physiological condition should be coded first. Posttraumatic organic brain syndrome is coded to **F07.81, Postconcussional syndrome,** with an additional code to identify any associated posttraumatic headache.

Organic Anxiety Disorder

Organic anxiety disorder is a transient organic psychosis characterized by clinically significant anxiety. It is considered to be the direct physiological effect of a general medical condition. The code for the general condition is sequenced first, with an additional code of **F06.4, Anxiety disorder due to known physiological condition.**

Dementia in Other Diseases Classified Elsewhere

Dementia is characterized by the development of multiple cognitive deficits such as memory impairment and cognitive disturbances including aphasia, apraxia, and agnosia. Subcategory F02.8, Dementia in other diseases classified elsewhere, specifically identifies the presence or absence of behavioral disturbances such as aggressive behavior, violent behavior, wandering off, or combative behavior. The dementia classified in subcategory F02.8 is due to direct physiological effects of a general medical condition and includes major neurocognitive disorders. When assigning codes F02.80 and F02.81, code first the underlying physiological condition associated with the dementia, such as Alzheimer's disease (G30.-) or Parkinson's disease (G20). When the cause of the dementia is not specified, the dementia is classified to subcategory F03.9, Unspecified dementia, with the fifth digit distinguishing without behavioral disturbance (F03.90) or with behavioral disturbance (F03.91). Unspecified dementia with behavior described as aggressive, combative, or violent is classified to code F03.91. If the patient has a tendency to wander off, code **Z91.83, Wandering in diseases classified elsewhere,** may be assigned in addition to code F02.81 or F03.91.

ALTERED MENTAL STATE

An alteration in level of consciousness not associated with delirium or another identified condition is classified to category R40 in chapter 18 of ICD-10-CM. Category R40 is further subdivided to indicate whether the alteration is identified as somnolence (R40.0), stupor (R40.1), coma (R40.2-), persistent vegetative state (R40.3), or transient alteration of awareness (R40.4). An altered mental status, or a change in mental status, of unknown etiology is coded to **R41.82, Altered mental status, unspecified.** If the condition causing the change in mental status is known, do not assign code R41.82; code the condition instead.

TRANSIENT GLOBAL AMNESIA

Transient global amnesia is a distinct form of amnesia of unknown etiology, characterized by a sudden loss of memory function. During an episode, the patient is unable to form memories or remember recent events and may ask the same question over and over because no memories of previous answers are formed. The episode usually lasts for a few hours, followed by total or near-total resolution of the memory loss, although the patient will remain amnesic for the event itself. Transient global amnesia is not psychotic in nature, and it is not considered to be due to ischemia; rather, it is a distinct cerebrovascular condition with its own code, G45.4.

SCHIZOPHRENIC DISORDERS

Schizophrenia is a severe mental illness characterized by a variety of symptoms including, but not limited to, the following:

* Bizarre behavior
* Disorganized thinking
* Disorganized speech
* Decreased emotional expressiveness
* Diminished or loss of contact with reality
* Diminished to total social withdrawal

Schizophrenic disorders are classified in category F20, with a fourth character indicating the type of schizophrenia as follows:

F20.0 Paranoid schizophrenia
Patients with this type of schizophrenia are preoccupied with delusions about being punished or persecuted by others.

F20.1 Disorganized schizophrenia
A type of schizophrenia whereby patients are usually confused and illogical; behavior is disorganized, emotionless, and inappropriate. It may lead to the patient having a limited ability to perform normal activities of daily living.

F20.2 Catatonic schizophrenia
A type of schizophrenia whereby patients become unresponsive and have limited physical response.

F20.3 Undifferentiated schizophrenia
A form of schizophrenia that is characterized by a number of schizophrenic symptoms, such as delusion(s), disorganized behavior, disorganized speech, flat affect, or hallucinations, but does not meet the criteria for any other type of schizophrenia.

F20.5 Residual schizophrenia

A type of schizophrenia characterized by decreased severity of symptoms of schizophrenia. Delusion, hallucinations, and other symptoms may be present, but they are far less severe than when originally diagnosed.

F20.8 Other schizophrenia

This subcategory is further subdivided as follows:

F20.81 Schizophreniform disorder

This is a short-term type of schizophrenia that distorts the way a person thinks, acts, expresses emotions, perceives reality, and relates to others. Schizophreniform disorder generally lasts less than six months, whereas schizophrenia is a life-long illness.

F20.89 Other schizophrenia

This code includes cenesthopathic schizophrenia (a subgroup of schizophrenia with marked and dominating abnormal bodily sensations) and simple schizophrenia (a disorder characterized by an insidious but progressive development of oddities of conduct, inability to meet the demands of society, and decline in total performance).

F20.9 Schizophrenia, unspecified

This code is used when the type of schizophrenia is not specified or when ICD-10-CM codes do not differentiate severity or acute exacerbation. For example, assign code F20.9 for acute exacerbation of chronic schizophrenia.

AFFECTIVE DISORDERS

Affective disorders are common mental diseases with multiple aspects, including biologic, behavioral, social, and psychological factors. Major depressive disorder (MDD), bipolar disorders, and anxiety disorders are the most common affective disorders. Affective disorders can result in symptoms ranging from the mild and inconvenient to the severe and life threatening. Affective disorders are characterized by mood disturbance. Mood [affective] disorders are classified under categories F30–F39 in ICD-10-CM.

Major depressive disorder is also known as monopolar depression or unipolar affective disorder. MDD causes prolonged periods of emotional, mental, and physical exhaustion. Patients with this condition have a considerable risk of self-destructive behavior, sometimes leading to suicide. MDD is classified in ICD-10-CM as:

F32.-   Major depressive disorder, single episode

F33.-   Major depressive disorder, recurrent

Categories F32 and F33 are further subdivided with fourth characters, and sometimes fifth characters, to provide information about the current severity of the disorder, as follows:

0   Mild

1   Moderate

2   Severe, without psychotic features

3   Severe with psychotic features

4   In remission (Category F32 uses the fourth character 4 to indicate in partial remission; category F33 uses the fourth character 4 to indicate remission and is further subdivided with fifth characters to indicate unspecified remission, partial remission, or full remission.)

5   In full remission (Used only for category F32.)

8   Other

9   Unspecified

Fourth characters 1 through 8 are assigned only when provider documentation of severity is included in the medical record.

Bipolar affective diseases are divided into various types according to the symptoms displayed. Other names for bipolar affective diseases include manic-depressive disorder, cyclothymia, manic-depressive illness, and bipolar disorder. Patients with bipolar diseases experience periods of manic (hyper-excitable) episodes alternating with periods of deep depression. These disorders are chronic and recurrent with varying degrees of severity. Severe crises can lead to suicide attempts during depressive episodes or to physical violence against oneself or others during manic episodes. In many patients, however, episodes are mild and infrequent. Mixed states may also occur with elements of mania and depression simultaneously present. Some people with bipolar affective disorders show a rapid cycling between manic and depressive states.

ICD-10-CM classifies bipolar disorders under the following categories/codes:

F30.-   Manic episode (includes bipolar disorder, single manic episode, and mixed affective episode)

F31.-   Bipolar disorder (includes manic-depressive illness, manic-depressive psychosis, and manic-depressive reaction)

F34.-   Persistent mood [affective] disorders (includes cyclothymic disorder and dysthymic disorder)

F39   Unspecified mood [affective] disorder (includes affective psychosis not otherwise specified)

Category F30, Manic episode, is further subdivided to identify the severity of the current episode and to indicate whether psychotic symptoms are involved. Category F31, Bipolar disorder, is further subdivided to specify the severity of the current episode; whether the current episode is hypomanic, manic, depressed, or mixed; and whether psychotic features are involved. When a patient with bipolar disorder has major depressive disorder, assign a code for bipolar disorder. Do not report the depression separately; bipolar disorder includes both depression and mania. Additionally, for patients with bipolar disorder currently in remission (F31.7-), fifth characters are available to specify whether the patient is in full or partial remission and whether the most recent episode was hypomanic, manic, depressed, mixed, or unspecified.

EXERCISE 15.1

Code the following diagnoses. Do not assign External cause of morbidity codes.

1.   Schizoaffective psychosis, depressive type

2.   Schizophrenia, catatonic type

3.   Schizophrenia, paranoid type

4.   Severe depressive disorder, recurrent, current episode severe with psychotic symptoms

5.   Reactive depressive psychosis

6. Bipolar disorder, in manic phase, mild

_____

7. Bipolar affective disorder, most recent episode mixed,

in partial remission

_____

NONPSYCHOTIC MENTAL DISORDERS

A variety of anxiety, dissociative, stress-related, somatoform, and other nonpsychotic mental disorders are classified in categories F40 through F48. These include such conditions as phobic anxiety disorders, reaction to stress, dissociative and conversion disorders, somatoform disorders, and other nonpsychotic mental disorders.

Anxiety Disorders

Anxiety disorders are common psychiatric disorders and are considered to be one of the most undertreated and overlooked health problems. Among their common manifestations are panic disorders, phobias, chronic generalized anxiety disorder, obsessive-compulsive disorder, and posttraumatic stress disorder. A phobia is a persistent and irrational fear of a particular type of object, animal, activity, or situation. Anxiety disorders are classified in ICD-10-CM under the following categories:

F40   Phobic anxiety disorders
F41   Other anxiety disorders
F42   Obsessive-compulsive disorder

Reactions to Stress

ICD-10-CM provides category F43 for coding reaction to severe stress and adjustment disorders. Code **F43.0, Acute stress reaction,** classifies acute reaction to stress, including acute crisis reaction, combat fatigue, crisis state, and psychic shock. Acute stress reaction is the result of a person experiencing or witnessing a traumatic event that causes the individual to experience extreme, disturbing, or unexpected fear, stress, or pain and that involves or threatens serious injury, perceived serious injury, or death to self or someone else.

Posttraumatic stress disorder (PTSD) is classified in ICD-10-CM to subcategory F43.1, with fifth characters for unspecified, acute, or chronic. PTSD is a severe anxiety disorder that can develop after exposure to any event resulting in psychological trauma. As an effect of psychological trauma, PTSD is less frequent and more enduring than the more commonly seen acute stress response. Symptoms of PTSD include re-experiencing the original trauma(s) through flashbacks or nightmares; avoiding stimuli associated with the trauma; and experiencing increased arousal, such as difficulty falling or staying asleep, anger, and hypervigilance. These symptoms last more than one month and cause significant impairment in social, occupational, or other important areas of functioning. When PTSD occurs as a result of war, a code from category Y36, Operations of war, may be assigned to describe the external cause of the condition.

An adjustment disorder is a psychological response to an identifiable stressor or group of stressors that cause(s) significant emotional or behavioral symptoms. Compared to acute stress disorder and PTSD, adjustment disorder is usually associated with a less-intense stressor. Adjustment disorders are classified to subcategory F43.2, with the fifth-character axis being the nature of the reaction—for example, anxiety, depression, disturbance of conduct, or other symptoms. The following situations fall into this category:

F43.21   Patient depressed over death of son

F43.24   Child adopted from a foreign country, suffering from culture shock with conduct disturbance

F43.21   Complicated bereavement (grief)

Dissociative and Conversion Disorders

ICD-10-CM classifies dissociative and conversion disorders to category F44. Dissociative disorders are conditions that involve disruptions or breakdowns of memory, awareness, identity, and/or perception. Four codes are available for dissociative disorders, as follows:

F44.0   Dissociative amnesia

F44.1   Dissociative fugue

F44.2   Dissociative stupor

F44.81   Dissociative identity disorder

Conversion disorder is a condition whereby the patient presents with neurological symptoms but with the exclusion of neurological disease or feigning, and the determination of a psychological mechanism. The symptoms can vary from weakness/paralysis of a limb or the entire body to impaired hearing or vision, loss of sensation, impairment of speech, seizures, syncope, and other neurological findings. The following codes are used to describe conversion disorder:

F44.4   Conversion disorder with motor symptom or deficit

F44.5   Conversion disorder with seizures or convulsions

F44.6   Conversion disorder with sensory symptom or deficit

F44.7   Conversion disorder with mixed symptom presentation

In addition, two codes are available for other (F44.89) and unspecified (F44.9) dissociative and conversion disorders.

Examples of conditions that are classified in category F44 include the following:

F44.4   Psychogenic paralysis

F44.4   Abnormal hysterical gait

F44.0   Hysterical amnesia

F44.6   Emotional blindness

Somatoform Disorders

Somatoform disorders are mental disorders characterized by physical symptoms that mimic physical disease or injury for which there is no identifiable physical cause. Instead, the symptoms are caused by mental factors. A diagnosis of a somatoform disorder implies that mental factors are a large contributor to the symptoms' onset, severity, and duration. ICD-10-CM classifies somatoform disorders to category F45. Examples of conditions classified in category F45 include the following:

F45.8   Psychogenic diarrhea

F45.8   Psychogenic dysmenorrhea

F45.20   Hypochondriacal disorder

In assigning codes from categories F44 and F45, it is important to make the distinction between these conditions and similar conditions that fall under the categories for neurotic disorders, psychoses, or organic disorders.

For pain that is exclusively related to psychological factors, assign code **F45.41, Pain disorder exclusively related to psychological factors.** A code from category G89, Pain, not elsewhere classified, should not be assigned with code F45.41. When the documentation reflects a psychological component for a patient's acute or chronic pain, assign code **F45.42, Pain disorder with related psychological factors,** with a code from category G89.

BEHAVIORAL SYNDROMES ASSOCIATED WITH PHYSIOLOGICAL DISTURBANCES AND PHYSICAL FACTORS

Categories F50 through F59 are devoted to behavioral syndromes associated with physiological disturbances and physical factors. These codes are not assigned when the conditions are present due to a mental disorder classified elsewhere or are of organic origin. This grouping includes the following conditions:

F50.- Eating disorders (such as anorexia nervosa and bulimia nervosa)

F51.- Sleep disorders not due to a substance or known physiological condition

F52.- Sexual dysfunction not due to a substance or known physiological condition

F53.- Mental and behavioral disorders associated with the puerperium, not elsewhere classified

F54 Psychological and behavioral factors associated with disorders or diseases classified elsewhere

F55.- Abuse of nonpsychoactive substances

F59 Unspecified behavioral syndromes associated with physiological disturbances and physical factors

Code F54 classifies psychological and behavioral factors associated with diseases classified elsewhere. Typical conditions that are often associated with code F54 include asthma, ulcerative colitis, and dermatitis. If such a condition is considered to be psychogenic in origin, the associated physical disorder is coded first, followed by code F54. For example:

J45.20 + F54 Mild intermittent psychogenic asthma

I47.1 + F54 Psychogenic paroxysmal atrial tachycardia

DISORDERS OF ADULT PERSONALITY AND BEHAVIOR

Categories F60 through F69 are devoted to disorders of adult personality and behavior. This grouping includes the following conditions:

F60.- Specific personality disorders

F63.- Impulse disorders

F64.- Gender identity disorders

F65.- Paraphilias

F66.- Other sexual disorders

F68.- Other disorders of adult personality and behavior

It is important to distinguish between two types of factitious disorders classified to category F68. Subcategory F68.1, Factitious disorder imposed on self, also referred to as Munchausen's syndrome, is a disorder in which a person falsely reports or causes his or her own physical or psychological signs or symptoms. Subcategory F68.1 is further subdivided as unspecified (F68.10), with predominantly psychological signs and symptoms (F68.11), with predominantly physical signs and symptoms (F68.12), and with combined psychological and physical signs and symptoms (F68.13).

On the other hand, Munchausen's syndrome by proxy (MSBP) is a disorder in which a caregiver (perpetrator) falsely reports or causes an illness or injury in another person (victim) under his or her care, such as a child, an elderly adult, or a person who has a disability. The condition is also referred to as "factitious disorder imposed on another" or "factitious disorder by proxy." The perpetrator, not the victim, receives this diagnosis. Code **F68.A, Factitious disorder imposed on another,** is assigned to the perpetrator's record. For the victim of a patient with MSBP, assign the appropriate code from category T74, Adult and child abuse, neglect and other maltreatment, confirmed, or T76, Adult and child abuse, neglect and other maltreatment, suspected.

EXERCISE 15.2

Code the following diagnoses.

1. Acute delirium resulting from pneumonia
   due to *Hemophilus influenzae*

2. Passive-aggressive personality disorder

3. Depression anxiety
   Conversion disorder (convulsions)

4. Adolescent adjustment reaction, with severe
   disturbance of conduct

5. Severe depression, recurrent

6. Acute stress reaction, psychomotor

SUBSTANCE ABUSE DISORDERS

Substance abuse and dependence are classified as mental disorders in ICD-10-CM. Contrary to the concept that these disorders are separate, scientific evidence shows they exist on a spectrum based on use; codes for abuse are assigned for mild substance use disorder, and codes for dependence are assigned for moderate and severe use disorder based on the inclusion terms in the Tabular List. There are codes for "in remission" for both substance dependence and substance abuse.

Alcohol Dependence and Abuse

Alcohol-related disorders are classified in ICD-10-CM to category F10. An additional code for blood alcohol level (Y90.-) may be assigned, if applicable. Alcohol abuse refers to the recurring use of alcoholic beverages despite negative consequences. Alcohol dependence may be differentiated from alcohol abuse by the presence of symptoms such as tolerance. Both alcohol dependence and alcohol abuse are sometimes referred to by the less-specific term "alcoholism."

Alcohol abuse is classified in ICD-10-CM under subcategory F10.1, Alcohol abuse, whereas alcohol dependence is classified under subcategory F10.2, Alcohol dependence. Both subcategories are further subdivided to specify the presence of intoxication or intoxication delirium. Additional characters are also provided to specify alcohol-induced mood disorder, psychotic disorder, and other alcohol-induced disorders.

Codes **F10.130, Alcohol abuse with withdrawal, uncomplicated; F10.131, Alcohol abuse with withdrawal delirium; F10.132, Alcohol abuse with withdrawal with perceptual distur-bance;** and **F10.139, Alcohol abuse with withdrawal, unspecified,** are assigned for withdrawal symptoms in alcohol abuse. Codes in subcategory F10.23- are assigned for alcohol dependence with withdrawal. The sixth-character provides additional detail regarding withdrawal symptoms such as delirium and perceptual disturbance.

Code **F10.129, Alcohol abuse with intoxication, unspecified,** is assigned for a diagnosis of simple drunkenness. However, acute drunkenness in alcoholism is indexed to **F10.229, Alcohol dependence with intoxication, unspecified;** chronic drunkenness is indexed to **F10.20, Alco-hol dependence, uncomplicated;** and chronic drunkenness in remission is indexed to **F10.21, Alcohol dependence, in remission.** Code F10.21 includes moderate and severe alcohol use in early and sustained remission. Selection of code F10.21 for "in remission" requires the provider's clinical judgment, as defined by the *ICD-10-CM Official Guidelines for Coding and Reporting*, rather than nursing or other documentation. Alcohol abuse in remission is indexed to **F10.11, Alco-hol abuse, in remission.** Code F10.11 includes mild alcohol use disorder in early or sustained remission. If alcohol use is documented without further specificity as to abuse or dependence, and without documentation of mental or behavioral disorders, it is classified to **Z72.89, Other prob-lems related to lifestyle.** Note that toxic effect of alcohol is not classified to category F10; instead, it is classified to subcategory T51.0-.

Drug Dependence and Abuse

ICD-10-CM classifies drug dependence and abuse in the following categories according to the class of drug:

F11   Opioid related disorders
F12   Cannabis related disorders
F13   Sedative, hypnotic or anxiolytic related disorders
F14   Cocaine related disorders
F15   Other stimulant related disorders
F16   Hallucinogen related disorders
F17   Nicotine dependence
F18   Inhalant related disorders
F19   Other psychoactive substance related disorders

In most cases, fourth characters indicate whether the disorder is nondependent abuse (1), dependence (2), or unspecified use (9). Additional characters are also provided to specify intoxication, intoxication delirium, and intoxication with perceptual disturbance. Patients with substance abuse or dependence often develop related physical complications or psychotic symptoms. These complica-tions are classified to the specific drug abuse or dependence, with the fifth or sixth characters pro-viding further specificity regarding any associated drug-induced mood disorder, psychotic disorder, withdrawal, and other drug-induced disorders (such as sexual dysfunction or sleep disorder).

Withdrawal most commonly refers to the group of symptoms that occurs upon the abrupt dis-continuation/separation or a decrease in dosage of the intake of medications, recreational drugs, and/ or alcohol. Symptoms and signs of withdrawal can vary based on the substance and from individual to individual. They include tremulousness, agitation, irritability, disturbed sleep, anorexia, autonomic hyperactivity, seizures, and hallucinations. A severe form of withdrawal known as delirium tremens is characterized by fever, tachycardia, hypertension or hypotension, hallucinations, agitation, confusion, fluctuating mental states, and seizures.

ICD-10-CM provides combination codes that include both the alcohol or substance abuse/dependence and any associated complications. Examples include:

F10.251   Alcohol-induced psychotic disorder with hallucinations due to alcohol dependence
F10.180   Alcohol-induced anxiety disorder due to alcohol abuse
F11.250   Heroin dependence with heroin-induced psychosis and delusions

Category F19, Other psychoactive substance related disorders, may be used when the specific drug class is not specified. A code from subcategory F19.13, is assigned for withdrawal in abuse of other psychoactive substance.

Similar to code **F10.21, Alcohol dependence, in remission,** the selection of codes for "in remission" for categories F11–F19 with -.21 requires the provider's clinical judgment. Coding professionals should assign the appropriate codes for "in remission" only on the basis of provider documentation (as defined in the *ICD-10-CM Official Guidelines for Coding and Reporting*), unless otherwise instructed by the classification. Mild substance use disorders in early or sustained remission are classified to substance abuse in remission. Moderate and severe substance use in early or sustained remission is classified to dependence in remission.

Psychoactive Substance Use

In addition to the codes for psychoactive substance abuse and dependence, ICD-10-CM provides codes for psychoactive substance use (F10.9-, F11.9-, F12.9-, F13.9-, F14.9-, F15.9-, F16.9-). As with all other diagnoses, these codes should only be assigned based on provider documentation and when they meet the definition of a reportable diagnosis per Section III, Reporting Additional Diagnoses, of the *ICD-10-CM Official Guidelines for Coding and Reporting*. The codes are to be used only when the psychoactive substance use is associated with a physical, mental, or behavioral disorder and such a relationship is documented by the provider. A "physical disorder" refers to conditions such as sexual dysfunction and sleep disorder that are not mental disorders but are included in chapter 5.

Alcohol withdrawal occurs in alcohol dependence and alcohol abuse, but it may also develop in patients with patterns of use that are not described as dependence or abuse. Codes **F10.930, Alcohol use, unspecified with withdrawal, uncomplicated; F10.931, Alcohol use, unspecified with withdrawal delirium; F10.932, Alcohol use, unspecified with withdrawal with perceptual disturbance; and F10.939, Alcohol use, unspecified with withdrawal, unspecified,** are assigned for withdrawal symptoms in alcohol use.

Psychoactive Substance Use, Abuse, and Dependence Code Hierarchy

When the provider documentation refers to use, abuse, and dependence of the same substance (e.g., alcohol, opioid, cannabis), only one code should be assigned to identify the pattern of use, based on the following hierarchy:

- If both use and abuse are documented, assign only the code for abuse.
- If both abuse and dependence are documented, assign only the code for dependence.
- If use, abuse, and dependence are all documented, assign only the code for dependence.
- If both use and dependence are documented, assign only the code for dependence.

Selection of the Principal Diagnosis

The designation of the principal diagnosis for patients with either substance abuse or substance dependence is determined by the circumstances of the admission, as defined in the following examples:

1. When a patient is admitted for detoxification or rehabilitation for both drug abuse or dependence and alcohol abuse or dependence, and both are treated, either condition may be designated as the principal diagnosis.

2. When a patient with a diagnosis of substance abuse or dependence is admitted for treatment or evaluation of a physical complaint related to the substance use, follow the directions in the Alphabetic Index for conditions described as alcoholic or due to drugs; sequence the physical condition first, followed by the code for abuse or dependence.

3. When a patient with a diagnosis of alcohol or drug abuse or dependence is admitted because of an unrelated condition, follow the usual guidelines for selecting a principal diagnosis.

Substance Abuse Therapy

Treatment for patients with a diagnosis of substance abuse or dependence consists of detoxification, rehabilitation, or both. The abuse or dependence is the principal diagnosis for a patient admitted for such programs.

Detoxification is the management of withdrawal symptoms for a patient who is physically dependent on alcohol or drugs. The process is more than simple observation; it involves active management. Treatment may involve evaluation, observation and monitoring, and administration of thiamine and multivitamins for nutrition as well as other medications (such as methadone, long-acting barbiturates or benzodiazepines, or carbamazepine) as needed. The detoxification program for patients with alcohol dependence is usually continued over a four- or five-day period, although it can also be provided on an outpatient basis depending on the severity of the withdrawal symptoms. Detoxification takes longer for opiates and sedatives/hypnotics, usually lasting from three weeks to a period of months, and may be carried out in either a residential or an outpatient setting. If the medical record documents detoxification as having been carried out, the code can be assigned even when no medications were administered.

Rehabilitation is a structured program carried out with the goal of establishing strict control of drinking and drug use. A variety of rehabilitation modalities may be utilized. These include methadone maintenance, therapeutic residential communities, and long-term outpatient drug- or alcohol-free treatments. When a patient with drug dependence is on medications for detoxification or as part of a maintenance program to prevent withdrawal symptoms (e.g., methadone maintenance for opiate dependence), the appropriate code for the drug dependence should be assigned, rather than code **Z79.891, Long-term (current) use of opiate analgesic,** or **Z79.899, Other long-term (current) drug therapy.**

EXERCISE 15.3

Code the following diagnoses.

---

1. Paranoid alcoholic psychosis with alcohol dependence

---

2. Alcoholic cirrhosis of liver
   Chronic alcoholism

---

3. Acute alcoholic intoxication
   Blood alcohol level of 59 mg/100 mL

---

4. Marijuana dependence

---

5. Acute alcohol intoxication and dependence

_____

6. Barbiturate abuse with sleep disorder

_____

7. Cocaine dependence

_____

8. Amphetamine abuse

_____

9. Dependence on barbiturate and heroin

_____

_____

10. Admitted because of syndrome of inappropriate
    secretion of antidiuretic hormone secondary
    to chronic alcoholism

_____

MENTAL HEALTH AND SUBSTANCE ABUSE TREATMENT PROCEDURE CODING

Mental disorders other than substance abuse disorders are commonly treated with psychodynamic ("talk") therapy, drug therapy, electroconvulsive therapy, or a combination of therapeutic modes. Because the diagnosis alone does not always explain the length of stay or the level of resource utilization for such patients, therapy codes are helpful in analyzing patterns of care.

ICD-10-PCS provides two sections for procedures related to mental health and substance abuse, as follows:

G   Mental Health
H   Substance Abuse Treatment

Mental Health Procedures

The Mental Health Section of ICD-10-PCS contains specific values in the third and fourth characters to describe mental health procedures. The most important character in this section is the root type (the third character), while the type qualifier (the fourth character) further specifies the procedure type as needed. The remaining characters (second, fifth, sixth, and seventh) only function as placeholders and do not represent specific information about the procedure. The value Z is used as the placeholder for these characters. The following example demonstrates the structure of ICD-10-PCS codes in the Mental Health Section.

Electroconvulsive therapy, unilateral-multiple seizure

Character 1 Section	Character 2 Body System	Character 3 Root Type	Character 4 Type Qualifier	Character 5 Qualifier	Character 6 Qualifier	Character 7 Qualifier
G	Z	B	1	Z	Z	Z
Mental health	None	Electroconvulsive therapy	Unilateral-multiple seizure	None	None	None

Table 15.1 lists the 12 values representing mental health root types, along with their corresponding definitions.

TABLE 15.1 Root Type Values in the Mental Health Section

Value	Description	Definition
1	Psychological tests	The administration and interpretation of standardized psychological tests and measurement instruments for the assessment of psychological function
2	Crisis intervention	Treatment of a traumatized, acutely disturbed or distressed individual for the purpose of short-term stabilization
3	Medication management	Monitoring and adjusting the use of medications for the treatment of a mental health disorder
5	Individual psychotherapy	Treatment of an individual with a mental health disorder by behavioral, cognitive, psychoanalytic, psychodynamic, or psychophysiological means to improve functioning or well-being
6	Counseling	The application of psychological methods to treat an individual with normal developmental issues and psychological problems in order to increase function, improve well-being, alleviate distress, address maladjustment, or resolve crises
7	Family psychotherapy	Treatment that includes one or more family members of an individual with a mental health disorder by behavioral, cognitive, psychoanalytic, psychodynamic, or psychophysiological means to improve functioning or well-being
B	Electroconvulsive therapy	The application of controlled electrical voltages to treat a mental health disorder
C	Biofeedback	Provision of information from the monitoring and regulating of physiological processes in conjunction with cognitive-behavioral techniques to improve patient functioning or well-being
F	Hypnosis	Induction of a state of heightened suggestibility by auditory, visual, and tactile techniques to elicit an emotional or behavioral response
G	Narcosynthesis	Administration of intravenous barbiturates in order to release suppressed or repressed thoughts
H	Group psychotherapy	Treatment of two or more individuals with a mental health disorder by behavioral, cognitive, psychoanalytic, psychodynamic, or psychophysiological means to improve functioning or well-being
J	Light therapy	Application of specialized light treatments to improve functioning or well-being

Examples of commonly performed mental health procedures in the inpatient setting include:

GZB1ZZZ   ECT (electroconvulsive therapy), unilateral, multiple seizure

GZ2ZZZZ   Crisis intervention

GZHZZZZ   Group psychotherapy

Substance Abuse Treatment

The Substance Abuse Treatment Section of ICD-10-PCS is structured as a smaller version of the Mental Health Section. Once again, the most important character in these codes is the third character, which describes the root type, while the fourth character is a qualifier that further classifies the root type. The remaining characters (second, fifth, sixth, and seventh) only function as placeholders and do not represent specific information about the procedure. The value Z is used as the placeholder for these characters. The following example demonstrates the structure of ICD-10-PCS codes in the Substance Abuse Treatment Section.

Methadone maintenance medication management

Character 1 Section	Character 2 Body System	Character 3 Root Type	Character 4 Type Qualifier	Character 5 Qualifier	Character 6 Qualifier	Character 7 Qualifier
H	Z	8	1	Z	Z	Z
Substance abuse treatment	None	Medication management	Methadone maintenance	None	None	None

Table 15.2 lists the seven values that represent substance abuse treatment root types, along with their corresponding definitions.

TABLE 15.2   Root Type Values in the Substance Abuse Treatment Section

Value	Description	Definition
2	Detoxification services	Detoxification from alcohol and/or drugs
3	Individual counseling	The application of psychological methods to treat an individual with addictive behavior
4	Group counseling	The application of psychological methods to treat two or more individuals with addictive behavior
5	Individual psychotherapy	Treatment of an individual with addictive behavior by behavioral, cognitive, psychoanalytic, psychodynamic, or psychophysiological means
6	Family counseling	The application of psychological methods that includes one or more family members to treat an individual with addictive behavior
8	Medication management	Monitoring and adjusting the use of replacement medications for the treatment of addiction
9	Pharmacotherapy	The use of replacement medications for the treatment of addiction

Examples of commonly provided substance abuse treatments in the inpatient setting include:

HZ2ZZZZ	Detoxification from alcohol and/or drugs
HZ83ZZZ	Medication management with Antabuse
HZ81ZZZ	Medication management with methadone
HZ41ZZZ	Behavioral group counseling

Detoxification services for substance abuse treatment (code HZ2ZZZZ) typically includes the active management of withdrawal symptoms. Medication management includes monitoring and adjusting the use of replacement medications for the treatment of addiction. Typically, pharmacotherapy involves replacing the substance of abuse over a longer period to wean the patient. For example, if a patient receives methadone to treat heroin dependence, the monitoring and adjustment of the methadone dosage is coded to **HZ81ZZZ, Medication management for substance abuse treatment, methadone maintenance.** If a patient receives methadone as part of long-term methadone maintenance for heroin dependence, that treatment is coded to **HZ91ZZZ, Pharmacotherapy for substance abuse treatment, methadone maintenance.**

EXERCISE 15.4

Code the following procedures.

1. Individual supportive psychotherapy

2. Crisis intervention

3. Substance abuse behavioral group counseling

4. Electroconvulsive therapy, bilateral, multiple seizures

5. Alcohol abuse detoxification

6. Nicotine patch management of tobacco dependence

7. Group counseling 12-step program

Coding OF Diseases OF THE Blood AND Blood-Forming Organs, Certain Disorders Involving THE Immune Mechanism, AND Diseases OF THE Nervous System

Diseases of the Blood and Blood-Forming Organs and Certain Disorders Involving the Immune Mechanism

CHAPTER OVERVIEW

- Diseases of the blood and blood-forming organs are classified in chapter 3 of ICD-10-CM.
- Anemia is the condition most commonly encountered in chapter 3.
  - It can be caused by chronic or acute blood loss, chronic disease, or the use of chemotherapy. Acute blood-loss anemia may occur after surgery or trauma.
  - The use of precise terminology is important in classifying anemias.
- A variety of codes are associated with sickle-cell anemia.
  - It is important to distinguish between sickle-cell anemia and sickle-cell trait.
  - Other conditions classified as sickle-cell disorders include Hb-SS disease and sickle-cell thalassemia.
- Coagulation defects are another type of disease of the blood.
  - They affect clotting time and ability.
  - Hypercoagulation is also a possible condition.
- Diseases may decrease or increase the production of white blood cells (leukocytes). These diseases are classified according to whether the white blood cell count is low or elevated.
- Various immune disorders are also classified in chapter 3 of ICD-10-CM. However, HIV is classified elsewhere.

LEARNING OUTCOMES

After studying this chapter, you should be able to:

Code the various types of anemia.

Understand when and when not to code a coagulation defect because certain drug therapies are being used.

Distinguish among the various diseases of the white blood cells and the various types of white blood cells.

Understand where disorders of the immune system are classified.

TERMS TO KNOW

Anemia
a condition in which blood is deficient in the amount of hemoglobin in red blood cells or in the volume of red blood cells

Aplastic anemia
a condition in which there is a deficiency of blood cells because the bone marrow is failing to produce them

Pancytopenia
a type of aplastic anemia in which red blood cells, white blood cells, and platelets are all deficient

Sickle-cell anemia
a hereditary disease of the red blood cells passed to a child when both parents carry the genetic trait

Sickle-cell trait
a condition that occurs when a child receives the genetic trait from only one parent

Thrombocytopenia
a deficiency of platelets, the cells that are important in blood clotting

REMEMBER . . .

A variety of conditions can be classified as an anemia. Be sure to check with the diagnosing physician if the terminology in the medical report is nonspecific or misleading.

INTRODUCTION

CHAPTER 16

Diseases of the
Blood and
Blood-Forming
Organs and
Certain
Disorders
Involving the
Immune
Mechanism

Diseases of the blood and blood-forming organs—including bone marrow, lymphatic tissue, platelets, and coagulation factors—are classified in chapter 3 of ICD-10-CM. Chapter 3 also includes certain disorders involving the immune mechanism, such as immunodeficiency disorders, although human immunodeficiency virus (HIV) disease is classified to chapter 1. Neoplastic diseases, such as leukemia, are classified in chapter 2 of ICD-10-CM along with other neoplastic diseases. Diseases of the blood and blood-forming organs complicating pregnancy, childbirth, or the puerperium are reclassified in chapter 15 of ICD-10-CM. For example, anemia of pregnancy is coded O99.01-, with an additional code from chapter 3 assigned to indicate the specific type of anemia. Hematological disorders of the fetus and newborn are classified as perinatal conditions in chapter 16 of ICD-10-CM.

ANEMIA

The condition coding professionals encounter most often in chapter 3 of ICD-10-CM is anemia. Anemia refers to either a reduction in the quantity of hemoglobin or a reduction in the volume of packed red blood cells, a condition that occurs whenever the equilibrium between red blood cell loss and red blood cell production is disturbed. A decrease in production can result from a variety of causes, including aging, bleeding, and cell destruction.

The use of precise terminology is important in classifying anemias. When a diagnostic statement of anemia is not qualified in any way, review the medical record to determine whether more information can be located in laboratory or pathology reports or in a hematology consultation before the code for an unspecified type of anemia is assigned. Remember, however, that a code should not be assigned on the basis of a diagnostic report alone; when it appears that a more specific type of anemia is present, check with the physician for concurrence.

Deficiency Anemias

Iron deficiency anemias are classified in category D50. This type of anemia may be due to a chronic blood loss (D50.0) from conditions such as chronic hemorrhagic gastrointestinal conditions or menorrhagia, or it may be caused by inadequate intake of dietary iron (D50.8). If the cause is unspecified, code D50.9 is assigned. Note, however, that iron deficiency anemia specified as secondary to acute blood loss is assigned to code **D62, Acute posthemorrhagic anemia,** rather than to category D50. Other deficiency anemias are coded according to the type of deficiency, such as vitamin B12 (category D51), folate (category D52), or other nutritional deficiencies (category D53), with a fourth character indicating the specific type of deficiency, such as dietary folate deficiency anemia or B12 vitamin deficiency due to intrinsic factor deficiency. In addition, code **D52.1, Drug-induced folate deficiency anemia,** requires that a code from T36–T50 be coded with fifth or sixth character 5 to identify the drug.

EXERCISE 16.1

Code the following diagnoses. Do not assign External cause of morbidity codes.

1. Anemia, hypochromic, microcytic, with iron deficiency,
   cause unknown

   _____

2. Macrocytic anemia secondary to selective vitamin B12
   malabsorption with proteinuria

   _____

Anemia due to Acute Blood Loss

CHAPTER 16

*Diseases of the
Blood and
Blood-Forming
Organs and
Certain
Disorders
Involving the
Immune
Mechanism*

It is important to distinguish between anemia due to chronic blood loss and anemia due to acute blood loss, because the two conditions have entirely different codes in ICD-10-CM. Acute blood-loss anemia results from a sudden, significant loss of blood over a brief period of time. It may occur due to trauma, such as laceration, or a rupture of the spleen or other injury of abdominal viscera, where no external blood loss is noted. A diagnosis of acute blood-loss anemia should be supported by documented evidence of the condition, such as a sustained, significant lowering of the hemoglobin and/or hematocrit level. However, these abnormal findings are not coded and reported unless the physician indicates their clinical significance. If findings are outside the normal range, and the physician has ordered other tests to evaluate the condition or prescribed treatment, it is appropriate to ask the physician whether the diagnosis should be added.

Acute blood-loss anemia may occur following surgery, but it is not necessarily a complication of the procedure and should not be coded as a postoperative complication unless the physician identifies it as such. Many surgical procedures, such as hip replacement, routinely involve a considerable amount of bleeding as an expected part of the operation. This may or may not result in anemia; a code for anemia should be assigned only when the anemia is documented by the physician. If, in the physician's clinical judgment, surgery results in an expected amount of blood loss and the physician does not describe the patient as having anemia or a complication of surgery, do not assign a code for the blood loss. If a postoperative blood count is low enough to suggest anemia, it is appropriate to ask the physician whether a diagnosis of anemia should be added. It should not be assumed, however, that mention of blood loss and/or transfusion during surgery is an indication that anemia is present. Blood replacement is sometimes carried out as a preventive measure. When postoperative anemia is documented without specification of acute blood loss, code **D64.9, Anemia, unspecified,** is the default. Code **D62, Acute posthemorrhagic anemia,** should be assigned when postoperative anemia is due to acute blood loss. When neither the diagnostic statement nor review of the medical record indicates whether a blood-loss anemia is acute or chronic, code **D50.0, Iron deficiency anemia secondary to blood loss (chronic),** should be assigned.

EXERCISE 16.2

Code the following diagnoses and procedures. Do not assign External cause of morbidity codes.

1. Anemia due to blood loss from chronic gastric ulcer

2. Anemia, chronic, secondary to blood loss due to adenomyosis

3. Posthemorrhagic anemia due to acute blood loss following perforation of chronic bleeding duodenal ulcer
   Esophagogastroduodenoscopy with clips applied to control hemorrhage

Anemia of Chronic Disease

CHAPTER 16

Diseases of the

Blood and

Blood-Forming

Organs and

Certain

Disorders

Involving the

Immune

Mechanism

Patients with chronic illnesses often have anemia, which may be the cause of the health care admission or encounter. Treatment is often directed at the anemia, not the underlying condition. Codes for this type of anemia are classified as follows:

- Anemia in chronic kidney disease: Code first the underlying chronic kidney disease (CKD) with a code from category N18 to indicate the stage of CKD, and code D63.1.
- Anemia in neoplastic disease: Code first the neoplasm (C00–D49) responsible for the anemia and code D63.0. Code D63.0 is for anemia in, due to, or with the malignancy. It is not for anemia due to the antineoplastic chemotherapy drugs, which is an adverse effect. If anemia in neoplastic disease and anemia due to antineoplastic chemotherapy (D64.81) are both documented, assign codes for both conditions.
- Anemia of other chronic disease: Code first the underlying chronic disease, followed by code D63.8.

Anemia due to Chemotherapy

Antineoplastic chemotherapy–induced anemia is classified to code **D64.81, Anemia due to antineoplastic chemotherapy.** This type of anemia is rarely a hemolytic process and is not truly an aplastic process. Antineoplastic chemotherapy–induced changes are generally short term and do not usually reduce the marrow cellularity to a point of aplasia. When the admission/encounter is for management of an anemia associated with an adverse effect of chemotherapy, and the only treatment is for anemia, the anemia code should be sequenced first, followed by the appropriate codes for the adverse effect and the neoplasm.

Anemia due to chemotherapy should not be confused with aplastic anemia due to antineoplastic chemotherapy, which is coded to **D61.1, Drug-induced aplastic anemia,** with an additional code to identify the adverse effect of a drug (T36–T50), and with a fifth or sixth character 5. Anemia due to a drug, where the drug is not specified, is coded to the type of anemia (or to code D64.9 if the type of anemia is not specified).

Aplastic Anemia and Pancytopenia

Aplastic anemia (D60.- and D61.-) is caused by a failure of the bone marrow to produce blood cells. The condition may be congenital, but it is usually idiopathic or acquired. It may be due to an underlying disease such as an autoimmune disorder or an infection (for example, viral hepatitis). It may also be caused by exposure to ionizing radiation, chemicals, or drugs, and it often results from treatment for malignancy. Aplastic anemia due to drugs is coded to **D61.1, Drug-induced aplastic anemia.** Aplastic anemia that is toxic or due to infection, radiation, or other external agents is coded to D61.2. Idiopathic aplastic anemia is coded to D61.3.

Pancytopenia (D61.81-) is a deficiency of all three elements of the blood. When a patient has anemia (deficiency of red blood cells), leukopenia (deficiency of white blood cells), and thrombocytopenia (deficiency of platelets), only the code for pancytopenia (D61.81-) should be assigned. When the pancytopenia is drug induced, ICD-10-CM distinguishes whether it is due to antineoplastic chemotherapy (D61.810) or other drug (D61.811). Code **D61.09, Other constitutional aplastic anemia,** is assigned if the pancytopenia is congenital rather than due to chronic disease. Do not assign a code from subcategory D61.81 if the pancytopenia is due to, or with, aplastic anemia (D61.9), bone marrow infiltration (D61.82), congenital (pure) red cell aplasia (D61.01), hairy cell leukemia (C91.4-), HIV disease (B20), leukoerythroblastic anemia (D61.82), myelodysplastic syndromes (D46.-), or myeloproliferative disease (D47.1).

CHAPTER 16

*Diseases of the
Blood and
Blood-Forming
Organs and
Certain
Disorders
Involving the
Immune
Mechanism*

EXERCISE 16.3

Code the following diagnoses and procedures.

1. Aplastic anemia due to accidental benzene exposure
   (subsequent encounter)

   _____

2. Myelophthisic anemia

   _____

3. Initial encounter for anemia due to chemotherapy treatment
   correctly administered

   _____

4. Pancytopenia related to methotrexate therapy for
   rheumatoid arthritis (initial encounter)

   _____

Sickle-Cell Anemia and Thalassemia

In coding sickle-cell disorders, it is important to understand the difference between sickle-cell anemia or disease (D57.0-, D57.1, D57.2-, D57.4-, and D57.8-) and sickle-cell trait (D57.3). Sickle-cell disease is a hereditary disease of the red blood cells; the disease is passed to a child when both parents carry the genetic trait. Sickle-cell trait occurs when a child receives the genetic trait from only one parent. Patients with sickle-cell trait do not generally develop sickle-cell disease; they are carriers of the trait. When a medical record contains both the terms "sickle-cell trait" and "sickle-cell disease," only the code for the sickle-cell disease is assigned.

A code from subcategory D57.0, Hb-SS disease with crisis, or subcategory D57.21, Sickle-cell/Hb-C disease, is assigned when vaso-occlusive crises or other crises are present. These subcategories are further subdivided to specify the type of crisis, such as acute chest syndrome (D57.01 or D57.211) or splenic sequestration (D57.02 or D57.212). If a condition such as cerebrovascular embolism occurs, a code for cerebral vascular involvement should be assigned with an additional code to indicate the presence of the embolism.

Another possible type of sickle-cell disease is sickle-cell thalassemia. There are two distinct types of sickle cell-thalassemia: sickle cell-thalassemia beta zero (HbS-β^0) and sickle cell-thalassemia beta plus (HbS-β^+). Sickle-cell thalassemia beta zero is clinically similar to sickle cell-SS disease in terms of degree of frequency and severity of complications. Sickle-cell thalassemia beta plus is significantly less severe with little or no anemia. Specific codes are available for unspecified sickle-cell thalassemia with crisis (D57.41-) or without crisis (D57.40); sickle-cell thalassemia beta zero with crisis (D57.43-) or without crisis (D57.42); and sickle-cell thalassemia beta plus with crisis (D57.45-) or without crisis (D57.44). Codes in subcategories D57.41, D57.43, and D57.45 have an additional sixth character to specify the type of crisis.

Other sickle-cell disorders include Hb-SD disease and Hb-SE disease, which are classified to subcategory D57.8. Codes in subcategory D57.8 have additional characters to specify whether there is crisis and the type of crisis when present.

Thalassemia is a genetic blood disorder resulting from a defect in a gene that controls production of one of the hemoglobin proteins. There are many forms of thalassemia. Each type has many different subtypes. The defective gene must be inherited from both parents in order for a person to

CHAPTER 16

Diseases of the
Blood and
Blood-Forming
Organs and
Certain
Disorders
Involving the
Immune
Mechanism

develop thalassemia major. Thalassemia minor occurs when the defective gene is inherited from only one parent. Persons with this form of the disorder are carriers of the disease and usually do not have symptoms. ICD-10-CM provides unique codes for different types of thalassemia, such as alpha thalassemia (D56.0), beta thalassemia (D56.1), delta-beta thalassemia (D56.2), thalassemia minor (D56.3), hemoglobin E-beta thalassemia (D56.5), and other thalassemia (D56.8). Code **D56.9, Thalassemia, unspecified,** is reported when the type of thalassemia is not identified. However, thalassemia trait, not otherwise specified, is assigned to code **D56.3, Thalassemia minor.**

EXERCISE 16.4

Code the following diagnoses. Do not assign External cause of morbidity codes.

1. Classical hemophilia

2. Sickle-cell Hb-SS disease

3. Hereditary spherocytic, hemolytic anemia

4. Thalassemia

5. Sickle-cell crisis with acute chest syndrome

COAGULATION DEFECTS

Coagulation defects are characterized by prolonged clotting time. Some are congenital in origin; others are acquired. Conditions in subcategory D68.31, Hemorrhagic disorder due to intrinsic circulating anticoagulants, antibodies, or inhibitors, result from the presence of circulating anticoagulants in the blood that interfere with normal clotting. These anticoagulants are usually inherent or intrinsic in the blood, like other coagulation defects. Autoimmune hemophilia, autoimmune inhibitors to clotting factors, and secondary and acquired hemophilia are assigned to code D68.311. Lupus anticoagulant (LAC) with hemorrhagic disorder, systemic lupus erythematosus [SLE] inhibitor with hemorrhagic disorder, and antiphospholipid antibody with hemorrhagic disorder are assigned to code D68.312. Code D68.318 includes hemorrhagic disorders due to increases in antithrombin, anti-VIIIa, anti-IXa, and other intrinsic circulating anticoagulants, antibodies, or inhibitors.

An increased risk of bleeding is an adverse effect associated with anticoagulation therapy. For bleeding in a patient who is being treated with warfarin (Coumadin), heparin, anticoagulants, or other antithrombotics as a part of anticoagulation therapy, assign code **D68.32, Hemorrhagic disorder due to extrinsic circulating anticoagulants.** To report the adverse effect of the properly administered anticoagulant, assign either code **T45.515-, Adverse effect of anticoagulant,** or code **T45.525-, Adverse effect of antithrombotic drugs.**

Heparin-induced thrombocytopenia (D75.82) is one of the most severe adverse effects of heparin therapy. Heparin therapy is widely used to prevent and treat clotting disorders. In some people, heparin triggers autoimmune conditions of severe platelet deficiency with severe thrombotic (clot-related) complications.

Hypercoagulable states are a group of acquired and inherited disorders caused by increased thrombin generation. There is an increased tendency for blood clotting, and there may be fibrin

CHAPTER 16

*Diseases of the
Blood and
Blood-Forming
Organs and
Certain
Disorders
Involving the
Immune
Mechanism*

deposition in the small blood vessels. These disorders are divided into primary and secondary hypercoagulable states. Primary hypercoagulable states (D68.5-) are inherited disorders of specific anticoagulant factors. Secondary hypercoagulable states (D68.6-) are primarily acquired disorders that predispose a person to thrombosis through complex and multifactorial mechanisms involving blood flow abnormalities or defects in blood composition and of vessel walls. Examples of conditions that can cause secondary hypercoagulable states are malignancy, pregnancy, trauma, myeloproliferative disorders, and antiphospholipid antibody syndrome.

Prolonged prothrombin time or other abnormal coagulation profiles should not be coded as a coagulation defect. If the patient is receiving warfarin (Coumadin) therapy, has an abnormal coagulation profile, and does not have a hemorrhage due to the medication, code **R79.1, Abnormal coagulation profile,** is assigned with code **Z79.01, Long term (current) use of anticoagulants.**

Examples of appropriate code assignments include the following:

D68.32 + K26.4 + T45.515A   Duodenal ulcer with hemorrhage due to Coumadin
                             therapy, initial encounter
D68.32 + K29.01 + T45.515D   Acute gastritis with hemorrhage due to anticoagulant
                             therapy, subsequent encounter

Following are case examples demonstrating code assignments:

* A 50-year-old man receiving Coumadin therapy is seen to monitor his Coumadin levels. A prolonged prothrombin time is reported, secondary to the anticoagulant effects of the Coumadin therapy. Assign codes **Z51.81, Encounter for therapeutic drug level monitoring; R79.1, Abnormal coagulation profile;** and **Z79.01, Long term (current) use of anticoagulants.**

* A patient is admitted following multiple episodes of hematemesis secondary to Coumadin therapy. No significant pathology was discovered. The Coumadin is discontinued, and no recurrence of the bleeding occurs. To indicate Coumadin as the responsible external agent, assign codes **K92.0, Hematemesis; D68.32, Hemorrhagic disorder due to extrinsic circulating anticoagulants;** and **T45.515A, Adverse effect of anticoagulants, initial encounter.** Drug-induced hemorrhagic disorder is an inclusion term at D68.32.

DISEASES OF PLATELET CELLS

Thrombocytopenia is a deficiency in the blood cells that help the blood to clot. Posttransfusion purpura is the recipient's response to produce anti-HPA (human platelet antigen) antibodies that destroy the platelets following a transfusion of blood products from an HPA-positive donor. The alloantibody destroys the transfused platelets as well as the recipient's own platelets to produce a severe thrombocytopenia in HPA-negative women who were immunized during previous pregnancy or transfusion. Code **D69.51, Posttransfusion purpura,** is assigned for this rare condition. Code **D69.59, Other secondary thrombocytopenia,** is assigned for secondary thrombocytopenia that is due to dilutional causes, drugs, extracorporeal circulation of blood, massive blood transfusion, platelet alloimmunization, and other secondary thrombocytopenia.

DISEASES OF WHITE BLOOD CELLS

White blood cells (leukocytes) play an important role in the body's immune system by fighting off infection. Many different diseases can affect white blood cells. There are several different types of normal leukocytes, including neutrophils, lymphocytes, monocytes, eosinophils, and basophils.

Production of white blood cells may be decreased due to conditions including drug toxicity, vitamin deficiencies, blood diseases, infections (viral diseases, tuberculosis, typhoid), or abnormalities

CHAPTER 16

*Diseases of the
Blood and
Blood-Forming
Organs and
Certain
Disorders
Involving the
Immune
Mechanism*

FIGURE 16.1   Four Major Types of Blood Cells

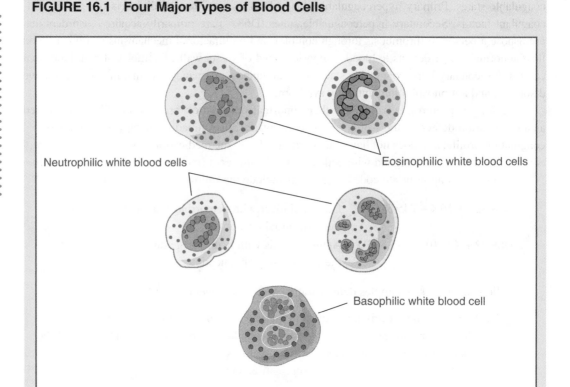

Neutrophilic white blood cells

Eosinophilic white blood cells

Basophilic white blood cell

Red blood cells

of the bone marrow; or the decrease could be cyclic (varying in severity, possibly due to biorhythm changes). Antibodies may attack leukocytes as a result of a disease or because of medications stimulating the immune system. Pooling of white blood cells occurs with some overwhelming infections, heart-lung bypass during heart surgery, and hemodialysis.

Some diseases increase the production of leukocytes. If all types of white blood cells are affected, leukocytosis occurs. Leukocytosis can be caused by infection, inflammation, allergic reaction, malignancy, hereditary disorders, or other miscellaneous causes—for example, medications such as cortisone-like drugs (prednisone), lithium, and nonsteroidal anti-inflammatory drugs. Other illnesses such as neutrophilia, lymphocytosis, and granulocytosis involve elevated levels of specific types of white blood cells.

Diseases of the white blood cells are primarily classified on the basis of whether the leukocyte count is low or elevated. In addition, more specific codes are available depending on the type of white blood cell affected, as shown by the examples that follow.

- Low neutrophil count or neutropenia (category D70) is further subdivided as follows: congenital neutropenia (D70.0); agranulocytosis secondary to cancer chemotherapy (D70.1); other drug-induced agranulocytosis (D70.2); neutropenia due to infection (D70.3); cyclic neutropenia (D70.4); other neutropenia (D70.8); and unspecified neutropenia (D70.9).

201

CHAPTER 16

Diseases of the
Blood and
Blood-Forming
Organs and
Certain
Disorders
Involving the
Immune
Mechanism

- Decreased white blood cell counts (subcategory D72.81) are classified as follows: decreased lymphocytes or lymphocytopenia (D72.810); other decreased white blood cell count, including basophils, eosinophils, monocytes, or plasmacytes (D72.818); unspecified decreased white blood cell count (D72.819).

- Elevated white blood cell counts (subcategory D72.82) are classified as follows: elevated lymphocytes or lymphocytosis (D72.820); monocytosis (D72.821); plasmacytosis (D72.822); leukemoid reaction, including basophilic, lymphocytic, monocytic, myelocytic, or neutrophilic leukemoid reaction (D72.823); basophilia (D72.824); bandemia (D72.825); other elevated white blood cell count (D72.828); and unspecified leukocytosis (D72.829).

It is important to remember that these codes should not be assigned on the basis of laboratory findings alone. Physician concurrence regarding the significance of the laboratory results should be confirmed before assigning these codes.

DISORDERS OF THE IMMUNE SYSTEM

Categories D80 through D89 classify various disorders of the immune system, with the exception of conditions associated with or due to HIV, which are classified to code B20 (see chapter 13 of this handbook for more information on HIV). The immune disorders discussed in this chapter include the following categories:

D80 Immunodeficiency with predominantly antibody defects
D81 Combined immunodeficiencies
D82 Immunodeficiency associated with other major defects
D83 Common variable immunodeficiency
D84 Other immunodeficiencies
D86 Sarcoidosis
D89 Other disorders involving the immune mechanism, not elsewhere classified

Immunodeficiency

An immunocompromised state is when a person's immune system is suppressed or weakened and less capable of battling infections. A patient may be immunocompromised due to a specific condition or external factors such as medications or exposure to radiation therapy, or a combination of both clinical conditions and external factors. Conditions within category D80–D89, Certain disorders involving the immune mechanism, are generally specific to the type of immune deficiency. Codes **D84.81, Immunodeficiency due to other conditions classified elsewhere; D84.821, Immunodeficiency due to drugs; D84.822, Immunodeficiency due to external causes;** and **D84.89, Other immunodeficiencies,** are assigned to report immunodeficiency that places a patient at greater health risk.

Sarcoidosis

Sarcoidosis is a disease of gradual onset in which abnormal collections of inflammatory cells (granulomas) form as nodules in many organs of the body. Sarcoidosis may be asymptomatic or chronic, and its etiology is unknown. The current working hypothesis is that sarcoidosis is caused in genetically susceptible individuals through alteration in immune response after exposure to an environmental, occupational, or infectious agent. The granulomas most often appear in the lungs or the lymph nodes, but any organ can be affected. ICD-10-CM provides unique codes within category D86, Sarcoidosis, for the most common sites affected, such as lungs (D86.0), lymph nodes (D86.1), lung with lymph nodes (D86.2), skin (D86.3), meninges (D86.81), cranial nerves (D86.82), eye uvea

(D86.83), kidney and ureters (D86.84), myocardium (D86.85), joints (D86.86), muscles (D86.87), and other sites, such as liver (D86.89), as well as a code for unspecified sarcoidosis (D86.9).

Cytokine Release Syndrome

Cytokine release syndrome (CRS) is a widespread inflammatory response caused by a large and rapid release of cytokines into the blood from immune cells that have been affected by immunotherapy treatment. CRS is the most common reaction after chimeric antigen receptor T-cell (CAR-T) therapy, which is used to treat relapsed or refractory acute lymphoblastic leukemia. When cytokines are released, symptoms range from low-grade constitutional symptoms to high-grade syndrome associated with life-threatening organ dysfunction. Mild to moderate symptoms include fever, weakness, headache, rash, rapid heartbeat, low blood pressure, and respiratory distress. Severe reactions include fluid overload and renal insufficiency. Subcategory D89.83, Cytokine release syndrome, is assigned for CRS with a sixth character to identify the grade of the condition, when documented by the provider.

EXERCISE 16.5

Code the following diagnoses.

1. Pancytopenia, congenital

2. Cyclic neutropenia

3. Hereditary thrombocytopenia

4. Anemia

   Neutropenia

   Thrombocytopenia

5. Autoerythrocyte sensitization purpura

6. Cell-mediated immune deficiency with thrombocytopenia and eczema

7. Sarcoidosis of lung and lymph nodes

8. Pernicious anemia, Addison type

9. Acute gastritis with hemorrhage, exacerbated by heparin therapy, initial encounter

10. Autoimmune lymphoproliferative syndrome

Diseases of the Nervous System and Sense Organs

CHAPTER OVERVIEW

- Nervous system diseases can be found in chapter 6 of ICD-10-CM.

- Diseases of the eye and adnexa can be found in chapter 7 of ICD-10-CM, and diseases of the ear and mastoid process are found in chapter 8.

- Dual coding is often required for infectious diseases of the central nervous system.

- Pain can be coded by recording the site of the pain.

  — Codes for pain, not elsewhere classified (G89), can be used for coding pain control or management.

  — If the cause is known but not treated during the encounter, code the cause as an additional diagnosis.

- Coding professionals must be careful when coding seizures to epilepsy. Seizures may be caused by a variety of conditions and should be coded accordingly.

- Other diseases of the central nervous system covered in this chapter of the handbook are hemiplegia, Parkinson's disease, autonomic dysreflexia, and narcolepsy.

- Many problems of the peripheral nervous system are manifestations of other conditions.

  — These problems are assigned as additional codes.

  — Critical illness polyneuropathy and critical illness myopathy, for example, are complications of sepsis.

- Eye diseases are extremely complicated to code, and understanding the terminology and diagnostic statement completely is vital to proper coding.

- Eye diseases and conditions covered in this handbook include corneal injuries (from both light and wounding), conjunctivitis, cataracts, and glaucoma.

- Hearing loss may be coded as conductive, sensorineural, or a combination of the two.

LEARNING OUTCOMES

After studying this chapter, you should be able to:

Explain the difference between the central and peripheral nervous systems and locate the two areas in ICD-10-CM.

Understand how to code for pain.

Explain what is needed before a code of epilepsy is assigned.

Code for a variety of conditions of the nervous system.

Code disorders of the eye and ear.

TERMS TO KNOW

Central nervous system
the brain and spinal cord

Conductive hearing loss
hearing loss due to a problem with a part of the ear

Peripheral nervous system
all elements of the nervous system except the brain and spinal cord

Sensorineural hearing loss
hearing loss due to a problem with the sensory part of the ear or the nerves associated with hearing

REMEMBER . . .

For legal and personal reasons, a code for epilepsy cannot be assigned unless epilepsy is clearly diagnosed by a physician.

INTRODUCTION

Diseases of the nervous system are classified in chapter 6 of ICD-10-CM. Eye and adnexa diseases can be found in chapter 7 of ICD-10-CM, and diseases of the ear and mastoid process are found in chapter 8. Because the nervous system is complex and difficult to comprehend, thinking of it as a two-level system may help to simplify the coding process:

G00–G47; G80–G99   Central nervous system (brain and spinal cord)

G50–G73   Peripheral nervous system (all other neural elements in the rest of the body)

Cerebral degeneration, Parkinson's disease, and meningitis are conditions affecting the central nervous system. Polyneuropathy, myasthenia gravis, and muscular dystrophies affect the peripheral nerves. The peripheral nervous system includes the autonomic nervous system, which regulates the activity of the cardiac muscle, smooth muscle, and glands.

FIGURE 17.1   The Nervous System

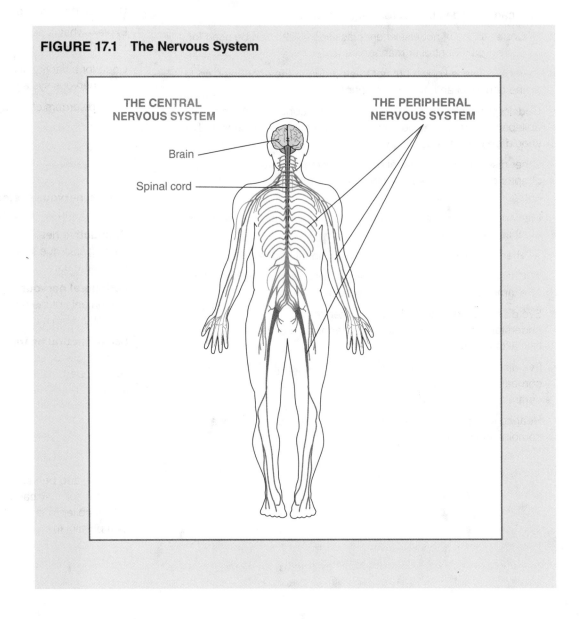

INFLAMMATORY DISEASES OF THE CENTRAL NERVOUS SYSTEM

Inflammatory diseases of the central nervous system include meningitis and encephalitis. The etiology of such conditions can be infectious or noninfectious. Infectious diseases of the central nervous system are classified in several ways, and it is imperative to carefully follow the directions provided by the Alphabetic Index and Tabular List. Dual coding is frequently required, with the code for the underlying condition sequenced first, followed by a manifestation code. For example, meningitis due to poliovirus is classified as **A80.9, Acute poliomyelitis, unspecified,** with a manifestation code of **G02, Meningitis in other infectious and parasitic diseases classified elsewhere.** Bacterial meningitis due to certain organisms such as *Pneumococcus, Streptococcus,* and *Staphylococcus* is classified in category G00, with a fourth character indicating the responsible organism. Codes G00.2–G00.8 also require an additional code to further specify the organism. Care should be exercised to determine whether the condition should be coded to the nervous system, or if there are combination codes in the Infectious Disease chapter that include the condition as well as the infectious organism. For example, candidal meningitis is coded to B37.5 and meningitis due to Lyme disease is coded to A69.21 rather than to categories G01 or G02.

EXERCISE 17.1

Code the following diagnoses.

1. Candidal meningitis

2. Poliovirus encephalitis

3. Encephalitis due to rubella

4. Herpes zoster with meningitis

5. *Staphylococcus aureus* meningitis

PARKINSON'S DISEASE

Parkinson's disease is a progressive disorder of the nervous system, which typically affects middle-aged adults. It is associated with degeneration of the basal ganglia and a deficiency of the neurotransmitter dopamine. Parkinson's disease affects movement, and tremors are a well-known sign of the disease. Parkinsonism refers to symptoms characteristic of Parkinson's disease (e.g., slow movements and tremors), regardless of the cause, and is typically caused by another condition or external agent, such as drugs.

Parkinson's disease is assigned to code G20 and includes primary parkinsonism. Secondary Parkinson's disease (G21.-) can be an adverse effect of the therapeutic use of medication, in which case a code from category G21 (e.g., G21.0, G21.11, G21.19) is assigned first, followed by code T43.3X5-, T43.4X5-, T43.505-, T43.595-, or a code from T36–T50 with fifth or sixth character 5 as an additional code to identify the responsible drug. Secondary parkinsonism may also be postencephalitic (G21.3), vascular (G21.4), other (G21.8), or unspecified (G21.9). Parkinson's disease is sometimes caused by syphilis; in that case, it is coded to **A52.19, Other symptomatic neurosyphilis.** For Parkinson's disease with dementia, assign code **G20, Parkinson's disease,** followed by code **F02.80, Dementia in other diseases classified elsewhere without behavioral disturbance.**

ALZHEIMER'S DISEASE

Alzheimer's disease is a process of progressive atrophy involving the degeneration of nerve cells. This degeneration leads to mental changes that range from subtle intellectual impairment to dementia with loss of cognitive functions and failure of memory. Alzheimer's disease is coded to category G30 and is further subdivided to specify early onset (G30.0), late onset (G30.1), other (G30.8), or unspecified (G30.9). Dementia is an inherent part of Alzheimer's disease. The provider does not need to document the condition separately for a patient with Alzheimer's disease. A code from subcategory F02.8-, Dementia in conditions classified elsewhere, is assigned as an additional diagnosis per the Alphabetic Index instructions to specify the presence or absence of behavioral disturbance. For example:

G30.9 + F02.80   Alzheimer's disease

G30.1 + F02.81   Dementia with behavioral disturbance due to late onset Alzheimer's disease

EPILEPSY

Epilepsy is a paroxysmal disorder of cerebral function characterized by recurrent seizures. It should not be assumed, however, that any diagnostic statement describing convulsions or seizures should be coded to epilepsy; these conditions also occur in a number of other diseases, such as brain tumor, cerebrovascular accident, alcoholism, electrolyte imbalance, and febrile conditions. Grand mal seizures, for example, can be due to causes other than epilepsy. Because a diagnosis of epilepsy can have serious legal and personal implications for the patient, such as the inability to obtain a driver's license, a code for epilepsy must not be assigned unless the physician clearly identifies the condition as such in the diagnostic statement. When the diagnosis is stated only in terms of convulsion or seizure without any further identification of the cause, code **R56.9, Unspecified convulsions,** should be assigned. When the physician mentions a history of seizure in the workup but does not include any mention of seizures in the diagnostic statement, no code should be assigned unless clear documentation indicates that the criteria for reporting the condition have been met and the physician agrees that a code should be added. Please note that the ICD-10-CM classification assigns seizure disorder and recurrent seizures to epilepsy, code G40.909, whereas the main term **Seizure(s)** is indexed to R56.9.

ICD-10-CM provides a fifth-character subclassification for category G40, Epilepsy and recurrent seizures, that permits identification of epilepsy as intractable when so described by the physician. Terms such as "pharmacoresistant (pharmacologically resistant)," "poorly controlled," "refractory (medically)," and "treatment resistant" are considered to be equivalent to intractable. That the condition is intractable should not be assumed from general statements in the medical record. In addition, a sixth character is used to identify whether status epilepticus is present.

207

CHAPTER 17

Diseases of the
Nervous
System and
Sense Organs

EXERCISE 17.2

Code the following diagnoses. Do not assign External cause of morbidity codes.

1. Parkinson's disease

2. Secondary parkinsonism due to prescribed Thorazine (neuroleptic drug), initial encounter

3. Intractable epilepsy, grand mal type, status epilepticus

4. Poorly controlled generalized idiopathic epilepsy

5. Intractable focal epilepsy

6. Febrile convulsions, recurrent

7. Alzheimer's disease with delirium

HEADACHE AND MIGRAINE

A diagnosis of headache without any further specificity is classified to chapter 18 of ICD-10-CM and coded to **R51.9, Headache, unspecified.** Migraines are classified to category G43, whereas specific headaches are classified to category G44, Other headache syndromes, in chapter 6, Diseases of the Nervous System.

Migraine is a neurological syndrome characterized by altered bodily perceptions, severe headaches, and nausea and vomiting. Approximately one-third of people who have migraine headaches perceive an aura—unusual visual, olfactory, or other sensory experiences that signal the migraine will soon occur. The following terms are considered equivalent to intractable: "pharmacoresistant (pharmacologically resistant)," "treatment resistant," "refractory (medically)," and "poorly controlled." Status migrainosus generally refers to a severe migraine attack that lasts for more than 72 hours. However, the designation of status migrainosus should be confirmed by the physician.

ICD-10-CM classifies migraines to category G43 as follows:

G43.0-   Migraine without aura
G43.1-   Migraine with aura
G43.4-   Hemiplegic migraine
G43.5-   Persistent migraine aura without cerebral infarction
G43.6-   Persistent migraine aura with cerebral infarction
G43.7-   Chronic migraine without aura
G43.A-   Cyclical vomiting
G43.B-   Ophthalmoplegic migraine
G43.C-   Periodic headache syndromes in child or adult

208

CHAPTER 17

Diseases of the
Nervous
System and
Sense Organs

G43.D-   Abdominal migraine

G43.8-   Other migraine

G43.9-   Migraine, unspecified

Specific headaches are classified in chapter 6 of ICD-10-CM under category G44, Other headache syndromes, as follows:

G44.0-   Cluster headaches and other trigeminal autonomic cephalgias

G44.1   Vascular headache, not elsewhere classified

G44.2-   Tension-type headache

G44.3-   Posttraumatic headache

G44.4-   Drug-induced headache, not elsewhere classified

G44.5-   Complicated headache syndromes

G44.8-   Other specific headache syndromes

Headache following lumbar puncture is assigned to code **G97.1, Other reaction to spinal or lumbar puncture.**

NARCOLEPSY

Narcolepsy is a chronic neurological disorder characterized by the inability to regulate sleep and wakefulness normally. Symptoms are excessive daytime sleepiness, sleep paralysis (paralysis upon falling asleep or waking up), cataplexy (sudden, brief episodes of paralysis or muscle weakness), and vivid hallucinations (vivid dreamlike images that occur at sleep onset). Other possible symptoms are disturbed nighttime sleep, leg jerks, nightmares, and frequent awakenings. Irresistible sleep attacks may occur throughout the day regardless of the amount or quality of prior nighttime sleep. Affected individuals may fall asleep at work or school or while eating, talking, or driving.

ICD-10-CM distinguishes between subcategory G47.41- (narcolepsy) and G47.42- (narcolepsy in conditions classified elsewhere). Sixth characters distinguish between narcolepsy with cataplexy (G47.411, G47.421) and without cataplexy (G47.419, G47.429).

HEMIPLEGIA/HEMIPARESIS

Hemiplegia is paralysis of one side of the body. It is classified to category G81, with a fifth character to indicate the side affected and whether the affected side is dominant or nondominant.

When information is not available regarding whether the affected side is dominant or nondominant, and when the classification does not provide a default, code selection is as follows: For ambidextrous patients, the default should be dominant. If the left side is affected, the default is nondominant. If the right side is affected, the default is dominant. This guideline applies to codes from category G81, Hemiplegia and hemiparesis, and subcategories G83.1, Monoplegia of lower limb; G83.2, Monoplegia of upper limb; and G83.3, Monoplegia, unspecified.

Hemiplegia occurring in connection with a cerebrovascular accident (CVA) often clears quickly and is sometimes called a transient hemiplegia. Hemiplegia is not inherent to an acute CVA; therefore, a code from category G81, Hemiplegia and hemiparesis, is assigned as an additional code when it occurs. Even if hemiplegia associated with CVA resolves without treatment, it affects the patient's care. Any neurological deficits caused by CVA should be reported even when they have resolved at the time of discharge.

Unilateral weakness clearly documented as associated with stroke is also synonymous with hemiparesis and hemiplegia. Likewise, weakness of one extremity associated with a stroke is synonymous with monoplegia. Weakness outside of this clear association cannot be assumed to be hemiparesis/hemiplegia or monoplegia unless it is associated with some other brain disorder or injury.

209

CHAPTER 17

Diseases of the

Nervous

System and

Sense Organs

When the patient is admitted at a later time with hemiplegia/hemiparesis or weakness of one extremity (upper or lower) due to sequela of cerebrovascular disease, a code from category I69 is assigned to indicate that the condition is a late effect of a CVA. (See chapter 27 of this handbook for more discussion of cerebrovascular disease.)

Examples of appropriate coding for hemiplegia follow:

I66.9 + G81.91	Cerebral thrombosis with transient right hemiplegia that has cleared by discharge
I66.9 + G81.91	Cerebral thrombosis with hemiplegia right dominant side
I69.352	Hemiplegia of left dominant side due to previous CVA
G81.90 + S34.109S	Hemiparesis due to old lumbar spinal cord injury

PAIN

Pain may be coded by reporting the site of pain. These codes may be found in the symptom chapter (e.g., headache, R51.9) or in the appropriate body system chapter (e.g., pain in limb, M79.609) of ICD-10-CM. Unless otherwise indicated below, codes from category G89, Pain, not elsewhere classified, may be used in conjunction with the site of pain codes if the category G89 code provides more detail about acute or chronic pain and neoplasm-related pain.

The determination of whether the pain is acute, chronic, or chronic pain syndrome is dependent on the provider's documentation. There is no time frame defining when pain becomes chronic. If the pain is not specified as acute or chronic, post-thoracotomy, postprocedural, or neoplasm related, do not assign codes from category G89. A code from category G89 should not be assigned if the underlying (definitive) diagnosis is known, unless the reason for the encounter is pain control/ management and not management of the underlying condition.

When an admission or encounter is for a procedure aimed at treating the underlying condition, such as a spinal fusion for treatment of pain associated with a vertebral fracture, a code for the underlying condition (e.g., vertebral fracture) should be assigned as the principal diagnosis. No code from category G89 should be assigned.

Encounter/Admission for Pain Control/Management

Category G89 codes may be used as the principal diagnosis or first-listed code when pain control or pain management is the reason for the admission/encounter. These encounters are typically not for diagnostic workup or treatment of the underlying condition but for management of pain. In these situations, if the underlying cause of the pain is known, report it as an additional diagnosis. An example is a patient with displaced intervertebral disc, nerve impingement, and severe back pain who presents for injection of steroid into the spinal canal. The injection is intended to relieve the pain, but it does not treat the displaced disc.

If the admission is for control of pain related to, associated with, or due to a malignancy, code **G89.3, Neoplasm related pain (acute) (chronic),** should be assigned. The underlying neoplasm is reported as an additional diagnosis. Because the neoplasm code will provide information regarding the specific site, an additional code for the site of pain should not be assigned. When the reason for the admission/encounter is management of the neoplasm and the pain associated with the neoplasm is also documented, code G89.3 may be assigned as an additional diagnosis. It is not necessary to assign an additional code for the site of the pain.

If the admission or encounter is for a procedure to treat the underlying condition, the underlying condition should be assigned as the principal or first-listed diagnosis. For example, if a patient is admitted for a spinal fusion to treat lumbar spinal stenosis with neurogenic claudication, assign code **M48.062, Spinal stenosis, lumbar region, with neurogenic claudication,** as the principal diagnosis. No code from category G89 should be assigned.

Patients with chronic pain whose conservative therapies have failed may undergo insertion of neurostimulators for pain control. In such cases, the appropriate pain code is assigned as the principal or first-listed diagnosis. When an admission or encounter is for a procedure aimed at treating the underlying condition, and a neurostimulator is inserted for pain control during the same admission/encounter, a code for the underlying condition should be assigned as the principal diagnosis with the pain code as a secondary diagnosis.

If the encounter is for any other reason except pain control or pain management and a related, definitive diagnosis for the pain has not been established (confirmed) by the provider, the code for the specific site of pain should be assigned first, followed by the appropriate code from category G89. If the definitive diagnosis has been established, assign the code for the definitive diagnosis.

Postoperative Pain

Post-thoracotomy pain and other postoperative pain are classified to subcategories G89.1 and G89.2, depending on whether the pain is acute or chronic. The default for post-thoracotomy and other postoperative pain not specified as acute or chronic is the code for the acute form. Postoperative pain associated with a specific postoperative complication (such as painful wire sutures) or associated with devices, implants, or grafts left in a surgical site (such as a painful hip prosthesis) is assigned to the appropriate code(s) found in chapter 19 of ICD-10-CM, Injury, Poisoning, and Certain Other Consequences of External Causes. A code from category G89 is assigned as an additional code to identify acute or chronic pain (G89.18 or G89.28).

Postoperative pain may be reported as the principal or first-listed diagnosis when the reason for the encounter or admission is postoperative pain control/management. Postoperative pain may be reported as a secondary diagnosis code when a patient has outpatient surgery and develops an unusual or inordinate amount of postoperative pain. Please note that routine or expected postoperative pain immediately after surgery should not be coded.

AUTONOMIC DYSREFLEXIA

Autonomic dysreflexia is a syndrome characterized by an abrupt onset of excessively high blood pressure caused by an uncontrolled sympathetic nervous system discharge in persons with spinal cord injury, usually at or above the T6 level. Anything that would ordinarily cause pain below this level may trigger a parasympathetic response resulting in bradycardia, blurred vision, and sweating. True autonomic dysreflexia is potentially life threatening and is considered a medical emergency. Code **G90.4, Autonomic dysreflexia,** is used to report this condition. It is not necessary to code each manifestation or symptom separately. In most dual coding scenarios, the underlying condition is listed first; however, in this case, the code for the dysreflexia is sequenced first, followed by an additional code for the underlying chronic condition that has precipitated this life-threatening condition (e.g., pressure ulcer, fecal impaction, urinary tract infection).

HYDROCEPHALUS

Normal pressure hydrocephalus (NPH) or secondary NPH can be caused by any condition in which the flow of cerebrospinal fluid (CSF) is blocked, such as subarachnoid hemorrhage, head trauma, cerebral infarction, infection, tumor, or complications of surgery. Assign code **G91.0, Communicating hydrocephalus,** for secondary NPH. Obstructive hydrocephalus develops secondary to a blockage in the normal circulation of CSF in the brain. In most instances, the blockage affects the third and fourth ventricles at the level of the aqueduct of Sylvius, also referred to as an aqueductal obstruction, which can result from scarring or tumor. Assign code **G91.1, Obstructive hydrocephalus,** for this acquired condition. Idiopathic normal pressure hydrocephalus (INPH) can occur without any identifiable cause. Code **G91.2, (Idiopathic) normal pressure hydrocephalus**

211

CHAPTER 17

*Diseases of the
Nervous
System and
Sense Organs*

(INPH), is assigned for this type of acquired hydrocephalus. If the medical record documentation does not specify whether the hydrocephalus is congenital or acquired, code **G91.9 Hydrocephalus, unspecified,** should be assigned.

ENCEPHALOPATHY

Encephalopathy is a general term used to describe any disorder of cerebral function. It is a very broad term and, in most cases, will be preceded by various terms describing the reason, cause, or special conditions leading to the brain disorder. It is important to carefully note these additional terms, as they will affect code assignment. More than 150 different terms modify or precede "encephalopathy" in the medical literature—not all of them are classified to chapter 6 of ICD-10-CM. Some of the more common encephalopathies are noted below:

- *Anoxic encephalopathy* refers to brain damage due to lack of oxygen. This type of encephalopathy is assigned to **G93.1, Anoxic brain damage, not elsewhere classified.**

- *Alcoholic encephalopathy* is a serious complication of alcoholic liver disease usually caused by excessive drinking for several years. It results in a loss of specific brain function (damage of brain tissue) caused by a thiamine deficiency. Alcoholic encephalopathy is classified to **G31.2, Degeneration of nervous system due to alcohol.**

- *Hepatic encephalopathy* is brain damage due to liver disease, and it is classified to code **K72.90, Hepatic failure, unspecified, without coma,** when the etiology is not specified or is unknown. At the Index entry "Failure, hepatic," there are subentries for codes to specifically describe different etiologies and for hepatic failure with or without coma. Hepatic encephalopathy is not synonymous with hepatic coma. The default for hepatic failure is without coma.

- *Metabolic encephalopathy* is temporary or permanent damage to the brain due to lack of glucose, oxygen, or other metabolic agent, or caused by organ dysfunction. Symptoms include an altered state of consciousness, usually characterized as delirium, confusion, or agitation, and changes in behavior or personality. There may also be muscle stiffness or rigidity, tremor, stupor, or coma. Symptoms can develop quickly and may resolve when the condition is reversed. Assign code **G93.41, Metabolic encephalopathy,** for this condition. Code G93.41 also includes septic encephalopathy.

- *Toxic encephalopathy* is also known as *toxic metabolic encephalopathy.* This type of encephalopathy is a degenerative neurological disorder caused by exposure to toxic substances or as an adverse effect of medication. It is characterized by an altered mental status, and symptoms can include memory loss, small personality changes, lack of concentration, involuntary movements, nausea, fatigue, seizures, arm strength problems, and depression. ICD-10-CM classifies this condition to code **G92, Toxic encephalopathy.** The appropriate reporting and sequencing of toxic encephalopathy due to drugs is based on whether the drug toxicity qualifies as an adverse effect or poisoning. When coding an adverse effect of a drug that has been correctly prescribed and properly administered, assign the appropriate code for the nature of the adverse effect followed by the appropriate code for the adverse effect of the drug (T36–T50). The code for the drug will have a fifth or sixth character 5 (e.g., T36.0x5-) to indicate adverse effect. If the toxic encephalopathy is due to a poisoning from a toxic agent, a code from categories T51–T65 is assigned first to identify the causative toxic agent.

- *Wernicke's encephalopathy* involves damage to the central nervous system and the peripheral nervous system and is caused by disorders of the liver such as cirrhosis, hepatitis, malnutrition, and conditions in which blood circulation bypasses the liver entirely. The symptoms can range from mild to severe and consist of various neurological symptoms including changes in consciousness, reflexes, and behavior. ICD-10-CM classifies this condition to **E51.2, Wernicke's encephalopathy.**

212

CHAPTER 17

Diseases of the

Nervous

System and

Sense Organs

- *Encephalopathy associated with cerebrovascular accident and stroke* is not inherent to the conditions; assign code **G93.49, Other encephalopathy**, in addition to the codes for cerebrovascular accident and stroke. Please note code **G93.49, Other encephalopathy**, is assigned when encephalopathy is linked to a condition (e.g., encephalopathy due to urinary tract infection) but a specific encephalopathy (e.g., metabolic, toxic, or hypertensive) is not documented.
- *Unspecified encephalopathy* is assigned to code **G93.40, Encephalopathy, unspecified**.

Code **G94, Other disorders of brain in diseases classified elsewhere**, should only be assigned for those conditions with Alphabetic Index entries that directly point to G94 for certain etiologies.

EXERCISE 17.3

Code the following diagnoses and procedures. Do not assign External cause of morbidity codes.

1. Chronic intractable tension-type headache

2. Cerebrovascular accident with left-sided weakness

3. Severe hypertension and pounding headache due to autonomic dysreflexia due to fecal impaction

4. Severe chronic low back pain due to displaced lumbar disc with neuritis due to previous trauma. Epidural injection of steroid (anti-inflammatory) for pain

5. Metabolic encephalopathy

6. Toxic metabolic encephalopathy due to accidental carbon monoxide asphyxiation, utility gas, initial encounter

---

DISORDERS OF THE PERIPHERAL NERVOUS SYSTEM

Disorders of the peripheral nervous system are classified to categories G50 through G73 according to the condition and the nerves involved. Many codes in this section are manifestations of other diseases and are assigned as additional codes, with the underlying condition listed first.

CRITICAL ILLNESS POLYNEUROPATHY

Critical illness polyneuropathy is commonly associated with complications of sepsis and multiple organ failure. It is considered to be secondary to systemic inflammatory response syndrome. Synonyms for critical illness polyneuropathy include neuropathy of critical illness, intensive care unit neuropathy, and intensive care polyneuropathy. Patients with this condition show abnormal electrophysiological changes consistent with primary axonal degeneration of motor fibers. They also demonstrate severe weakness, making it difficult to wean them from mechanical ventilation. Assign code **G62.81, Critical illness polyneuropathy,** for this condition.

CRITICAL ILLNESS MYOPATHY

Critical illness myopathy is associated with sepsis, the use of neuromuscular blocking agents and corticosteroids (in asthma and organ transplant patients), and neuropathy. It is a cause of difficulty in weaning patients from mechanical ventilation and prolonged recovery after illness. Code **G72.81, Critical illness myopathy,** is used to report this condition.

CEREBROSPINAL FLUID LEAK

Cerebrospinal fluid leaks occur when a tear in the dura allows the escape of the fluid that surrounds and protects the brain or spinal cord. Spontaneous cerebrospinal fluid leak that occurs for no known reason is assigned to code G96.01 (cranial) or G96.02 (spinal). Other cerebrospinal fluid leak is assigned to code G96.08 (cranial) or G96.09 (spinal). Code G96.00 is assigned for unspecified cerebrospinal fluid leak.

INTRACRANIAL HYPOTENSION

The reduction of cerebrospinal fluid volume and pressure results in intracranial hypotension. Intracranial hypotension is most often associated with a cerebrospinal fluid leak at the spinal level. Headache is the most common symptom; however, there are other signs and symptoms caused by the effects of the leak on surrounding nerve roots and other structures. Spontaneous intracranial hypotension is assigned to code G96.811. Other intracranial hypotension is assigned to code G96.819. Unspecified intracranial hypotension is assigned to code G96.810.

Intracranial hypotension caused by a procedure is included in subcategory G97.8, Other intraoperative and postprocedural complications and disorders of nervous system. When the condition is due to a shunting device, assign code **G97.83, Intracranial hypotension following lumbar cerebrospinal fluid shunting.** Assign code **G97.84, Intracranial hypotension following other procedure,** when it is due to another procedure.

EXERCISE 17.4

Code the following diagnoses and procedures.

1. Amyloid polyneuropathy

2. Morton's neuroma, 3–4 and 4–5 interspaces, left foot
   Excision of Morton's neuroma, left foot

214

CHAPTER 17

Diseases of the
Nervous
System and
Sense Organs

3. Tardy palsy due to entrapment of right ulnar nerve

_____

4. Peripheral polyneuritis, severe, due to chronic alcoholism

_____

5. Nutritional polyneuropathy

_____

6. Tic douloureux

_____

DISORDERS OF THE EYE AND ADNEXAE

The classification for diseases of the eye is very detailed, and understanding the terminology used is especially important for the coding professional. Terms that seem similar may have entirely different meanings. Be sure to fully understand the diagnostic statement in the medical record before assigning a code.

Visual impairment (H54) is classified according to severity, with the status of the lesser eye listed first and the better eye listed second in the code title. If the associated underlying cause of the blindness or visual loss is known, it should be coded first. ICD-10-CM includes a table with the classification of severity of visual impairment recommended by a World Health Organization study group. The term "low vision" in category H54 comprises categories 1 and 2 of the table; the term "blindness," categories 3, 4, and 5; and the term "unqualified visual loss," category 9. The information is intended to provide "clues" to identify possible gaps in documentation where provider query may be necessary. It is not intended to replace the need for specific provider documentation to substantiate code assignment. Sample codes include the following:

H54.1141   Blindness, right eye category 4, low vision left eye category 1
H54.413A   Blindness, right eye category 3, normal vision left eye

Assign code **H54.3, Unqualified visual loss, both eyes,** when "blindness" or "low vision" of both eyes is documented but the visual impairment category is not documented. Assign a code from subcategory H54.6, Unqualified visual loss, one eye, if "blindness" or "low vision" in one eye is documented but the visual impairment category is not documented. Assign code **H54.7, Unspecified visual loss,** when "blindness" or "visual loss" is documented without information about whether one or both eyes are affected by the condition.

Occasionally, visual problems can cause tilting of the head, resulting in ocular torticollis or ocular-induced torticollis. Torticollis refers to abnormal head posture. Palsy of the superior or inferior oblique muscles causes the patient to hold the head at an angle to compensate for the visual disturbance. Ocular torticollis is coded by assigning first the appropriate code for the ocular condition causing the torticollis, e.g., nystagmus (H55.-), strabismus (H50.9), or fourth nerve palsy (H49.1-), followed by code **R29.891, Ocular torticollis.**

Corneal Injury

Code **H16.13-, Photokeratitis,** is assigned for a corneal flash burn, generally referred to as ultraviolet keratitis. The condition typically occurs at high altitudes on highly reflective snow fields or, less often, with a solar eclipse. Artificial sources of ultraviolet light can also cause photokeratitis. These sources include sun-tanning beds, a welder's arc (flash burn, welder's flash, or arc eye), carbon arcs, photographic flood lamps, lightning, electric sparks, and halogen desk lamps. It is always an injury, and the appropriate External cause of morbidity code should be assigned as an additional code, such as codes from category W89, Exposure to man-made visible and ultraviolet light, or code **X32.-, Exposure to sunlight.**

215

CHAPTER 17

Diseases of the
Nervous
System and
Sense Organs

FIGURE 17.2 The Eye

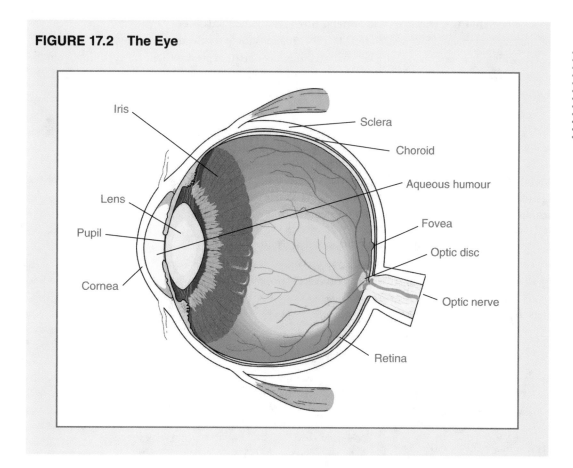

Corneal or corneoscleral lacerations are classified in category S05, Injury of eye and orbit. The fourth characters are assigned to indicate whether there is contusion of eyeball and orbital tissues, whether there is associated prolapse or loss of intraocular tissue, whether the laceration is a penetrating injury, whether the laceration is with or without a foreign body, whether there is avulsion of the eye, and whether the laceration is related to other conditions. The fifth characters indicate unspecified eye, right eye, or left eye. An External cause of morbidity code is assigned for the external cause. Corneal repair is classified as **08Q8XZZ, Repair right cornea, external approach,** or **08Q9XZZ, Repair left cornea, external approach.**

Conjunctivitis

Conjunctivitis (category H10) is an inflammation of the conjunctiva, which may be due to infection, allergy, or other cause.

Giant papillary conjunctivitis, also called contact lens–induced papillary conjunctivitis, is a common complication of contact lens wear. It is an inflammation resulting from an allergic reaction to contact lenses. Chronic giant papillary conjunctivitis is classified to subcategory H10.41-. Vernal conjunctivitis (H10.44) is due to an allergic reaction to pollen. When the cause of acute conjunctivitis is a chemical or toxic agent, code H10.21- is used, with a code from categories T51–T65 assigned first to identify the chemical agent and intent (e.g., accidental, assault). Conjunctivitis due to chlamydia is classified to A74.0 or to A71.1 when designated as due to trachoma.

Disorders of conjunctivochalasis are reported using code H11.82-. With these disorders, the redundant conjunctiva lies over the lower eyelid margin and covers the lower punctum. This situation can create a variety of symptoms, from aggravation of a dry eye at the mild stage to disruption of the normal flow of tears at the moderate stage to exposure problems at the severe stage. Treatment consists of a simple local surgical excision to relieve the symptoms.

216

CHAPTER 17

*Diseases of the
Nervous
System and
Sense Organs*

Code **H04.12-, Dry eye syndrome,** is provided by the Index for dry eye syndrome, a disorder of the lacrimal gland. However, code H04.12- is inappropriate for the dry eye associated with Bell's palsy, which does not involve the lacrimal gland but is due to exposure to the air resulting from the inability to close the eye as a result of the acute severe facial paralysis of Bell's palsy. Code **H16.21-, Exposure keratoconjunctivitis,** is assigned for dry eye related to Bell's palsy.

Corneal Dystrophies

Corneal dystrophies are genetic eye disorders that are caused by the accumulation of abnormal material on the cornea. These disorders are classified based on the clinical presentation of the lesion (resembling the overlapping pattern of a lattice) and the layer of the cornea affected by the lesion. Several subcategories identify corneal dystrophy with seventh characters for laterality:

H18.50-	Unspecified hereditary corneal dystrophies
H18.51-	Endothelial corneal dystrophy
H18.52-	Epithelial (juvenile) corneal dystrophy
H18.53-	Granular corneal dystrophy
H18.54-	Lattice corneal dystrophy
H18.55-	Macular corneal dystrophy
H18.59-	Other hereditary corneal dystrophies

EXERCISE 17.5

Code the following diagnoses. Do not assign External cause of morbidity codes.

1. Intermittent monocular esotropia right eye

2. Senile entropion, left upper eyelid

3. Blepharoptosis, congenital, bilateral

4. Ectropion due to cicatrix left upper eyelid

5. Conjunctivochalasis, bilateral

Cataracts

When coding cataracts, avoid making assumptions about the type of cataract based on the patient's age or other conditions. A cataract in an older patient is not necessarily senile or mature; be alert to the terminology used in the diagnostic statement. ICD-10-CM presumes a causal relationship between diabetes and cataracts based on the linkage in the Alphabetic Index by the subterms "with" and "in." Diabetes and cataracts should be coded as related even in the absence of provider documentation explicitly linking them. For example, if a patient with diabetes is documented as having an "age-related cataract" or "senile cataract," the cataract should be coded as a diabetic cataract.

EXERCISE 17.6

Code the following diagnoses. Do not assign External cause of morbidity codes.

1. Diabetic cataract in type 1 diabetes mellitus

2. Incipient senile cataract, right eye

   Diabetes mellitus, type 2

3. Myotonic cataract with Thomsen's disease

4. Steroid-induced cataract, bilateral

   Long-term use of Prednisone for chronic

   obstructive asthma, severe persistent asthma

5. Trauma to the left eye six years ago,

   causing left cataract and mydriasis

Glaucoma

Glaucoma is an eye disease characterized by increased intraocular pressure that causes pathological changes in the optic disk and defects in the field of vision. Codes in category H40, Glaucoma, use either the fourth character or the fourth and fifth characters to classify glaucoma by type; most codes in this category also use a fifth or sixth character to identify the affected eye. In addition, codes in subcategories H40.1-, H40.20-, H40.22-, H40.3-, H40.4-, H40.5-, and H40.6- require a seventh character for the stage (unspecified, mild, moderate, severe, or indeterminate). Assign as many codes from category H40 as needed to identify the type of glaucoma, the affected eye, and the glaucoma stage.

It is possible for a patient to have bilateral glaucoma, with each eye being of the same or different types, and the same or different glaucoma stages in each eye. Specific guidelines have been created to address the coding of these situations. The guidelines largely vary on the basis of whether or not the classification distinguishes laterality; subcategories H40.10- and H40.20- do not distinguish laterality; the other subcategories do. Table 17.1 summarizes these guidelines.

When a patient is admitted with glaucoma and the stage of the glaucoma progresses during the admission, only the code for the highest stage documented is coded. Care should be taken not to confuse a glaucoma in which the stage is unspecified or not documented (seventh character 0) with a glaucoma stage documented as indeterminate (seventh character 4). The assignment of the indeterminate stage should be based on clinical documentation and is reserved for glaucoma whose stage cannot clinically be determined.

TABLE 17.1   Coding of Glaucoma

Bilateral Glaucoma	Classification Distinguishes Laterality	Classification Does Not Distinguish Laterality
Same type and stage	Assign one code for the type of glaucoma, bilateral, with the seventh character for the stage. **Example:** Bilateral chronic angle-closure glaucoma, mild stage H40.2231	Assign one code for the type of glaucoma, with the seventh character for the stage. **Example:** Bilateral open-angle glaucoma, mild stage H40.10x1
Same type, but different stage	Assign codes for the type of glaucoma for each eye, with the seventh character for the specific stage rather than the code for bilateral glaucoma. **Example:** Bilateral chronic angle-closure glaucoma, mild stage right eye, moderate stage left eye H40.2211 + H40.2222	Assign codes for the type of glaucoma for each eye, with seventh character for the specific stage. **Example:** Bilateral open-angle glaucoma, mild stage right eye, moderate stage left eye H40.10x1 + H40.10x2
Different type, but same stage	Assign the appropriate code for each eye rather than the code for bilateral glaucoma. **Example:** Chronic-angle closure glaucoma, mild stage left eye, low tension open-angle glaucoma, mild stage right eye H40.2221 + H40.1211	Assign codes for the specific type of glaucoma for each eye, with the seventh character for the stage. **Example:** Open-angle glaucoma, mild stage right eye, primary angle-closure glaucoma, mild stage left eye H40.10x1 + H40.20x1

Category H42, Glaucoma in diseases classified elsewhere, requires that the underlying condition be coded first, such as amyloidosis (E85.-), aniridia (Q13.1), or specified metabolic disorder (E70–E88). Glaucoma in diabetes mellitus is classified to the type of diabetes (E08–E13) with -.39. Note that glaucoma in syphilis is coded to **A52.71, Late syphilitic oculopathy,** and tuberculous glaucoma is classified to **A18.59, Other tuberculosis of eye.**

Aqueous misdirection was formerly known as malignant glaucoma. No true malignancy is associated with this type of glaucoma. Aqueous misdirection is characterized by fluid buildup in the back of the eye, pushing the lens and iris forward, blocking off the drain, and thereby increasing the intraocular pressure. This condition is extremely difficult to treat and often requires surgical intervention. Code **H40.83-, Aqueous misdirection,** is used to report this condition.

EXERCISE 17.7

Code the following diagnoses. Do not assign External cause of morbidity codes.

1. Glaucoma secondary to posterior dislocation of lens, right eye

2. Exophthalmos secondary to thyrotoxicosis

3. Acute narrow-angle glaucoma, right eye
   Chronic severe stage narrow-angle glaucoma, left eye

4. Primary open-angle glaucoma, moderate stage, bilateral

DISEASES OF THE EAR AND MASTOID PROCESS

Chapter 8 of ICD-10-CM, Diseases of the Ear and Mastoid Process, includes diseases of the external ear (H60–H62), diseases of the middle ear and mastoid (H65–H75), diseases of the inner ear (H80–H83), other disorders of the ear (H90–H94), and intraoperative and postprocedural complications and disorders of the ear and mastoid process not elsewhere classified (H95).

Otitis

Otitis is a general term for infection or inflammation of the ear. Symptoms may include chills, drainage from the ear, earache, buzzing, hearing loss, malaise, irritability, itching or discomfort in the ear or ear canal, nausea, and vomiting. Otitis can affect the inner or outer parts of the ear.

ICD-10-CM classifies otitis to the following categories on the basis of whether it affects the external or middle ear and whether it occurs suddenly and for a short time (acute) or repeatedly over a long period of time (chronic):

H60   Otitis externa
H61   Other disorders of external ear
H62   Diseases of external ear in diseases classified elsewhere
H65   Nonsuppurative otitis media
H66   Suppurative and unspecified otitis media
H67   Otitis media in diseases classified elsewhere

For otitis externa (category H60), additional characters provide further specificity regarding the condition, such as infective and noninfective (chemical, actinic, reactive, or eczematoid). Category H65, Nonsuppurative otitis media, is further divided to provide specificity for acute, subacute, or chronic, whether serous, allergic, or mucoid. Category H66, Suppurative and unspecified otitis media, is further subdivided to identify whether the condition is acute or chronic and whether there is spontaneous rupture of the ear drum.

FIGURE 17.3   The Ear

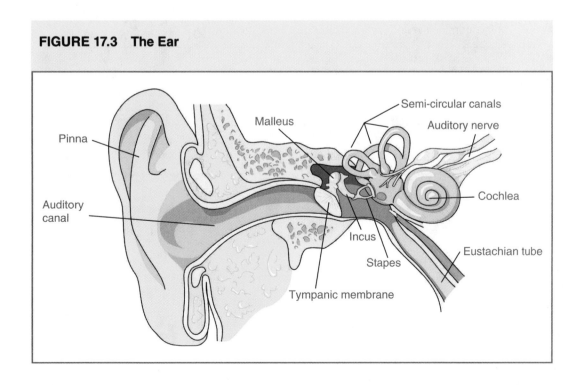

Deafness and Hearing Loss

Hearing loss may be unilateral or bilateral. Most hearing loss is classified in one of three ways:

• Conductive (H90.0–H90.2, H90.A11, and H90.A12), with the hearing loss due to a defect in the conductive apparatus of the ear (also called conduction deafness)

• Sensorineural (H90.3–H90.5, H90.A21, and H90.A22), with the hearing loss due to a defect in the sensory mechanism of the ear or nerves

• Mixed conductive and sensorineural hearing loss (H90.6–H90.8, H90.A31, and H90.A32)

Other classifications of hearing loss are related to the underlying cause, such as the following:

• Ototoxic hearing loss (H91.0-) caused by ingestion of toxic substances. When this type of hearing loss results from poisoning, it requires that a code from T36–T65 with fifth or sixth character 1–4 or 6 be assigned first. A code from T36–T50 with fifth or sixth character 5 is assigned as an additional code when the hearing loss is an adverse effect.

• Presbycusis (H91.1-), or age-related hearing loss with gradually progressing inability to hear. It is considered a sensorineural hearing loss.

• Sudden idiopathic hearing loss (H91.2-), or sudden, unexplained hearing loss.

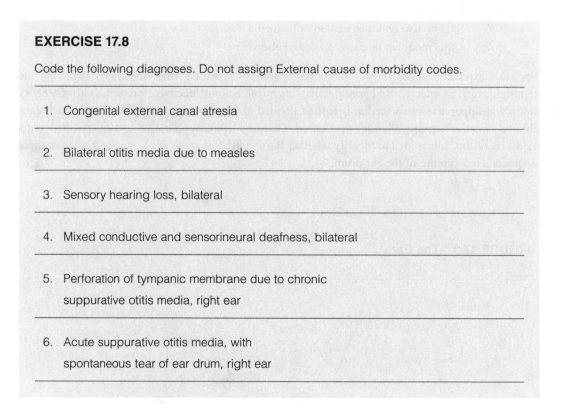

EXERCISE 17.8

Code the following diagnoses. Do not assign External cause of morbidity codes.

1. Congenital external canal atresia

2. Bilateral otitis media due to measles

3. Sensory hearing loss, bilateral

4. Mixed conductive and sensorineural deafness, bilateral

5. Perforation of tympanic membrane due to chronic
   suppurative otitis media, right ear

6. Acute suppurative otitis media, with
   spontaneous tear of ear drum, right ear

Coding of Diseases
of the Respiratory, Digestive, and Genitourinary Systems

CHAPTER 18

Diseases of the Respiratory System

CHAPTER OVERVIEW

- Respiratory diseases are classified in chapter 10 of ICD-10-CM.
- Pneumonia is a common infection that is coded several ways.
  - It is coded in combination with the responsible organism.
  - It is coded as a dual classification.
- Influenza may be coded alone or in combination with other codes.
- Chronic obstructive pulmonary disease (COPD) is always caused by another condition.
- Asthma is classified with a fourth character to indicate type and a fifth character to indicate exacerbation or status asthmaticus.
- Respiratory failure is always due to an underlying condition. Therefore, it is important to be sure that the principal diagnosis and secondary diagnosis are properly assigned.
- Acute pulmonary edema is divided into two categories.
  - Acute pulmonary edemas of cardiogenic origin take codes that are related to heart failure.
  - Those of noncardiogenic origin take a variety of codes, such as for drowning.
- Procedures involving the respiratory system have a large section of codes. Some of these procedures include biopsies of the bronchus and lung, ablation, mechanical ventilation, and respiratory assistance not considered mechanical.

LEARNING OUTCOMES

After studying this chapter, you should be able to:

- Classify the variety of types of pneumonia that you will encounter as a coding professional.
- Determine the correct coding of COPD based on the documented diagnosis.
- Know when to code for respiratory failure as the principal or secondary diagnosis.
- Know how to classify both cardiogenic and noncardiogenic acute pulmonary edemas.
- Code procedures commonly used to treat respiratory system diseases.

TERMS TO KNOW

Acute pulmonary edema
excessive fluid in the tissue and alveolar spaces of the lung

Atelectasis
a collapse of lung tissue; an integral part of pulmonary disease

Bronchospasm
a sudden constriction of the muscles in the walls of the bronchioles

COPD
chronic obstructive pulmonary disease; a general term describing conditions (e.g., emphysema, asthma, chronic bronchitis) that result in an airway obstruction

Pleural effusion
accumulation of fluid within the pleural spaces

REMEMBER . . .

Coding professionals should only code for avian influenza or other novel influenza A if the case is confirmed. Modifiers such as "suspected" are not adequate to establish a classification.

INTRODUCTION

Except for neoplastic diseases and some major infectious diseases, respiratory diseases are classified in categories J00 through J99 in chapter 10 of ICD-10-CM. Note that *Streptococcus* and *Neisseria* bacteria are normal flora for the respiratory system; therefore, their presence does not indicate an infection unless they are seriously out of control. A respiratory infection cannot be assumed from a laboratory report alone; physician concurrence and documentation are necessary. Remember also that infectious organisms are not always identified by laboratory examination, particularly when antibiotic therapy has been started; an infection code may be assigned without laboratory evidence when it is supported by clinical documentation.

PNEUMONIA

Pneumonia is a common respiratory infection that is coded in several ways in ICD-10-CM. Combination codes that account for both pneumonia and the responsible organism are included in chapters 1 and 10 of ICD-10-CM. Examples of appropriate codes for pneumonia include the following:

J15.0	Pneumonia due to *Klebsiella*
J15.211	Pneumonia due to *Staphylococcus aureus*
A02.22	Salmonella pneumonia
B05.2	Post measles pneumonia
J11.08 + J12.9	Viral pneumonia with influenza

FIGURE 18.1   The Respiratory System

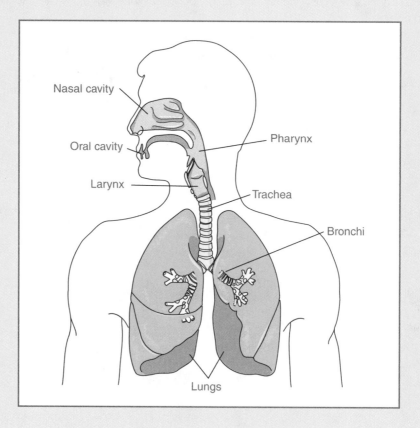

Other pneumonias are coded as manifestations of underlying infections classified in chapter 1, and two codes are required in such cases. Examples of this dual classification coding include the following:

I00+J17   Pneumonia in rheumatic fever
B65.9+J17 Pneumonia due to schistosomiasis

When the diagnostic statement is pneumonia without any further specification, review laboratory reports for mention of the causative organism and check with the physician to determine whether there is support for a more definitive diagnosis. When the organism is not identified, code **J18.9, Pneumonia, unspecified organism,** is assigned.

Pneumocystis pneumonia

Pneumocystis pneumonia (PCP) is a serious infection caused by the fungus *Pneumocystis jirovecii* (which used to be called *Pneumocystis carinii*). The condition is coded as **B59, Pneumocystosis.** It is frequently seen in patients with weakened immune systems, such as those with HIV disease or AIDS. Prior to the availability of antiretroviral therapy, this condition was a major cause of death among AIDS patients. When associated with AIDS, code B20 is sequenced first with an additional code of B59. However, this type of pneumonia is not limited to patients with AIDS. It may develop in patients with immunocompromised states due to other causes, such as cancer, severe malnutrition, or debility. It may also occur in patients treated with certain types of immunosuppressive drugs after undergoing organ transplantation or cancer treatment.

Lobar Pneumonia

A diagnosis of "lobar pneumonia" typically involves consolidation of one or more lobes of the lung, meaning there is consolidation of an entire lobe rather than the presence of infiltrates in a lobe. The various types of pneumonia usually have different patterns on radiological imaging. Lobar pneumonia should be coded according to the responsible organism, if known. Examples include:

J13   Left lobar pneumococcal pneumonia
J15.211 Multilobar *Staphylococcus aureus* pneumonia

If the provider is unable to identify the organism causing the lobar or multilobar pneumonia, assign code **J18.1, Lobar pneumonia, unspecified organism.** When the specific organism causing the pneumonia is documented, assign the combination code to indicate the specific pneumonia with the responsible organism. Lobar pneumonia should be coded based on specific provider documentation rather than based on an imaging report that specifies pneumonia in a specific lobe, part of a lobe, or multiple lobes.

Interstitial Lung Diseases

Interstitial lung diseases are a group of scarring diseases of the lung of unknown etiology with distinctive presentation, pathophysiology, and clinical course. Subcategories J84.1–J84.9 provide codes for several specific types. For example:

J84.112 Idiopathic pulmonary fibrosis
J84.113 Idiopathic non-specific interstitial pneumonitis
J84.114 Acute interstitial pneumonitis
J84.115 Respiratory bronchiolitis interstitial lung disease
J84.116 Cryptogenic organizing pneumonia

J84.2   Lymphoid interstitial pneumonia

J84.89   Bronchiolitis obliterans organized pneumonia

Childhood interstitial lung disease (subcategory J84.84) is rarer than interstitial lung disease in adults and is typically associated with respiratory distress, diffuse infiltrates on chest imaging, and abnormal lung histology. Codes for childhood interstitial lung disease include:

J84.841   Neuroendocrine cell hyperplasia of infancy

J84.842   Pulmonary interstitial glycogenosis

J84.843   Alveolar capillary dysplasia with vein misalignment

J84.848   Other interstitial lung diseases of childhood

If not more specifically identified, interstitial pneumonia is classified in ICD-10-CM as **J84.9, Interstitial pulmonary disease, unspecified.**

Lymphoid interstitial pneumonia (J84.2) is a rare disorder with lymphocytic infiltration of the alveolar interstitium and air spaces. It is the most common cause of pulmonary disease after *Pneumocystis* infection in HIV-positive children. It most often occurs in children with HIV infection and in people of any age with an autoimmune disorder.

Legionnaires' Disease

Legionnaires' disease (A48.1) is a type of pneumonia that is almost always caused by inhalation of aerosols that come from a water source contaminated with *Legionella* bacteria. This disease usually occurs as single, isolated cases not associated with any recognized outbreak. The fatality rate of Legionnaires' disease has ranged from 5 percent to 30 percent during various outbreaks.

Gram-Negative Pneumonia

Gram-negative pneumonia not elsewhere classified is classified as **J15.6, Pneumonia due to other aerobic Gram-negative bacteria,** or as **J15.8, Pneumonia due to other specified bacteria,** when it is specified as anaerobic. When the organism has been identified, the Alphabetic Index may provide a more specific code. Gram-negative organisms develop a particular type of stain on testing and are considered part of a group of organisms that require careful management. Gram-positive pneumonia, not otherwise qualified, is classified as **J15.9, Unspecified bacterial pneumonia.** Gram-positive pneumonia is far easier to treat, and requires the expenditure of fewer resources, than gram-negative pneumonia.

Gram-negative pneumonia most often affects people who are hospitalized, infants, the elderly, people with alcoholism, and patients with chronic diseases, particularly immune system disorders. These bacteria rarely infect the lungs of healthy adults. The symptoms of gram-negative bacterial pneumonia are similar to those for gram-positive pneumonia. However, patients with gram-negative pneumonia tend to be sicker, and their condition deteriorates quickly because the bacteria can rapidly destroy lung tissue. About 25 percent to 50 percent of patients with gram-negative pneumonia die, in spite of treatment.

A diagnosis of gram-negative or other bacterial pneumonia cannot be assumed on the basis of the presence of laboratory or clinical findings alone; only the physician can determine the diagnosis. Such findings can, however, help document a diagnosis or serve as the basis for a query to the doctor.

Aspergillosis

Pneumonia due to infectious aspergillosis is classified as code **B44.9, Aspergillosis, unspecified.** However, code **B44.81, Allergic bronchopulmonary aspergillosis,** is assigned to allergic bronchopulmonary or pulmonary aspergillosis. This eosinophilic pneumonia is caused by an allergic reaction to the aspergillosis fungus, commonly found on dead leaves, bird droppings, compost stacks, or other decaying vegetation.

Aspiration Pneumonia

Aspiration pneumonia is a severe type of pneumonia resulting from the inhalation of foods, liquids, oils, vomitus, or microorganisms from the upper respiratory tract or the oropharyngeal area. Pneumonitis due to inhalation of foods or vomitus is coded to J69.0, that due to inhalation of oils and essences to J69.1, and that due to inhalation of other solids or liquids to J69.8. Pneumonia due to aspiration of microorganisms is classified to bacterial or viral pneumonia in category J15 or J12. Patients transferred from a nursing home to an acute care hospital because of pneumonia often have aspiration pneumonia due to aspirated organisms, usually gram-negative bacteria.

Ventilator Associated Pneumonia

Pneumonia associated with the use of a ventilator is assigned to code **J95.851, Ventilator associated pneumonia.** If the organism is known, a code to identify it (B95.-, B96.-, B97.-) should also be assigned. Do not assign an additional code from categories J12 through J18 to identify the type of pneumonia. For example, ventilator associated pneumonia (VAP) due to *Staphylococcus aureus* is coded to J95.851 and B95.61.

Code J95.851 should be assigned only when the provider has documented VAP. As with all procedural or postprocedural complications, code assignment is based on the provider's documentation of the relationship between the condition and the procedure. J95.851 should not be assigned for cases where the patient has pneumonia and is on mechanical ventilation, unless the provider has specifically stated that the pneumonia is VAP. The provider should be queried when the documentation is unclear.

It is clinically possible for a patient to be admitted with one type of pneumonia and to develop VAP later. The principal diagnosis is the type of pneumonia diagnosed at the time of admission (J12–J18), and code J95.851 is a secondary diagnosis.

EXERCISE 18.1

Code the following diagnoses and procedures. Do not assign External cause of morbidity codes.

1. Lobar pneumonia with influenza

2. Pneumonia, bacterial, left upper lobe

3. *Klebsiella* pneumonia

4. Postinfectional pneumonia

5. Acute pneumococcal lobar pneumonia

6. Perihilar viral pneumonia

7. Pneumonia due to chlamydia

Intermittent positive-pressure breathing (IPPB),

4 hours

_____

8. Aspiration pneumonia due to aspiration of vomitus

_____

9. Pneumocystis pneumonia due to AIDS

_____

10. Pneumonia due to pulmonary coccidioidomycosis

_____

INFLUENZA

ICD-10-CM classifies influenza due to certain identified influenza viruses to category J09. The Centers for Disease Control and Prevention (CDC) National Center for Health Statistics (NCHS) has confirmed that subcategory J09.X is used to report a specific strain of influenza (such as "novel" influenza A) that includes avian (bird) influenza, influenza A/H5N1, influenza of other animal origin (not bird or swine), and swine influenza virus. Category J10, Influenza due to other identified influenza virus, is used to report ordinary seasonal influenza A (non-novel), influenza B, and influenza C; and category J11 is used for influenza due to unidentified influenza virus.

Influenza in combination with any form of pneumonia or bronchopneumonia is assigned to influenza with pneumonia (J09.X1, J10.00–J10.08, and J11.00–J11.08). For codes J09.X1, J10.08, and J11.08, code also the other specified type of pneumonia. Influenza with other types of respiratory manifestations such as upper respiratory infection, laryngitis, pharyngitis, and pleural effusion are classifiable to J09.X2, J10.1, and J11.1. Influenza may also involve body systems other than the respiratory system, such as the gastrointestinal tract (J09.X3, J10.2, and J11.2), and other manifestations such as encephalopathy, myocarditis, and otitis media (J09.X9, J10.81–J10.89, and J11.81–J11.89).

Similar to the guidelines for coding HIV infection, codes from categories J09 and J10 should be assigned only for confirmed cases of avian flu or other novel influenza A, or for other identified influenza virus. In this context, "confirmation" does not require documentation of positive laboratory testing; however, it does require provider documentation of avian influenza or other novel influenza A.

A code from categories J09 or J10 is not assigned when the diagnostic statement indicates that the infection is "suspected," "possible," "likely," or "?". This advice is an exception to the general guideline that directs the coding professional to assign a code for an inpatient diagnosis qualified as "suspected" or "possible" as if it were established. Instead, a code from category J11, Influenza due to unidentified influenza virus, should be assigned.

COVID-19

On January 30, 2020, the World Health Organization (WHO) declared the 2019 novel coronavirus (2019-nCoV) disease (COVID-19) a public health emergency of international concern. On March 13, 2020, the COVID-19 outbreak was declared a national emergency in the United States. Given the urgent need to capture the reporting of this condition in claims and surveillance data, the CDC under the National Emergencies Act Sections 201 and 301 announced the effective date of April 1, 2020, for a new diagnosis code: **U07.1, COVID-19.** See chapter 13 of this handbook, Infectious and Parasitic Diseases, for discussion of coding COVID-19.

VAPING-RELATED DISORDER

Code **U07.0, Vaping-related disorder,** was implemented effective April 1, 2020, in response to the occurrences of respiratory illnesses associated with the use of electronic nicotine delivery systems. Electronic cigarette devices resemble traditional cigarettes and produce an inhalable aerosol that may contain nicotine, tetrahydrocannabinol (TCH) and cannabinoid (CBD) oils, flavoring, and other chemicals.

Code U07.0 is assigned for "vaping" or "dabbing" injuries. For patients presenting with condition(s) related to vaping, assign code **U07.0, Vaping-related disorder,** as the principal diagnosis. For lung injury due to vaping, assign only code U07.0. Assign additional codes for other manifestations, such as acute respiratory failure (subcategory J96.0-) or pneumonitis (code J68.0). Associated respiratory signs and symptoms due to vaping, such as cough, shortness of breath, etc., are not coded separately, because a definitive diagnosis has been established. However, it would be appropriate to code separately any gastrointestinal symptoms, such as diarrhea and abdominal pain. For patients with documented substance use, abuse, or dependence, additional codes identifying the substance(s) used should be assigned.

LARYNGITIS AND TRACHEITIS

Category J04, Acute laryngitis and tracheitis, has unique subcategories for laryngitis, tracheitis, and laryngotracheitis. Acute laryngitis and laryngotracheitis, with and without obstruction, are identified at the code level.

Supraglottitis is an infection of the supraglottic structures that affects the lingual tonsillar areas, epiglottic folds, false vocal cords, and the epiglottis. It is an acute, life-threatening upper respiratory infection, which seems to occur primarily in children but can be rapidly fatal to individuals in all age groups. This fatal event appears to result from an edematous epiglottis that is obstructing the airway.

Because the infection covers all of the supraglottic structures, the term "supraglottitis" is nonspecific, and the diagnosis of supraglottitis may represent any of the codes within category J04. The codes for the conditions affecting the supraglottic structures are as follows:

J04.0   Acute laryngitis

J04.1   Acute tracheitis

      J04.10   Acute tracheitis without obstruction

      J04.11   Acute tracheitis with obstruction

J04.2   Acute laryngotracheitis

J04.3   Supraglottitis, unspecified

      J04.30   Supraglottitis, unspecified, without obstruction

      J04.31   Supraglottitis, unspecified, with obstruction

Subcategory J04.3 is used for supraglottitis when the term is used and a specific site of infection is not identified; a fifth character is used to indicate the presence or absence of obstruction.

Acute obstructive laryngitis, or croup (J05.0), occurs in young children, usually between the ages of six months and three years. The manifestations are a high-pitched cough and difficulty in breathing, due to a spasm or swelling of the larynx. It can be caused by an acute infection (especially by the influenza virus or diphtheria bacterium), an allergy, a tumor of the larynx, or obstruction by a swallowed object.

Acute epiglottitis refers to a severe, rapidly progressing bacterial infection of the upper respiratory tract. Symptoms include sore throat, croupy stridor, and inflamed epiglottis, which may result in sudden respiratory obstruction and possibly death. The infection is generally caused by *Haemophilus influenzae,* type B, although streptococci may occasionally be the causative agents. Acute epiglottitis is coded to subcategory J05.1, with a fifth character to indicate the presence or absence of obstruction. Both categories J04 and J05 use an additional code (B95–B97) to specifically identify the infectious agent. In addition, for both categories J04 and J05, if influenza is also present, also assign a code for influenza with other respiratory conditions (i.e., J09.X2, J10.1 or J11.1).

CHRONIC OBSTRUCTIVE PULMONARY DISEASE

Chronic obstructive pulmonary disease (COPD) is a general term used to describe a variety of conditions that result in obstruction of the airway. ICD-10-CM classifies these conditions to category J44, Other chronic obstructive pulmonary disease. Category J44 includes the following conditions:

- Asthma with chronic obstructive pulmonary disease
- Chronic asthmatic (obstructive) bronchitis
- Chronic bronchitis with airways obstruction
- Chronic bronchitis with emphysema
- Chronic emphysematous bronchitis
- Chronic obstructive asthma
- Chronic obstructive bronchitis
- Chronic obstructive tracheobronchitis

Category J44 is further subdivided to specify whether there is an acute lower respiratory infection (J44.0) and whether there is an exacerbation of the condition (J44.1). If applicable, a code from category J45 is assigned to specify the type of asthma. In the case of code **J44.0, Chronic obstructive pulmonary disease with (acute) lower respiratory infection,** a code should also be assigned to identify the infection. Code J44.0 is assigned for COPD with acute bronchitis or pneumonia, but not for COPD with influenza, because influenza involves both upper and lower respiratory infections. The codes in category J44 distinguish between uncomplicated cases (J44.9) and those with acute exacerbation (J44.1). An acute exacerbation is a worsening or a decompensation of a chronic condition. An acute exacerbation is not equivalent to an infection superimposed on a chronic condition, although an exacerbation may be triggered by an infection. For example, COPD with acute bronchitis should be coded to J44.0, rather than J44.1. Examples of the terms classified to **J44.1, Chronic obstructive pulmonary disease with (acute) exacerbation,** are "exacerbation," "in exacerbation," "decompensated," "acute exacerbation," "exacerbated," or "uncompensated." When the diagnosis is stated only as COPD, review the medical record to determine whether a more definitive diagnosis is documented. Code **J44.9, Chronic obstructive pulmonary disease, unspecified,** is assigned only when a more specific code cannot be assigned.

In addition to codes in category J44, codes may also be assigned to identify exposure to environmental tobacco smoke (Z77.22), history of tobacco dependence (Z87.891), occupational exposure to environmental tobacco smoke (Z57.31), tobacco dependence (F17.-), or tobacco use (Z72.0).

Note that emphysema without chronic bronchitis is coded to J43.-, and chronic bronchitis not otherwise specified is classified to J42.

Asthma

Asthma is a bronchial hypersensitivity characterized by mucosal edema, constriction of bronchial musculature, and excessive viscid edema. Manifestations of asthma are wheezing, dyspnea out of proportion to exertion, and cough. A diagnosis of wheezing alone is not classified as asthma; code R06.2 is assigned in such a case. Asthma is classified into category J45, with a fourth character indicating the severity (mild intermittent, mild persistent, moderate persistent, severe persistent, other, and unspecified) and a final character indicating whether the condition is uncomplicated or whether status asthmaticus or exacerbation is present.

Status asthmaticus is defined in slightly different ways by different authorities, but, in general, it represents a patient who continues to have extreme wheezing in spite of conventional therapy or who has suffered from an acute asthmatic attack in which the degree of obstruction is not relieved by the usual therapeutic measures. Early status asthmaticus represents patients who are refractory to treatment or who fail to respond to the usual therapies; advanced status asthmaticus represents patients who show full development of an asthma attack that could result in respiratory failure, with signs and symptoms of hypercapnia (excess carbon dioxide in the blood). The final character 2 is assigned for both types of status asthmaticus. Use of this final character usually indicates a medical emergency for treatment of acute, severe asthma. Other terms used to describe status asthmaticus include the following:

- Intractable asthma attack
- Refractory asthma
- Severe, intractable wheezing
- Airway obstruction not relieved by bronchodilators
- Severe, prolonged asthmatic attack

It should never be assumed that status asthmaticus is present without a specific statement from the provider. However, asthma described as acute, characterized by prolonged or severe intractable wheezing, or asthma being treated by the administration of adrenal corticosteroids should alert the coding professional that status asthmaticus may exist and that the provider should be asked whether the diagnosis is to be added.

Exacerbations of asthma are acute or subacute episodes of progressively worsening shortness of breath, cough, wheezing, and chest tightness—or some combination of these symptoms. The final character 1 is used for asthma referred to as "exacerbated" or in "acute exacerbation." An asthma code with a final character 1, with acute exacerbation, may *not* be assigned with an asthma code with a final character 2, with status asthmaticus. When there is documentation of both acute exacerbation and status asthmaticus, only the code with the final character 2 should be assigned.

Asthma characterized as obstructive or diagnosed in conjunction with COPD is classified to category J44, Other chronic obstructive pulmonary disease. Code also the type of asthma (J45.-) only when the specific type of asthma is documented by the provider. If the documentation does not specify the type of asthma, do not assign code J45.909, Unspecified asthma, uncomplicated. "Unspecified" is not a type of asthma.

A diagnosis of asthmatic bronchitis without further specification is coded as J45.9-. If the diagnosis is stated as exacerbated or acute chronic asthmatic bronchitis, code J44.1 is assigned. A diagnosis of asthmatic bronchitis with COPD or chronic asthmatic bronchitis is coded to J44.9. Examples of coding for asthma include the following:

J45.902	Asthmatic bronchitis with status asthmaticus
J45.909	Childhood asthma
J44.9 + J45.40	Moderate persistent asthma with COPD
J44.1 + J45.901	Chronic asthmatic bronchitis with acute exacerbation
J45.909 + F54	Psychogenic asthma

Bronchospasm

Bronchospasm is an integral part of asthma or any other type of chronic airway obstruction; therefore, no additional code is assigned to indicate its presence when an asthma or other chronic airway obstruction is diagnosed. Code J98.01, Acute bronchospasm, is assigned only when the underlying cause has not been identified.

EXERCISE 18.2

Code the following diagnoses. Do not assign External cause of morbidity codes.

1. Bronchial asthma, allergic, due to house dust

2. Chronic bronchitis with decompensated COPD

3. Acute exacerbation of chronic asthmatic bronchitis

4. Emphysema

5. Chronic obstructive lung disease with acute exacerbation

6. Emphysema with chronic obstructive bronchitis

7. Mild intermittent asthma with status asthmaticus

8. Acute bronchitis with acute bronchiectasis

9. Perforated right tympanic membrane due to influenza
   with otitis media

10. Exacerbation of severe persistent asthma

ATELECTASIS

Atelectasis is a very common finding in chest X-rays and other radiological studies. It is a condition where the alveoli are deflated. It may be caused by normal exhalation or by several medical conditions. Atelectasis reduces the ventilatory function. Pulmonary collapse can be a severe problem, but mild atelectasis usually has little effect on the patient's condition or the therapy provided. Slight strands of atelectasis are often noted on X-ray reports, but this finding is generally of little clinical importance and is usually not further evaluated or treated. Code **J98.11, Atelectasis,** should not be assigned on the basis of an X-ray finding alone; it should be coded only when the physician identifies it as a clinical condition that meets the criteria for a reportable diagnosis.

PLEURAL EFFUSION

Pleural effusion is an abnormal accumulation of fluid within the pleural spaces. It occurs in association with pulmonary disease and certain cardiac conditions, such as congestive heart failure, or certain diseases involving other organs. Pleural effusion is almost always integral to the underlying disease and is usually addressed only by treatment of that condition. In these cases, it should not be coded. However, occasionally the effusion is addressed separately, with additional diagnostic studies such as decubitus X-ray or diagnostic thoracentesis. The effusion may be treated by therapeutic thoracentesis (chest-tube drainage). It is appropriate to report pleural effusion (J91.8) as an additional diagnosis when the condition requires either therapeutic intervention or diagnostic testing. A code is assigned first for the underlying condition, followed by code **J91.8, Pleural effusion in conditions classified elsewhere.** Pleural effusion noted only on an X-ray report is not reported.

Pleural effusion due to tuberculosis is classified to A15.6 unless it is due to primary progressive tuberculosis (A15.7). Pleural effusion due to systemic lupus erythematosus is coded to **M32.13, Lung involvement in systemic lupus erythematosus.** Influenzal pleural effusion is coded to influenza, with respiratory manifestations (J09.X2, J10.1, or J11.1), with code **J91.8, Pleural effusion in other conditions classified elsewhere,** assigned to specify the associated pleural effusion.

Malignant pleural effusion can occur due to impaired pleural lymphatic drainage from a mediastinal tumor (especially in lymphomas) and not because of direct tumor invasion into the pleura. Malignant pleural effusion is coded to J91.0 with the underlying neoplasm assigned as the first-listed or principal diagnosis.

RESPIRATORY FAILURE

Respiratory failure is a life-threatening condition that is always due to an underlying condition. It may be the final pathway of a disease process or a combination of different processes. Respiratory failure can result from either acute or chronic diseases that cause airway obstruction, parenchymal infiltration, or pulmonary edema. It can arise from an abnormality in any of the components of the respiratory system, central nervous system, peripheral nervous system, respiratory muscles, and chest wall muscles. The diagnosis is based largely on findings from arterial blood gas analysis, which vary from individual to individual, depending on several factors. Never assume a diagnosis of respiratory failure without a documented diagnosis by the physician. Respiratory failure is classified as acute (J96.0-), chronic (J96.1-), acute and chronic combined (J96.2-), or unspecified (J96.9-), and a fifth character is used to specify whether hypoxia or hypercapnia is present.

Careful review of the medical record is required for the coding and sequencing of respiratory failure. Review the circumstances of admission to determine the principal diagnosis. Code **J96.00, Acute respiratory failure, unspecified whether with hypoxia or hypercapnia,** or code **J96.20, Acute and chronic respiratory failure, unspecified whether with hypoxia or hypercapnia,** may be assigned as a principal diagnosis when the respiratory failure is the condition established after study to be chiefly responsible for occasioning the admission to the hospital, and the selection is supported by the Alphabetic Index and Tabular List. Respiratory failure may be listed as a secondary diagnosis if it develops after admission. When respiratory failure follows surgery, code **J95.821, Acute postprocedural respiratory failure,** or code **J95.822, Acute and chronic postprocedural respiratory failure,** is assigned.

When a patient is admitted with respiratory failure and another acute condition (e.g., myocardial infarction, aspiration pneumonia, cerebrovascular accident), the principal diagnosis will depend on the individual patient's situation and what caused the admission of the patient to the hospital. This guideline applies regardless of whether the other acute condition is a respiratory or nonrespiratory condition. The physician should be queried for clarification if the documentation is unclear as to which one of the two conditions was the reason for the admission. The guideline regarding two or more diagnoses equally meeting the definition of principal diagnosis (Section II, C) may be applied in situations when both the respiratory failure and the other acute condition are equally responsible for occasioning the admission to the hospital. Examples are the following.

EXAMPLE 1: A patient with chronic myasthenia gravis goes into acute exacerbation and develops acute respiratory failure. The patient is admitted due to the respiratory failure.

Principal diagnosis:	J96.00	Acute respiratory failure, unspecified whether with hypoxia or hypercapnia
Secondary diagnosis:	G70.01	Myasthenia gravis with (acute) exacerbation

EXAMPLE 2: A patient with emphysema develops acute respiratory failure. The patient is admitted through the emergency department for treatment of the respiratory failure.

Principal diagnosis:	J96.00	Acute respiratory failure, unspecified whether with hypoxia or hypercapnia
Secondary diagnosis:	J43.9	Emphysema, unspecified

EXAMPLE 3: A patient arrived in the hospital in acute respiratory failure and hypoxia. The patient was intubated, and the physician documents that the patient is being admitted to the hospital for treatment of the acute respiratory failure with hypoxia. The patient also has congestive heart failure.

Principal diagnosis:	J96.01	Acute respiratory failure with hypoxia
Secondary diagnosis:	I50.9	Heart failure, unspecified

Some ICD-10-CM chapter-specific coding guidelines (e.g., obstetrics, poisoning, HIV, newborn) provide sequencing directions. If a patient has respiratory failure associated with a condition from one of these chapters, follow the chapter-specific guidelines when assigning code J96.0- or J96.2-. Examples are the following.

EXAMPLE 4: A patient is admitted to the hospital postpartum as a result of developing pulmonary embolism leading to acute respiratory failure.

Principal diagnosis:	O88.23	Thromboembolism in the puerperium
Secondary diagnosis:	J96.00	Acute respiratory failure, unspecified whether with hypoxia or hypercapnia

In example 4, the obstetric code is sequenced first because a chapter-specific guideline (Section I, C, 15, a, 1) provides sequencing directions specifying that chapter 15 codes have sequencing priority over codes from other chapters.

EXAMPLE 5: A patient who is diagnosed as accidentally overdosing on crack cocaine is admitted to the hospital with acute respiratory failure.

Principal diagnosis:	T40.5x1A	Poisoning by cocaine, accidental, initial encounter
Secondary diagnoses:	J96.00	Acute respiratory failure, unspecified whether with hypoxia or hypercapnia
	F14.10	Cocaine abuse, uncomplicated

In example 5, poisoning is sequenced first because a chapter-specific guideline (Section I, C, 19, e, 5, b) provides sequencing directions specifying that the poisoning code is sequenced first, followed by a code for the manifestation. The acute respiratory failure is a manifestation of the poisoning.

EXAMPLE 6:	A patient is admitted with acute respiratory failure due to *Pneumocystis jirovecii* due to AIDS.		
	Principal diagnosis:	B20	Human immunodeficiency virus [HIV] disease
	Secondary diagnoses:	J96.00	Acute respiratory failure, unspecified whether with hypoxia or hypercapnia
		B59	Pneumocystosis

In example 6, HIV disease is sequenced first because a chapter-specific guideline (Section I, C, 1, a, 2, a) provides sequencing directions specifying that if a patient is admitted for an HIV-related condition (in this case, the *Pneumocystis jirovecii* infection), the principal diagnosis should be B20, followed by additional diagnosis codes for all reported HIV-related conditions.

In the event that instructional notes in the Tabular List provide sequencing direction, the sequencing of respiratory failure is dependent on these notes. An example follows.

EXAMPLE 7:	A patient is admitted to the hospital with severe *Staphylococcus aureus* sepsis and acute respiratory failure.		
	Principal diagnosis:	A41.01	Sepsis due to methicillin susceptible *Staphylococcus aureus*
	Secondary diagnoses:	R65.20	Severe sepsis without septic shock
		J96.00	Acute respiratory failure, unspecified whether with hypoxia or hypercapnia

Sepsis is sequenced first in this case because an instructional note under subcategory R65.2- indicates to code first the underlying infection. In addition, subcategory R65.2- has a "use additional code" note to specify acute organ dysfunction and lists acute respiratory failure (J96.0-). Following this instruction, respiratory failure is given as a secondary diagnosis.

ACUTE RESPIRATORY DISTRESS SYNDROME

Acute respiratory distress syndrome (ARDS) is a lung condition that leads to low oxygen levels in the blood. ARDS can be life threatening because organs such as the kidneys and brain need oxygen-rich blood for proper functioning. ARDS can occur within 24 to 48 hours of an injury (trauma, burns, aspiration, massive blood transfusion, drug/alcohol abuse) or an acute illness (infectious pneumonia, sepsis, acute pancreatitis). ARDS patients usually present with shortness of breath and tachypnea, and occasionally present with confusion. Long-term illnesses, such as malaria, can also trigger ARDS, which may then occur sometime after the onset of a particularly acute case of the infection. ARDS is coded to **J80, Acute respiratory distress syndrome.**

ACUTE PULMONARY EDEMA

Acute pulmonary edema is a pathological state in which there is excessive, diffuse accumulation of fluid in the tissues and the alveolar spaces of the lung. It is broadly divided into two categories that reflect the origin of the condition: cardiogenic and noncardiogenic.

Cardiogenic

Acute pulmonary edema of cardiac origin is a manifestation of heart failure and as such is included in the following code assignments:

I01.-	Rheumatic heart disease, acute
I09.81	Rheumatic heart failure
I11.-	Hypertensive heart disease
I50.-	Heart failure

Pulmonary edema is not included in the codes for acute myocardial infarction (I21.01–I22.9), acute ischemic heart disease (I24.0–I24.9), or chronic ischemic heart disease (I25.-). When pulmonary edema is present along with a heart condition or failure, the pulmonary edema is assumed to be associated with left ventricular failure (I50.1) unless the heart failure is described as congestive or decompensated, in which case a code for the more-specific congestive heart failure (I50.2–I50.9) is assigned. Pulmonary edema is included in codes I50.-; no additional code is assigned for pulmonary edema associated with conditions in this category.

Noncardiogenic

Noncardiogenic acute pulmonary edema occurs in the absence of heart failure or other heart disease. It is coded in a variety of ways depending on the cause. When the cause is not specified, code **J81.0, Pulmonary edema,** is assigned. When the cause of the pulmonary edema is known, it is coded as follows:

- Postradiation pulmonary edema (postradiation pneumonia) is an inflammation of the lungs due to the adverse effects of radiation. It is coded as **J70.0, Acute pulmonary manifestations due to radiation.**
- Pulmonary edema due to chemicals, gas fumes, or vapors is coded as J68.1.
- Pulmonary edema due to aspiration of water in a near-drowning is coded to **T75.1-, Unspecified effects of drowning and nonfatal submersion.**
- Pulmonary edema due to high altitude is coded as **T70.29-, Other effects of high altitude.**
- Acute pulmonary edema in cases of drug overdose is classified as poisoning, with code J81.0 assigned as an additional code. Any mention of drug dependence or abuse should also be coded.

External cause of morbidity codes should be assigned with any of these codes to indicate the external circumstances involved.

Chronic pulmonary edema or pulmonary edema not otherwise specified that is not of cardiac origin is coded as **J81.1, Chronic pulmonary edema,** unless the Alphabetic Index or the Tabular List instructs otherwise.

Pulmonary edema caused by congestive overloads, such as pulmonary fibrosis (J84.10), congenital stenosis of the pulmonary veins (Q26.8), or pulmonary venous embolism (I26.99), is noncardiogenic. When such conditions are described as acute, they are assigned to code J81.0; code J81.1 is assigned when the condition is described as chronic or not otherwise specified. Be careful not to confuse this condition with edema associated with heart disease.

SURGICAL PROCEDURES

When assigning ICD-10-PCS codes for procedures performed in the respiratory system, it is important to ensure that the documentation provides information regarding the site where the procedure was performed. Body part values include the specific lobe of the lung (when available) or, at a minimum, whether the site is the right or left lung, or bilateral lungs. Many of the root operations commonly performed do not provide "unspecified" body part values for when the left or right side is not stated for the lungs, pleura, or diaphragm. Examples of these root operations include "Destruction," "Drainage," "Excision," "Insertion," and "Extirpation."

It is also important to understand the surgical approaches in order to select the correct ICD-10-PCS codes. (For illustrations of such approaches, please refer to figure 7.5 on pages 74–75.) For example, thoracoscopic procedures involve the creation of small incisions into the chest wall and insertion of a thoracoscope through the incision. Thoracoscopic procedures are coded to the approach "percutaneous endoscopic." Procedures stated as "bronchoscopic" involve passing the bronchoscope through the nose (or sometimes the mouth), down the throat, and into the airway. The approach character for bronchoscopic procedures is "via natural or artificial opening endoscopic" because the procedure involves entering via a natural opening (nose or mouth) and then using an endoscope. A mini-thoracotomy is a minimally invasive procedure that requires only a small incision; however, it is still an open procedure and is coded as an open approach.

BIOPSIES OF BRONCHUS, PLEURA, AND LUNG

An endoscopic biopsy of the bronchus involves passing an endoscope into the lumen of the trachea and bronchus, where a bit of tissue is removed for pathological study. An endoscopic biopsy of the lung is performed by passing the endoscope through the main bronchus into the smaller bronchi and lung alveoli. Either type of endoscopic biopsy can be performed independently, or both may be performed in the same operative episode, in which case both codes are assigned. The root operation "Excision" is assigned for the excision of tissue, with the approach character "via natural or artificial opening endoscopic." For example, endoscopic excisional biopsy of the right middle lobe of the lung is coded to **0BBD8ZX, Excision of right middle lung lobe, via natural or artificial opening endoscopic, diagnostic.**

Another type of lung biopsy is the thoracoscopic biopsy. In this procedure, small incisions are made into the chest wall and a thoracoscope is inserted through them to remove specimens for pathological examination. The approach for this type of biopsy is "percutaneous endoscopic" because it requires entering through the skin and inserting a scope. For example, thoracoscopic excisional wedge biopsy of the right lung is coded to **0BBK4ZX, Excision of right lung, percutaneous endoscopic approach, diagnostic.**

A bronchial brush biopsy utilizes the bronchoscope and a small brush with stiff bristles to remove cells from the airways. A brush biopsy fits the definition of the root operation "Extraction," pulling or stripping out or off all or a portion of a body part by the use of force. For example, brush biopsy of the right upper lobe bronchus is coded to **0BD48ZX, Extraction of right upper lobe bronchus, via natural or artificial opening endoscopic, diagnostic.**

When fluid (as opposed to tissue) is removed for the purpose of a biopsy, the root operation "Drainage" is assigned with the qualifier for "diagnostic." For example, a fine needle biopsy removing fluid from the right pleura is coded to **0B9N3ZX, Drainage of right pleura, percutaneous approach, diagnostic.**

Bronchoalveolar lavage (BAL), also called "liquid biopsy," is a diagnostic procedure performed via a bronchoscope under local anesthesia. It involves washing out alveoli tissue of the lung and peripheral airways to obtain a small sampling of tissue. BAL is coded to the root operation "Drainage" because it involves removing fluids. The body part (lung) captures the objective of the procedure. For example, bronchoalveolar lavage of the right lower lobe of the lung is coded to **0B9F8ZX, Drainage of right lower lung lobe, via natural or artificial opening endoscopic, diagnostic.**

BAL should not be confused with whole lung lavage. Whole lung lavage is a therapeutic procedure performed for pulmonary alveolar proteinosis. The procedure is performed under general anesthesia and mechanical ventilation. The lungs are lavaged by filling and emptying one lung at a time with saline solution. The second lung is usually lavaged three to seven days after the first lung has been lavaged. Report whole lung lavage using code **3E1F88Z, Irrigation of respiratory tract using irrigating substance, via natural or artificial opening endoscopic.** Assign also a code for the mechanical ventilation provided.

ABLATION OF LUNG AND PLEURODESIS

Tumor ablation is an alternative to surgical removal of lung lesions. Ablation can be achieved using extreme heat, freezing chemicals (cryoablation), focused ultrasound, microwaves, or radiofrequency. These procedures are typically performed by interventional radiologists using imaging guidance—such as computerized tomography (CT), ultrasound, or fluoroscopy—and inserting a probe directly to the lesion.

ICD-10-PCS classifies ablation procedures under the root operation "Destruction," meaning "physical eradication of all or a portion of a body part by the direct use of energy, force, or a destructive agent." ICD-10-PCS codes for ablation do not distinguish between the different energy sources used to ablate the tumor. Examples include the following:

0B5G0ZZ	Open ablation left upper lung lobe
0B5L3ZZ	Percutaneous ablation left lung
0B5J4ZZ	Thoracoscopic ablation left lower lung lobe

Bronchoscopic ablation (or bronchial thermoplasty ablation) of airway smooth muscle of the lung is a procedure to treat asthmatic patients in which a bronchoscope and a catheter are used to deliver radiofrequency energy into the airways to reduce constricted airway smooth muscle. This reduction lessens the area that narrows in response to external stimuli such as dust and other allergens. For example, bronchial thermoplasty ablation of the right main bronchus is coded as **0B538ZZ, Destruction of right main bronchus, via natural or artificial opening endoscopic.**

Pleurodesis is a procedure performed to prevent recurrent pneumothorax or recurrent pleural effusion by artificially obliterating the pleural space. There are two main types of pleurodesis: surgical (mechanical) and chemical. Mechanical or surgical pleurodesis is performed via thoracotomy or thoracoscopy. The procedure consists of surgically abrading the parietal pleura using a rough pad, gauze, or a mechanical rotary brush. Mechanical (surgical) pleurodesis is coded to the root operation "Destruction" (for example, **0B5N0ZZ, Destruction of right pleura, open approach**).

Chemical pleurodesis may use substances such as bleomycin, povidone-iodine, tetracycline, and nitrogen mustard, but the most popular substance is talc. One method for talc pleurodesis uses video-assisted thoracoscopic surgery (VATS), a minimally invasive procedure that may be performed to treat diseases of the lung, pleura, and mediastinum. A small camera is delivered through several small chest incisions. The camera transmits images to guide the surgeon in performing the procedure. When talc pleurodesis is performed via VATS to treat recurrent spontaneous pneumothorax, talc is injected into the pleural cavity to cause adhesions between the pleura and the chest wall that seal the space and prevent recurrence of pneumothorax (the collapse of the lung due to leakage of air). The root operation "Destruction" is not appropriate for this procedure. Assign code **3E0L3GC, Introduction of other therapeutic substance into pleural cavity, percutaneous approach,** because "percutaneous endoscopic" is not available on Table 3E0.

For inspection of the pleura, assign code **0BJQ4ZZ, Inspection of pleura, percutaneous endoscopic approach,** to capture the endoscopic component of the procedure.

Other examples of common lung procedures include:

0BBD4ZZ	Thoracoscopic excision of lesion right middle lobe
0BBC0ZZ	Open segmental resection of right upper lobe
0BTG0ZZ	Open lobectomy, left upper lobe
0B9N30Z	Percutaneous drainage of right pleura

MECHANICAL VENTILATION

Mechanical ventilation is a process by which the patient's own effort to breathe is augmented or replaced by the use of a mechanical device. ICD-10-PCS classifies mechanical ventilation to the Extracorporeal or Systemic Assistance and Performance Section (first character 5).

Mechanical ventilation may be described as noninvasive or invasive. Noninvasive mechanical ventilation is delivered via a noninvasive interface like a face mask, a nasal mask, a nasal pillow, an oral mouthpiece, or an oronasal mask. ICD-10-PCS classifies this type of mechanical ventilation to the root operation "Assistance" because it meets the definition of "taking over a portion of a physiological function by extracorporeal means." Character 5 in this section provides the value for the duration of the ventilation: less than 24 consecutive hours (value = 3), 24–96 consecutive hours (value = 4), or greater than 96 consecutive hours (value = 5). Character 7, qualifier, specifies the type of ventilation with the following values:

7   Continuous positive airway pressure

8   Intermittent positive airway pressure

9   Continuous negative airway pressure

A   High nasal flow/velocity

B   Intermittent negative airway pressure

Z   No qualifier

Coding examples follow:

5A09357	Assistance with respiratory ventilation, less than 24 consecutive hours, continuous positive airway pressure
5A09457	Assistance with respiratory ventilation, 24–96 consecutive hours, continuous positive airway pressure
5A09458	Assistance with respiratory ventilation, 24–96 consecutive hours, intermittent positive airway pressure
5A09559	Assistance with respiratory ventilation, greater than 96 consecutive hours, continuous negative airway pressure
5A0955Z	Assistance with respiratory ventilation, greater than 96 consecutive hours

Mechanical ventilation is considered invasive when the ventilatory assistance is provided via an invasive interface, such as endotracheal intubation or tracheostomy, and the patient receives mechanical ventilation in an uninterrupted fashion. Endotracheal intubation requires nonsurgical placement of the tracheal tube, either orally or nasally. Assign code **0BH17EZ, Insertion of endotracheal airway into trachea, via natural or artificial opening,** or code **0BH18EZ, Insertion of endotracheal airway into trachea, via natural or artificial opening endoscopic.** If either intubation or tracheostomy is performed after admission or in the emergency department of the same hospital immediately before admission, it should be reported. Intubation or tracheostomy carried out elsewhere prior to admission or in an ambulance prior to arrival at the hospital cannot be reported even though the ambulance may be operated by the same facility.

Codes for invasive mechanical ventilation are classified to the root operation "Performance" because these procedures completely take over the physiological function of breathing by extracorporeal means. Similar to the root operation "Assistance," character 5 in this section provides values for the duration of the ventilation: less than 24 consecutive hours (value = 3), 24–96 consecutive hours (value = 4), or greater than 96 consecutive hours (value = 5).

Examples include the following codes:

5A19054   Respiratory ventilation, single, nonmechanical

5A1935Z   Respiratory ventilation, less than 24 consecutive hours

5A1945Z   Respiratory ventilation, 24–96 consecutive hours

5A1955Z   Respiratory ventilation, greater than 96 consecutive hours

Duration of Mechanical Ventilation

The starting time for calculating the duration begins with one of these events:

- Endotracheal intubation performed in the hospital or hospital emergency department, followed by initiation of mechanical ventilation

- Initiation of mechanical ventilation through tracheostomy performed in the hospital or hospital emergency department

- At the time of admission of a previously intubated patient or a patient with a tracheostomy who is on mechanical ventilation

When a patient receives mechanical ventilation over an extended period, a tracheostomy may be created in the anterior cervical trachea. A tracheal tube is often inserted to keep the tracheostomy open for attachment to the mechanical ventilator. Start counting hours on ventilation only after mechanical ventilation has actually been initiated.

It is occasionally necessary to replace an endotracheal tube because of a problem such as a leak; removal with immediate replacement is considered part of the duration, and counting of hours should continue. Patients who are started on mechanical ventilation by means of an endotracheal tube may later receive a tracheostomy through which the ventilation continues. Continue counting the number of hours the patient is on ventilation from the time the original intubation was initiated.

Once a patient's condition has stabilized and the patient no longer needs continuous ventilatory assistance, various weaning methods may be employed to allow the patient to gradually resume the work of breathing. During weaning, the patient is monitored for any evidence of cardiopulmonary instability. The entire period of weaning is counted during the process of withdrawing the patient from ventilatory support. The duration ends when the patient is extubated and the mechanical ventilation is turned off (after the weaning period). Note that some patients do not require this weaning process. For patients being weaned from intermittent ventilation, calculate the entire weaning trial, including the time the patient is on the ventilator and the weaning period up until the patient is extubated and the ventilator is turned off. If the patient is on mechanical ventilation only at night and is not being weaned, count the duration as the time the patient is actually put on the ventilator. For overnight use, assign code **5A1935Z, Respiratory ventilation, less than 24 consecutive hours.**

Duration of mechanical ventilation ends with one of the following events:

- Removal of the endotracheal tube (extubation)

- Discontinuance of ventilation for patients with tracheostomy after any weaning period is completed

- Discharge or transfer while still on mechanical ventilation

Occasionally, the condition of a patient who has been on ventilation earlier in the hospital stay deteriorates and a subsequent period of mechanical ventilation may be required. In such cases, two codes should be assigned to represent each episode of continuous mechanical ventilation.

Mechanical ventilation used during surgery is not coded when it is considered a normal part of the surgery. However, in the event that the physician documents that the patient has a specific problem and is maintained on the mechanical ventilator longer than expected or if the patient requires mechanical ventilation for an extended period of time postoperatively, it may be coded. If the postoperative mechanical ventilation continues for more than two days, or if the physician has clearly documented an unexpected extended period of mechanical ventilation, the mechanical ventilation may be reported separately. The hours of mechanical ventilation should be counted starting from the point of intubation.

When a patient who is dependent on oxygen is admitted to the hospital while connected to his or her own ventilator equipment, it is appropriate to report the mechanical ventilation assistance while the patient is being evaluated and monitored in the hospital. Ownership of the equipment has no bearing on code assignment for the ventilator assistance. Count the hours according to the guidelines stated above.

Sequencing of Mechanical Ventilation

The sequencing of mechanical ventilation with other procedures follows the guidelines for selection of the principal procedure, as noted in chapter 8 of this handbook. The following examples help illustrate the application of these guidelines:

- A patient with a history of endocarditis is admitted with severe acute meningitis, which is causing respiratory decompensation. A diagnostic lumbar puncture is performed, and mechanical ventilation is provided. The mechanical ventilation code is sequenced as a secondary procedure because the lumbar puncture is the diagnostic procedure performed for the principal diagnosis of severe acute meningitis.

- A patient is admitted with an acute ischemic cerebral vascular accident and is started on tissue plasminogen activator (tPA) infusion. Four hours after admission, the patient suffers a second, massive infarction. Cardiopulmonary resuscitation is successfully carried out, but the patient requires mechanical ventilation. The thrombolytic therapy was directed at the principal diagnosis of cerebrovascular accident; therefore, the tPA administration is the principal procedure and the mechanical ventilation is sequenced as a secondary procedure.

- A premature newborn requires mechanical ventilation for respiratory distress syndrome and therapeutic lumbar puncture for relief of intracranial pressure. In this case, there are no procedures (definitive or nondefinitive treatment) related to the principal diagnosis. Both the mechanical ventilation and the therapeutic lumbar puncture are performed for the secondary diagnoses. Select the most significant procedure addressing the secondary diagnoses. When the documentation is unclear regarding which is the most significant procedure, query the physician for clarification.

- A patient is admitted with severe sepsis. To treat the sepsis, a central venous catheter is inserted to administer intravenous antibiotics. The patient is also placed on mechanical ventilation. The documentation states that the patient has no underlying respiratory condition, and the respiratory decompensation is due to the severity of the sepsis. Sequence the code for the insertion of the catheter as the principal procedure. The mechanical ventilation code is sequenced as a secondary procedure.

- A patient is admitted with sepsis and placed on mechanical ventilation. The documentation states that the patient's initial respiratory decompensation is due to the sepsis, and that the presumed cause of the sepsis is spontaneous bacterial peritonitis. Percutaneous drainage of the peritoneal cavity is performed, and the fluid is sent for cultures. The paracentesis is the principal procedure because it is the procedure most related to the principal diagnosis. The mechanical ventilation code is sequenced as an additional procedure.

Tracheostomy Complications

Complications of a tracheostomy are classified to subcategory J95.0 in chapter 10 of ICD-10-CM. Infection of a tracheostomy stoma is classified to code J95.02, with an additional code to identify the type of infection and/or a code from category B95–B97 to identify the organism. If an infection is specified as sepsis, assign a code from A40.- or A41.-. Hemorrhage from tracheostomy is coded to J95.01; tracheostomy malfunction complications are coded to J95.03; trachea-esophageal fistula following tracheostomy is assigned to J95.04; unspecified complication is classified to J95.00; other complications are coded to J95.09.

EXERCISE 18.3

Code the following diagnoses and procedures. Do not assign External cause of morbidity codes.

1. Chronic left maxillary sinusitis

   Open left total maxillary sinusectomy

2. Acute upper respiratory infection due to *Pneumococcus*

   Febrile convulsions

3. Deviated nasal septum

   Allergic rhinitis

   Ethmoidal sinusitis

   Excision of nasal septum, percutaneous

4. Chronic pulmonary edema

5. Allergic rhinitis due to tree pollen

6. Congestive heart failure with pleural effusion

7. Acute respiratory failure due to intracerebral hemorrhage

8. Acute pharyngitis due to *Staphylococcus aureus* infection

9. Chronic chemical bronchitis due to accidental inhalation

   of chlorine fumes 2 years ago

   Bronchoscopy with excisional biopsy of right lower bronchus

10. Total tension pneumothorax, spontaneous, recurrent, left

    Video-assisted thoracoscopic surgical pleurodesis, left pleura

11. Admitted in acute respiratory failure due to acute exacerbation of chronic obstructive bronchitis

_____

12. Acute tracheobronchitis due to respiratory syncytial virus infection

_____

13. Gram-negative pneumonia, anaerobic

_____

14. Acute pulmonary insufficiency, due to shock

_____

15. Acute respiratory distress syndrome due to hantavirus infection

_____

16. Infected tracheostomy due to staphylococcal abscess of the neck

_____

CHAPTER 19

Diseases of the Digestive System

CHAPTER OVERVIEW

- Diseases of the digestive system are found in chapter 11 of ICD-10-CM.

- Many types of gastrointestinal (GI) hemorrhage can be classified. Sometimes, documentation may point to bleeding in multiple locations.

- Esophagitis is classified to the digestive system codes, but esophageal varices are coded as a disease of the circulatory system.

- Combination codes are provided for ulcers that indicate bleeding, perforation, or both. Coding professionals should review the medical record for any indication of site.

- Special notice should be given to conditions involving diverticula because of the similarity of the conditions and names.

- Coding diseases of the biliary system involves determining the presence and location of the calculus.

- Certain biliary system conditions revolve around removal of the gallbladder.

- Codes for adhesions include both intestinal and peritoneal adhesions. However, minor adhesions are usually not coded.

- Hernias are classified by type and site, and combination codes are used to indicate associated issues.

- Diarrhea can be related to a variety of conditions. It is important to check the Alphabetic Index carefully before coding.

- Other common digestive system issues classified in this chapter include appendicitis and constipation.

- Coding gastric bypass procedures requires the understanding of the body part bypassed from and the body part bypassed to.

LEARNING OUTCOMES

After studying this chapter, you should be able to:

- Classify a variety of conditions that affect the GI tract.

- Differentiate the various terms associated with diverticula.

- Classify diseases of the biliary system.

- Classify common digestive system conditions such as diarrhea, constipation, and appendicitis.

- Correctly code bariatric surgeries and any possible complications related to these procedures.

TERMS TO KNOW

Biliary system
a network including the gallbladder and bile ducts

Calculus
a stone composed of minerals that forms in an organ or duct of the body

Diverticulitis
the inflammation of existing diverticula

Diverticulosis
the presence of one or more diverticula of the designated site

Diverticulum
a small pouch or sac opening from a tubular or saccular organ; considered a medical condition; the plural term is diverticula

Esophageal varices
abnormally enlarged veins in the lower part of the esophagus

Esophagitis
an inflammation of the lining of the esophagus

GI
gastrointestinal; of the stomach and/or intestines

REMEMBER . . .

Many combination codes and exclusion notes are used in chapter 11 of ICD-10-CM.

INTRODUCTION

Diseases of the digestive system are classified in chapter 11 of ICD-10-CM. The coding principles presented in previous chapters of this handbook apply throughout chapter 11. In addition, particular attention should be given to the use of combination codes and to the many exclusion notes in chapter 11.

GASTROINTESTINAL HEMORRHAGE

Gastrointestinal (GI) bleeding manifests itself in several ways:

- Hematemesis (vomiting of blood), which indicates acute upper GI hemorrhage
- Melena (presence of dark-colored blood in stool), which indicates upper or lower GI hemorrhage
- Occult bleeding (presence of blood in stool that can be seen only on laboratory examination), which indicates upper or lower GI bleeding
- Hematochezia (presence of bright-colored blood in stool), which indicates lower GI bleeding

FIGURE 19.1 The Digestive System

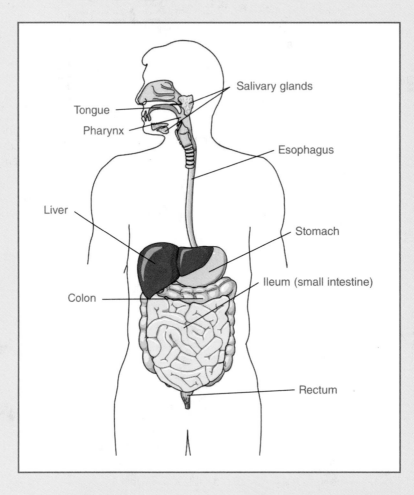

The most common causes of GI bleeding are gastric and intestinal ulcers and diverticular disease of the intestine. A diverticular hemorrhage stops spontaneously in approximately 80 percent of cases, with the other 20 percent experiencing a second or third bleeding episode. ICD-10-CM provides specific codes for GI tract ulcers, gastritis, angiodysplasia, duodenitis, gastroduodenitis, Crohn's disease, ulcerative colitis, diverticulosis, and diverticulitis to indicate whether there is associated hemorrhage or bleeding. Examples include the following:

K29.01	Acute gastritis with hemorrhage
K57.13	Diverticulitis of small intestine with hemorrhage
K31.811	Angiodysplasia of duodenum with hemorrhage

As stated in Section I. A. 15 of the Official Coding Guidelines, the classification presumes a causal relationship between the two conditions linked by the terms "with" or "in" in the Alphabetic Index or Tabular List. ICD-10-CM provides such a linkage for bleeding with certain GI conditions such as ulcers, gastritis, duodenitis, ulcerative esophagitis, and diverticulosis. Unless the provider documents a different cause of the bleeding or states that the conditions are unrelated, it is appropriate to report the combination code for these conditions. When codes for bleeding of any of the conditions mentioned above are available, do not assign codes **K92.0, Hematemesis; K92.1, Melena;** or **K92.2, Gastrointestinal hemorrhage, unspecified.** These codes are acceptable only when the classification does not presume a linkage between bleeding and the condition, or when the physician's diagnostic statement clearly indicates that the bleeding is due to another condition. Patients with a recent history of GI bleeding are sometimes seen for an endoscopy to determine the site of the bleeding but do not demonstrate any bleeding during the examination. If the physician documents a clinical diagnosis based on the history or other evidence, the fact that no bleeding occurs during the episode of care does not preclude the assignment of a code that includes mention of hemorrhage, or a code from K92.0 through K92.2 when the cause of bleeding could not be determined.

Patients may present for a colonoscopy because of rectal bleeding. If the findings include internal and external hemorrhoids with no statement as to whether the rectal bleeding is due to the hemorrhoids, the physician should be queried to determine whether the rectal bleeding is secondary to the hemorrhoids or the hemorrhoids are an incidental finding. If the hemorrhoids are incidental findings and unrelated to the rectal bleeding, code **K62.5, Hemorrhage of anus and rectum,** should be assigned followed by codes for the hemorrhoids without mention of complication. If, however, the physician establishes a causal relationship between the bleeding and the internal and external hemorrhoids, assign codes **K64.8, Other hemorrhoids,** and **K64.4, Residual hemorrhoidal skin tags.** "Bleeding" is a nonessential modifier under "hemorrhoids" in the Alphabetic Index and in the inclusion terms for codes K64.0–K64.3; therefore, bleeding is included in the code assignment for the hemorrhoids and should not be coded separately.

DISEASES OF THE ESOPHAGUS

Esophagitis is classified to category K20, with several different specific conditions. Eosinophilic esophagitis is coded to K20.0, other esophagitis is coded to K20.8-, and unspecified esophagitis is coded to K20.9-. Esophagitis with gastroesophageal reflux disease is coded to K21.0-. Esophagitis with other diseases of the esophagus are classified to category K22 as follows: Ulcerative esophagitis without bleeding is classified to **K22.10, Ulcer of esophagus without bleeding;** ulcerative esophagitis with bleeding is classified to **K22.11, Ulcer of esophagus with bleeding.** Other esophageal conditions classified to category K22 are dyskinesia of esophagus and spasm of esophagus, both of which are classified to K22.4. Barrett's esophagus (codes K22.70 and K22.71-) is a precancerous condition in which the normal cells of the lining of the esophagus are replaced by columnar cells.

Bleeding of the esophagus is coded as **K22.8, Other specified diseases of esophagus,** unless the bleeding is due to esophageal varices. Esophageal varices are not classified as a disease of the digestive system but as a disease of the circulatory system. They are coded as follows:

I85.00   Esophageal varices without bleeding

I85.01   Esophageal varices with bleeding

When esophageal varices are associated with alcoholic liver disease, cirrhosis of the liver, schistosomiasis, toxic liver disease, or portal hypertension, dual coding is required, with the underlying condition coded first and an additional code for the esophageal varices (I85.10 or I85.11).

Examples include:

K74.60+I85.11   Bleeding esophageal varices with cirrhosis of liver

K76.6+I85.11   Bleeding esophageal varices in portal hypertension

Therapy for esophageal varices consists primarily of ligation of the esophageal vein (rather than the esophagus), which ICD-10-PCS classifies to the root operation "Occlusion," meaning "completely closing an orifice or the lumen of a tubular body part." This procedure may be performed via open approach, percutaneous approach, percutaneous endoscopic approach, natural or artificial opening approach, or natural or artificial opening endoscopic approach. Examples follow:

06L30ZZ   Occlusion of esophageal vein, open approach

06L33ZZ   Occlusion of esophageal vein, percutaneous approach

06L34ZZ   Occlusion of esophageal vein, percutaneous endoscopic approach

A related procedure is endoscopic banding (or ligation) of esophageal varices. The procedure involves the placement of rubber bands around the esophageal varices through a flexible endoscope. Code **06L38CZ, Occlusion of esophageal vein with extraluminal device, via natural or artificial opening endoscopic,** is assigned for this procedure.

Another treatment for esophageal varices is the endoscopic injection of a sclerosing agent or sclerotherapy, which ICD-10-PCS classifies to the root operation "Introduction." For example, endoscopic injection of sclerosing agent into varix of the lower esophagus is coded to **3E0G8TZ, Introduction of destructive agent into upper GI, via natural or artificial opening endoscopic.**

ULCERS OF THE STOMACH AND SMALL INTESTINE

Combination codes are provided for gastric, gastrojejunal, and duodenal ulcers that indicate whether there is associated bleeding, associated perforation, or both. These combination codes also distinguish between acute and chronic ulcers.

Ulcers of the stomach and the small intestine are often described as peptic without any further identification of the site. Review the medical record for any indication of the site involved; codes from category K27, Peptic ulcer, site unspecified, should not be used when a more specific code can be assigned. Examples of appropriate coding include the following:

K25.5   Chronic or unspecified gastric ulcer with perforation

K26.3   Acute duodenal ulcer without hemorrhage or perforation

K25.6   Chronic or unspecified gastric ulcer with hemorrhage and perforation

DIEULAFOY LESIONS

Dieulafoy lesions are a rare cause of major GI bleeding. When GI bleeding is present with Dieulafoy lesions, a separate code for the bleeding is not assigned because the bleeding is an integral part of the disease. Assign code K31.82 for Dieulafoy lesion of the stomach and duodenum and code K63.81 for Dieulafoy lesion of the intestine.

Code K22.8 is assigned for Dieulafoy lesions of the esophagus. Dieulafoy lesions of the esophagus typically cause severe bleeding. Endoscopic adrenaline injections can be used to control the bleeding. An injection that is performed in the inpatient setting or during a procedure is not coded separately. However, when the injection is the only therapeutic portion of an endoscopic procedure, the injection may be coded separately to report that the procedure was more than a diagnostic endoscopy. For example, when adrenaline is injected to control bleeding at the gastric fundus during esophagogastroduodenoscopy, assign code **3E0G8GC, Introduction of other therapeutic substance into upper GI, via natural or artificial opening endoscopic.**

COMPLICATIONS OF ARTIFICIAL OPENINGS OF THE DIGESTIVE SYSTEM

Complications of colostomy, enterostomy, gastrostomy, or esophagostomy are classified to category K94, Complications of artificial openings of the digestive system, rather than complications of surgical and medical care (categories T80–T88).

Complications of Colostomy and Enterostomy

Complications of colostomy and enterostomy are classified to subcategory K94.0, Colostomy complications. Additional codes are assigned to specify the type of infection, such as cellulitis of abdominal wall (L03.311) or sepsis (A40.-, A41.-), if that information is available in the medical record. Examples include:

K94.01   Colostomy hemorrhage
K94.03   Malfunction of colostomy
K94.12 + L03.311   Cellulitis of abdominal wall due to complication of enterostomy

Complications of Gastrostomy and Esophagostomy

Code K94.22 is assigned for an infection of the gastrostomy or gastrojejunostomy. Additional codes are assigned to specify the type of infection, if that information is available in the medical record. The mechanical complication of a gastrostomy or gastrojejunostomy, such as a clogged tube, is assigned code K94.23.

Code K94.32 is assigned for an infection of the esophagostomy. An additional code is assigned to specify the infection, if documented. Code K94.33 is assigned for a malfunction of the esophagostomy, such as a mechanical complication.

DIVERTICULOSIS AND DIVERTICULITIS

A diverticulum is a small pouch or sac opening from a tubular or saccular organ, such as the esophagus, intestine, or urinary bladder. Diverticulosis indicates the presence of one or more diverticula of the designated site; diverticulitis is the inflammation of existing diverticula. A diagnosis of diverticulitis assumes the presence of diverticula; only the code for diverticulitis is assigned, even when both diverticulitis and diverticulosis are mentioned in the physician's diagnostic statement. Examples of appropriate coding include the following:

K57.10   Diverticulosis of duodenum
K57.12   Diverticulosis and diverticulitis of duodenum

K57.13   Diverticulitis of jejunum with hemorrhage

K57.20   Diverticulitis of cecum with abscess

ICD-10-CM assumes diverticulosis, not otherwise specified, to be a condition of the intestine.

Congenital versus Acquired Diverticula

Diverticula may be either acquired or congenital. For certain sites, ICD-10-CM assumes that the condition is congenital unless specified otherwise; in other sites, the presumption is that the diverticula are acquired. For example, diverticula of the colon are assumed to be acquired unless specified as congenital; but diverticula of the esophagus are assumed to be congenital unless otherwise specified. The Alphabetic Index lists the following entries for diverticula of the colon and the esophagus:

> **Diverticulum, diverticula** ... K57.90 ...
> -colon—see Diverticulosis, intestine, large ...
> --congenital Q43.8 ...
> -esophagus (congenital) Q39.6
> --acquired (epiphrenic) (pulsion) (traction) K22.5 ...
> -Meckel's (displaced) (hypertrophic) Q43.0

Acquired diverticula of the esophagus are often described by the type of diverticulum (pulsion or traction) or by the portion of the esophagus involved (pharyngoesophageal, midesophageal, or epiphrenic). These qualifications do not affect the code assignment; all are coded **K22.5, Diverticulum of esophagus, acquired.** For example:

K22.5   Epiphrenic diverticula of esophagus

K22.5   Midesophageal traction diverticula of esophagus

COLON POLYPS

Colon polyps are growths that form on the lining of the colon. The type of polyp is used to predict whether the growth will develop into a malignancy. Adenomatous polyps, or adenomas, are the most common type of polyp and are the most likely to become malignant. Category D12, Benign neoplasm of colon, rectum, anus and anal canal, is assigned according to anatomical location for adenomatous (neoplastic) polyps. Sessile serrated polyp is a type of adenoma that is also known as sessile serrated adenoma. Assign a code from category D12 for a sessile serrated polyp. Code **D12.8, Benign neoplasm of the rectum,** is assigned for hyperplastic rectal polyp with focal adenomatous changes. This is a mixed polyp that is clinically treated as an adenoma, requiring stricter surveillance and follow-up.

Hyperplastic polyps are the second most common type of colon polyp. They have little potential to become malignant, so they are followed on a different surveillance protocol than adenomatous polyps. Code **K63.5, Polyp of colon,** is the default code assignment when the polyp is not documented by the provider as adenomatous or neoplastic, even if the specific site is known and indexed (e.g., sigmoid or transverse colon).

Code **Z87.19, Personal history of other diseases of the digestive system,** is assigned for a personal history of hyperplastic colon polyp and for history of rectal polyp. A code from subcat-

egory Z86.01, Personal history of benign neoplasm, is assigned for history of adenoma or neoplastic polyp. Code **Z86.010, Personal history of colonic polyps,** is assigned for history of unspecified colon polyp.

DIGESTIVE SYSTEM PROCEDURES

Two ICD-10-PCS guidelines are important to consider when coding procedures of the GI system. The first guideline relates to the general body part values "upper intestinal tract" and "lower intestinal tract" provided for the root operations "Change," "Inspection," "Removal," and "Revision." Upper intestinal tract includes the portion of the GI tract from the esophagus down to and including the duodenum. The lower intestinal tract includes the portion of the GI tract from the jejunum down to and including the rectum and anus. For example, in the root operation "Inspection" (Table 0DJ), inspection of the jejunum is coded using the body part "lower intestinal tract."

The second guideline of note (not limited to the GI system) is a reminder that anastomosis of a tubular body part is not coded separately. As noted in chapter 9 of this handbook, the directive states that "procedural steps necessary to reach the operative site and close the operative site" are not coded separately. For example, when a resection of the sigmoid colon is performed with anastomosis of the descending colon to the rectum, the anastomosis is not coded separately.

Stoma reversal surgery is also known as stoma closure or stoma takedown. During an ileostomy closure, an incision is made around the stoma, the intestine is pulled out of the abdominal cavity, both ends of the intestine are excised, and an anastomosis is done using sutures or staples. Ileostomy closure is coded using the root operation "Excision." The anastomosis of the intestinal ends is inherent to the surgery and is not coded separately.

Similarly, during reversal of a transverse or loop colostomy, an incision is made around the stoma to access the abdomen and the distal colon. The ends of the intestine are excised and an end-to-end anastomosis is performed. "Excision" is the root operation for a transverse loop colostomy takedown. If the colon ends are sutured together without excision of the colon, the procedure is coded as a "Repair."

Closure of a Hartmann (end stoma) is complex and requires a more invasive approach to access two ends of the bowel that are not in proximity. The stoma end and the distal end of the bowel are mobilized to reach each other and are connected. After the anastomosis, the bowel is returned to its proper anatomical location. "Reposition" is the root operation for a Hartmann closure. Reposition captures the objective of the procedure: moving some or all of a body part to a normal or other suitable location.

The Index entry under "Takedown, Stoma" directs the user to "see Excision" or "see Reposition." Coding professionals should note that there are various types of procedures with different root operations for stoma takedown. ICD-10-PCS procedure codes should not be assigned based solely on where the Index directs. Further review of the documentation should be done to determine what was actually performed during the procedure.

Fine needle aspiration introduces a needle through tissue. Suction is applied and aspirated for biopsy. The Index to Procedures classifies fine needle aspiration as "Drainage" when fluid or gas is aspirated, and as "Excision" when tissue is removed. When the documentation does not specify whether fluid or tissue was removed, assign the root operation "Excision" with the appropriate body part.

Brush biopsies to obtain samples of cells are reported with the root operation "Extraction" of the body part and with the qualifier "diagnostic." For example, brush biopsy of the stomach performed via esophagogastroduodenoscopy is coded as **0DD68ZX, Extraction of stomach, via natural or artificial opening endoscopic, diagnostic.**

EXERCISE 19.1

Code the following diagnoses and procedures. Do not assign External cause of morbidity codes.

1. Acute gastric ulcer with massive gastrointestinal hemorrhage
   Exploratory laparotomy with gastric resection, pylorus, with end-to-end anastomosis

2. Duodenal ulcer, with perforation and hemorrhage

3. Penetrating gastric ulcer
   Open resection of esophageal junction (subtotal gastrectomy) with esophageal anastomosis
   Vagotomy

4. Bleeding gastric ulcer

5. Gastrointestinal ulcerative mucositis due to high-dose chemotherapy for multiple myeloma, subsequent encounter

6. Hemorrhage from Dieulafoy lesion of the duodenum
   Esophagogastroduodenoscopy with placement of clips to control bleeding

7. Clogged feeding jejunostomy. Nonincisional change of feeding jejunostomy catheter

DISEASES OF THE BILIARY SYSTEM AND THE LIVER

Acute and chronic cholecystitis without associated calculus is classified into category K81, with additional characters indicating whether the cholecystitis is acute (K81.0), chronic (K81.1), both acute and chronic (K81.2), or unspecified (K81.9). Combination codes are assigned for cholecystitis, cholelithiasis, and choledocholithiasis to permit reporting these related conditions with a single code. These codes are presented in three groups: calculus of gallbladder (K80.0- through K80.2-), calculus of bile duct (K80.3- through K80.5-), and calculus of both gallbladder and bile ducts (K80.6- through K80.7-).

Within the K80.0-, K80.1-, K80.2-, K80.4-, K80.6-, and K80.7- groups, the fourth character indicates whether there is associated cholecystitis. In subcategory K80.3, the fourth character indicates whether there is cholangitis, rather than cholecystitis, whereas the fourth character in subcategory K80.5 indicates that there is neither cholangitis nor cholecystitis. Codes K80.66 and K80.67 are combination codes that include calculus of gallbladder and bile duct with both acute and chronic cholecystitis. Fifth characters in category K80, Cholelithiasis, indicate whether there is associated obstruction.

Codes **K82.0, Obstruction of gallbladder,** and **K83.1, Obstruction of bile duct,** are assigned only when there is obstruction but no calculi are present.

Cholesterolosis

Cholesterolosis is a condition characterized by abnormal deposits of cholesterol and other lipids in the lining of the gallbladder. In its diffuse form, it is known as strawberry gallbladder. This diagnosis is usually made by the pathologist on the basis of tissue examination and is ordinarily an incidental finding without clinical significance. It should not be coded when other gallbladder pathology is present.

Postcholecystectomy Syndrome

Postcholecystectomy syndrome (K91.5) is a condition in which symptoms suggestive of biliary tract disease either persist or develop following cholecystectomy with no demonstrable cause or abnormality found on workup. A postoperative complication code from the T80–T88 series is not assigned with code K91.5.

Hepatic Encephalopathy

Care should be exercised when coding hepatic encephalopathy because the condition is not synonymous with hepatic coma. Hepatic encephalopathy refers to the loss of brain function resulting when the liver is unable to remove toxins from the blood. The toxic buildup in the brain can advance to the point of resulting in hepatic coma. It is the physician's responsibility to document whether or not the patient has hepatic encephalopathy "with" coma. When coding hepatic encephalopathy, the default is "without coma." The ICD-10-CM Index to Diseases and Injuries entry for "Encephalopathy, hepatic" states "see Failure, hepatic." At the Index entry "Failure, hepatic," there are subentries for codes to specifically describe hepatic failure with or without coma. The appropriate code assignment for hepatic encephalopathy would depend on the underlying cause, such as due to drugs or toxic liver disease (K71.10), due to alcohol (K70.40), postprocedural (K91.82), or due to viral hepatitis (B15–B19). Code **K72.90, Hepatic failure, unspecified without coma,** should be assigned if the only documentation in the medical record is "hepatic encephalopathy," without any further specification of the underlying cause.

Cholecystectomy

A cholecystectomy (excision of the gallbladder) can be total (root operation "Resection") or partial (root operation "Excision") and can be performed either as an open procedure (open approach); through a minor incision (percutaneous approach); through a small, less-invasive laparoscopic incision (percutaneous endoscopic approach); or through a transorifice endoscopic approach (via natural or artificial opening endoscopic). (For illustrations of Medical and Surgical Section approaches, please refer to figure 7.5 on pages 74–75.) When coding a cholecystectomy, review the operative report to determine whether exploration or incision of the bile ducts was also performed for removal of stones or for other relief of obstruction, as well as whether an intraoperative cholangiogram was performed.

FIGURE 19.2   Excerpt from ICD-10-PCS Table for Hepatobiliary System Extirpation

Section   **0**   Medical and Surgical
Body System   **F**   Hepatobiliary System and Pancreas
Operation   **C**   Extirpation: Taking or cutting out solid matter from a body part

Body Part	Approach	Device	Qualifier
0 Liver 1 Liver, Right Lobe 2 Liver, Left Lobe	0 Open 3 Percutaneous 4 Percutaneous Endoscopic	Z No Device	Z No Qualifier
4 Gallbladder G Pancreas	0 Open 3 Percutaneous 4 Percutaneous Endoscopic 8 Via Natural or Artificial Opening Endoscopic	Z No Device	Z No Qualifier
5 Hepatic Duct, Right 6 Hepatic Duct, Left 7 Hepatic Duct, Common 8 Cystic Duct 9 Common Bile Duct C Ampulla of Vater D Pancreatic Duct F Pancreatic Duct, Accessory	0 Open 3 Percutaneous 4 Percutaneous Endoscopic 7 Via Natural or Artificial Opening 8 Via Natural or Artificial Opening Endoscopic	Z No Device	Z No Qualifier

Removal of Biliary Calculi

Biliary stones are removed in several ways. A cholecystectomy automatically removes any gallbladder calculus. Alternatively, a cholecystotomy can be carried out for the removal of gallbladder stones without removing the gallbladder. ICD-10-PCS classifies the removal of biliary stones to the root operation "Extirpation" with unique body part (character 4) values for the biliary ducts as shown in figure 19.2.

Stones in the biliary duct can be removed via the open approach, percutaneously, via percutaneous endoscopic approach, via natural or artificial opening, or via natural or artificial opening endoscopic.

Extracorporeal shock wave lithotripsy (ESWL) destroys biliary stones without invasive surgery. The advantages of lithotripsy over conventional surgery for removal of stones include a shorter hospital stay and avoidance of the potential complications associated with surgical intervention. A physician may opt to perform fragmentation of the stones as a stand-alone procedure to allow for spontaneous expulsion of the fragments, or she may perform additional procedures to physically remove the fragments. ICD-10-PCS classifies lithotripsy without fragment removal to the root operation "Fragmentation" with the approach being "external." For example, extracorporeal lithotripsy of the left hepatic duct is coded to **0FF6XZZ, Fragmentation in left hepatic duct, external approach.** However, if the lithotripsy involves removal of the fragments, the procedure is classified to the root operation "Extirpation" instead. Examples of procedures performed with ESWL include endoscopic retrograde cholangiopancreatography (ERCP) and endoscopic pancreatic sphincterotomy.

EXERCISE 19.2

Code the following diagnoses and procedures. Do not assign External cause of morbidity codes.

1. Acute cholecystitis with calculus of gallbladder

   and bile duct

   Total laparoscopic cholecystectomy

2. Chronic cholecystitis with calculus in common duct

   Total open cholecystectomy

   Open common bile duct exploration with removal of

   common bile duct stone

   Intraoperative cholangiogram (gallbladder and

   bile ducts with high osmolar contrast)

   Incidental open total appendectomy

3. Biliary obstruction, extrahepatic

4. Cholecystitis, acute and chronic, with cholesterolosis

   Total laparoscopic cholecystectomy

5. Acute cholecystitis with choledocholithiasis

6. Calculi in gallbladder and bile duct

7. Acute and chronic cholecystitis with gallbladder

   and bile duct calculus and obstruction

ADHESIONS

Intestinal and peritoneal adhesions are classified as code **K56.50, Intestinal adhesions [bands], unspecified as to partial versus complete obstruction; K56.51, Intestinal adhesions [bands], with partial obstruction; K56.52, Intestinal adhesions [bands], with complete obstruction; or K66.0, Peritoneal adhesions (postprocedural) (postinfection); or with codes in subcategory K56.6, Other and unspecified intestinal obstruction.** These codes do not include pelvic peritoneal adhesions; such adhesions are classified as code **N73.6, Female pelvic peritoneal adhesions (postinfective).**

Usually, minor adhesions do not cause symptoms or increase the difficulty of performing an operative procedure. When minor adhesions are easily lysed as part of another procedure, coding a diagnosis of adhesions and a lysis procedure is inappropriate. For example, minor adhesions around the gallbladder may be lysed during gallbladder surgery; coding of adhesions and/or lysis is not appropriate in such situations. Sometimes, however, a strong band of adhesions can cause obstruction or prevent the surgeon from gaining access to the organ to be removed, and a surgical lysis is required before the operation can proceed. In such cases, coding both the adhesions and lysis is appropriate when both the clinical significance of the adhesions and the complexity of the lysis of adhesions are documented by the provider. Do not code adhesions, and lysis thereof, based solely on mention of adhesions or lysis in an operative report. Documentation of clinical significance by the surgeon may include, but is not limited to, the following language: numerous adhesions requiring a long time to lyse, extensive adhesions involving tedious lysis, extensive lysis, and so forth. If there is any question, the determination of whether the adhesions and the lysis are significant enough to merit coding must be made by the physician.

Lysis of adhesions procedures are classified in ICD-10-PCS to the root operation "Release." In the root operation "Release," the body part value coded is the body part being freed and not the tissue being manipulated or cut to free the body part. For example, open lysis of small intestine adhesions is coded to the "small intestine" body part value (8) and reported as 0DN80ZZ.

HERNIAS OF THE ABDOMINAL CAVITY

Hernias are classified by type and site, with combination codes used to indicate any associated gangrene or obstruction. With inguinal and femoral hernias, the codes further subdivide the hernia as unilateral or bilateral and whether it is specified as recurrent (that is, whether it had been repaired during a previous surgery). An incisional hernia is classified as a ventral hernia. Hernias described as incarcerated or strangulated are classified as obstructed. A hernia with both gangrene and obstruction is classified to hernia with gangrene. Careful review of the medical record and attention to instructional notes are important steps in coding these conditions. Coding examples include the following:

K40.00	Bilateral inguinal hernia with obstruction (no mention of gangrene)
K40.41	Unilateral recurrent inguinal hernia with gangrene
K41.11	Gangrenous femoral hernia, recurrent, bilateral
K44.1	Diaphragmatic hernia with gangrene
K42.0	Umbilical hernia with obstruction
K41.30	Incarcerated femoral hernia

Hernia repairs (herniorrhaphies) can be performed with a laparoscope inserted through a small incision or through a traditional open surgical approach. When coding hernia repairs, be careful not to use a bilateral repair code when the hernia itself is described as unilateral. A unilateral repair may be performed even though bilateral hernias are present, but, obviously, it is impossible to repair bilateral hernias when only one hernia exists.

Care should be taken to understand how the hernia repair is performed because ICD-10-PCS classifies herniorrhaphy procedures to two different root operations. Herniorrhaphies are classified to the root operation "Repair," unless the repair is accomplished with the use of a biologic or synthetic material such as a mesh or graft, in which case the root operation "Supplement" is used. In addition, herniorrhaphies are classified to the body systems "anatomical regions, lower extremities," or "general" and the appropriate body part where the hernia is located. For example, an open repair of a bilateral inguinal hernia is coded to 0YQA0ZZ, while an open repair of a ventral hernia is coded to 0WQF0ZZ.

Coding examples include:

0YQ50ZZ	Open repair of right inguinal hernia
0YU54JZ	Laparoscopic repair of right inguinal hernia with mesh prosthesis
0YQA3ZZ	Percutaneous repair of bilateral inguinal hernias

EXERCISE 19.3

Code the following diagnoses and procedures. Do not assign External cause of morbidity codes.

1. Right direct inguinal hernia and left indirect sliding inguinal hernia
   Open repair of bilateral inguinal hernias

2. Incarcerated left inguinal hernia
   Laparoscopic left inguinal herniorrhaphy with mesh prosthesis

3. Recurrent left inguinal hernia
   Percutaneous repair of inguinal hernia, left

4. Gangrenous umbilical hernia
   Open repair of umbilical hernia

5. Strangulated umbilical hernia
   Laparoscopic repair of umbilical hernia with mesh prosthesis

6. Reflux esophagitis secondary to sliding
   esophageal hiatal hernia
   Repair of right esophageal hiatus hernia, open abdominal
   approach

7. Recurrent ventral incisional hernia with obstruction
   and gangrene

APPENDICITIS

Category K35, Acute appendicitis, uses a fourth character to indicate the presence of either generalized peritonitis (K35.2) or localized peritonitis (K35.3). A fifth character reports whether there is perforation, gangrene, or abscess. Unspecified acute appendicitis is coded to K35.80. Occasionally, an appendix ruptures during an appendectomy; this is not classified as a complication of surgery.

Category K37, Unspecified appendicitis, is a vague category that should not be used in an acute care facility. Additional information is almost always available in the medical record.

Surgical removal of the appendix is coded to the root operation "Resection." Incidental appendectomy refers to a procedure performed to remove the appendix as a routine prophylactic measure in the course of other abdominal surgery. ICD-10-PCS does not distinguish between an incidental appendectomy and an appendectomy to remove a diseased appendix.

DIARRHEA

A code from categories A00 through A09 is assigned for infectious diarrhea when the organism has been identified. Code A09 is assigned for infectious diarrhea not otherwise specified, or described only as dysenteric diarrhea, endemic diarrhea, or epidemic diarrhea. Check the Alphabetic Index carefully before coding, because diarrhea can be related to a variety of conditions. Symptom code R19.7 is assigned for diarrhea for which no appropriate subterm can be located. Examples of appropriate code assignments include the following:

A04.71	Diarrhea due to *Clostridium difficile,* recurrent
R19.7	Acute diarrhea
A07.3	Coccidial diarrhea
K52.9	Chronic diarrhea
R19.7	Infantile diarrhea
K59.1	Functional diarrhea

CONSTIPATION

Slow transit constipation (K59.01) results from a delay in transit of fecal material throughout the colon secondary to smooth muscle. Outlet dysfunction constipation (K59.02) results from difficulty evacuating the rectum during attempts at defecation. Treatments for these two types of constipation are very different. The slow transit type is treated with either laxatives or surgery. Biofeedback is taught for relaxation for outlet dysfunction constipation. Medications may alter nerve input to the GI tract and inhibit bowel movement. Constipation that is a side effect of medication is reported with code **K59.03, Drug induced constipation.** An additional code from T36–T50 is assigned with the fifth or sixth character 5 to identify the adverse effect of the drug. For example, opioid-induced constipation is coded to K59.03 followed by **T40.2X5-, Adverse effect of other opioids.** Chronic idiopathic constipation or functional constipation (K59.04) is constipation in the absence of physiological abnormality. Unspecified constipation is coded to K59.00.

BARIATRIC SURGERY AND COMPLICATIONS

Bariatric surgery refers to procedures performed on morbidly obese patients for the purpose of weight loss. Several types of malabsorptive and restrictive gastric procedures are performed for weight loss when other methods have failed for severely obese patients. (See figure 19.3 for illustrations of bariatric procedures.)

Malabsorptive operations, such as gastric bypass surgery, are the most common types of bariatric procedures. They achieve weight loss by removing a portion of the stomach or by resecting and rerouting the small intestines to a small stomach pouch, which restricts food intake and the amount of calories and nutrients the body absorbs. When coding bypass procedures, it is important to understand the body part bypassed from and the body part bypassed to. The ICD-10-PCS fourth character body part specifies the body part bypassed from (for example, the stomach), and the seventh character qualifier specifies the body part bypassed to (for example, the jejunum).

Restrictive operations, such as adjustable gastric banding and vertical banded gastroplasty, restrict food intake by reducing the size of the stomach with an implanted device, but they do not interfere with the normal digestive process. Restrictive operations such as gastric banding are classified to the root operation "Restriction."

FIGURE 19.3   Illustrations of Bariatric Surgery

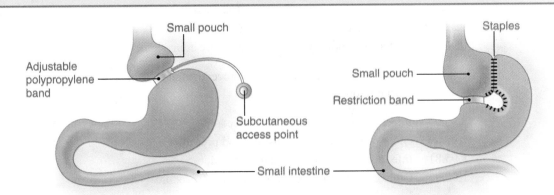

ADJUSTABLE GASTRIC BANDING

VERTICAL BANDED GASTROPLASTY

Adjustable gastric banding and *vertical banded gastroplasty* are gastric surgeries used to restrict and decrease food intake. The adjustable polypropylene band may be tightened or loosened over time to change the size of the gastric passage. The vertical banded gastroplasty utilizes a restriction band and staples to create a small stomach pouch. The band delays the emptying of food from the pouch, causing a feeling of fullness.

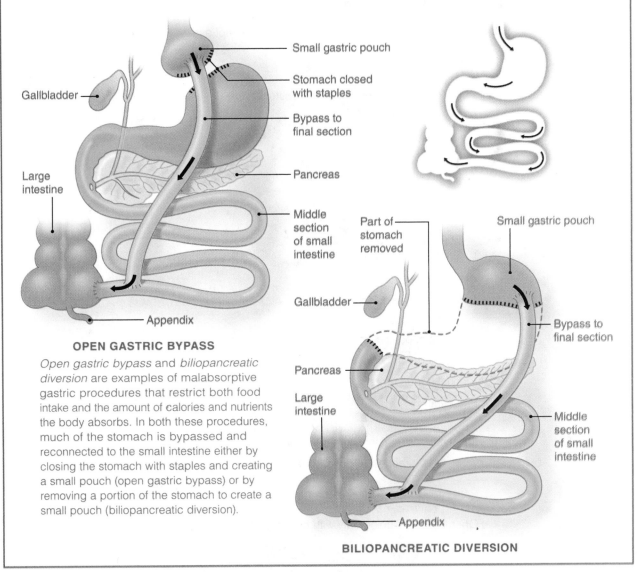

OPEN GASTRIC BYPASS

Open gastric bypass and *biliopancreatic diversion* are examples of malabsorptive gastric procedures that restrict both food intake and the amount of calories and nutrients the body absorbs. In both these procedures, much of the stomach is bypassed and reconnected to the small intestine either by closing the stomach with staples and creating a small pouch (open gastric bypass) or by removing a portion of the stomach to create a small pouch (biliopancreatic diversion).

BILIOPANCREATIC DIVERSION

Coding examples include:

0DV64CZ	Laparoscopic gastric restrictive procedure
0DW64CZ	Laparoscopic revision of gastric band
0D160ZB	Open gastric bypass (stomach to ileum)
0DB64Z3	Laparoscopic vertical (sleeve) gastrectomy

Category K95, Complications of bariatric procedures, has been created to uniquely identify complications of bariatric procedures:

K95.01	Infection due to gastric band procedure
K95.09	Other complications of gastric band procedure
K95.81	Infection due to other bariatric procedure
K95.89	Other complications of other bariatric procedure

In the case of infections, additional codes are used to specify the type of infection, such as cellulitis of abdominal wall (L03.311) or sepsis (A40.-, A41.-), and the organism, such as a bacterial or viral infectious agent (B95.-, B96.-).

EXERCISE 19.4

Code the following diagnoses and procedures. Do not assign External cause of morbidity codes.

---

1. Acute ruptured appendicitis with postoperative

   intestinal obstruction

   Open appendectomy

---

2. Acute hepatitis and early cirrhosis of the liver

   due to chronic alcoholism

---

3. Perirectal abscess

   Atony of colon

   Percutaneous incision and drainage of perirectal abscess

---

4. Alcoholic hepatic coma with massive ascites secondary

   to Laennec's cirrhosis

   Alcohol dependence

   Paracentesis

---

5. Intestinal obstruction due to peritoneal adhesive band

   Open lysis of adhesive band large intestine

---

6. Diverticulosis and diverticulitis of right colon

   Open right hemicolectomy with end-to-end anastomosis

---

7. Infection of gastrostomy with abscess of abdominal wall
   due to *Streptococcus* B

   _____

8. Polyp of rectum
   Colonoscopy with polypectomy

   _____

9. Neurogenic bowel

   _____

10. Morbid obesity
    Laparoscopic gastric bypass to ileum

   _____

CHAPTER 20

Diseases of the Genitourinary System

CHAPTER OVERVIEW

- Most diseases of the genitourinary system are classified in chapter 14 of ICD-10-CM.

  — Genitourinary diseases are not found in chapter 14 if they are classified by etiology.

  — The genitourinary diseases classified by etiology include transmissible infections; neoplastic diseases; and conditions complicating pregnancy, childbirth, and the puerperium.

- The term "urinary tract infection" is often used by physicians when referring to conditions such as urethritis, cystitis, or pyelonephritis.

- There are different codes for urinary incontinence depending on the type of incontinence (e.g., stress, functional). When the underlying cause is known, that should be sequenced first.

- Chronic kidney disease develops in conjunction with other conditions. The instructions for sequencing of the kidney disease code in conjunction with other codes are found in the Tabular List.

- A relationship is presumed when a patient has both hypertension and kidney disease. Codes extend to the fifth character to cover this condition.

- Renal dialysis codes range from admission codes to codes for the insertion of catheter without the performance of dialysis. Dialysis codes cover complications such as dialysis dementia.

- Conditions involving the prostate involve a fourth and fifth character. Neoplasms of the prostate are not included within this category of codes.

- Other related codes covered in this chapter are prostatectomy, endometriosis, genital prolapse, dysplasia of the cervix and vulva, and endometrial ablation.

- Neoplasms of the breast are classified in chapter 2 of ICD-10-CM. However, not all conditions and procedures involving the breast are related to neoplasms.

LEARNING OUTCOMES

After studying this chapter, you should be able to:

Distinguish among the different conditions often referred to as urinary tract infections.

Code for a variety of kidney diseases and their treatments.

Explain coding for kidney disease in conjunction with hypertension and diabetes.

Classify conditions that affect male and female genitalia.

TERMS TO KNOW

Acute kidney failure
sudden failure of renal function following a severe insult to the kidneys

Chronic kidney disease
long-term disability of the renal function

Nephropathy
general term indicating that renal disease is present

Ureter
carries urine from the kidneys to the bladder

Urethra
carries urine from the bladder to the outside of the body

REMEMBER . . .

It is important to distinguish between chronic kidney disease, acute kidney failure, and acute kidney injury.

INTRODUCTION

Chapter 14 of ICD-10-CM classifies diseases of the genitourinary system, except those that are classified by etiology, such as certain easily transmissible infections; neoplastic diseases; and conditions complicating pregnancy, childbirth, and the puerperium. Subterms should be checked carefully in the Alphabetic Index, and special attention should be given to the terms "urethra" and "ureter," which are often confused by coding professionals.

INFECTIONS OF THE GENITOURINARY TRACT

Physicians often use the term "urinary tract infection" (UTI) when referring to conditions such as urethritis, cystitis, or pyelonephritis. Urethritis and cystitis are lower urinary tract infections; pyelonephritis is an infection of the upper urinary tract. The main term for the specific condition in the Alphabetic Index should be reviewed before checking the main term **Infection.** For example, under the main term **Cystitis,** subterms are located for diphtheritic (A36.85) and chlamydial (A56.01) infection. When there is no subterm for the organism, the code for the condition is assigned, with an additional code from categories B95–B97 to indicate the organism. For example, there is no subterm for *Escherichia coli* under the main term **Cystitis;** therefore, codes N30.90 and B96.20 are assigned for cystitis due to *E. coli*.

The following examples indicate complete coding for such infections:

A59.03	Cystitis due to trichomonas
N30.00 + B96.4	Acute cystitis due to proteus infection
N11.9 + B96.20	Chronic pyelonephritis due to *E. coli*

Urinary tract infections that develop following surgery are rarely true postoperative infections and are not usually classified as such. When the operative procedure involves the urinary tract, how-

---

FIGURE 20.1   The Urinary System

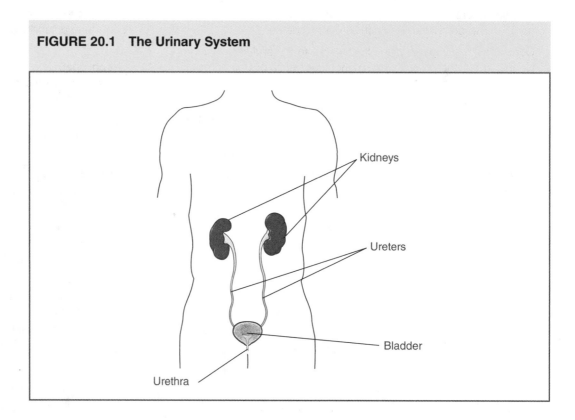

ever, it may be appropriate to ask the physician whether the infection is related to the procedure. As with all postprocedural complications, code assignment is based on the provider's documentation of the relationship between the infection and the procedure. In the absence of documentation indicating that the infection is due to the surgical procedure, code **N39.0, Urinary tract infection, site not specified,** should be assigned. When the infection is related to the presence of an implant, a graft, or a device (such as an indwelling or a suprapubic catheter), code T83.5- or T83.6- is assigned. An additional code may be included to identify the infection. If the provider states that the UTI is secondary to the indwelling urethral catheter, assign code **T83.511-, Infection and inflammatory reaction due to indwelling urethral catheter,** and code **N39.0, Urinary tract infection, site not specified.**

EXERCISE 20.1

Code the following diagnoses and procedures. Do not assign External cause of morbidity codes.

1. Urethral stricture due to gonorrheal infection
   Urethral dilation via cystoscope

   _____

2. Abscess of right scrotum due to group B
   Streptococcus
   Percutaneous incision and drainage of scrotal abscess

   _____

3. Acute pyelonephritis due to *Helicobacter pylori*
   infection

   _____

4. Chronic cystitis with hematuria
   Pseudomonas infection

   _____

5. Chronic cystitis due to *Monilia* infection

   _____

6. Urinary tract infection due to candidiasis

   _____

HEMATURIA

Hematuria refers to blood in the urine. Gross hematuria refers to hematuria that is so plentiful that it is visible to the naked eye. Microscopic hematuria refers to blood in the urine visible only under a microscope. ICD-10-CM provides separate codes for gross hematuria (R31.0), benign essential microscopic hematuria (R31.1), asymptomatic microscopic hematuria (R31.21), other microscopic hematuria (R31.29), and unspecified hematuria (R31.9). Many genitourinary conditions have hematuria as an integral associated symptom. For example, if the medical record has a diagnostic statement of hematuria due to renal calculus, only a code of **N20.0, Calculus of kidney,** is assigned. Because the hematuria is integral to this condition, no additional code is assigned for the symptom. A certain amount of hematuria is expected following a urinary tract procedure or a prostatectomy.

This is not considered a postoperative complication, and no code is assigned unless the bleeding is excessive or persistent.

Microscopic hematuria should not be confused with hemoglobinuria, which is coded as R82.3. Hemoglobinuria is an abnormal finding and refers to the presence of free hemoglobin in the urine on laboratory examination of the urine. It is reported only when the physician has indicated its clinical significance.

Codes in category N30, Cystitis, provide combination codes with a fifth character identifying whether hematuria is present or not.

URINARY INCONTINENCE

Stress incontinence causes involuntary urine loss with physical strain such as coughing or sneezing. Although it occurs in both male and female patients, it occurs more frequently in women, typically as a result of physical changes brought on by earlier childbearing. Prostate surgery is the primary cause of incontinence in men. Stress incontinence is coded as **N39.3, Stress incontinence (female) (male).** Urge incontinence is the sudden, intense urge to urinate followed by an involuntary loss of urine. It is sometimes referred to as "overactive bladder" or "spastic bladder." Urge incontinence is coded as **N39.41, Urge incontinence.** Urinary incontinence due to cognitive impairment, severe physical disability, or immobility is coded to **R39.81, Functional urinary incontinence.** Urinary incontinence of nonorganic origin is coded to **F98.0, Enuresis not due to a substance or known physiological condition.**

Other types of incontinence are classified in subcategory N39.4, Other specified urinary incontinence. When both urge and stress incontinence are present, the condition is coded as **N39.46, Mixed incontinence (male) (female).** Code N39.46 is not used when stress incontinence occurs with nocturnal enuresis, or when any other types of incontinence are present in combination. Report these conditions as separate codes. When the underlying cause of incontinence is known, the code for that condition should be sequenced first. Code N32.81 should also be assigned for any overactive bladder associated with conditions classified to codes N39.3 and N39.4-.

Treatment for incontinence depends, to a large extent, on the particular type of incontinence present. If it is due to an intrinsic sphincter deficiency, collagen injections are sometimes carried out. Code **3E0K3GC, Introduction of other therapeutic substance into genitourinary tract, percutaneous approach,** is assigned for this therapy.

Other treatments for incontinence are surgical in nature. Codes for repair of incontinence depend on the procedure performed. Typically, these procedures are classified to the root operation "Repair," "Reposition," or "Supplement." Examples of these procedure codes are:

0TSC0ZZ	Reposition bladder neck, open approach
0TSD4ZZ	Reposition urethra, percutaneous endoscopic approach
0TUC7KZ	Supplement bladder neck with nonautologous tissue substitute, via natural or artificial opening
0TQDXZZ	Repair urethra, external approach

RENAL DISEASE

Renal disease is classified into categories N00 through N29. Glomerulonephritis is a type of nephritis in which there is bilateral inflammatory change without infection. Nephrotic syndrome is a complex clinical state characterized by edema, albuminuria, and increased permeability of the glomerular capillary basement membrane. The syndrome may result from an unknown cause or from glomerulonephritis or diseases such as diabetes, systemic lupus erythematosus, hypertension, and amyloidosis. Nephropathy is a general term that indicates that renal disease is present. Infection of the kidney not otherwise specified is classified to code N15.9. Kidney disease complicating pregnancy, childbirth, and the puerperium is classified in chapter 15 of ICD-10-CM.

Chronic Kidney Disease and End-Stage Renal Disease

Chronic kidney disease (CKD) is considered a more current and precise term than chronic renal failure or chronic renal insufficiency. CKD develops as a complication of other diseases, such as diabetes mellitus, primary hypertension, glomerulonephritis, nephrosis, interstitial nephritis, systemic lupus erythematosus, obstructive uropathy, and polycystic kidney disease. The sequencing of the CKD code in relationship to codes for other contributing conditions is based on the conventions of the Tabular List.

Patients usually live for many years with CKD. When kidney involvement becomes so extensive that kidney function can no longer keep up with the body's needs, dialysis is usually required.

ICD-10-CM classifies CKD on the basis of severity. Based on the glomerular filtration rate (GFR), CKD has been categorized into five stages. Category N18, Chronic kidney disease (CKD), has been expanded to the fourth-character subcategory level for further specification of the varying stages of the disease. Subcategory N18.3 uses fifth characters to identify stage 3a, stage 3b, and unspecified stage 3 CKD. The fourth-character subcategory codes are as follows:

N18.1 Chronic kidney disease, stage 1
N18.2 Chronic kidney disease, stage 2 (mild)
N18.3- Chronic kidney disease, stage 3 (moderate)
N18.4 Chronic kidney disease, stage 4 (severe)
N18.5 Chronic kidney disease, stage 5
N18.6 End stage renal disease
N18.9 Chronic kidney disease, unspecified

End-stage renal disease (ESRD) (N18.6) is a complex syndrome characterized by a variable and inconsistent group of biochemical and clinical changes that affect volume regulation, acid-base balance, electrolyte balance, excretion of waste products, and several endocrine functions. It is a progression of CKD and is defined by clinicians as the point at which regular dialysis sessions or a kidney transplant is required to maintain life. For patients with end-stage renal disease, code Z99.2, Dependence on renal dialysis, should be assigned as an additional code to report dialysis status. Note that a patient with chronic kidney disease, stage 5, documented as requiring chronic dialysis, is to be coded to N18.6 and Z99.2, instead of N18.5, as instructed by the "excludes1" note at code N18.5. If both a stage of CKD and ESRD are documented for the same patient, only code N18.6 is assigned.

Chronic renal failure, not otherwise specified, chronic renal disease, and chronic renal insufficiency are assigned to code N18.9, Chronic kidney disease, unspecified.

Kidney transplant may be recommended for patients with severe CKD caused by severe, uncontrollable hypertension, infections, diabetes mellitus, or glomerulonephritis. Patients who have undergone kidney transplant may still have some form of CKD because the kidney transplant may not fully restore kidney function. Code Z94.0, Kidney transplant status, may be assigned with the appropriate CKD code to indicate that a CKD patient is status post–kidney transplant. It is incorrect to assume that mild or moderate CKD following a transplant is a transplant failure unless it is documented as such in the medical record.

If a transplant failure or rejection, or other transplant complication, is documented in a patient with severe CKD or ESRD, code T86.1-, Complications of kidney transplant, is assigned. If a post–kidney transplant patient has CKD and the documentation is unclear whether there is transplant failure or rejection, it is necessary to query the provider because the CKD or ESRD alone is not a transplant complication.

Acute Kidney Failure

Acute kidney failure (N17.-) is very different from chronic kidney disease; it is not a phase of the same condition. Chronic kidney disease is a long-term inability of the kidneys to function adequately; acute kidney failure is the sudden cessation of renal function following severe insult to normal kidneys. Toxic agents, traumatic or surgical shock, tissue destruction due to injury or surgery, or a variety of other conditions can cause acute kidney failure.

Acute renal insufficiency (N28.9) is considered an early stage of renal impairment, evidenced by diminished creatinine clearance or mildly elevated serum creatinine or blood urea nitrogen (BUN). Clinical symptoms or other abnormal laboratory findings may or may not be present but are usually minimal. Treatment varies, depending on the underlying cause, but serious attention is given to prevent the condition's progression to renal failure. Code **N99.89, Other postprocedural complications and disorders of genitourinary system,** is assigned if renal insufficiency is due to a procedure.

Physicians sometimes use the terms "renal insufficiency" and "renal failure" interchangeably, but ICD-10-CM classifies these terms to different codes when the conditions are acute. ICD-10-CM classifies unspecified and acute renal insufficiency to code N28.9, whereas acute kidney failure is assigned to category N17. It is important to be guided by the classification. If the physician uses both terms in the medical record, the physician should be queried for clarification as to the correct diagnosis. Unspecified renal failure is identified with code **N19, Unspecified kidney failure.**

Acute kidney injury is a phrase used by some physicians to refer to acute kidney failure. Care should be taken to determine whether the documentation refers to a traumatic injury to the kidney (which is assigned to a code in subcategory S37.0) or to a nontraumatic event, which is actually acute kidney failure. Nontraumatic acute kidney injury is assigned to **N17.9, Acute kidney failure, unspecified.** The default for acute kidney injury, unspecified as to traumatic or nontraumatic, is code N17.9.

Kidney Disease with Hypertension

ICD-10-CM presumes a causal relationship between hypertension and heart involvement and between hypertension and kidney involvement as the two conditions are linked by the term "with" in the Alphabetic Index. These conditions should be coded as related even in the absence of provider documentation explicitly linking them, unless the documentation clearly states the conditions are unrelated and/or the provider has specifically documented a different cause for the kidney or heart disease. Assign a code from combination category I12, Hypertensive chronic kidney disease, when both hypertension and a condition classifiable to category N18, Chronic kidney disease (CKD), are present. Assign a code from combination category I13, Hypertensive heart and chronic kidney disease, when there is hypertension with both heart and kidney involvement. The fourth or fifth character indicates the stage of CKD as follows:

- Category I12

  —Fourth character 0 is for "chronic kidney disease stage 5 or end-stage renal disease."

  —Fourth character 9 is for "chronic kidney disease stage 1 through stage 4, or unspecified chronic kidney disease."

- Category I13

  —Fourth character 0 is for "with heart failure and chronic kidney disease, stage 1 through 4, or unspecified chronic kidney disease."

  —Fourth character 1 is for CKD without heart failure, with the fifth character indicating the CKD stage as follows:

    –Fifth character 0 is for "chronic kidney disease stage 1 through stage 4, or unspecified."

    –Fifth character 1 is for "chronic kidney disease stage 5 or end-stage renal disease."

  —Fourth character 2 is for "with heart failure and chronic kidney disease, stage 5, or end-stage renal disease."

TABLE 20.1 Hypertensive Chronic Kidney Disease and Hypertensive Heart and Chronic Kidney Disease and the Applicable CKD Stages

Category I12–I13 Code	Additional CKD Stage Code Required	
	N18.1–N18.4 or N18.9	N18.5 or N18.6
I12.0		X
I12.9	X	
I13.0	X	
I13.10	X	
I13.11		X
I13.2		X

Codes from categories I12 and I13 require additional codes to identify the stage of CKD, as shown in table 20.1.

Acute kidney failure is not caused by hypertension and is not included in the hypertensive kidney disease codes. When acute kidney failure and hypertension are both present, assign a code from category N17, Acute kidney failure, with an additional code for the hypertension.

The use of codes from categories I12 and I13 does not apply in the following situations:

- The renal condition is acute kidney failure.
- The hypertension is described as secondary.
- The kidney disease is specifically stated as unrelated to the hypertension.

Examples of appropriate codes for kidney disease with hypertension include the following:

I12.9 + N18.9	Hypertensive kidney disease with chronic kidney disease
I13.10 + N18.32	Hypertensive heart and kidney disease with chronic kidney disease, stage 3b
I13.2 + N18.5 + I50.9	Hypertensive heart and kidney disease with stage 5 chronic kidney disease and congestive heart failure
N17.9 + I10	Acute kidney failure; hypertension

Kidney Disease with Diabetes Mellitus

Diabetic kidney complications are coded to E08–E13 with .21 for diabetic nephropathy, .22 for chronic kidney disease, and .29 for other kidney complication. Kidney disease sometimes results from both hypertension and diabetes mellitus. In this situation, the combination code from category I12 or category I13 and a code from subcategory E08–E13 with .2- are assigned. A code from category N18 is assigned to specify the stage of chronic kidney disease.

Examples of appropriate codes for kidney disease due to diabetes include the following:

E11.21	Diabetic nephrosis
I12.9 + E10.22 + N18.4	Chronic kidney disease stage 4 due to hypertension and type 1 diabetes mellitus
E10.22	Chronic kidney disease, unspecified, due to type 1 diabetes

RENAL DIALYSIS

When the kidneys are impaired and unable to function normally, renal dialysis may be started to replace the function of the kidneys. There are basically two types of kidney dialysis to remove waste and excess water from the blood: peritoneal dialysis and hemodialysis.

Patients with end-stage renal disease require a regular schedule of dialysis treatments to manage the symptoms arising from kidney disease. Typically, dialysis is performed as an outpatient service. When the encounter is for dialysis, assign the code for the underlying condition necessitating the dialysis as the reason for the encounter. Periodically, it may be necessary for care to be provided to the renal dialysis catheter, such as toilet or cleansing, or replacement of the catheter. These situations are coded to **Z49.01, Encounter for fitting and adjustment of extracorporeal dialysis catheter,** or code **Z49.02, Encounter for fitting and adjustment of peritoneal dialysis catheter.** Other encounters may be related to adequacy testing for dialysis, which are classified to codes **Z49.31, Encounter for adequacy testing for hemodialysis,** or **Z49.32, Encounter for adequacy testing for peritoneal dialysis.**

If the patient is admitted for other reasons but continues to receive dialysis therapy during the hospital stay or is known to be maintained on renal dialysis, code **Z99.2, Dependence on renal dialysis,** may be assigned as an additional code; the condition responsible for the admission is designated as the principal diagnosis. If the patient is known to be noncompliant with renal dialysis, code **Z91.15, Patient's noncompliance with renal dialysis,** may be assigned.

Peritoneal Dialysis

Peritoneal dialysis is accomplished by instilling a prepared fluid into the peritoneal cavity and removing the uremic toxins along with the prepared fluid. In peritoneal dialysis, a tube is inserted into the peritoneal cavity. Placement of a peritoneal catheter for dialysis is coded to insertion of infusion device. For example, if the procedure is performed using a percutaneous approach, it is coded to **0WHG33Z, Insertion of infusion device into peritoneal cavity, percutaneous approach.** In some cases, a peritoneal dialysis catheter may be placed with the external portion of the catheter left buried under the skin in anticipation of future dialysis. This technique allows the external cuff to heal in a sterile environment and reduces peritonitis. The embedded catheter also allows the patient to be prepared for peritoneal dialysis when there is the potential for a rapid decline in kidney function that produces the sudden need for dialysis. When it is time to externalize the cuff for dialysis, assign a code with the root operation "Revision." Revision is "correcting, to the extent possible, a portion of a malfunctioning device or the position of a displaced device." Although the device was not corrected or malfunctioning, it is considered displaced and nonfunctional until it is externalized. The catheter is repositioned in order to be used properly in the correct position. For example, assign code **0JWT33Z, Revision of infusion device in trunk subcutaneous tissue and fascia, percutaneous approach,** for the percutaneous externalization of a peritoneal dialysis catheter that was placed in a subcutaneous pocket several months before it was needed for dialysis. Code **3E1M39Z, Irrigation of peritoneal cavity using dialysate, percutaneous approach,** is assigned for the associated dialysis.

Hemodialysis

In hemodialysis, blood is removed from the body and filtered through a dialyzer, or artificial kidney, after which the filtered blood is returned to the body. There are three types of hemodialysis access: catheter, arteriovenous (AV) graft, and AV fistula. The associated dialysis is coded to the Extracorporeal or Systemic Assistance and Performance Section, "physiological systems" body system, and root operation "Performance" (completely taking over a physiological function by extracorporeal means). A fifth character is assigned for duration (less than 6 hours per day, 6–18 hours per day, or more than 18 hours per day) and continuity (intermittent, prolonged, or continuous).

Intermittent hemodialysis is the type of hemodialysis conventionally performed for ESRD. It usually involves four-hour sessions performed three times a week. Such intermittent hemodialysis encounters are coded to **5A1D70Z, Performance of urinary filtration, intermittent, less than 6 hours per day.**

Renal replacement therapy (RRT) represents two other forms of hemodialysis: prolonged intermittent renal replacement therapy (PIRRT) and continuous renal replacement therapy (CRRT). These treatments may be delivered to critically ill patients with acute renal failure or acute renal injury in intensive care. PIRRT is also known as sustained low-efficiency dialysis (SLED) and extended daily dialysis (EDD). It may be delivered for 6–18 hours per day with lower blood-pump speeds and lower dialysate flow rates to help maintain hemodynamic stability. CRRT is a slower form of hemodialysis that is delivered for 18–24 hours a day. It is often called continuous veno-venous hemofiltration (CVVH).

Hemodialysis via Catheter

Hemodialysis access via catheter is usually short-term access, although a catheter may be used for permanent access in some instances. The catheter is inserted into a large vein in either the neck or the chest. Compared with arteriovenous access, catheters have a greater tendency to become infected, and the blood may not be cleaned as thoroughly.

The coding of hemodialysis catheter access depends on whether the procedure requires the insertion of a venous catheter (assign the ICD-10-PCS code for insertion of infusion device, percutaneous approach), a tunneled catheter (assign codes for the infusion device catheter and for the tunneled vascular access device), or a totally implantable vascular access device (assign the codes for the totally implantable vascular access device and the infusion device catheter). Selection of the body part value for insertion of a vascular access device is based on the end placement of the infusion device, not the point of entry. For example, when a dialysis catheter is inserted via a micropuncture through the right internal jugular vein into the cavoatrial junction, where the superior vena cava joins the wall of the right atrium, assign code **02HV33Z, Insertion of infusion device into superior vena cava, percutaneous approach.**

A tunneled dialysis catheter is placed through a small incision at the neck where the catheter tip is advanced into the superior vena cava or right atrium. The opposite end of the catheter is tunneled through subcutaneous tissue and exits the body through a small incision at the chest wall. For a tunneled hemodialysis catheter that is placed into the right atrium, assign code **02H633Z, Insertion of infusion device into right atrium, percutaneous approach,** for the central venous catheter, and code **0JH63XZ, Insertion of tunneled vascular access device into chest subcutaneous tissue and fascia, percutaneous approach,** for the vascular access device.

When a tunneled hemodialysis catheter is exchanged by placing a new access catheter through the existing tunnel and into the right atrium using fluoroscopic guidance, the root operation "Change" is assigned for placing the catheter into the same exact position as the previous catheter. "Change" is defined as taking out or off a device from a body part and putting back an identical or similar device in or on the same body part without cutting or puncturing the skin or a mucous membrane. The approach is external. All "Change" procedures are coded by using the approach "external."

A totally implantable central vascular access device may be referred to as an implanted port, venous access port, or port-a-cath. It consists of two parts: an injection port and a catheter system. No part of the catheter system is brought out through the skin. The subcutaneous port is placed in a pocket created on the chest wall. The port is accessed percutaneously using a needle. The catheter is inserted into one of the main veins of the upper chest and is tunneled through the subcutaneous tissue. The tip of the catheter is advanced into the superior vena cava or the atrium. When a totally implantable central venous access device is placed via the right subclavian vein with the tip in the superior vena cava, and a pocket is created in the subcutaneous tissue of the chest to hold the port, assign code **02HV33Z, Insertion of infusion device into superior vena cava, percutaneous**

approach, for placement of the catheter, and code **0JH60WZ, Insertion of totally implantable vascular access device into chest subcutaneous tissue and fascia, open approach,** for placement of the subcutaneous port.

Patients are sometimes admitted for insertion of a catheter or a vascular access device, but no dialysis is performed during the admission. When dialysis is performed during the same episode of care, a procedure code for the dialysis is assigned to specify that dialysis was actually performed during the encounter. When the admission is for fitting or adjustment of the dialysis catheter, code Z49.01 is assigned for an extracorporeal catheter and code Z49.02 is assigned for a peritoneal catheter. Some coding examples follow:

N18.6 + Z99.2 + 0JH60WZ + 02H633Z   Patient with end-stage renal disease admitted for insertion of a totally implantable port-a-cath; the port was anchored in a subcutaneous pocket in the chest, and the catheter tip rested in the right atrium

Z49.01 + N18.6 + Z99.2 + 5A1D70Z   Patient with chronic kidney disease, stage 5, on chronic dialysis, admitted for cleansing of hemodialysis catheter, hemodialysis performed for five hours

Arteriovenous Graft

When a tubular graft is used to connect the artery and vein, the connection is known as an arteriovenous graft. After the graft has healed, hemodialysis is performed by puncturing the actual graft to provide access to the blood vessels. One needle is placed in the arterial side of the graft and one in the venous side. When coding the creation of an AV graft, the root operation is "Bypass," with the sixth character assigned to identify the type of graft. For example, for a left brachiocephalic arteriovenous graft, assign code **03180JD, Bypass left brachial artery to upper arm vein with synthetic substitute, open approach.**

Arteriovenous Fistula

Arteriovenous fistulas are indicated when permanent vascular access is required. An artery is surgically joined directly to a vein when creating an AV fistula. As the connection matures, the vein grows larger and stronger until it becomes a reliable point of access, allowing for frequent puncture for hemodialysis.

The AV fistula has fewer complications and lasts longer than other types of access for hemodialysis. When coding the creation of an AV fistula in ICD-10-PCS, the root operation is "Bypass." The fourth-character body part represents the body part bypassed "from"; the qualifier specifies the body part bypassed "to." In the context of hemodialysis access, blood flow is generally bypassed from the artery to the vein (high-pressure system to low-pressure system). For example, for a left brachiocephalic arteriovenous fistula, assign code **03180ZD, Bypass left brachial artery to upper arm vein, open approach.**

It normally takes two to three months for an AV fistula to mature. A nonmaturing or nondeveloping fistula is considered a mechanical complication and is coded to **T82.590-, Other mechanical complication of surgically created arteriovenous fistula.** Primary causes of a nonmaturing fistula are narrowing of a vein or multiple competing veins. Treatment may consist of performing an arteriovenostomy to create a new AV fistula. Other treatment options may be performed by interventional radiologists—such as balloon angioplasty; revision of AV fistula; and/or closing off competing veins, which can be performed using various techniques.

Other mechanical complications related to the AV fistula are breakdown (T82.510-), displacement (T82.520-), and leakage (T82.530-). Mechanical complications of the vascular dialysis catheter are coded to subcategory T82.4.

COMPLICATIONS OF CYSTOSTOMY

Complications of cystostomy are classified as N99.51-. Code N99.511 is assigned for an infection of the cystostomy. An additional code is assigned to specify the type of infection, such as abscess of the abdominal wall (L02.211) or cellulitis of the abdominal wall (L03.311), with an additional code to identify the organism. Malfunction of cystostomy is coded as N99.512; other complications of cystostomy, such as fistula, hernia, or prolapse, are coded as N99.518. Note that mechanical complication of urinary catheter is classified to T83.0- rather than N99.51-.

EXERCISE 20.2

Code the following diagnoses and procedures. Do not assign External cause of morbidity codes.

---

1. End-stage renal disease
   Peritoneal dialysis

---

2. Chronic kidney disease, stage 5, requiring chronic dialysis
   Catheter insertion into the superior vena cava via the left subclavian vein for renal dialysis
   Intermittent hemodialysis performed for four hours

---

3. Stenosis of dialysis arteriovenous fistula, initial encounter
   Percutaneous balloon angioplasty right radial artery

---

4. Hypertensive end-stage renal disease, dialysis maintenance
   Intermittent hemodialysis treatments provided for four hours
   per day

CYSTOSCOPY AS OPERATIVE APPROACH

Cystoscopy is used as the approach for many procedures performed in diagnosing and treating urinary tract conditions and is not coded separately when it is the procedural approach. ICD-10-PCS classifies the cystoscopic approach as "via natural or artificial opening endoscopic." (For illustrations of Medical and Surgical Section approaches, please refer to figure 7.5 on pages 74–75.) Procedures described as transurethral should be coded to the approach "via natural or artificial opening," while those described as transurethral ureteroscopic are classified to the "via natural or artificial opening endoscopic" approach. When a cystoscopy is performed to visually and/or manually explore the bladder (without performing another procedure), it is coded to the root operation "Inspection" with code **0TJB8ZZ, Inspection of bladder, via natural or artificial opening endoscopic.**

REMOVAL OF URINARY CALCULUS

Urinary calculi are relatively common and often pass without surgery. Several types of surgical techniques are used when intervention is necessary. Extracorporeal shock wave lithotripsy (ESWL) of the kidney, ureter, and/or bladder (ICD-10-PCS root operation "Fragmentation," external approach) uses shock waves to reduce the stones to a slush that can more easily pass through the urinary tract and be excreted over a short period of time. For example, ESWL of the right ureter is coded to **0TF6XZZ, Fragmentation in right ureter, external approach.**

For stones that are poor candidates for ESWL, endoscopic therapy is indicated. Ureteroscopy is the most common means of visualizing an upper urinary tract calculus. In addition, percutaneous techniques (e.g., percutaneous endourology) can be used.

Ultrasonic lithotripsy requires a rigid endoscope and is commonly performed via a percutaneous renal approach. Ultrasonic lithotriptors are used to treat large bladder stones. Because the ultrasound requires a relatively large, rigid instrument to perform, most stones treated are limited to the lower ureter or the bladder. Lithotripsy with removal of fragments is coded to the root operation "Extirpation." Fragmentation would not be coded separately because it is inherent to the "Extirpation." Extirpation is the removal of solid matter, such as calculus or other abnormal physiological byproduct from a body part, and includes any previous fragmentation of the solid matter prior to its removal. For example, ureteroscopic fragmentation of a stone of the left ureter with basket removal is coded to **0TC78ZZ, Extirpation of matter from left ureter, endoscopic approach.**

When the kidney stones are quite large, or in a location that does not allow for effective lithotripsy, the stones can be removed by percutaneous nephrostomy. The procedure is performed with a small incision in the back; a tunnel is created directly into the kidney, and a tube is inserted. The stone is removed through the tube. Percutaneous nephrostomy is coded to the root operation "Extirpation" with percutaneous or percutaneous endoscopic approach.

Kidney stones can migrate through the urinary system, passing through the kidney and ureter toward the bladder. When coding "Extirpation" of a calculus, the body part value is based on the location of the stone at the beginning of the procedure. For example, if a patient is readmitted for removal of a stone from the bladder following a previous admission for removal of a stone from the kidney, the kidney stone is reported for the first admission while the bladder stone is reported for the second admission.

EXERCISE 20.3

Code the following diagnoses and procedures. Do not assign External cause of morbidity codes.

---

1. Right ureteral calculus

   Right calyceal diverticulum

   Left renal cyst, solitary (acquired)

---

2. Impacted renal calculus with medullary sponge
   kidney

   Extracorporeal shock wave lithotripsy of left kidney

   calculus

---

3. Calculus in bladder

   Lithotripsy of urinary bladder with ultrasonic

   fragmentation and removal of fragments via

   percutaneous endoscopic approach

PROSTATE DISEASE AND THERAPY

Diseases of the male genital organs are classified in categories N40 through N53, with conditions of the prostate using categories N40 through N42. Neoplasms of the prostate are classified elsewhere, as follows:

C61   Malignant neoplasm of the prostate

D29.1   Benign neoplasm of the prostate

D07.5   In situ neoplasm of the prostate

Hyperplasia of the prostate is classified to category N40, Benign prostatic hyperplasia, with fourth characters providing additional specificity regarding the presence or absence of lower urinary tract symptoms. As indicated by the "use additional code" note under code N40.1, an additional code should be assigned to identify associated symptoms when specified, such as incomplete bladder emptying (R39.14), nocturia (R35.1), straining on urination (R39.16), urinary frequency (R35.0), urinary hesitancy (R39.11), urinary incontinence (N39.4-), urinary obstruction (N13.8), urinary retention (R33.8), urinary urgency (R39.15), or weak urinary stream (R39.12).

Category N41 classifies inflammatory disease of the prostate as follows:

N41.0   Acute prostatitis

N41.1   Chronic prostatitis

N41.2   Abscess of prostate

N41.3   Prostatocystitis

N41.4   Granulomatous prostatitis

N41.8   Other inflammatory diseases of prostate

N41.9   Inflammatory disease of prostate, unspecified

Category N42 classifies other disorders of the prostate with such conditions as follows:

N42.0   Calculus of prostate

N42.1   Congestion and hemorrhage of prostate

N42.3   Dysplasia of prostate

N42.81   Prostatodynia syndrome

N42.82   Prostatosis syndrome

N42.83   Cyst of prostate

N42.89   Other specified disorders of prostate

N42.9   Disorder of prostate, unspecified

To code a prostatectomy, it is necessary to determine whether the complete prostate was removed (root operation "Resection"), or only a portion of the prostate was removed (root operation "Excision"), as well as surgical approach (open, percutaneous endoscopic, via natural or artificial opening, or via natural or artificial opening endoscopic). (For illustrations of Medical and Surgical Section approaches, please refer to figure 7.5 on pages 74–75.) For example:

FIGURE 20.2 The Male Reproductive System

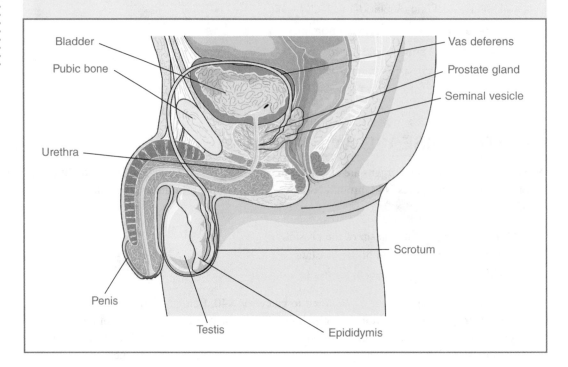

- Total transurethral prostatectomy via cystoscope: 0VT08ZZ, Resection of prostate, via natural or artificial opening endoscopic
- Suprapubic prostatectomy: 0VT00ZZ, Resection of prostate, open approach

In a radical prostatectomy, the seminal vesicles and vas ampullae are excised along with the prostate. This procedure requires two codes: one code for the prostate resection, and a separate code for the resection of bilateral seminal vessels. A prostatectomy performed with a radical cystectomy involves removal of the bladder, prostate, and seminal vessels. Thus, it requires three codes: one for the prostate resection, another for the bladder resection, and a third for the resection of bilateral seminal vessels.

Different types of energy sources may be utilized for the destruction of prostatic tissue, such as microwave thermotherapy, radiofrequency thermotherapy, ablation, and cryotherapy. All these different types of energy sources are coded to the same root operation, "Destruction."

ENDOMETRIOSIS

Endometriosis is a condition in which aberrant tissue that almost perfectly resembles the mucous membrane of the uterus is found in various other sites within the pelvic cavity. (See figure 20.3 for common sites of endometriosis implantation.) A code from category N80, Endometriosis, is assigned for this condition, with a fourth character indicating the site in which the aberrant tissue is found. For example:

N80.1   Endometriosis of the ovary

N80.5   Endometriosis of the colon

N80.2   Endometriosis of fallopian tube

GENITAL PROLAPSE

Prolapse of the vagina and/or the uterus is a relatively common condition. In coding genital prolapse, it is first necessary to determine whether the condition involves the vaginal wall, the uterus, or both, and whether the prolapse is complete or incomplete. For example:

N81.2   Incomplete uterovaginal prolapse (uterus descends into introitus, and cervix
protrudes slightly beyond)

N81.3   Complete uterovaginal prolapse (entire cervix and uterus protrude beyond the
introitus, and vagina is inverted)

Code N99.3 is assigned for prolapse of vaginal vault occurring after hysterectomy; it is not classified as a surgical complication. This condition may be due to the surgical technique or to the relaxation of supporting structures following surgery. Pelvic or vaginal enterocele, a herniation of the intestine through intact vaginal mucosa, is coded **N81.5, Vaginal enterocele,** whether it is

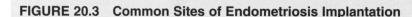

FIGURE 20.3   Common Sites of Endometriosis Implantation

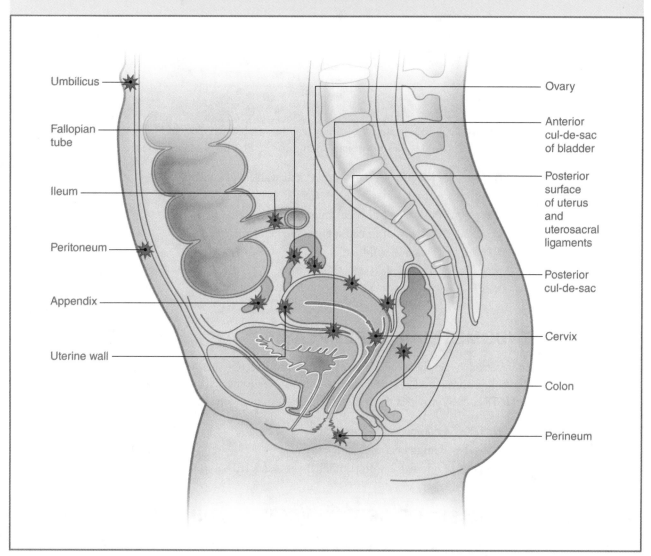

FIGURE 20.4 The Female Reproductive System

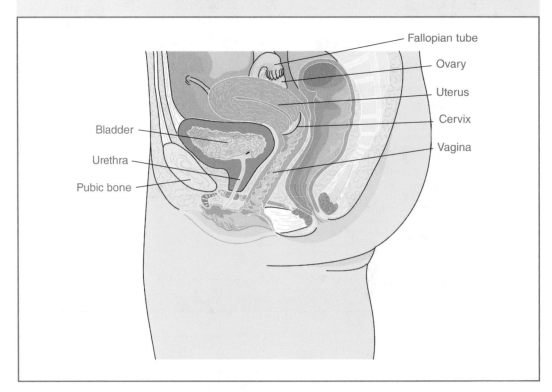

congenital or acquired. Prolapse of the uterus in an obstetric patient is classified in chapter 15 of ICD-10-CM. Examples of appropriate coding for genital prolapse include the following:

N81.4	Prolapse of uterus (no vaginal wall involvement)
N81.5	Vaginal enterocele
N81.85	Prolapse of cervical stump
O34.522	Prolapse of gravid uterus (second trimester)
N81.11	Cystocele, midline
N81.0	Urethrocele
N81.6	Rectocele

ENDOMETRIAL HYPERPLASIA

Endometrial hyperplasia refers to excessive proliferation of the cells of the inner lining of the uterus. It is considered a significant risk factor for endometrial cancer and requires careful monitoring. ICD-10-CM provides the following codes for endometrial hyperplasia:

N85.00	Endometrial hyperplasia, unspecified
N85.01	Benign endometrial hyperplasia
N85.02	Endometrial intraepithelial neoplasia [EIN]

DYSPLASIA OF CERVIX, VAGINA, AND VULVA

Cervical intraepithelial neoplasia (CIN), also known as cervical dysplasia, is the potentially premalignant transformation and abnormal growth (dysplasia) of squamous cells on the surface of the cervix. CIN I is coded to **N87.0, Mild cervical dysplasia,** and CIN II is coded to **N87.1, Moderate cervical dysplasia.** However, dysplasia of the cervix specified as CIN III, or severe dysplasia of cervix uteri, is carcinoma in situ of the cervix, and code **D06.-, Carcinoma in situ of cervix uteri,** is assigned.

Vaginal intraepithelial neoplasia (VAIN) refers to premalignant histological findings in the vagina characterized by dysplastic changes. It is a rare, generally asymptomatic disorder. Similar to CIN, it is classified in three stages: VAIN I, VAIN II, and VAIN III. Code **N89.0, Mild vaginal dysplasia,** is assigned for VAIN I, whereas VAIN II is classified to code **N89.1, Moderate vaginal dysplasia.** Similar to CIN III, VAIN III—or severe vaginal dysplasia—is considered to be carcinoma in situ; VAIN III is coded to **D07.2, Carcinoma in situ of vagina.**

Vulvar intraepithelial neoplasia (VIN) refers to changes that can occur in the skin covering the vulva. In some cases, VIN may disappear without treatment. VIN is classified as follows:

- VIN I, or mild dysplasia of vulva: N90.0, Mild vulvar dysplasia
- VIN II, or moderate dysplasia of vulva: N90.1, Moderate vulvar dysplasia
- VIN III, or severe dysplasia of vulva: D07.1, Carcinoma in situ of vulva

A diagnosis of CIN III, VAIN III, or VIN III can be made only on the basis of pathological examination of tissues. Codes from **R87.61-, Abnormal cytological findings in specimens from cervix uteri,** or **R87.62-, Abnormal cytological findings in specimens from vagina,** are assigned for abnormal results from a cervical or vaginal cytologic examination without histologic confirmation. For similar findings for the vulva, code **R87.69, Abnormal cytological findings in specimens from other genital organs,** is assigned.

HYSTERECTOMY

A hysterectomy to remove the uterus may be performed for different conditions, including symptomatic uterine fibroids, uterine prolapse, endometriosis, and malignant neoplasms of the uterus, cervix, or ovaries. Depending on the indications for surgery, the surgeon may opt to remove all or only part of the uterus. When coding hysterectomies, it is important to clarify whether the cervix is removed, as some of the ICD-10-PCS Tables in the "Female Reproductive System" (e.g., Table 0UT, resection) contain anatomical subdivisions with separate values for "uterus" and "cervix."

- In a supracervical or subtotal hysterectomy, only the upper part of the uterus is removed, keeping the cervix intact. This procedure is coded to the root operation "Resection" and body part value "uterus." For example, for a subtotal laparoscopic hysterectomy, code **0UT94ZL, Resection of uterus, supracervical, percutaneous endoscopic approach,** is assigned.
- A total hysterectomy removes the whole uterus and cervix. For example, a total laparoscopic hysterectomy is coded as **0UT94ZZ, Resection of uterus, percutaneous endoscopic approach.**

ENDOMETRIAL ABLATION

Endometrial ablation is used as an alternative to hysterectomy for women with dysfunctional bleeding that does not respond to hormone therapy. It can also be used to treat women with fibroid tumors or endometrial polyps. A scope equipped with either a roller ball or a u-shaped wire is inserted into the uterus. The lining of the uterus is ablated by laser, radiofrequency electromagnet energy, or electrocoagulation. Endometrial ablation is classified to the root operation "Destruction." For example, **0U5B8ZZ, Destruction of endometrium, via natural or artificial opening, endoscopic,** is assigned for a vaginal endometrial ablation.

DISEASES OF THE BREAST

Neoplasms of the breast are classified in chapter 2 of ICD-10-CM. Coding professionals should be aware, however, that terms such as "growth," "cyst," and "lump" do not necessarily refer to neoplastic disease. When surgery is performed, the pathology report provides more specific information to assist in code assignment. Examples of appropriate coding include the following:

N60.11	Fibrocystic disease of the right breast
D24.9	Benign neoplasm of female breast
D23.5	Benign neoplasm of skin of breast
N62	Gynecomastia
C50.929	Carcinoma of the male breast
C50.919	Carcinoma of the female breast
N63.24	Lump of lower inner quadrant of left breast

Providers often document the location of a lump in terms related to the positions on a clock. Facilities may choose to develop a facility-specific coding guideline addressing the correlation of clock positions and breast quadrants that allow for code selection based on this type of documentation. These facility guidelines should not conflict with the ICD-10-CM Official Coding Guidelines, and they should not replace physician documentation that is necessary to support code assignment.

ICD-10-PCS classifies breast procedures to the body system "skin and breast" with the second-character value of "H." Biopsies of the breast are classified to the root operations "Drainage" (value of "9") or "Excision" (value of "B") depending on whether the biopsy involves fluid removal ("Drainage"), as in the case of a cyst, or tissue ("Excision"), as in the case of a mass or lump. Biopsies are coded in ICD-10-PCS with a seventh-character qualifier of "X" for diagnostic. When the procedure is described as an excisional biopsy, it usually refers to excision of the entire lesion rather than a simple biopsy, in which case it is coded to the root operation "Excision." The term "lumpectomy" also describes a local excision of a breast lesion.

When surgery on the breast is performed for possible neoplasm, it is customary to perform a biopsy before the definitive surgery begins. A rapid-frozen section is reviewed by a pathologist to determine whether malignancy is present. The code for the definitive procedure is sequenced first, followed by the code for the biopsy. If a diagnostic excision, extraction, or drainage procedure (biopsy) is followed by a more definitive procedure, such as destruction, excision, or resection at the same procedure site, both the biopsy and the more definitive procedure are coded. For example, if a biopsy of the breast is performed first, followed by a partial mastectomy at the same procedure site during the same surgical episode, both the biopsy and the partial mastectomy procedures are coded. The partial mastectomy is sequenced as the principal procedure because it is the procedure performed for definitive treatment most related to the principal diagnosis.

With advances in cancer therapy, radical mastectomy is not performed as often as in the past because a lumpectomy or a modified radical mastectomy appears to be equally effective in most cases. The main distinction between a radical and a modified mastectomy is that all or part of the pectoralis major and all of the pectoralis minor are removed in a radical mastectomy, whereas the pectoralis major is preserved in a modified radical mastectomy. ICD-10-PCS requires separate codes for all components involved in a radical mastectomy. For example, a left radical mastectomy is coded to **0HTU0ZZ, Resection of left breast, open approach; 07T60ZZ, Resection of left axillary lymphatic, open approach;** and **0KTJ0ZZ, Resection of left thorax muscle, open approach.** On the other hand, a left modified radical mastectomy is coded as **0HTU0ZZ, Resection of left breast, open approach,** and **07T60ZZ, Resection of left axillary lymphatic, open approach.** A skin-sparing mastectomy, an alternative to traditional mastectomy, preserves the outer skin of the breast with removal of the underlying breast tissue, nipple, and areola. A left skin-sparing mastectomy is coded as **0HTU0ZZ, Resection of left breast, open approach.** A separate code is not assigned for the resection of the nipple. When coding these surgeries, review the operative report carefully before assigning the procedure codes.

Insertion of tissue expander is another procedure frequently carried out in conjunction with breast surgery. This tissue insertion permits a flap closure of the site, making it unnecessary for the patient to undergo a skin graft. Saline is usually injected into the breast expander at regular intervals following the expander's insertion to gradually enlarge the size of the expander. ICD-10-PCS classifies these procedures to the root operation "Insertion" with the device value of "N" for tissue expander; for example, **0HHT0NZ, Insertion of tissue expander into right breast, open approach.**

BREAST RECONSTRUCTION

Reconstructive breast surgery (figure 20.5) is performed for a variety of reasons. If the purpose of reconstruction is to increase breast size for improved appearance, prosthetic implants are usually used. Prostheses are also often implanted for patients who have undergone mastectomies.

Breast reconstruction can be performed immediately after the mastectomy or delayed to a later time. When breast reconstruction follows immediately after the mastectomy, both resection and replacement of the breast are coded. This is supported by the ICD-10-PCS guideline B3.18, which states "if an excision or resection of a body part is followed by a replacement procedure, code both procedures to identify each distinct objective, except when the excision or resection is considered integral and preparatory for the replacement procedure." When it is known that a patient will undergo postoperative radiation therapy, breast reconstruction is usually delayed. When a patient undergoes a mastectomy and the reconstruction is delayed, code **Z42.1, Encounter for breast reconstruction following mastectomy,** is assigned as the principal or first-listed diagnosis for the return admission for each encounter for a stage of the breast reconstruction.

Coding examples for reconstruction include the following:

0HRT0JZ	Replacement of right breast with synthetic substitute, open approach
0HRU075	Replacement of left breast using latissimus dorsi myocutaneous flap, open approach
0HRV077	Replacement of bilateral breast using deep inferior epigastric artery perforator flap, open approach
0KXH0ZZ	Transfer right thorax muscle, open approach
0KXL0Z6	Transfer left abdomen muscle, transverse rectus abdominis myocutaneous, open approach
0HRV079	Replacement of bilateral breast using gluteal artery perforator flap, open approach
0HRW0JZ	Replacement of right nipple with synthetic substitute, open approach

Note that care should be exercised when coding breast reconstruction procedures because the main term **Reconstruction** in the Index to Procedures of ICD-10-PCS only references the root operations "Repair," "Replacement," and "Supplement." The root operation "Transfer" is the appropriate root operation for a transverse rectus abdominis muscle (TRAM) flap reconstruction when a portion of the abdominal muscle is moved to the breast and the muscle remains connected to its vascular and nervous supply. The root operation "Transfer" is moving, without taking out, all or a portion of a body part to another location to take over the function of all or a portion of a body part.

Problems related to deformity and disproportion post–breast reconstruction may require patients to seek further medical care. Contour irregularity, excess tissue in reconstructed breast, or misshapen reconstructed breast are assigned to code **N65.0, Deformity of reconstructed breast.** Breast asymmetry, or disproportion between native breast and reconstructed breast, and ptosis (sagging) of native breast in relation to reconstructed breast are assigned to **N65.1, Disproportion of reconstructed breast.**

Sometimes complications develop in patients who have breast implants, making removal of the implants advisable. In such cases, the code for the principal diagnosis depends on the nature of the complication. For example, if the reason for the surgery is that the implant has ruptured, the principal diagnosis is code **T85.41x-, Breakdown (mechanical) of breast prosthesis and implant.** When the reason for removal is that the patient has a capsular contracture of the right breast implant, code **T85.44x-, Capsular contracture of breast implant,** is assigned as the principal

FIGURE 20.5 Breast Reconstruction Surgery

FRONTAL VIEW

BACK LATERAL VIEW

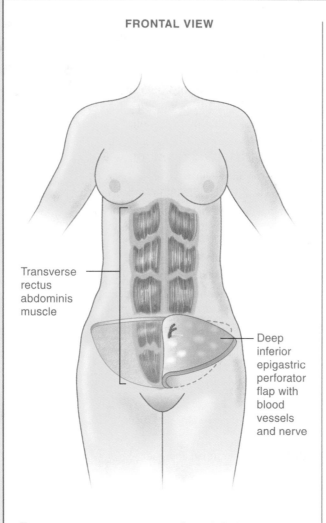
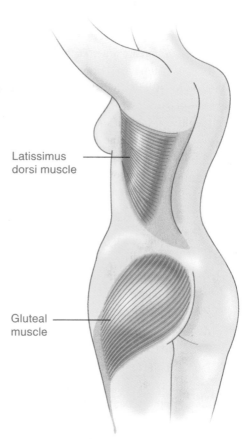

Transverse rectus abdominis muscle

Deep inferior epigastric perforator flap with blood vessels and nerve

Latissimus dorsi muscle

Gluteal muscle

Transverse rectus abdominis muscle (TRAM) flap:

Skin, fat, and transverse rectus abdominis muscle are moved to the chest.

Deep inferior epigastric perforator (DIEP) flap:

Abdominal skin and fat are removed along with the perforator vessel and transplanted to the chest using microsurgery.

Latissimus dorsi flap:

Skin, fat, and latissimus dorsi muscle from the upper back are pulled under the skin to the chest area.

Gluteal free flap:

Skin, fat, and gluteal muscle are removed and transplanted to the chest.

diagnosis. Other codes related to problems with breast implants include **T85.42x-, Displacement of breast prosthesis and implant,** which includes malposition of breast prosthesis and implant, and **T85.43x-, Leakage of breast prosthesis and implant.** Removal of the breast implant is classified to the root operation "Removal" and the device "synthetic substitute"; for example, **0HPT0JZ, Removal of synthetic substitute from right breast, open approach.**

Patients sometimes request removal of an implant because they are concerned that a complication might occur in the future, although there is no problem at present. In this case, assign **Z45.81-, Encounter for adjustment or removal of breast implant.**

The following are examples of diagnoses and procedures related to breast reconstruction:

- A patient experiences a ruptured breast implant on the left side and is admitted for open removal of the implant and insertion of a new implant.

Principal diagnosis:	T85.41xA	Breakdown (mechanical) of breast prosthesis and implant, initial encounter
Surgery performed:	0HPU0JZ	Removal of synthetic substitute from left breast, open approach
	0HRU0JZ	Replacement of left breast with synthetic substitute, open approach

- A patient who had undergone a previous right mastectomy with a breast implant inserted at the time of surgery suffers from a painful capsule. She is admitted for removal and reinsertion of the implant.

Principal diagnosis:	T85.848A	Pain due to other internal prosthetic devices, implants and grafts, not elsewhere classified, initial encounter
Surgery performed:	0HPT0JZ	Removal of synthetic substitute from right breast, open approach
	0HRT0JZ	Replacement of right breast with synthetic substitute, open approach

- A patient had undergone bilateral breast implantation three years ago and is now admitted for elective implant removal. She had no related problems but had become concerned because of newspaper reports describing illnesses associated with breast implants.

Principal diagnosis:	Z45.811	Encounter for adjustment or removal of right breast implant
	Z45.812	Encounter for adjustment or removal of left breast implant
Surgery performed:	0HPT0JZ	Removal of synthetic substitute from right breast, open
	0HPU0JZ	Removal of synthetic substitute from left breast, open

Reduction mammoplasty is sometimes performed for patients whose large breast size interferes with normal daily activities or causes significant discomfort, as well as for cosmetic reasons. When mammoplasty is performed to reduce breast size, code **N62, Hypertrophy of breast,** is assigned as the principal diagnosis. When the purpose of the mammoplasty is cosmetic, code **Z41.1, Encounter for cosmetic surgery,** is assigned as the principal diagnosis.

REVIEW EXERCISE 20.4

Code the following diagnoses and procedures. Do not assign External cause of morbidity codes.

1. Hydronephrosis with chronic pyelitis
   Pyelonephritis, focal, chronic, left

2. Rapidly progressive glomerulonephritis

3. Syphilitic epididymitis

4. Chronic prostatitis due to proteus

5. Phimosis and balanoposthitis

6. Encysted right hydrocele, male
   Open hydrocelectomy of hydrocele of spermatic cord

7. Benign prostatic hypertrophy with urinary
   obstruction Total transurethral prostatectomy via cystoscope

8. Acute and chronic cervicitis
   Total vaginal hysterectomy

9. Chronic pelvic inflammatory disease
   Dysmenorrhea

10. Menometrorrhagia
    Endometrial polyp
    Corpus luteum cysts of both ovaries
    Total abdominal hysterectomy
    Bilateral salpingo-oophorectomy

11. Cystocele with incomplete uterine prolapse
    and stress incontinence

Cystocele repair (open approach)

Vaginal suspension of uterus (open approach)

12. Pelvic peritoneal endometriosis

13. Dermoid cyst of left ovary

Laparoscopic wedge resection of ovarian cyst

14. Infertility due to pelvic peritoneal adhesions blocking tubes

Hysterosalpingogram, radiopaque dye

15. Psychogenic dysmenorrhea

16. Adhesions of ovary and fallopian tubes

Laparoscopic lysis of adhesions

17. Menorrhagia

Dilatation and curettage with vaginal endometrial ablation

18. Submucous fibroid of uterus

Laparoscopically assisted partial vaginal hysterectomy

(leaving cervix intact)

Coding OF Diseases OF THE Skin AND Diseases OF THE Musculoskeletal System

CHAPTER 21

Diseases of the Skin and Subcutaneous Tissue

CHAPTER OVERVIEW

- Diseases of the skin and subcutaneous tissue can be found in chapter 12 of ICD-10-CM.

- Categories L23–L25 classify dermatitis due to plants, food, drugs, and medications in contact with skin.

- Category L27 classifies dermatitis caused by medications taken internally.

  — The coding professional must determine whether the condition is an adverse effect of proper administration or a poisoning due to the incorrect use of the drug.

  — Codes from categories T36 through T65 are used to classify the causation.

- Chronic ulcers of the skin are classified using the fifth character to specify the site.

- The sequencing of the code for cellulitis depends on the severity of the wound and the primary goal of the treatment (for cellulitis or for the wound).

- Debridement is classified as either excisional or non-excisional (brushing, irrigating, scrubbing, or washing).

LEARNING OUTCOMES

After studying this chapter, you should be able to:

Know how to classify dermatitis due to contact, food, and ingestion of drug (both correct and incorrect usage).

Code ulcers of the skin.

Explain how to classify cellulitis based on location and the primary goal of the treatment.

Code procedures done on the skin, such as excisions, debridement, and grafting.

TERMS TO KNOW

Cellulitis
an infection of the skin and soft tissues resulting from some sort of break in the skin

Debridement
removal of dead, damaged, or infected tissue

REMEMBER . . .

Chapter 12 of ICD-10-CM includes more than just conditions of the skin. It also includes conditions of the nails, sweat glands, hair, and hair follicles.

INTRODUCTION

Chapter 12 of ICD-10-CM deals with conditions affecting the skin and subcutaneous tissue. The chapter is organized around the following subdivisions:

L00–L08	Infections of skin and subcutaneous tissue
L10–L14	Bullous disorders
L20–L30	Dermatitis and eczema
L40–L45	Papulosquamous disorders
L49–L54	Urticaria and erythema
L55–L59	Radiation-related disorders of the skin and subcutaneous tissue
L60–L75	Disorders of skin appendages
L76	Intraoperative and postprocedural complications of skin and subcutaneous tissue
L80–L99	Other disorders of the skin and subcutaneous tissue

Conditions affecting the nails, sweat glands, hair, and hair follicles are included in this chapter. Congenital conditions of skin, hair, and nails are classified in categories Q80–Q84. Neoplasms of skin are classified in chapter 2 of ICD-10-CM.

DERMATITIS DUE TO DRUGS

ICD-10-CM uses the terms "dermatitis" and "eczema" synonymously and interchangeably in the L20–L30 category range. There are several types of dermatitis, such as atopic (L20.-), seborrheic (L21.-), diaper (L22), allergic contact (L23.-), irritant contact (L24.-), and exfoliative (L26).

Contact dermatitis is a localized rash or irritation of the skin caused by contact with allergens (allergic-contact dermatitis) or irritants (irritant-contact dermatitis). Category L23 is used to classify allergic-contact dermatitis due to metals, adhesives, cosmetics, drugs, dyes, chemical products, food, and plants in contact with skin. Category L24 is assigned for irritant-contact dermatitis caused by irritants, such as detergents, oils and greases, and solvents, in contact with skin. Category L25, Unspecified contact dermatitis, is used when the contact dermatitis is not specified as allergic- or irritant-contact dermatitis. Category L27 is for dermatitis due to substances taken internally.

To code dermatitis caused by medication, first determine whether the condition represents an adverse effect due to the proper administration of a drug or poisoning due to the incorrect use of the drug. When the dermatitis is due to a medication used correctly as prescribed, it is considered an adverse effect. When the dermatitis is due to incorrect use of the drug, it is classified as a poisoning by drugs, medicaments, and biological substances.

When coding allergic-contact dermatitis, irritant-contact dermatitis, unspecified contact dermatitis, or dermatitis due to substances taken internally, a code from categories T36 through T65 should be assigned to indicate the way in which the poisoning or adverse effect occurred (e.g., accidental, intentional self-harm) and the type of drug involved. The sequencing of the code from categories T36 through T65 will depend on the circumstances: When the condition is due to poisoning, the T36–T65 code is assigned first. However, the T36–T65 code is assigned as an additional code when the condition is due to adverse effect. (A more detailed discussion of the distinction between adverse effects and poisoning due to drugs and medications is provided in chapter 31 of this handbook.)

Correct coding examples include the following:

L27.0 + T36.0x5A	Initial encounter for dermatitis due to allergic reaction to penicillin tablets, taken as prescribed (adverse reaction)
T36.0x1A + L27.0	Initial encounter for dermatitis due to accidental ingestion of mother's penicillin tablets (poisoning)

FIGURE 21.1   The Skin and Subcutaneous Tissue

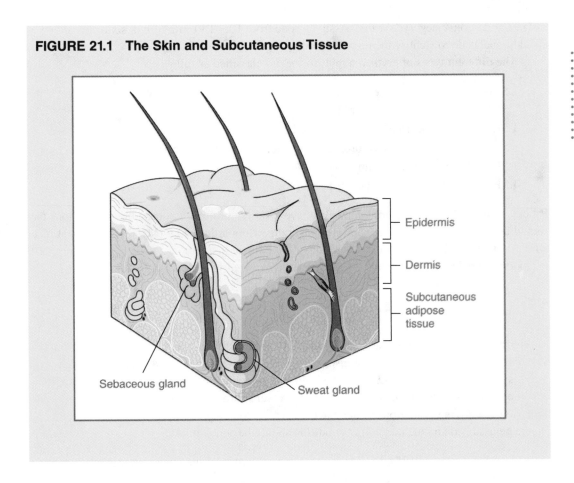

- Epidermis
- Dermis
- Subcutaneous adipose tissue
- Sebaceous gland
- Sweat gland

In the first example, which indicates an adverse reaction to a prescribed medication taken as directed, the code for the dermatitis is sequenced first, followed by the code for the adverse effect of the penicillin. In the second example, code **T36.0x1A, Poisoning by penicillin, accidental, initial encounter,** is sequenced first, with an additional code to indicate that the effect of the poisoning is dermatitis.

Palmar plantar erythrodysesthesia (PPE), also called hand foot syndrome, is an example of a specific dermatitis that occurs as an adverse reaction to antineoplastic or biologic drugs used for cancer treatment. After the administration of chemotherapy, small amounts of the drug can leak from the capillaries, damaging tissue in the palms of the hands and the soles of the feet. The leakage results in redness, tenderness, and peeling of the palms and soles. The affected area resembles sunburn and may become dry, peeled, and numb. This condition affects the hands and feet because of the increased friction and heat to which the extremities are exposed through normal use. Treatment involves reducing or stopping the drug therapy. Assign code **L27.1, Localized skin eruption due to drugs and medicaments taken internally,** followed by code **T45.1x5A, Adverse effect of antineoplastic and immunosuppressive drugs, initial encounter,** for the PPE due to antineoplastic antibiotics.

ERYTHEMA MULTIFORME

Erythema multiforme is a skin disorder resulting in symmetrical red, raised skin areas all over the body, often resembling targets because they are dark circles with purple-gray centers. In some cases, there are severe systemic symptoms. Erythema multiforme can occur in response to medications, infections, or illness. The exact cause is unknown. If the condition is a drug-induced adverse effect, assign a code from category L51 first. Assign a code from T36–T50 with fifth or sixth character 5 as an additional code to identify the responsible drug.

The different types of erythema multiforme are classified as follows:

L51.0   Nonbullous erythema multiforme
L51.1   Stevens-Johnson syndrome
L51.2   Toxic epidermal necrolysis [Lyell]
L51.3   Stevens-Johnson syndrome-toxic epidermal necrolysis overlap syndrome
L51.8   Other erythema multiforme
L51.9   Erythema multiforme, unspecified

Patients with erythema multiforme may also have a variety of other associated manifestations that should be coded separately. The manifestations range from arthropathy (M14.8-) to corneal ulcer (H16.0.-) to stomatitis (K12.-) and several other conditions. In addition, a code from category L49 is reported to reflect the percentage of body surface involved with skin exfoliation.

ULCERS OF THE SKIN

Most chronic ulcers of the skin are classified in categories L89, Pressure ulcer, and L97, Nonpressure chronic ulcer of lower limb, not elsewhere classified, with code I96 assigned first when gangrene is present. A code from L97 may be used as a principal or first-listed code if no underlying condition is documented as the cause of the nonpressure chronic ulcer of lower limb. If one of the following underlying conditions is documented with a lower-extremity ulcer, a causal condition should be assumed and the underlying condition should be coded first:

I70.23-, I70.24-, I70.33-, I70.34-, I70.43-, I70.44-, I70.53-, I70.54-, I70.63-, I70.64-, I70.73-, I70.74-	Atherosclerosis of the lower extremities
I87.31-, I87.33-	Chronic venous hypertension
E08.621, E08.622, E09.621, E09.622, E10.621, E10.622, E11.621, E11.622, E13.621, E13.622	Diabetic ulcers
I87.01-, I87.03-	Postphlebitic syndrome
I87.01-, I87.03-	Postthrombotic syndrome
I83.0-, I83.2-	Varicose ulcer
I96	Any associated gangrene

Chronic ulcer of the skin, not otherwise specified, is classified to subcategory L98.4, Nonpressure chronic ulcer of skin, not elsewhere classified. Arteriosclerosis of the lower extremities is classified to subcategories I70.2 through I70.7 with fifth characters 3 or 4 when it is associated with ulceration. An additional code from category L97 is assigned to indicate the severity of the ulcer. If gangrene is present, assign code I70.26- or I70.36- with an additional code from L98.49- to identify the severity of any ulcer, if applicable.

Codes from category L89, Pressure ulcer, identify the site of the pressure ulcer as well as the stage of the ulcer. Category L89 provides fifth characters to identify the specific site of the ulcer, such as elbow (L89.0-); back (L89.1-); hip (L89.2-); buttock (L89.3-); contiguous site of back, buttock, and hip (L89.4-); ankle (L89.5-); heel (L89.6-); other site (L89.8-); and unspecified site (L89.9-). The sixth character for category L89 indicates the severity of the ulcer by identifying the stage of the pressure ulcers, such as unstageable, stage 1, stage 2, stage 3, stage 4, deep tissue damage, or unspecified stage.

293

CHAPTER 21

*Diseases of the
Skin and
Subcutaneous
Tissue*

The code assignment for the pressure ulcer stage may be based on nursing documentation; however, the associated diagnosis of pressure ulcer should be coded on the basis of the provider's documentation (namely, the physician or any qualified health care practitioner who is legally accountable for establishing the patient's diagnosis, as defined in the *ICD-10-CM Official Guidelines for Coding and Reporting*).

Care should be taken not to confuse a pressure ulcer in which the stage is unspecified or not documented (L89.- with a sixth character 9) with a pressure ulcer documented as unstageable (L89.- with a sixth character 0). The staging of pressure ulcers takes into account the depth of tissue loss and the depth of tissue exposed. "Unstageable" refers to full-thickness skin- and tissue-loss ulcers whose stage cannot be clinically determined (e.g., the ulcer is covered by eschar or slough). The true stage of an ulcer that is covered cannot be determined until the eschar or slough is removed from the ulcer. When eschar is removed to reveal the stage of the ulcer, assign a code for the highest stage reported during the encounter. The coding professional should be guided by the clinical documentation and the terms found in the Alphabetic Index when coding the stage of a pressure ulcer. The provider should be queried if the clinical term cannot be found in the Index or if there is no documentation of the stage.

Providers may refer to pressure ulcers as "pressure injury" or "deep tissue injury." This terminology more accurately describes pressure injuries of both intact and ulcerated skin of all stages. The Alphabetic Index entry for "Injury, pressure, injury" directs the user to "see Ulcer, pressure, by site." Deep tissue injury may be indexed under the term, "Damage, deep tissue, pressure-induced, see also L89 with final character .6." For example:

- Deep tissue injury of the left hip is assigned to code L89.226, Pressure-induced deep tissue damage of left hip
- Stage 3 pressure injury of left hip is assigned to code L89.223, Pressure ulcer of left hip, stage 3

Care should be taken to review the provider documentation to determine whether the term "injury" refers to a traumatic injury (such as contusion) or a pressure ulcer.

A Kennedy ulcer is a pressure ulcer that occurs at the end of life and is related to multiorgan failure. This type of ulcer does not typically respond to standard treatment. Assign the appropriate code from category L89, Pressure ulcer, for a Kennedy ulcer.

If a patient is admitted with a pressure ulcer of one stage, and it progresses to a higher stage, two separate codes should be assigned: one code for the site and stage of the ulcer on admission and a second code for the same ulcer site and the highest stage reported during the stay. For example, the condition of an individual admitted with stage 2 pressure ulcer of left heel that advances to stage 3 during the encounter should be coded to **L89.622, Pressure ulcer of left heel, stage 2,** and **L89.623, Pressure ulcer of left heel, stage 3.**

Care should be taken to distinguish between pressure ulcers documented as "healed" (no code assigned) and "healing" (assign the appropriate code for the stage documented). For ulcers that were present on admission but healed at the time of discharge, the code for the site and stage of the pressure ulcer at the time of admission should be assigned. If the documentation does not provide information about the stage of the healing pressure ulcer, assign the appropriate code for unspecified stage.

Examples of correct coding for chronic ulcers of the skin include the following:

L89.154	Pressure ulcer, sacral area, stage 4
I96 + L89.153	Pressure ulcer, sacral area, stage 3 with gangrene
L97.909	Ulcer of lower limb, except pressure ulcer
L89.210	Unstageable pressure ulcer of the right hip
L89.149	Pressure ulcer left lower back
L98.499	Chronic ulcer of skin, unspecified site

Stasis ulcers are ordinarily due to varicose veins of the lower extremities and are coded to category I83, Varicose veins of lower extremities, rather than to the categories for conditions of the skin.

294

CHAPTER 21

*Diseases of the
Skin and
Subcutaneous
Tissue*

When the physician has used the term "stasis ulcer" but has identified a cause other than varicose veins, code the condition to **I87.2, Venous insufficiency (chronic) (peripheral).** A basic rule of coding is that further research must be done when the title of the code suggested by the Alphabetic Index clearly does not identify the condition correctly. In this case, even though the Index directs you to a code involving varicose veins, the code should not be used when no varicosities are present.

CELLULITIS OF THE SKIN

Cellulitis is an acute, diffuse infection of the skin and soft tissues that commonly results from a break in the skin, such as a puncture wound, a laceration, or an ulcer. Occasionally, the break is so small that it cannot be identified by either the patient or the examining physician. Clinically, cellulitis usually presents as an abrupt onset of redness, swelling, pain, or heat in the infected area. Do not assume, however, that a reference to redness at the edges of a wound or an ulcer represents cellulitis. The normal hyperemia associated with a wound usually extends a small distance beyond the edges of the wound rather than extending to the diffuse pattern that characterizes cellulitis.

Coding of cellulitis secondary to superficial injury, burn, or frostbite requires two codes, one for the injury and one for the cellulitis. Sequencing of codes depends on the circumstances of the admission. When the patient is seen primarily for treatment of an open wound, the appropriate code for open wound is assigned, with an additional code for the cellulitis. When the wound itself is trivial or when it was treated earlier and the patient is now being seen for treatment of the cellulitis, the code for the cellulitis may be sequenced first, with an additional code for the open wound. For example:

- A patient suffered laceration of the right lower leg while on a hiking trip two days ago and comes to the hospital on his return. By the time he is seen, cellulitis is beginning to develop. The wound is cleansed of the foreign material, non-excisional debridement is carried out, and antibiotics are started for the cellulitis.

Principal diagnosis:	S81.821A	Laceration with foreign body, right lower leg, initial encounter
Additional diagnosis:	L03.115	Cellulitis of right lower limb
Procedure:	0HDKXZZ	Extraction of right lower leg skin, external approach

- A patient suffers a minor puncture injury to a finger on the right hand when removing a staple at the office. Five days later, he is admitted to the hospital because of cellulitis of the finger and is treated with intravenous antibiotics. The wound itself does not require treatment; therefore, no code for injury is assigned.

Principal diagnosis:	L03.011	Cellulitis of right finger

Both cellulitis and lymphangitis of skin are included in category L03. However, separate codes are available for cellulitis and lymphangitis. An additional code should be assigned to indicate the organism responsible (B95–B96), if this information is available. The responsible organism is usually *Streptococcus.*

Cellulitis may also present as a postoperative wound infection or as a result of the penetration of the skin involved in intravenous therapy. For example:

- A patient had an appendectomy six days ago and is now readmitted with evidence of staphylococcal cellulitis of the superficial incision site.

Principal diagnosis:	T81.41xA	Infection following procedure, superficial incisional surgical site, initial encounter
Additional diagnosis:	L03.311	Cellulitis of abdominal wall
Additional diagnosis:	B95.8	*Staphylococcus*

295

CHAPTER 21

*Diseases of the
Skin and
Subcutaneous
Tissue*

Cellulitis frequently develops as a complication of chronic skin ulcers, in which case it is assigned to a code from category L89 or L97 or subcategory L98.4. These codes do not include any associated cellulitis, so two codes are required to describe these conditions. Designation of the principal diagnosis depends on the circumstances of the admission.

Cellulitis described as gangrenous is classified to code I96, Gangrene, not elsewhere classified. When gangrene is present with an ulcer or injury, the gangrene is coded first, with the code for the injury or ulcer assigned as an additional code. This practice follows the instructional notes in the Tabular List to code first any associated gangrene.

OTHER CELLULITIS

Although cellulitis most commonly occurs in the skin and subcutaneous tissue, it also occurs in other areas. In such cases, codes from other chapters of ICD-10-CM are assigned as appropriate.

Cellulitis of female external genital organs is classified as an inflammatory condition and assigned code N76.4. Pelvic cellulitis in women is classified as an inflammatory condition and assigned to category N73. Occasionally, pelvic cellulitis occurs following abortion, delivery, or molar or ectopic pregnancy, in which case it is classified to chapter 15 of ICD-10-CM. In male patients, pelvic cellulitis is coded as K65.0, Generalized (acute) peritonitis.

EXCISION OF LESION

To correctly assign a procedure code for the removal of lesions, it is important to first determine whether the procedure was performed on the skin (body system "skin and breast"), or subcutaneous tissue and fascia (body system "subcutaneous tissue and fascia"). Next, determine whether the root operation performed is "Excision" (cutting out or off, without replacement, a portion of a body part) or "Destruction" (physical eradication of all or a portion of a body part by the direct use of energy, force, or a destructive agent). For most skin excisions and destructions, the approach used will be external. For example:

- A simple excision involving only the skin of the face is classified to the root operation "Excision" and coded to 0HB1XZZ, Excision of face skin, external approach.

- Removal of lesions carried out by cauterization, cryosurgery, fulguration, or laser beam is classified to the root operation "Destruction"; for example, fulguration of a skin tag of the chest is coded to 0H55XZZ, Destruction of chest skin, external approach.

When the removal of the lesion goes beyond the skin and involves underlying and/ or adjacent tissue such as subcutaneous tissue and fascia, the procedure is classified to the "subcutaneous tissue and fascia" body system. The surgeon's description should be followed carefully when assigning these codes to determine whether the root operation is "Excision" or "Destruction" and whether the approach was open (cutting through the skin or mucous membrane) or percutaneous (by puncture or minor incision through the skin or mucous membrane). For example:

- Excision of Kaposi's sarcoma of the subcutaneous tissue, right thigh, is classified to the root operation "Excision" and coded to 0JBL0ZZ, Excision of right upper leg subcutaneous tissue and fascia, open approach.

- Open fulguration of a benign subcutaneous tissue lesion of the right upper arm is classified to the root operation "Destruction" and coded to 0J5D0ZZ, Destruction of right upper arm subcutaneous tissue and fascia, open approach.

DEBRIDEMENT

Debridement of the skin and subcutaneous tissue is a procedure by which foreign material and devitalized or contaminated tissue are removed from a traumatic or infected lesion until the surrounding healthy tissue is exposed.

Excisional debridement of the skin or subcutaneous tissue is the surgical removal or cutting away of such tissue, necrosis, or slough; these procedures are classified to the root operation "Excision." Depending on the availability of a surgical suite or the extent of the area involved, excisional debridement can be performed in the operating room, in the emergency department, or at the patient's bedside. Excisional debridement may be performed by a physician and/or another health care provider and involves an excisional, as opposed to a mechanical (brushing, scrubbing, washing), debridement. Use of a sharp instrument does not always indicate that an excisional debridement was performed. Minor removal of loose fragments with scissors or using a sharp instrument to scrape away tissue is not an excisional debridement. Excisional debridement involves the use of a scalpel to remove devitalized tissue. Documentation of excisional debridement should be specific regarding the type of debridement. If the documentation is not clear or if there is any question about the procedure, the provider should be queried for clarification.

Non-excisional debridement of the skin is the nonoperative brushing, irrigating, scrubbing, or washing of devitalized tissue, necrosis, slough, or foreign material. Most non-excisional debridement procedures are classified to the root operation "Extraction" (pulling or stripping out or off all or a portion of a body part by the use of force), except when the procedure is performed by irrigating the devitalized tissue. In that case, the debridement is coded to the Administration Section, root operation "Irrigation." Non-excisional debridement may be performed by a physician or by other health care personnel. Examples of non-excisional debridement include Versajet and ultrasonic debridement. The Versajet consists of an ultra-high-pressure generator with a console and disposable attachments. A natural vacuum created by the jet stream removes tissue fragments. Specialized features allow physicians to debride traumatic wounds, chronic wounds, or other soft-tissue lesions and aspirate and remove contaminants or other debris.

When coding for debridement of areas other than skin, the procedure is coded to the root operation "Excision" (for excisional debridement) or "Extraction" (for non-excisional debridement) of the specific body part. For non-excisional debridement of a joint, there is no body part value for "joint" for the root operation "Extraction"; therefore, report the root operation "Release."

When coding multiple-layer debridements of the same site, assign a code only for the deepest layer of debridement. For example, open excision and debridement of a coccyx wound including bone is coded to **0QBS0ZZ, Excision of coccyx, open approach.** Debridement carried out in conjunction with another procedure is often, but not always, included in the code for the procedure.

When excisional and non-excisional debridements are both performed at the same site, report only the code for excisional debridement.

DERMAL REGENERATIVE GRAFT

Several new technologies that permanently regenerate or replace skin layers are now being used to treat severe burns. Procedures involving the application of grafts are classified to the root operation "Replacement" (putting in or on biological or synthetic material that physically takes the place and/ or function of all or a portion of a body part). The approach for all the skin replacement procedures is "external." The root operation "Replacement" identifies through the device character the use of synthetic substitutes (sixth character "J"), autologous tissue substitutes (sixth character 7), and nonautologous tissue substitutes (sixth character "K"). The following guidance should be followed when selecting the device character for grafts:

- If the material used is derived from a living or biologic basis, it should be coded as "nonautologous tissue substitute"; otherwise, it is considered synthetic.

297

CHAPTER 21

Diseases of the
Skin and
Subcutaneous
Tissue

- If living or biologic material is mixed with synthetic material, the graft should be coded as "nonautologous tissue substitute."
- If two separate products are used (synthetic and biologic), code each separately.

Examples of skin synthetic substitutes include:

- Artificial skin, not otherwise specified
- Creation of "neodermis"
- Decellularized allodermis
- Integumentary matrix implants
- Prosthetic implant of dermal layer of skin
- Regenerate dermal layer of skin

Code **T85.693-, Other mechanical complication of artificial skin graft and decellularized allodermis,** is assigned for failure or rejection of these systems. Codes **T86.820, Skin graft (allograft) rejection,** and **T86.821, Skin graft (allograft) (autograft) failure,** are assigned for complication of other skin graft. Status code **Z96.81, Presence of artificial skin,** is assigned to indicate that the patient has an artificial skin graft.

EXERCISE 21.1

Code the following diagnoses and procedures.

1. Varicose ulcer, lower right leg with severe inflammation

2. Pilonidal fistula with abscess
   Excision of pilonidal sinus

3. Large cutaneous abscess of trunk due to
   Staphylococcus aureus

   Incision and drainage of abscess, trunk (chest)

4. Hard corn deformity, right little toe
   Soft corn deformities, third, fourth, and fifth toes, right

5. Keloid scar on left hand from previous burn

   Excision of scar, left hand

6. Chronic purulent inflamed acne rosacea of lower lip
   Wide excision of chronic acne rosacea of
   lower lip (external) with full-thickness autologous
   graft over defect, lower lip

7. Giant urticaria, initial encounter

8. Contact dermatitis of eyelid

9. Seborrheic keratosis underlying the second
    metatarsal head, right foot

10. Cellulitis of anus

11. Acute lymphangitis, right upper arm, due to group A
    streptococcal infection

12. Gangrenous diabetic ulcer of right foot due to
    peripheral circulatory disorder

13. Surgical (excisional) debridement of skin and fascia
    of right foot

14. Infected ingrown toenail, right great toe
    Ablative electrocauterization of toenail

15. Cellulitis, buttock

16. Cellulitis of left upper eyelid

17. Non-excisional debridement of right diabetic heel ulcer

CHAPTER 22 — Diseases of the Musculoskeletal System and Connective Tissue

CHAPTER OVERVIEW

- Diseases of the musculoskeletal system and connective tissue are covered in chapter 13 of ICD-10-CM.

- Most of the codes within chapter 13 have site and laterality designations referring to the bone, joint, or muscle involved.

- If more than one bone, joint, or muscle is involved and there is no "multiple sites" code provided, separate codes should be used to indicate the different sites involved.

- Coding back pain is often dependent on the distinction between degeneration and displacement and on the presence or absence of myelopathy or radiculopathy.

- Arthritis may occur independently or be a manifestation of another condition.

  — When arthritis is due to another condition, combination codes should be used when available.

  — Arthritis is assigned a separate code if it is an independent condition or if it is a manifestation of another condition and no combination code is available.

- Osteoarthritis can be further classified based on whether it is primary or secondary.

- Fractures are considered to be stress fractures, pathological fractures, or traumatic fractures.

  — Fractures that are spontaneous are always considered pathological.

  — A traumatic fracture should never be coded on the same bone as a pathological fracture.

- Coding joint replacements requires knowledge of the joint involved.

- Coding joint revisions requires information on the removal of any joint-replacement components.

- Coding spinal fusion requires knowing the anatomical portion (column) fused, the approach used (anterior, posterior, or lateral transverse), and whether two or more vertebrae are fused.

- Coding spinal disc prostheses requires knowledge of the type of prosthesis and the segment treated.

- Other conditions coded in chapter 13 include plica syndrome and fasciitis.

LEARNING OUTCOMES

After studying this chapter, you should be able to:

Explain the different types of arthritis and what to look for when coding arthritis.

Explain the difference between pathological and traumatic fractures.

Code joint replacements and revisions.

Code back disorders and the variety of procedures for correcting spinal problems.

TERMS TO KNOW

Joint revision
procedure that adjusts, removes, or replaces a joint-replacement component

Myelopathy
damage to the myelinated fiber tracts that carry information to the brain

Osteoarthritis
the most common form of arthritis; a degenerative joint disease

Pathological fracture
fracture that occurs in a bone weakened by disease

REMEMBER . . .

Separate codes are assigned to indicate different bone, joint, or muscle sites when no "multiple sites" code is provided.

CHAPTER 22

*Diseases of the
Musculoskeletal
System and
Connective
Tissue*

INTRODUCTION

Chapter 13 of ICD-10-CM is governed by the general coding guidelines already discussed in this handbook. An understanding of the following terms may be helpful to the coding professional in assigning codes from chapter 13:

- Arthropathy: disorder of the joint
- Arthritis: inflammation of the joint
- Dorsopathy: disorder of the back
- Myelopathy: disorder of the spinal cord
- Radiculopathy: problem in which one or more nerves are affected, resulting in pain (radicular pain), weakness, numbness, or difficulty controlling specific muscles.

Most arthropathies are classified in categories M00 through M25 in ICD-10-CM, and most dorsopathies in categories M40 through M54.

Site and Laterality

Most of the codes within chapter 13 have site and laterality designations. The site refers to the bone, joint, or muscle involved. For some conditions in which more than one bone, joint, or muscle is usually involved (e.g., osteoarthritis), a code is available for "multiple sites." If no "multiple sites" code is provided and if more than one bone, joint, or muscle is involved, separate codes should be used to indicate the different sites involved.

Bone versus Joint

For certain conditions, such as avascular necrosis of bone (M87) and osteoporosis (M80, M81), the bone may be affected at the upper or lower end. Although the portion of the bone affected may be at the joint, the site designation will be the bone, not the joint.

Acute Traumatic versus Chronic or Recurrent Musculoskeletal Conditions

Many musculoskeletal conditions are a result of previous injury or trauma to a site, or are recurrent conditions. Chapter 13 of ICD-10-CM contains bone, joint, or muscle conditions that are the result of a healed injury as well as recurrent conditions of these sites. ICD-10-CM classifies current, acute injuries to chapter 19. Chronic or recurrent conditions should generally be coded with a code from chapter 13. If it is difficult to determine from the documentation in the medical record which code is best to describe a condition, query the provider.

BACK DISORDERS

Back pain described as lumbago or low back pain, without further qualification, is coded **M54.5, Low back pain.** Back pain not otherwise specified is coded **M54.9, Dorsalgia, unspecified.** Psychogenic back pain is assigned codes M54.9 and **F45.41, Pain disorder exclusively related to psychological factors.**

Intervertebral disc disorders are classified in categories M50, Cervical disc disorders, and M51, Thoracic, thoracolumbar, and lumbosacral intervertebral disc disorders. Careful attention to the terminology is important in coding these conditions. Degeneration of the disc is not the same condition as displacement (herniation) of the disc, and each requires a different code. For cervical disc disorders (category M50), the code for the most superior (highest) level affected should be

CHAPTER 22

*Diseases of the
Musculoskeletal
System and
Connective
Tissue*

FIGURE 22.1 The Human Skeleton

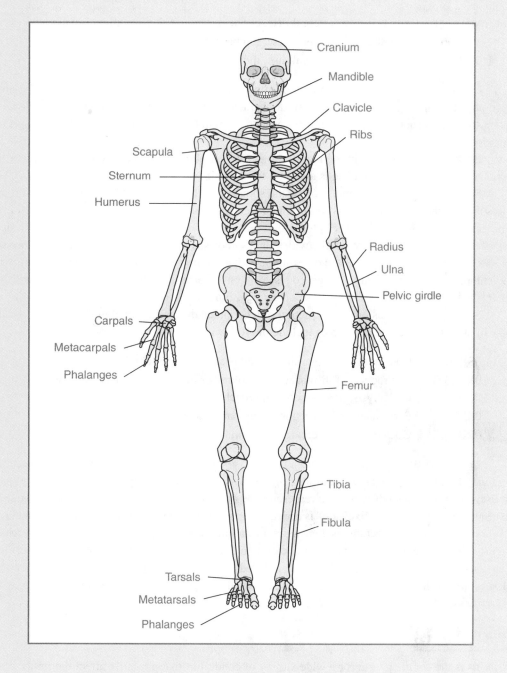

used. For example, when there is myelopathy of C3–C4 and C5–C6, assign code **M50.01, Cervical disc disorder with myelopathy, high cervical region,** for C3–C4, the most superior level.

The presence or absence of myelopathy is an important distinction to be made in assigning codes for certain back disorders. Myelopathy is a functional disorder and/or pathological change in the spinal cord that often results from compression. Codes for back disorders such as spondylosis and herniation of the intervertebral disc differentiate between conditions with and without myelopathy. Codes for a herniated disc without myelopathy include those with paresthesia but not paralysis. Terms included in intervertebral disc disorders with myelopathy are classified into

CHAPTER 22

Diseases of the
Musculoskeletal
System and
Connective
Tissue

subcategories M50.0 and M51.0, with a fifth or sixth character used to indicate the site involved. Examples include the following:

M50.222   Herniated intervertebral disc, cervical region, C5–C6, without myelopathy
M51.06   Herniated intervertebral disc, lumbar region, with myelopathy
M51.24   Herniated intervertebral disc, thoracic region, without myelopathy

Categories M50 and M51 also include subcategories M50.1 and M51.1 to identify the presence of radiculopathy, with the fifth or sixth character indicating the site involved. Radiculopathy refers to a nerve root problem resulting in weakness, numbness, or difficulty controlling specific muscles.

Back pain associated with herniation of an intervertebral disc is included in the code for the herniated disc. No additional code is assigned for the pain.

Spinal stenosis with compression of the spinal canal that contains the spinal cord and nerve roots is assigned to subcategory M48.0, Spinal stenosis. Spinal stenosis with radiculopathy of the cervical spine is assigned to codes **M48.02, Spinal stenosis, cervical region,** and **M54.12, Radiculopathy, cervical region.** Myelopathy with spinal stenosis is assigned to code **G99.2, Myelopathy in diseases classified elsewhere.** For example, when coding stenosis of the lumbar spine with radiculopathy and myelopathy, assign codes **M48.061, Spinal stenosis, lumbar region without neurogenic claudication, M54.16, Radiculopathy, lumbar region,** and G99.2.

Surgery for the excision or destruction of a herniated disc is classified in ICD-10-PCS by the type of surgery performed. Examples include the following:

0SB40ZZ   Open excision of herniated lumbosacral intervertebral disc
0R5B3ZZ   Destruction of displaced thoracolumbar intervertebral disc by chemonucleolysis, percutaneous approach
0S523ZZ   Percutaneous destruction of lumbar vertebral disc
0RB10ZZ   Open excision of cervical vertebral joint

Code **00JU0ZZ, Inspection of spinal canal, open approach,** is assigned for a laminectomy performed for the purpose of exploration of the spinal canal. Laminectomy performed for the purpose of excision of herniated disc material represents the operative approach and is not coded separately. Instead, the root operation "Excision" is coded to report the excision of the disc. When a decompressive foraminotomy/laminectomy is done to treat foraminal stenosis by releasing pressure and freeing up the spinal nerve root, along with a discectomy to treat a lumbar disc herniation, each surgery has a distinct procedural objective and should be coded separately. The appropriate root operations are "Excision" for the discectomy and "Release" for the decompressive foraminotomy/laminectomy.

ARTHRITIS

Arthritis is the common term for a wide variety of conditions that primarily affect the joints, muscles, and connective tissue. The associated symptoms are inflammation, swelling, pain, stiffness, and mobility problems. Arthritis may occur independently, but it is also a common manifestation of a variety of other conditions. When arthritis is due to another condition, combination codes should be used when available, and dual-coding guidelines should be applied when combination codes are not available. Examples include the following:

M11.811   Arthritis of the right shoulder due to dicalcium phosphate crystals
E11.610   Charcot's arthritis due to type 2 diabetes
C95.90+M36.1   Arthritis due to leukemia
D66+M36.2   Hemophilic arthritis
A69.23   Arthritis associated with Lyme disease

FIGURE 22.2 The Spinal Column

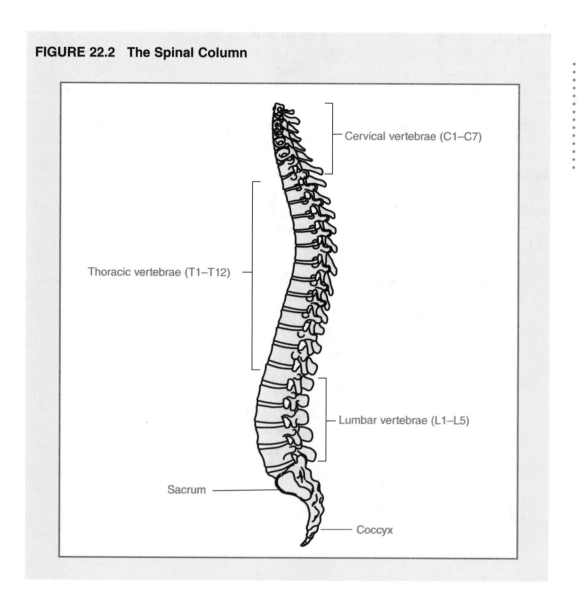

CHAPTER 22

*Diseases of the
Musculoskeletal
System and
Connective
Tissue*

Osteoarthritis is the most common form of arthritis; it is also called polyarthritis, degenerative arthritis, and hypertrophic arthritis. In the United States, "arthritis" is primarily meant to represent osteoarthritis, and defaults in ICD-10-CM were adjusted to recognize this distinction. It is a degenerative joint disease, usually occurring in older people, with chronic degeneration of the articular cartilage and hypertrophy of the bone. It is characterized by pain and swelling. Codes from categories M15 through M19 are assigned for osteoarthritis, except when the spine is involved, in which case a code from category M47, Spondylosis, is assigned.

In addition to coding osteoarthritis by site, codes also specify whether the condition is primary, secondary (for example, posttraumatic), or generalized. Primary osteoarthritis, also known as degenerative arthritis, affects joints in the spine, knee, and hip, as well as certain small joints of the hands and feet. Primary osteoarthritis is the most common form of osteoarthritis; it is usually caused by "wear and tear" related to age, resulting in damage to the cartilage. When the type of osteoarthritis is not specified, "primary" is the default. Secondary arthritis has a specific cause, such as injury, or is an effect of obesity, genetics, inactivity, or other diseases. It is confined to the joints of one area. When coding osteoarthritis, the Index may refer to an unspecified code. It is important to review the Tabular List for other codes in the related area to determine whether a more specific code may be located to capture the diagnostic statement. For example, for osteoarthritis of the left knee, assign code **M17.12, Unilateral primary osteoarthritis, left knee,** instead of code **M17.9,**

304

CHAPTER 22

Diseases of the
Musculoskeletal
System and
Connective
Tissue

Osteoarthritis of knee, unspecified. When the site of the osteoarthritis is not documented, assign code **M19.90, Unspecified osteoarthritis, unspecified site.** Osteoarthritis that involves multiple sites but is not specified as generalized is coded as **M15.9, Polyosteoarthritis, unspecified.**

Rheumatoid arthritis (categories M05 and M06), another fairly common type of arthritis, is an autoimmune disease that affects the entire body. Pyogenic arthritis (M00.-) is due to infection and is classified to the causative organism (*Staphylococcus*, *Pneumococcus*, *Streptococcus*, or other bacteria), with additional characters to indicate the joints involved. An additional code for the responsible organism should be assigned for staphylococcal arthritis (B95.61–B95.8), streptococcal arthritis (B95.0–B95.2, B95.4, B95.5), or other bacteria (B96). Category M01 is used to report direct infections of joints in infectious and parasitic diseases. The underlying disease, such as leprosy, mycoses, or parathyroid fever, should be coded first.

Gouty arthritis is a recurrent arthritis of the peripheral joints in which excessive uric acid in the blood is deposited in the joints. Gouty arthritis is classified to idiopathic gout. Category M10, Gout, is further subdivided to distinguish whether it is idiopathic (M10.0-), due to lead (M10.1-), drug induced (M10.2-), due to renal impairment (M10.3-), or other secondary gout (M10.4-). Unspecified gout is coded to M10.9. When the gout is specified to be chronic, it is classified to category M1A, Chronic gout, with seventh characters added to specify with or without tophus (crystallized uric acid deposit under the skin).

EXERCISE 22.1

Code the following diagnoses and procedures. Do not assign External cause of morbidity codes.

---

1. Acute gouty arthritis, right foot

---

2. Chronic nodular rheumatoid arthritis with
   polyneuropathy

---

3. Traumatic arthritis, left ankle, due to old
   traumatic dislocation
   Arthroscopic arthrodesis with internal fixation, left ankle

---

4. Herniated intervertebral disc, L4–L5
   Laminectomy with open excision of
   intervertebral disc, L4–L5

---

5. Chronic lumbosacral sprain, subsequent encounter

DERANGEMENT

Internal derangement of the knee is classified to category M23; derangement of other specific joints is classified to category M24, with additional characters indicating the site. Recurrent nontraumatic dislocation of the knee is classified to M22.0-, Recurrent dislocation of patella. Recurrent disloca-

305

CHAPTER 22

Diseases of the
Musculoskeletal
System and
Connective
Tissue

tion or subluxation of joints is classified to M24.4-, Recurrent dislocation of joint. Derangement of the knee due to current injury is classified to dislocation under S83.104-, S83.105-, or S83.106-. However, derangement of the meniscus or cartilage of the knee due to current injury is classified to subcategory S83.2, Tear of meniscus, current injury.

EXERCISE 22.2

Code the following diagnoses. Do not assign External cause of morbidity codes.

1. Recurrent derangement of left ankle

2. Recurrent derangement of knee

3. Derangement of right knee due to a current fall, initial encounter

---

OSTEOPOROSIS

Osteoporosis is a systemic condition that affects all bones of the musculoskeletal system and leads to an increased risk of pathological fractures. In osteoporosis, the bones are thinner and weaker than normal. Osteoporosis is classified to categories M80 and M81 depending on whether a current pathological fracture is present or not. Because osteoporosis is a systemic condition, site is not a component of the codes under category M81, Osteoporosis without current pathological fracture. The codes under category M80, Osteoporosis with current pathological fracture, identify the osteoporosis and the site of the pathological fracture.

PATHOLOGICAL FRACTURES

Pathological fractures occur in bones that are weakened by disease. These fractures are usually spontaneous but sometimes occur in connection with slight trauma (such as a minor fall) that ordinarily would not result in a fracture in normal, healthy bone. There are many different underlying causes for pathological fractures, including osteoporosis, metastatic tumor of the bone, osteomyelitis, Paget's disease, disuse atrophy, hyperparathyroidism, and nutritional or congenital disorders.

   Fractures described as spontaneous are always pathological fractures. When the fracture is described as a compression fracture, the record should be reviewed to determine whether any significant trauma has been experienced. A fall from a height, such as a diving board, with compression fracture of the spine is classified as an injury, but a compression fracture in an older patient resulting from a slight stumble or another minor injury is usually considered pathological, particularly when the patient also has an underlying condition that elevates the risk for such fractures. The physician should be asked for clarification if the medical documentation does not indicate whether a compression fracture is pathological or traumatic.

   All pathological fractures are classified to the following categories/subcategories according to the underlying cause:

- Category M80   Osteoporosis with current pathological fracture
- Subcategory M84.4   Pathological fracture, not elsewhere classified
- Subcategory M84.5   Pathological fracture in neoplastic disease (code also the underlying cause)

306

CHAPTER 22

Diseases of the
Musculoskeletal
System and
Connective
Tissue

- Subcategory M84.6   Pathological fracture in other disease (code also the underlying condition)
- Subcategory M84.7   Nontraumatic fracture, not elsewhere classified

Additional characters are used to indicate the bone involved. The following seventh-character values are required when coding pathological fractures:

A   Initial encounter for fracture
D   Subsequent encounter for fracture with routine healing
G   Subsequent encounter for fracture with delayed healing
K   Subsequent encounter for fracture with nonunion
P   Subsequent encounter for fracture with malunion
S   Sequela

The assignment of the seventh-character value for pathological fractures should be performed using the following guidelines:

- "A" is used when the patient is receiving active treatment for the pathological fracture. Examples of active treatment are surgical treatment, emergency department encounter, and evaluation and management of acute injuries. While the patient may be seen by a new or different provider over the course of treatment for a pathological fracture, assignment of the seventh character is based on whether the patient is undergoing active treatment— not on whether the provider is seeing the patient for the first time.
- "D" is used for encounters after the patient has completed active treatment and there is routine healing.
- "G," "K," and "P" are used for subsequent encounters for treatment of problems associated with the healing, such as delayed healing, malunions, and nonunions.
- "S" is to be used for encounters for the treatment of sequelae or the residual effect after the acute phase of the fracture has terminated.

Care for complications of surgical treatment for fracture repairs during the healing or recovery phase should be coded with the appropriate complication codes.

Sequencing of codes for pathological fractures depends on the circumstances of admission. A pathological fracture is designated as the principal diagnosis only when the patient is admitted solely for treatment of the pathological fracture. Ordinarily, the code for the underlying condition responsible for the fracture is listed first, with an additional code for the fracture. An example follows.

- Pathological fracture due to neoplasm: If the focus of treatment is the fracture, a code from subcategory M84.5, Pathological fracture in neoplastic disease, should be sequenced first, followed by the code for the neoplasm. If the focus of treatment is the neoplasm with an associated pathological fracture, the neoplasm code should be sequenced first, followed by a code from M84.5 for the pathological fracture.

Never assign codes for both a traumatic fracture and a pathological fracture of the same bone; only one type of fracture should be coded. (See chapter 29 of this handbook for a discussion of coding traumatic fractures.)

Appropriate coding examples include the following:

M80.061A + M89.761	Initial encounter for acute fracture of right tibia and major osseous defects due to senile osteoporosis
M84.559D + C79.51 + Z85.43	Subsequent encounter for healing pathological fracture of the hip due to metastatic carcinoma of bone; ovarian cancer five years ago

STRESS FRACTURES

Stress fractures are different from pathological fractures in that stress fractures are due to repetitive force applied before the bone and its supporting tissues have had enough time to absorb such force, whereas pathological fractures are always due to a physiological condition, such as cancer or osteoporosis, that results in damage to the bone. Typically, stress fractures initially test negative in an X-ray display, and days or weeks may pass before the fracture line is visible on an X-ray. Stress fractures are classified to subcategory M84.3. Additional External cause of morbidity codes are used to identify the cause of the stress fracture (for example, code **Y93.01, Activity, walking, marching and hiking**). Other terms classified to stress fractures are fatigue fracture, march fracture, and stress reaction fracture.

Atypical Femoral Fractures

Atypical femoral fractures are a form of stress fracture that is associated with osteoporosis. These fractures occur in patients receiving long-term bisphosphonate therapy or other medications such as glucocorticoids. Atypical femoral fractures occur in the subtrochanteric region of the hip or the femoral shaft. They may be complete and extend across both cortices, or they may be incomplete, involving only the lateral cortex. In addition to their location, atypical femoral fractures have several other distinctive features: (1) they can have a transverse or short oblique orientation; (2) there is minimal or no trauma associated with these fractures; (3) there is a lack of comminution; (4) there is cortical thickening that is either generalized or localized at the lateral cortex of the fracture site; (5) there is periosteal reaction of the lateral cortex; and (6) there is a medial spike when the fracture is complete.

Atypical femoral fractures are classified to subcategory M84.75, Atypical femoral fracture. The entire term "atypical femoral fracture" must be documented to assign a code from subcategory M84.75. Seventh characters are required for atypical femoral fractures to indicate initial encounter, subsequent encounter, or sequela. In addition, if the fracture is due to the patient's long-term use of bisphosphonates, code **Z79.83, Long term (current) use of bisphosphonates,** should also be assigned.

Periprosthetic Fractures

Periprosthetic fractures are fractures that occur around a prosthesis. Periprosthetic fractures are not complications of the prosthesis, but the result of the same conditions as other fractures—trauma or pathological conditions. These fractures can occur around any prosthesis, but the most common sites are the hip (M97.01-, M97.02-), knee (M97.11-, M97.12-), ankle (M97.21-, M97.22-), shoulder (M97.31-, M97.32-), and elbow (M97.41-, M97.42-). Assign code M97.8- for a periprosthetic fracture around "other" joint and code M97.9- for a periprosthetic fracture around an "unspecified" joint.

MUSCULOSKELETAL BODY PART GUIDELINES

Most ICD-10-PCS body part guidelines are covered in chapter 7 of this handbook, Introduction to ICD-10-PCS and ICD-10-PCS Conventions. However, there is a specific guideline describing tendons, ligaments, bursae, and fascia near a joint that pertains more closely to this chapter of the handbook.

Procedures performed on tendons, ligaments, bursae, and fascia supporting a joint are coded to the body part in the respective body system that is the focus of the procedure. Procedures performed on joint structures themselves are coded to the body part in the joint body systems. For example, repair of the anterior cruciate ligament of the knee is coded to the "knee bursae and ligaments" body part in the bursae and the "ligaments" body system. Knee arthroscopy with shaving of articular cartilage is coded to the "knee joint" body part in the "lower joints" body system.

REPLACEMENT OF A JOINT

CHAPTER 22

*Diseases of the
Musculoskeletal
System and
Connective
Tissue*

Replacement of a joint is classified in the Medical and Surgical Section to the root operation "Replacement." ICD-10-PCS guideline B3.18 indicates that if an excision or resection of a body part is followed by a replacement procedure, code both procedures to identify each distinct objective, except when the excision or resection is considered integral and preparatory for the replacement procedure. For example, resection of a joint as part of a joint replacement procedure is considered integral and preparatory for the replacement of the joint; therefore, the resection is not coded separately. Code assignment for the joint replacement procedure depends on the joint involved.

When coding hip replacements, the type of bearing surface is identified by the sixth-character qualifier using the following values:

0	Polyethylene
1	Metal
2	Metal on polyethylene
3	Ceramic
4	Ceramic on polyethylene
6	Oxidized zirconium on polyethylene
7	Autologous tissue substitute
E	Articulating spacer
J	Synthetic substitute
K	Nonautologous tissue substitute

When the bearing surface information is not available in the health record, assign the sixth character "J" (with "synthetic substitute") for the device or query the provider for clarification.

The seventh-character qualifier describes whether the prosthesis is cemented or uncemented. A cemented joint replacement attaches the joint to the bone with epoxy cement. An uncemented joint prosthesis has a mesh of holes on its surface that allows the growth of the patient's natural bone to hold the device in place. When it cannot be determined whether a cemented or uncemented prosthesis was placed, use "Z" for "no qualifier."

The patella is part of a total knee joint replacement. When reporting total knee replacements, assign either value "C" for "Knee joint, right" or "D" for "Knee joint, left" for the body part character at Table 0SR, Replacement, lower joint. These body part values include the femoral, tibial, and patellar portions of the total knee replacement.

If replacement also involves the placement of a bone-growth stimulator, it should be coded separately to the root operation "Insertion" and the device "bone-growth stimulator" (sixth character "M"). Other examples of joint replacement procedures include the following:

0SRA03Z	Replacement of right hip joint, acetabular surface with ceramic prosthesis
0SRG0J9	Total left ankle replacement with synthetic prosthesis, cemented
0SRS01Z	Replacement of left femoral head (metal)
0SRA00A	Partial replacement (acetabular, polyethylene) of right hip, uncemented
0RRL0JZ	Total right elbow replacement (synthetic)

ICD-10-PCS does not provide codes to indicate that a bilateral replacement has been carried out. The procedure code should be assigned twice when the same procedure is performed on bilateral joints unless individual codes are available to identify left and right joints; in that case, a code is assigned for each joint.

Occasionally, a prosthesis must be removed because of infection, with a new prosthesis placed after a month or two when the infection has completely cleared. The first admission for such a problem is coded **T84.5-, Infection and inflammatory reaction due to internal joint prosthesis,** with an additional code to identify the infection and a procedure code for removal of the prosthesis (e.g.,

0SP90JZ, Removal of synthetic substitute from right hip joint, open approach). Assign code
0SH908Z if a spacer is inserted. On the next admission for joint prosthesis insertion, the principal
diagnosis is assigned from subcategory Z47.3 (e.g., **Z47.32, Aftercare following explantation of
hip joint prosthesis**), with a procedure code for insertion of a new device.

CHAPTER 22

*Diseases of the
Musculoskeletal
System and
Connective
Tissue*

Any time a joint replacement is adjusted but not removed, the procedure is coded as a joint
revision. The definition for the root operation "Revision" is "correcting, to the extent possible, a
malfunctioning or misplaced device without taking out and putting a whole new device in its place."
Although the term *revision* may be documented by the surgeon, the full definition for the root operation "Revision" must be applied. An example of revision surgery is recementing of a prosthetic
joint. Codes for revision of hip replacements identify the specific joint components revised (e.g.,
acetabular surface, femoral surface).

When components of a joint prosthesis are removed and new components are inserted during the same encounter, code both the removal of the old components and placement of the new
components with the root operations "Removal" and "Replacement." A code for "Supplement" is
assigned if a new liner is placed. The liner is not functioning as a replaced body part. It is placed
to physically reinforce the replaced joint. If a joint spacer (e.g., cement) is removed, a code with
the root operation "Removal" is also assigned (e.g., **0SP908Z, Removal of spacer from right hip
joint, open approach**) for the removal of the spacer.

Any time a component of a joint has been previously replaced, the procedure is still considered
a replacement even though part of the component is being replaced for the first time. For example,
when a patient is admitted for conversion of a previous right hip hemiarthroplasty to a total metal-
on-polyethylene right hip replacement, open approach, it should be reported with codes **0SP90JZ,
Removal of synthetic substitute from right hip joint, open approach**, and **0SR902Z, Replacement of right hip joint with metal on polyethylene, synthetic substitute, open approach.**

If a malfunctioning joint replacement device is corrected, assign a code for the root operation
"Revision" (e.g., **0SW90JZ, Revision of synthetic substitute in right hip joint, open approach**).

Hip resurfacing involves grinding away the worn surfaces of the femoral head and acetabulum
while retaining the femoral neck and majority of the femoral head. The procedure concludes with
the placement of new bearing surfaces. Resurfacing arthroplasty is classified to the root operation "Supplement" because the procedure meets the definition of "putting in or on biological or
synthetic material that physically reinforces and/or augments the function of a portion of a body
part." In addition, character 4 (body part) identifies the specific joint components resurfaced (total
resurfacing involves both the acetabular and femoral components; partial involves femoral surface
or acetabular surface only), as follows:

0SU90BZ	Resurfacing right hip, total, acetabulum and femoral
0SUR0BZ	Resurfacing right hip, partial, femoral head
0SUA0BZ	Resurfacing right hip, partial, acetabulum

Subcategory Z96.6, Presence of orthopedic joint implants, can be assigned as an additional
code when the presence of a joint replacement is significant in terms of patient care.

EXERCISE 22.3

Code the following diagnoses and procedures. Do not assign External cause of morbidity
codes.

---

1. Primary osteoarthritis of right hip

   Replacement, total, of hip with ceramic-bearing surface, cemented

---

310

CHAPTER 22

Diseases of the
Musculoskeletal
System and
Connective
Tissue

2. Total right knee replacement (synthetic)

3. Partial replacement (synthetic) of left shoulder (humeral head)

SPINAL FUSION AND REFUSION

Spinal fusion is a surgical procedure whereby two or more vertebrae are fused to correct problems with the vertebrae. The vertebrae can be fused using bone grafting, genetically engineered bone substitute, and interbody fusion devices containing bone graft material. The goal of spinal fusion surgery is pain relief after conservative treatments have failed. The procedure is indicated for spinal vertebrae injuries such as protrusion and degeneration of the cushion between vertebrae, curvature of the spine, or weak spine caused by injections or tumors.

The failure of solid bone to develop between two or more levels of the spine after spinal fusion is called nonunion or pseudarthrosis. Symptoms may not occur until months or years after the original spinal fusion. Patients can often function relatively normally with pseudarthrosis unless they develop problems such as sharp localized pain and tenderness over the fusion, progression of the deformity or disease, or localized motion in the fusion mass. Treatment for symptomatic pseudarthrosis consists of refusion. The procedure involves thorough removal of fibrous tissue from the intended fusion area and the addition of new bone graft.

The structure of the spine is composed of the anterior and posterior columns. (See figures 22.3 and 22.4 for structures of the spine involved in spinal fusion.) The anterior column is composed of the anterior longitudinal ligament, vertebral body, intervertebral disc, annulus fibrosus, and posterior longitudinal ligament. The posterior column includes those spinal structures that are posterior to the posterior longitudinal ligament such as the pedicles, transverse process, lamina, facets, and spinous process.

Traditionally, three basic approaches have been used for spinal fusion or spinal refusion: anterior, posterior, and lateral transverse. The classic anterior approach requires an incision in the neck or the abdomen, and the fusion is carried out from the front of the vertebrae through the anterior annulus. In the classic posterior approach, the incision is made in the patient's back directly over the vertebrae. In the lateral transverse approach, an incision is made on the patient's side and the vertebrae are approached through the lamina.

During an anterior column fusion, the body (corpus) of adjacent vertebrae are fused (interbody fusion). The anterior column can be fused using an anterior, lateral, or posterior technique. For the posterior column fusion, posterior structures of adjacent vertebrae are fused (pedicle, lamina, facet, transverse process, or "gutter" fusion). A posterior column fusion can be performed using a posterior, posterolateral, or lateral transverse technique.

TABLE 22.1   Components of Each Column of the Spine

Anterior Column	Posterior Column
Anterior longitudinal ligament	Pedicles
Vertebral body	Transverse process
Intervertebral body	Lamina
Intervertebral disc	Facets
Annulus fibrosus	Spinous process
Posterior longitudinal ligament	

Spinal fusion and refusion procedures are coded to the root operation "Fusion"—joining together portions of an articular body part rendering the articular body part immobile. The body part coded for a spinal vertebral joint(s) rendered immobile by a spinal fusion procedure is classified by the level of the spine, namely, cervical, thoracic, lumbar, lumbosacral, or sacrococcygeal. There are distinct body part values for a single vertebral joint and for multiple vertebral joints at each spinal level. For example, body part values specify "lumbar vertebral joint," "lumbar vertebral joints, 2 or more," and "lumbosacral joint."

If multiple vertebral joints are fused, a separate procedure is coded for each vertebral joint that uses a different device and/or qualifier. For example, **Open fusion of lumbar vertebral joint with synthetic substitute, posterior approach, anterior column (0SG00JJ),** and **Open fusion of lumbar vertebral joint with synthetic substitute, posterior approach, posterior column (0SG00J1),** are coded separately because the procedures involve different portions of the column (anterior column versus posterior column).

No additional code is assigned for the insertion of fixation devices such as rods, plates, and screws. Insertion of these types of devices is a component of the root operation "Fusion."

FIGURE 22.3   Structure of the Spine Involved in Spinal Fusion

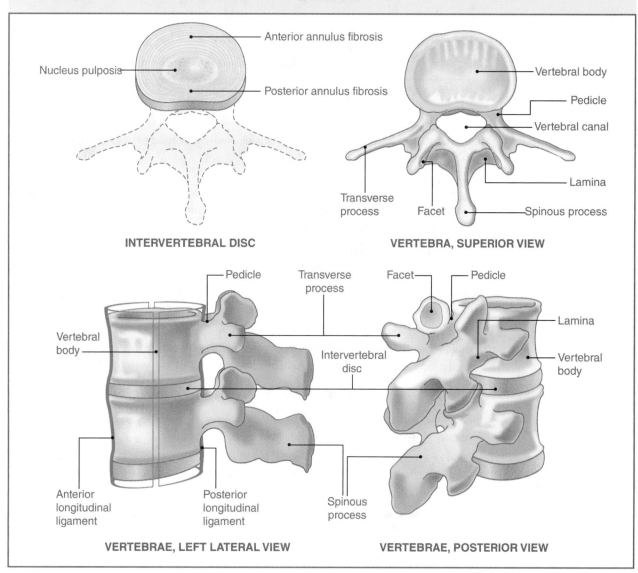

312

CHAPTER 22

Diseases of the
Musculoskeletal
System and
Connective
Tissue

FIGURE 22.4   Columns of the Spine, Lateral View

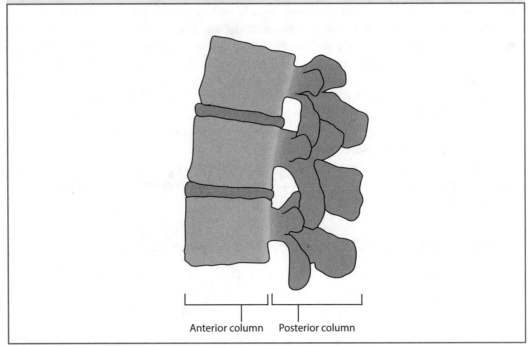

Anterior column   Posterior column

Occasionally, instruments called interbody fusion devices are used to stabilize and fuse degenerative disc spaces and to provide an immediately stable segment for fusion and relief of symptoms. These devices are also known as interbody fusion cages, BAK cages, ray-threaded fusion cages, synthetic cages, spacers, or bone dowels. Combinations of devices and materials are often used on a vertebral joint to render the joint immobile. When combinations of devices are used on the same vertebral joint, the device value for the procedure is coded using the following guidelines:

- *If an interbody fusion device is used to render the joint immobile (containing bone graft or bone graft substitute),* the procedure is coded with the device value "interbody fusion device."

- *If bone graft is the only device used to render the joint immobile,* the procedure is coded with the device value "nonautologous tissue substitute" or "autologous tissue substitute."

- *If a mixture of autologous and nonautologous bone graft (with or without biological or synthetic extenders or binders) is used to render the joint immobile,* code the procedure with the device value "autologous tissue substitute."

Examples include the following:

- Fusion of a vertebral joint using a cage-style interbody fusion device containing morsellized bone graft is coded to the device "interbody fusion device."

- Fusion of a vertebral joint using a bone dowel interbody fusion device made of cadaver bone and packed with a mixture of local morsellized bone and demineralized bone matrix is coded to the device "interbody fusion device."

- Fusion of a vertebral joint using both autologous bone graft and bone bank bone graft is coded to the device "autologous tissue substitute."

Synchronous harvesting of bone graft (e.g., iliac crest) to be used in a different part of the body (e.g., for spinal fusion) is reported separately (root operation "Excision"). However, in

ICD-10-PCS, locally harvested tissue (e.g., bone marrow harvested from the femur and used as a stem cell autograft) is not coded separately.

CHAPTER 22

Diseases of the
Musculoskeletal
System and
Connective
Tissue

If bone morphogenetic protein (BMP), a genetically engineered protein, is inserted to help create a bone graft substitute, it is identified with the device character in the fusion code. Reporting a code for placement of BMP is optional, and facilities may code it, if desired. When an open approach is used, assign code **3E0U0GB, Introduction of recombinant bone morphogenetic protein into joints, open approach.**

A 360-degree spinal fusion is a fusion of both the anterior and posterior portions of the spine. A 360-degree fusion may be performed through a single incision (usually via the lateral transverse approach) or via two incisions: an anterior incision for anterior fusion, followed by physically turning the patient over and then performing a posterior incision for posterior fusion. Two codes are required; for example, when lumbar interbody fusion of the posterior and anterior portions of the L3–L4 vertebrae is performed via a posterior open approach using autologous bone graft, assign codes **0SG0071, Fusion of lumbar vertebral joint with autologous tissue substitute, posterior approach, posterior column, open approach,** and **0SG00AJ, Fusion of lumbar vertebral joint with interbody fusion device, posterior approach, anterior column, open approach.**

See figure 22.5 for the types of spinal fusion surgeries. The following is a brief explanation of common fusion and refusion procedures:

- ALIF: The anterior lumbar interbody fusion (ALIF) is an interbody fusion of the anterior column of the spine through an anterior incision, either transperitoneal or retroperitoneal. It can also be done laparoscopically.

FIGURE 22.5 Types of Spinal Fusion Surgeries

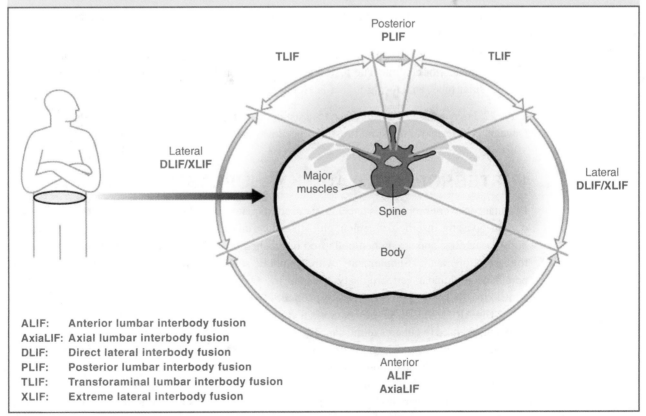

314

CHAPTER 22

Diseases of the
Musculoskeletal
System and
Connective
Tissue

TABLE 22.2   Common Fusion and Refusion ICD-10-PCS Qualifiers

Fusion Procedure	Approach and Column	ICD-10-PCS Qualifier (Seventh Character)
ALIF	Anterior approach, anterior column	0
AxiaLIF	Posterior approach, anterior column	J
DLIF	Anterior approach, anterior column	0
PLIF	Posterior approach, anterior column	J
TLIF	Posterior approach, anterior column	J
XLIF	Anterior approach, anterior column	0

- AxiaLIF: The axial lumbar interbody fusion (AxiaLIF®) is a percutaneous fusion of the anterior column at L5–S1. An AxiaLIF® 360° refers to the combination of an AxiaLIF® procedure of the anterior column performed along with a posterior column fusion, which may include the use of pedicle screws or facet screws. The AxiaLIF® 360° is described as providing a percutaneous 360-degree spinal fusion.

- DLIF: The direct lateral lumbar interbody fusion (DLIF) is a minimally invasive alternative to conventional spinal fusion. The DLIF is performed through a lateral approach, which allows for limited soft-tissue disruption. The procedure can only be performed at L4–L5 or at higher levels and requires dissection through the psoas muscle.

- PLIF: The posterior lumbar interbody fusion (PLIF) involves an anterior column fusion through a posterior approach.

- TLIF: The transforaminal lumbar interbody fusion (TLIF) involves a transverse lateral interbody fusion through a posterior approach.

- XLIF: The extreme lateral interbody fusion (XLIF®) is a less invasive spinal surgery of the anterior column. The fusion may be accomplished either percutaneously or via a circular tube retractor through a lateral approach.

Table 22.2 may be used as a reference to assist in determining the appropriate ICD-10-PCS qualifier (seventh character) for the spinal fusion procedures listed above.

VERTEBROPLASTY AND KYPHOPLASTY

Percutaneous vertebroplasty is a technique used to treat vertebral compression fractures. The procedure involves the insertion of cement glue–like material (polymethylmethacrylate) into the vertebral body to stabilize and strengthen collapsed or crushed bone. ICD-10-PCS classifies this procedure to the root operation "Supplement," with "synthetic substitute" for the device value. For example, percutaneous lumbar vertebroplasty is coded to **0QU03JZ, Supplement lumbar vertebra with synthetic substitute, percutaneous approach.**

The ARCUATE™ XP procedure is a variation of a percutaneous vertebroplasty in which an osteotome is used to cut arcs in the cancellous bone within the vertebral body. The arcs created with the osteotome allow for dispersion of bone cement material when it is subsequently injected into the vertebral body. No bone or bone marrow is removed from, or compacted within, the vertebral body. The ARCUATE™ XP procedure is also coded to the root operation "Supplement."

Percutaneous vertebral augmentation is a procedure using an inflatable balloon that is expanded to reestablish vertebral height in compression fractures. After the balloon is removed, the

315

CHAPTER 22

Diseases of the
Musculoskeletal
System and
Connective
Tissue

cavity is filled with polymethylmethacrylate, which hardens to further stabilize the bone. Coding of percutaneous vertebral augmentation requires two codes, one for the root operation "Reposition" and another for the root operation "Supplement." Other similar procedures coded in the same manner include arcuplasty, kyphoplasty, skyphoplasty, and spineoplasty. For example, percutaneous kyphoplasty of the lumbar spine should be coded to **0QS03ZZ, Reposition lumbar vertebra, percutaneous approach,** and **0QU03JZ, Supplement lumbar vertebra with synthetic substitute, percutaneous approach.**

While these procedures are similar to vertebroplasty, there is no balloon involved in the vertebroplasty, and it does not attempt to restore vertebral height to reduce the compression fractures of the vertebra. Therefore, only the root operation "Supplement" is coded for vertebroplasty.

If a vertebral biopsy is performed during a kyphoplasty of the lumbar vertebra, assign codes **0QS03ZZ, Reposition lumbar vertebra, percutaneous approach; 0QU03JZ, Supplement lumbar vertebra with synthetic substitute, percutaneous approach;** and **0QB03ZX, Excision of lumbar vertebra, percutaneous approach, diagnostic.** The biopsy is not an inherent part of the kyphoplasty and should be coded separately if performed.

SPINAL DISC PROSTHESES

Minimally invasive arthroplasty procedures may be an alternative to spinal fusion. These procedures are performed to replace the degenerated disc nucleus and restore or maintain the normal function of the disc by inserting artificial disc prostheses. The prostheses are used to replace the entire spinal disc or replace the disc nucleus.

The insertion of spinal disc prostheses is classified to the root operation "Replacement" and the spinal segment treated, for example, cervical (0RR30JZ), thoracic (0RR90JZ), or lumbosacral (0SR40JZ). The repair of a spinal disc prosthesis is reported using the root operation "Revision." For the removal of the artificial disc prosthesis with the synchronous insertion of a new prosthesis, assign two procedure codes, one for root operation "Removal" and another for "Replacement." The revision/replacement codes specify the part of the spine treated. However, ICD-10-PCS does not use unique codes to differentiate between partial and total disc prostheses.

SPINAL DECOMPRESSION

Patients with spinal stenosis or degenerative disc disease may be treated with conservative measures, including physical therapy and pain management. When conservative care does not provide relief, surgical decompression may be an alternative treatment. Surgical decompression involves removal of the bone and/or tissue causing pressure on the spinal cord or nerve root(s). Common surgical decompression procedures include laminotomy, laminectomy, discectomy, foraminotomy, and medial facetectomy. Care should be exercised to understand the objective of the procedure. For example, the main term **Laminectomy** in the ICD-10-PCS Alphabetic Index refers the user to "see Release, Central Nervous System and Cranial Nerve"; "see Release, Peripheral Nervous System"; "see Excision, Lower Bones"; and "see Excision, Upper Bones." When a decompressive surgery is performed to release pressure and free a body part (such as the nerve root) from constraint, the appropriate code from the root operation "Release," rather than the root operation "Excision," should be used. "Release" involves freeing a body part from an abnormal physical constraint by cutting or by use of force. Some of the restraining tissue may be taken out, but none of the body part is taken out.

SPINAL MOTION PRESERVATION

Depending on the extent of bone and tissue removed during a spinal decompression procedure, the spinal segment may be deemed unstable. Stabilization of the spinal segment is primarily accomplished

CHAPTER 22

Diseases of the

Musculoskeletal

System and

Connective

Tissue

with spinal fusion. However, new spinal motion preservation technologies have been developed to allow for spine stabilization without the motion restriction associated with fusion.

Motion preservation technologies placed in the posterior column of the spine include the following:

- Interspinous process devices (e.g., X-Stop®, Wallis®, and Coflex® systems)
- Pedicle screw dynamic stabilization devices (e.g., Dynesys® and M-Brace™)
- Facet replacement devices (e.g., Total Facet Arthroplasty System®)

The root operations "Insertion," "Revision," and "Replacement" are used for the insertion, revision, and replacement of posterior spinal motion preservation device(s), respectively. These codes include the dynamic stabilization device(s) and any synchronous facetectomy (partial, total) performed at the same level. For example:

0RH63BZ	Insertion of interspinous process spinal stabilization device into thoracic vertebral joint, percutaneous approach
0RW104Z	Revision of internal fixation device in cervical vertebral joint, open approach
0SH30CZ	Insertion of pedicle-based spinal stabilization device into lumbosacral joint, open approach
0RW634Z	Revision of internal fixation device in thoracic vertebral joint, percutaneous approach
0SR00JZ	Replacement of lumbar vertebral joint, with synthetic substitute, open approach
0SW30JZ	Revision of synthetic substitute in lumbosacral joint, open approach

If a synchronous surgical decompression (foraminotomy, laminectomy, laminotomy) is also performed, it is coded as an additional procedure.

PLICA SYNDROME

Plica syndrome occurs when the synovial bands that are present early in fetal development have not combined into one large synovial unit as they develop further. The condition almost always affects the knee, although it can occasionally be found in other areas. Patients with this syndrome often experience pain and swelling, weakness, and a locking and clicking sensation of the knee. The therapeutic goal is to reduce the inflammation of the synovium and the thickening of the plica. Usual treatment measures attempt to relieve symptoms within three months; if that does not occur, arthroscopic or open surgery to remove the plica may be required. Assign code **M67.5-, Plica syndrome,** for this condition and code for excision of knee joint for the surgery.

FASCIITIS

Necrotizing fasciitis is a fulminating infection that begins with severe or extensive cellulitis that spreads to the superficial and deep fascia, producing thrombosis of the subcutaneous vessels and gangrene of the underlying tissue. Group A *Streptococcus* is the most common organism responsible for this condition, but any bacteria may be the cause. Code M72.6 is assigned for this condition, with an additional code for the organism when this information is known.

CHAPTER 22

*Diseases of the
Musculoskeletal
System and
Connective
Tissue*

EXERCISE 22.4

Code the following diagnoses and procedures. Do not assign External cause of morbidity codes.

1. Acute polymyositis

   Mild thoracogenic scoliosis

   Percutaneous excisional biopsy of left trunk muscle

2. Sclerosing tenosynovitis, left thumb

   and middle finger

3. Acute osteomyelitis of left distal femur

   due to type 2 diabetes with diabetic arthropathy

   Sequestrectomy (percutaneous) and percutaneous

   excision of sinus tract, left distal femur

4. Adhesive capsulitis, left shoulder

   Arthroscopic release of coracohumeral ligament

5. Nonunion of traumatic fracture, left femoral neck,

   subsequent encounter

   Inlay-type iliac bone graft of nonunion

   of left femoral neck (open approach)

   Left iliac crest bone excised for graft (percutaneous)

6. Recurrent dislocation of patella

7. Deformity of left ring finger, due to old extensor muscle

   and tendon laceration of left ring finger

   Transfer of flexor tendon from distal

   phalanx to middle phalanx (open approach)

8. Cervical spondylosis, C5–C6, C6–C7

   Anterior column cervical spinal fusion, C5–C6, C6–C7

   open, anterior approach, with interbody device

9. Dupuytren's contracture (right hand)

   Incision and division of palmar fascia (open approach)

CHAPTER 22

*Diseases of the
Musculoskeletal
System and
Connective
Tissue*

10. Multiple compression fractures of vertebrae
    and major osseous defects due to senile osteoporosis
    (initial encounter)

---

11. Lumbar spinal stenosis with neuroclaudication
    Decompressive laminectomy with Dynesys stabilization
    system (open approach) to release spinal cord

---

12. Disc herniation and degenerative spondylosis C5–C6
    with C6 radiculopathy
    Arthrodesis C5–C6 anterior interbody fusion device
    with allograft

Coding OF Pregnancy AND Childbirth Complications, Abortion, Congenital Anomalies, AND Perinatal Conditions

CHAPTER 23

Complications of Pregnancy, Childbirth, and the Puerperium

CHAPTER OVERVIEW

- Conditions affecting pregnancy, childbirth, and the puerperium are found in chapter 15 of ICD-10-CM.
  - Codes from chapter 15 take precedence over codes from other chapters.
  - Codes from chapter 15 are never assigned to the newborn's record.
- Assignment of the final character for trimester should be based on the provider's documentation of the trimester for the current admission/encounter.
- The date of the admission should be used to determine weeks of gestation (category Z3A) for inpatient admissions that encompass more than one gestational week.
- Z codes are used to indicate the outcome of the delivery.
- A normal delivery is contingent on a variety of criteria.
- The Tabular List must be reviewed for assignment of the final character for trimester and the correct seventh character for multiple gestations for some chapter 15 codes.
- When deliveries are not deemed normal, the principal diagnosis code is the main circumstance or complication of the delivery.
- When assigning codes from chapter 15, it is important to assess whether a condition was pre-existing prior to pregnancy or developed during or due to the pregnancy in order to assign the correct code.
- Postpartum complications are any complications that occur throughout the six weeks following the delivery.
- There is a sequela code to use for complications that occur after the postpartum period. This code follows the codes for the condition.
- There are codes for delivery assistance procedures, such as induction of labor, artificial rupture of membranes, fetal head rotation, forceps delivery, vacuum extraction, episiotomy, and cesarean delivery.
- Contraceptive management and procreative management, through both admission and outpatient encounter, are covered by a series of Z codes. These codes can be supplemented by additional codes if an underlying condition is present.

INTRODUCTION

Conditions that affect the management of pregnancy, childbirth, and the puerperium are classified to categories O00 through O9A in chapter 15 of ICD-10-CM. Conditions from other chapters of ICD-10-CM are usually reclassified in chapter 15 when they are related to or aggravated by the pregnancy, childbirth, or the puerperium.

Should the provider document that the pregnancy is incidental to the encounter, code **Z33.1, Pregnant state, incidental,** is assigned in place of any chapter 15 codes. It is the provider's responsibility to state that the condition being treated is not affecting the pregnancy.

Chapter 15 codes take precedence over codes from other chapters, but codes from other chapters may be used as additional codes when needed to provide more specificity. Codes from chapter 15 of ICD-10-CM refer to the mother only and are assigned only on the mother's record. They are never assigned on the newborn's record; other codes are provided for that purpose. (See chapter 26 of this handbook.) Codes from categories O00 through O08 are assigned for pregnancy with abortive outcome, including ectopic pregnancy, molar pregnancy, and abortion. Code assignments for these conditions are discussed in chapter 24 of this handbook.

Codes from categories O09 through O9A are used to describe the entire obstetric experience, which begins at conception and ends six weeks (42 days) after delivery.

ICD-10-CM divides chapter 15 as follows:

O09	Supervision of high-risk pregnancy
O10–O16	Edema, proteinuria and hypertensive disorders in pregnancy, childbirth, and the puerperium
O20–O29	Other maternal disorders predominantly related to pregnancy
O30–O48	Maternal care related to the fetus and amniotic cavity and possible delivery problems
O60–O77	Complications of labor and delivery
O80, O82	Encounter for delivery
O85–O92	Complications predominantly related to the puerperium
O94–O9A	Other obstetric conditions not elsewhere classified

The process of labor and delivery includes three stages. The first stage begins with the onset of regular uterine contractions and ends when the cervical os is completely dilated. The second stage begins with complete dilation and continues until the infant has been completely expelled. The third stage begins with the expulsion of the infant and continues until the placenta and membranes have been expelled and contraction of the uterus is complete. The puerperium begins at the end of the third stage of labor and continues for six weeks.

Occasionally, a pregnancy continues for a longer term than usual gestation and is considered to be a long pregnancy. The following two codes are used when this occurs:

O48.0	Post-term pregnancy (40 completed weeks through any number of days in week 42)
O48.1	Prolonged pregnancy (43 or more weeks of gestation)

FINAL CHARACTER FOR TRIMESTER

The majority of codes in chapter 15 of ICD-10-CM have a final character indicating the trimester of pregnancy. Note that the Tabular List must be reviewed for assignment of the final character for trimester, as the codes in the Alphabetic Index of Diseases and Injuries do not include the complete code. The time frames for the trimesters are indicated at the beginning of chapter 15 and are defined by an instructional note as follows:

FIGURE 23.1   Primary Organs of the Female Reproductive System

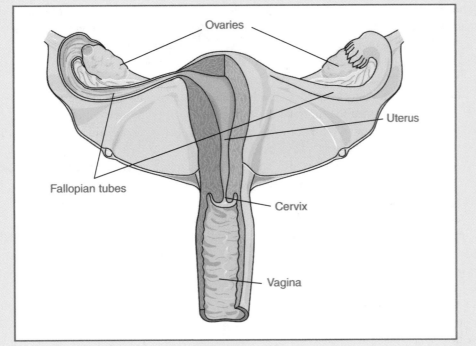

- First trimester—less than 14 weeks 0 days
- Second trimester—14 weeks 0 days to less than 28 weeks 0 days
- Third trimester—28 weeks 0 days until delivery

Assignment of the final character for trimester should be based on the provider's documentation of the trimester (or number of weeks) for the current admission/encounter. This definition applies to the assignment of trimester for pre-existing conditions as well as those that develop during or are due to the pregnancy. The provider is defined in the *ICD-10-CM Official Guidelines for Coding and Reporting* as "Physician or other qualified healthcare practitioner legally accountable for establishing the patient's diagnosis." The provider's documentation of the number of weeks may be used to assign the appropriate final character identifying the trimester. For example, if the documentation refers to the patient having completed 20 weeks of pregnancy, the appropriate code for second trimester may be selected; the provider does not have to explicitly document "second trimester."

Not every code in chapter 15 has a trimester component. If trimester is not a component of a code, it is because the condition always occurs in a specific trimester or the concept of trimester of pregnancy is not relevant. For example, category O48, Late pregnancy, does not include trimester because, by definition, this category is to be used for pregnancies longer than 40 completed weeks. Certain codes have characters for only certain trimesters because the condition does not occur in all trimesters, but it may occur in more than one. For example, category O60, Preterm labor, is for spontaneous onset of labor before 37 completed weeks of gestation, and therefore there are no codes for first trimester, which is less than 14 weeks.

If a condition complicating the pregnancy develops prior to the current admission/encounter or represents a pre-existing condition, the trimester character for the trimester at the time of the admission/encounter should be assigned. For example, a pregnant patient with pre-existing

324

CHAPTER 23

*Complications
of Pregnancy,
Childbirth, and
the Puerperium*

type 1 diabetes mellitus, at 16 weeks' gestation (second trimester) is admitted for an emergent transvaginal cerclage for cervical shortening. Assign code **O26.872, Cervical shortening, second trimester,** as the principal diagnosis. Code **O24.012, Pre-existing type 1 diabetes mellitus in pregnancy, second trimester,** is assigned for the diabetes along with a code from category E10 for any diabetic manifestations, as well as code Z3A.16 to identify weeks of gestation. Also assign code **0UVC7ZZ, Restriction of cervix, via natural or artificial opening,** for the placement of the cerclage. A cerclage is a suture used to restrict the opening of the cervix and is not considered a device in ICD-10-PCS.

Occasionally, an inpatient hospitalization may encompass more than one trimester, such as when a patient is admitted to a hospital for complications of pregnancy during one trimester and remains in the hospital into a subsequent trimester. In such instances, the trimester character for the antepartum complication code should be assigned on the basis of the trimester when the complication developed, not the trimester of the discharge. For example, a pregnant female is admitted to the hospital at 27 weeks of completed gestation with acute appendicitis complicating her pregnancy. She requires emergency laparoscopic appendectomy, which she tolerates well. She is kept in the hospital for two weeks postoperatively, with intravenous antibiotics administered due to postoperative fever. Because the acute appendicitis developed during the second trimester, code **O99.612, Diseases of the digestive system complicating pregnancy, second trimester,** is assigned rather than code O99.613. Assign also code **K35.80, Unspecified acute appendicitis,** to describe the specific condition, and code Z3A.27 to identify weeks of gestation.

The exception to the above guideline is when a delivery occurs during the current admission. Whenever delivery occurs during the current admission and there is an "in childbirth" option for the obstetric complication, the "in childbirth" code should be assigned. For example, a patient is admitted during the third trimester with malnutrition and stays in the hospital until she delivers. Code **O25.2, Malnutrition in childbirth,** should be assigned rather than code **O25.13, Malnutrition in pregnancy, third trimester,** for the malnutrition. If the specific type of malnutrition is documented, assign an additional code from category E40–E46; the appropriate code from category Z3A should also be assigned.

It is important to note that although each category in chapter 15 that includes codes for trimester has a code for "unspecified trimester," the "unspecified trimester" code should be used only in rare circumstances, such as when the documentation in the record is insufficient to determine the trimester and it is not possible to obtain clarification.

Codes in category Z3A, Weeks of gestation, may be used only on the maternal record to provide additional information about the pregnancy. Category Z3A codes refer to completed weeks of gestation. For example, for a patient admitted at 42 1/7 weeks of gestation for induction of labor and delivered at 42 2/7 weeks, code **Z3A.42, 42 weeks gestation of pregnancy,** is assigned, as it is the code for any number of days in week 42 up to 43 weeks. The date of the admission should be used to determine weeks of gestation for inpatient admissions that encompass more than one gestational week. Pregnancy is considered "at term" when gestation attains 37 complete weeks but is less than 42. Category Z3A codes should not be assigned for pregnancies with abortive outcomes (categories O00–O08), for elective termination of pregnancy (Z33.2), or for postpartum conditions—category Z3A is not applicable to these conditions.

OUTCOME OF DELIVERY

Because chapter 15 codes do not indicate the outcome of delivery, a code from category Z37 is assigned as an additional code to provide this information whenever the patient delivers in the hospital. To locate the code assignment for outcome of delivery, refer to the main term **Outcome of delivery** in the Alphabetic Index. Fourth characters indicate both whether the outcome was single or multiple and whether liveborn or stillborn. For multiple births with more than twins, additional characters indicate the number of outcomes (e.g., triplets, quadruplets) and whether they were all liveborn, some liveborn, or all stillborn. These codes are used only on the mother's

325

CHAPTER 23

*Complications
of Pregnancy,
Childbirth, and
the Puerperium*

record, not the record of the newborn, and are assigned only for the episode of care during which delivery occurred. No code from category Z37 is assigned when delivery occurs outside the hospital prior to admission. Examples of appropriate use of codes from category Z37 include the following:

O80 + Z37.0 + Z3A.40   40-week term pregnancy, spontaneous delivery, vertex presentation; liveborn male infant

O30.003 + O36.4xx2 +   39-week term pregnancy with spontaneous delivery; twin
Z3A.39 + Z37.3   pregnancy, with twin A liveborn and twin B stillborn

---

EXERCISE 23.1

For the following exercise, do not assign the delivery codes; assign only the Z codes for outcome of delivery. Remember that, in actual practice, the delivery code precedes the Z code.

1. Delivery of twins, both stillborn

2. Delivery of triplets, one stillborn

3. Delivery of liveborn, female infant

4. Delivery of single stillborn

FETAL SEVENTH CHARACTERS

The following subcategories/codes require a seventh character to identify the fetus for which the complication code applies:

O31.00–O31.8x9	Complications specific to multiple gestation
O32.0–O32.9	Maternal care for malpresentation of fetus
O33.3	Maternal care for disproportion due to outlet contraction of pelvis
O33.4	Maternal care for disproportion of mixed maternal and fetal origin
O33.5	Maternal care for disproportion due to unusually large fetus
O33.6	Maternal care for disproportion due to hydrocephalic fetus
O33.7	Maternal care for disproportion due to other fetal deformities
O35.0–O35.9	Maternal care for known or suspected fetal abnormality and damage
O36.011–O36.93	Maternal care for other fetal problems
O40.1–O40.9	Polyhydramnios
O41.00–O41.93	Other disorders of amniotic fluid and membranes

326

CHAPTER 23

*Complications
of Pregnancy,
Childbirth, and
the Puerperium*

O60.10–O60.14	Preterm labor with preterm delivery
O60.20–O60.23	Term delivery with preterm labor
O64.0–O64.9	Obstructed labor due to malposition and malpresentation of fetus
O69.0–O69.9	Labor and delivery complicated by umbilical cord complications

Seventh characters 1–9 are for cases of multiple gestations to identify the fetus to which the code applies. The seventh character 0, not applicable or unspecified, is used for the following situations:

- Single gestations
- When the documentation in the record is insufficient to determine the fetus affected and it is not possible to obtain clarification
- When it is not possible to clinically determine which fetus is affected

Note that the Tabular List must be reviewed for assignment of the correct seventh character for multiple gestations for chapter 15 codes, because the seventh characters are not included in the Alphabetic Index.

Some providers prefer to refer to each fetus in multiple gestation cases by alphabetical characters, such as fetus A, fetus B, etc., rather than numbers (fetus 1, fetus 2, etc.). In such cases, fetus A should be equated to fetus 1, fetus B should be equated to fetus 2, and so on. There is no expectation that the same fetus number or alphabetical character be consistently carried over from one admission to another. Identification of the fetus, whether by number or alphabetical character, is based on the provider documentation. If a condition affects all fetuses (e.g., preterm labor, post-term pregnancy, etc.), assign a separate code for each fetus. For example, a woman delivered preterm twins in the third trimester at 34 weeks of gestation. Assign code **O60.14X1, Preterm labor third trimester with preterm delivery third trimester, fetus 1,** and code **O60.14X2, Preterm labor third trimester with preterm delivery third trimester, fetus 2,** to indicate each fetus affected.

A code from category O30, Multiple gestation, is assigned to provide additional information such as the number of fetuses (e.g., triplet pregnancy), the number of amniotic sacs, and the number of placentas. The risk of complications increases with multiple gestations, and the treatment plan will differ, depending on the number of placentas and amniotic sacs.

SELECTION OF FIRST-LISTED AND PRINCIPAL DIAGNOSIS

The selection of first-listed diagnoses or principal diagnoses for encounters/admissions for normal deliveries and other obstetric care is based on the following guidelines.

Routine Outpatient Prenatal Visits

For routine outpatient prenatal visits when no complications are present, a code from category Z34, Encounter for supervision of normal pregnancy, should be used as the first-listed diagnosis. These codes should not be used in conjunction with chapter 15 codes.

Supervision of High-Risk Pregnancy

Codes from category O09 are intended for use only during the prenatal period. For complications during the labor or delivery episode resulting from a high-risk pregnancy, assign the applicable complication codes from chapter 15. If there are no complications during the labor or delivery episode, assign code **O80, Encounter for full-term uncomplicated delivery.**

ICD-10-CM provides codes for the supervision of the following types of high-risk pregnancies:

O09.00–O09.03	Pregnancy with history of infertility
O09.10–O09.13	Pregnancy with history of ectopic pregnancy
O09.A0–O09.A3	Pregnancy with history of molar pregnancy
O09.211–O09.299	Pregnancy with other poor reproductive or obstetric history
O09.30–O09.33	Pregnancy with insufficient antenatal care
O09.40–O09.43	Pregnancy with grand multiparity
O09.511–O09.529	Elderly (pregnancy for female age 35 years or older at expected date of delivery) primigravida and multigravida
O09.611–O09.629	Young (pregnancy for a female less than 16 years old at expected date of delivery) primigravida and multigravida
O09.70–O09.73	High risk pregnancy due to social problems
O09.811–O09.899	Other high risk pregnancies (includes pregnancy resulting from assisted reproductive technology [O09.81-] and pregnancy with history of in utero procedure during previous pregnancy [O09.82-])

Episodes When No Delivery Occurs

In episodes when no delivery occurs, the principal diagnosis should correspond to the principal complication of the pregnancy that necessitated the encounter. If multiple complications are treated or monitored, any of the complication codes may be sequenced first.

Admission with Normal Delivery

Code O80, Encounter for full-term uncomplicated delivery, is used only when the delivery is entirely normal with a single liveborn outcome. There can be no postpartum complications, and any antepartum complication experienced during pregnancy must have been resolved before the time of delivery. Code O80 is always the principal diagnosis. If there is any complication, code O80 cannot be assigned. Code O80 cannot be used if any other code from chapter 15 is needed to describe a current complication of the antenatal, delivery, or perinatal period. Codes from other chapters may be used as additional codes with code O80 only when the physician has documented that the conditions are not related to, and in no way complicate, the pregnancy.

All of the following criteria must be met in order for code O80 to be used correctly:

- The delivery is entirely normal (requiring minimal or no assistance, with or without episiotomy).
- There is no fetal manipulation (e.g., rotation version) or instrumentation (forceps).
- There is a spontaneous, cephalic, vaginal delivery.
- Presentation at delivery can be only cephalic (head) or occipital. Terms such as "right occipito-anterior (ROA)," "left occipito-anterior (LOA)," "right occipito-posterior (ROP)," "left occipito-posterior (LOP)," and "vertex" describe an occipital presentation. Any other presentation, such as breech, face, or brow, disallows the use of code O80.
- Any antepartum complication experienced during pregnancy must have been resolved before the time of delivery.
- No abnormalities of either labor or delivery can have occurred.
- No postpartum complications can be present.
- No procedures other than the following can have been performed: episiotomy without forceps, episiorrhaphy, amniotomy (artificial rupture of the membranes), manually assisted delivery without forceps, administration of analgesics and/or anesthesia, fetal monitoring, induction of labor (in the absence of medical indications), and sterilization. If any other procedure is performed, code O80 cannot be assigned.

328

CHAPTER 23

Complications
of Pregnancy,
Childbirth, and
the Puerperium

- Outcome of delivery must be single live birth, Z37.0. When there has been a multiple birth or stillbirth, code O80 cannot be assigned.

Examples include the following:

- A patient who had a completely normal delivery at 38 weeks' gestation suffers a postpartum hemorrhage several hours after delivery. Code **O72.1, Other immediate postpartum hemorrhage,** is assigned. Assign also codes Z3A.38 and Z37.0. Although the delivery itself was normal, complications were present during the episode of care; therefore, code O80 cannot be used.

- The prenatal history for a patient who had a completely normal delivery at 40 weeks' gestation of a live infant indicates that she had a urinary tract infection at three months' gestation. This was treated with Bactrim on an outpatient basis. There was no recurrence of the infection during the pregnancy, and the patient had no infection at the time of delivery. In this case, code **O80, Encounter for full-term uncomplicated delivery,** is assigned. Codes Z37.0 and Z3A.40 are also assigned to describe the outcome of delivery and the completed weeks of gestation.

EXERCISE 23.2

Write an "X" next to each of the following circumstances of delivery that is assigned code O80, Encounter for full-term uncomplicated delivery.

1. Liveborn, full-term, breech presentation   _____

2. Liveborn, premature, cephalic presentation   _____

3. Stillborn, full-term, vertex presentation   _____

4. Liveborn, full-term, cephalic presentation; episiotomy with repair   _____

5. Liveborn, full-term, vertex presentation; elective low forceps   _____

6. Liveborn, full-term, vertex presentation; postpartum breast abscess   _____

7. Liveborn, full-term, breech presentation changed to vertex presentation by version prior to delivery   _____

Admission with Other Delivery

When an obstetric patient is admitted and delivers during that admission, the condition that was the reason for the admission should be sequenced as the principal diagnosis. If multiple conditions prompted the admission, sequence the one most related to the delivery as the principal diagnosis. A code for any complication of the delivery should be assigned as an additional diagnosis. In cases of cesarean delivery, if the patient was admitted with a condition that resulted in the performance of a cesarean procedure, that condition should be selected as the principal diagnosis. If the reason for the admission was unrelated to the condition resulting in the cesarean delivery, the condition related to the reason for the admission/encounter should be selected as the principal diagnosis.

For example:

- A patient who had a previous low cesarean delivery is admitted for a second cesarean delivery at 39 weeks' gestation. She also has pre-existing type 1 diabetes mellitus. Cesarean delivery is accomplished without complication. Code **O34.211, Maternal care for low transverse scar from previous cesarean delivery,** is assigned as the principal diagnosis, with an additional code of **O24.02, Pre-existing type 1 diabetes mellitus, in childbirth.** To provide more specificity, the following codes are also assigned: **E10.9, Type 1 diabetes mellitus without complications; Z37.0, Single live birth;** and **Z3A.39, 39 weeks gestation of pregnancy.**

- A patient at 40 weeks' gestation is admitted to the hospital in obstructed labor due to a breech presentation. Version is unsuccessful, and the patient delivers by cesarean section (C-section) several hours later. The principal diagnosis code is **O64.1xx0, Obstructed labor due to breech presentation.** Assign also codes Z37.0 and Z3A.40. There is no need to assign code **O32.1xx0, Maternal care for breech presentation,** as an additional code per the guidance provided with the "excludes1" note at category O32. Code O64.1xx0 already identifies the breech presentation.

- A patient is admitted for treatment of preeclampsia, and fetal decelerations complicate the spontaneous vaginal delivery. The preeclampsia is sequenced as the principal diagnosis, rather than fetal decelerations.

Occasionally, a C-section may be performed without a medical indication; therefore, there will be no medical condition that resulted in the cesarean delivery. For example, a patient elected to have a low C-section due to fear of a vaginal delivery. Assign code **O82, Encounter for cesarean delivery without indication,** as the principal diagnosis.

Code O75.82 is assigned to describe a planned cesarean delivery when the onset of labor occurs after 37, but before 39, completed weeks of gestation. This code allows data to be collected for quality markers for elective cesarean delivery performed between 37 and 39 weeks.

Admission for Other Obstetric Care

When the admission or encounter is for obstetric care other than delivery, the principal diagnosis should correspond to the complication that necessitated the admission or encounter. If more than one complication is present, all of which are treated or monitored, any of the complication codes may be sequenced first. If no obstetric complications are present, the following guidelines govern selection of the principal diagnosis:

- If the reason for admission or encounter is not related to an obstetric condition but the patient is pregnant, code **Z33.1, Pregnant state, incidental,** is assigned as an additional code. This code is never assigned as the principal diagnosis, and it cannot be used when codes from chapter 15 are assigned.

- When a patient delivers outside a health care facility and is then admitted for routine postpartum care with no complications present, code **Z39.0, Encounter for care and examination of mother immediately after delivery,** is assigned as the principal diagnosis. When a postpartum complication is present, the code for that condition is designated as the principal diagnosis, and code Z39.0 is not assigned.

- For example, a woman is admitted following delivery in the parking lot of the hospital. On admission, it is noted that she had sustained a first-degree perineal laceration. Code **O70.0, First degree laceration during delivery,** is assigned rather than code Z39.0.

- Code **Z39.1, Encounter for care and examination of lactating mother,** is assigned for a visit related to lactation (e.g., supervision, counseling). However, if the patient presents postpartum with a condition associated with lactation, assign a code from category O92,

330

CHAPTER 23

*Complications
of Pregnancy,
Childbirth, and
the Puerperium*

Other disorders of breast and disorders of lactation associated with pregnancy and the puerperium.

- Occasionally, an expectant mother may visit a pediatrician to receive advice on childcare or to evaluate the pediatric office. This is not a visit related to a problem with the pregnancy. Code **Z76.81, Expectant parent(s) prebirth pediatrician visit,** may be assigned for these encounters.

EXERCISE 23.3

Code the following diagnoses.

---

1. Antepartum supervision of pregnancy in patient
   with history of three previous stillbirths, 12 weeks' gestation

---

2. Office visit for routine prenatal care, for primigravida
   patient with no complications, second trimester

---

3. Office visit for care of 40-year-old patient who is in the
   fourth month of her third pregnancy

---

4. Hospital admission of patient in good
   condition after delivering a single liveborn
   infant in taxi on the way to the hospital

---

5. Admission for intravenous antibiotic therapy of patient
   who delivered a single liveborn at home three days ago;
   patient now suffering an abscess of the breast

FETAL CONDITIONS AFFECTING MANAGEMENT OF PREGNANCY

Codes from categories O35, Maternal care for known or suspected fetal abnormality and damage, and O36, Maternal care for other fetal problems, are assigned only when the fetal condition is actually responsible for modifying the mother's care. Such an effect may be documented by additional diagnostic studies based on the fetal problem, additional observation, special care, or termination of the pregnancy. The existence of the fetal condition does not in itself justify assigning a code from these categories; code assignment is appropriate only when the condition affects the management of the mother's care. Codes from categories O35 and O36 are used when the listed condition in the fetus is the reason for hospitalization or other obstetric care to the mother, or for termination of pregnancy.

For example, when the mother receives care because of an abnormal fetal heart rate or rhythm, a code or codes from subcategory O36.83-, Maternal care for abnormalities of the fetal

331

CHAPTER 23

*Complications
of Pregnancy,
Childbirth, and
the Puerperium*

heart rate or rhythm, is assigned. Codes in this series specify the trimester and the affected fetus in a multiple gestation pregnancy. Assign a separate code for each fetus that has an abnormal heart rate or rhythm.

When decreased fetal movements result in a decision to perform a cesarean delivery or early induction of labor in the mother, a code from subcategory O36.81-, Decreased fetal movements, is assigned. On the other hand, if no change is made in the mother's care, a code from subcategory O36.81- is not assigned because the decreased fetal movement is not considered to have affected the management of the mother significantly.

Occasionally, it may be difficult to determine fetal viability or nonviability during early pregnancy. Patients previously confirmed as pregnant in the very early weeks may return weeks later for an evaluation. If the fetal heartbeat cannot be heard, an ultrasound may be necessary to confirm that the pregnancy is viable. Assign code O36.80- to describe an encounter to determine fetal viability.

Multiple Gestation

Category O30, Multiple gestation, is used to identify multiple gestation, such as twin (O30.001–O30.099), triplet (O30.101–O30.199), quadruplet (O30.201–O30.299), other specified multiple gestations (O30.801–O30.899), and unspecified (O30.90–O30.93). The risk of complications increases with multiple gestations, and the treatment plan will differ depending on the number of placentas and amniotic sacs. Fifth characters under category O30 indicate the number of placentas and amniotic sacs, while sixth characters indicate the trimester.

In Utero Surgery

Surgery performed on a fetus in utero (while the fetus is still in the womb) is considered an obstetric encounter. Codes from ICD-10-CM chapter 16, perinatal codes, should not be used on the mother's record to identify fetal conditions. Instead, when surgery is performed on the fetus in utero, a diagnosis code from category O35, Maternal care for known or suspected fetal abnormality and damage, should be assigned for the fetal condition. Assign the appropriate ICD-10-PCS code for the procedure performed.

Code **O35.7xx-, Maternal care for (suspected) damage to fetus by other medical procedures,** describes maternal and fetal complications resulting from in utero surgery performed during the current pregnancy. Code O35.7- is used for supervision of pregnancy affected by an in utero procedure during the current pregnancy. If the newborn experiences any problems or complications because of in utero procedures, assign code **P96.5, Complication to newborn due to (fetal) intrauterine procedure,** on the newborn record.

A code from subcategory O09.82-, Supervision of pregnancy with history of in utero procedure during previous pregnancy, can be used as an additional code assignment with code O35.7- if the patient also has a past history of in utero surgery during a previous pregnancy.

ICD-10-PCS classifies in utero surgeries to the Obstetrics Section, body system "pregnancy," root operation "Repair," body part "products of conception." For example, in utero surgical repair of herniated diaphragm for congenital diaphragmatic hernia is coded to **10Q00ZK, Repair respiratory system in products of conception, open approach.** The diaphragm is classified to the "respiratory" body system in the Medical and Surgical Section.

OTHER CONDITIONS COMPLICATING PREGNANCY, CHILDBIRTH, OR THE PUERPERIUM

Some conditions inevitably complicate the obstetric experience or are themselves aggravated by pregnancy. Certain categories in chapter 15 of ICD-10-CM distinguish between conditions of the mother that existed prior to pregnancy (pre-existing) and those that are a direct result of pregnancy.

When assigning codes from chapter 15, it is important to assess whether a condition was pre-existing prior to pregnancy or developed during or due to the pregnancy in order to assign the correct code. For example, hypertension complicating pregnancy, delivery, and the puerperium is classified to category O10 when it is pre-existing, to category O13 when it is gestational (pregnancy induced), and to category O16 when it is unspecified maternal hypertension.

Categories that do not distinguish between pre-existing and pregnancy-related conditions may be used for either. It is acceptable to use codes specifically for the puerperium with codes for complications of pregnancy and childbirth if a condition arises postpartum during the delivery encounter.

Designated conditions, such as edema, proteinuria, and hypertensive disorders in pregnancy, childbirth, and the puerperium are classified to categories O10 through O16. Other maternal disorders, such as hemorrhage, hyperemesis gravidarum, venous complications, genitourinary infections, diabetes mellitus, malnutrition, and liver disorders, are classified to categories O20 through O29 when they complicate the obstetric experience. Certain infectious diseases such as HIV disease, viral hepatitis, viral diseases (such as Zika infection), tuberculosis, and venereal disease are classified in category O98.

Some codes for such complications are very specific, and others are rather broad. When a code from chapter 15 describes the condition adequately, only that code is assigned. It is appropriate, however, to assign an additional code when it provides needed specificity. For example, a patient who has a history of genital herpes maintained on Valtrex is admitted to the hospital for delivery. At the time of delivery, she is symptom free with no outbreak. Nevertheless, herpes infection during pregnancy poses a risk to the fetus and is appropriately coded as a complication of the pregnancy. Code **O98.32, Other infections with a predominantly sexual mode of transmission complicating childbirth,** is assigned as the principal diagnosis. Codes **A60.09, Herpesviral infection of other urogenital tract,** and **Z79.899, Other long term (current) drug therapy,** should be assigned as additional diagnoses, along with Z codes for outcome of delivery and for weeks of gestation.

Codes from subcategory O22.3-, Deep thrombophlebitis complicating pregnancy, require an additional code to specify whether the deep thrombophlebitis is acute or chronic, and to specify the site. On the other hand, the code for varicose veins of the legs complicating pregnancy (O22.0-) or the puerperium (O87.4) provides complete information, and assignment of an additional code is redundant.

Other examples of the appropriate use of these codes follow.

O23.12 + Z3A.15	A pregnant patient at 15 weeks' gestation has a chronic cystitis and has had recurrent bouts of acute cystitis during her pregnancy, with an acute episode at time of admission
O26.611 + K76.2 + Z3A.10	Necrosis of liver, complicating pregnancy, 10 weeks' gestation

Hypertension

Hypertension in pregnancy is always considered a complicating factor in pregnancy, childbirth, or the puerperium. For correct code assignment, it is important to determine whether the hypertension is a pre-existing or gestational condition. Pre-existing hypertension is classified to category O10, Pre-existing hypertension complicating pregnancy, childbirth and the puerperium, as follows:

O10.01–O10.03	Essential hypertension
O10.111–O10.13	Hypertensive heart disease
O10.211–O10.23	Hypertensive chronic kidney disease
O10.311–O10.33	Hypertensive heart and chronic kidney disease

333

:   **CHAPTER 23**
:   *Complications*
:   *of Pregnancy,*
:   *Childbirth, and*
:   *the Puerperium*

O10.411–O10.43   Secondary hypertension

O10.911–O10.93   Unspecified

When assigning one of the O10 codes that includes hypertensive heart disease or hypertensive chronic kidney disease, it is necessary to add a secondary code from the appropriate hypertension category to specify the type of hypertensive heart disease (category I11), heart failure (category I50), chronic kidney disease (category I12), or hypertensive heart and chronic kidney disease (category I13).

Patients who do not have pre-existing hypertension may develop transient or gestational or pregnancy-induced hypertension during pregnancy. This condition is essentially an elevated blood pressure and clears relatively quickly once the pregnancy is over. This condition is coded to category O13, Gestational [pregnancy-induced] hypertension without significant proteinuria.

Hypertension in pregnancy sometimes leads to a pathological condition described as eclampsia or preeclampsia. Preeclampsia is a condition marked by high blood pressure accompanied with a high level of protein in the urine. Women with preeclampsia often also have swelling in the feet, legs, and hands. Eclampsia is the final and most severe phase of preeclampsia and occurs when preeclampsia is left untreated. Eclampsia usually results in seizures and causes coma and even death of the mother and baby, and it can occur before, during, or after childbirth. Preeclampsia can also occur in the postpartum period, although this is uncommon. When preeclampsia is superimposed on a pre-existing hypertension, a code from category O11, Pre-existing hypertension with pre-eclampsia, and an additional code from category O10 to identify the type of hypertension are assigned. When pre-eclampsia arises without any pre-existing hypertension, it is classified in category O14, Pre-eclampsia. When a patient is admitted with mild pre-eclampsia that progresses to severe pre-eclampsia during the stay, assign only a code from subcategory O14.1, Severe pre-eclampsia. The most severe stage is reported when a patient experiences deterioration or worsening of preeclampsia. Eclampsia, regardless of whether it is due to pre-existing hypertension, gestational hypertension, or unspecified material hypertension, is classified to category O15, Eclampsia.

Gestational hypertension associated with albuminuria (albumin in urine), edema (abnormal accumulation of fluid in body tissues), or both is generally considered to be preeclampsia or eclampsia. However, codes for eclampsia or preeclampsia are never assigned solely on the basis of an elevated blood pressure, an abnormal albumin level, or the presence of edema. The physician must specify the condition as eclampsia or preeclampsia before any of these codes may be assigned.

When gestational edema, gestational proteinuria, or both gestational edema and gestational proteinuria are present without hypertension, these conditions are classified to category O12, Gestational [pregnancy-induced] edema and proteinuria without hypertension.

Diabetes

Diabetes mellitus is a significant complicating factor in pregnancy. Pregnant women who are diabetic should first be assigned a code from category O24, Diabetes mellitus in pregnancy, childbirth, and the puerperium, followed by the appropriate diabetes code(s) (E08–E13) from chapter 4 of ICD-10-CM.

Similar to hypertension, category O24 distinguishes between pre-existing diabetes mellitus (including type 1, type 2, other, or unspecified), gestational diabetes, and unspecified diabetes as follows:

O24.011–O24.03   Pre-existing type 1 diabetes mellitus

O24.111–O24.13   Pre-existing type 2 diabetes mellitus

O24.311–O24.319   Unspecified pre-existing diabetes mellitus

O24.410–O24.439   Gestational diabetes mellitus

O24.811–O24.83   Other pre-existing diabetes mellitus

O24.911–O24.93   Unspecified diabetes mellitus

Gestational (pregnancy-induced) diabetes can occur during the second and third trimesters of pregnancy in women who were not diabetic prior to pregnancy. Gestational diabetes can cause complications in the pregnancy similar to those of pre-existing diabetes mellitus. Women with gestational diabetes are at increased risk to develop diabetes mellitus following delivery. Codes for gestational diabetes are in subcategory O24.4, Gestational diabetes mellitus. No other code from category O24, Diabetes mellitus in pregnancy, childbirth, and the puerperium, should be used with a code from O24.4. The codes under subcategory O24.4 classify gestational diabetes as diet controlled, insulin controlled, or controlled by oral hypoglycemic drugs. If a patient with gestational diabetes is treated with both diet and insulin, only the code for insulin controlled is required. If a patient with gestational diabetes is treated with both diet and oral hypoglycemic drugs, only the code for "controlled by oral hypoglycemic drugs" is required.

Code **Z79.4, Long-term (current) use of insulin,** should be assigned as an additional code if the pre-existing or unspecified diabetes mellitus is being treated with insulin. Code Z79.4 should not be assigned if insulin is used temporarily to bring the blood sugar under control in a patient with pre-existing type 2 diabetes. Code **Z79.84, Long-term (current) use of oral hypoglycemic drugs,** should be assigned if the pre-existing or unspecified diabetes mellitus is being treated with oral hypoglycemic drugs. However, neither code Z79.4 nor code Z79.84 should be assigned with codes from subcategory O24.4, Gestational diabetes. If a patient with gestational diabetes is medication controlled, the appropriate medication-controlled code (O24.414, O24.415, O24.424, O24.425, O24.434, or O24.435) should be assigned instead of Z79.4 or Z79.84. Code **Z86.32, Personal history of gestational diabetes,** is assigned to indicate that a patient has a history of gestational diabetes in a previous pregnancy.

A pregnant patient may have an abnormal glucose tolerance and not be diagnosed with gestational diabetes. In such cases, a code from subcategory O99.81, Abnormal glucose complicating pregnancy, childbirth, and the puerperium, should be assigned instead.

Examples include the following:

O24.113 + E11.620 + Z79.4 + Z3A.29	Pre-existing type 2 diabetes mellitus, with diabetic dermatitis, on insulin, intrauterine pregnancy, 29 weeks' gestation
O24.012 + E10.11 + Z3A.26	Pre-existing type 1 diabetes mellitus, ketoacidosis, and in coma; intrauterine pregnancy, 26 weeks' gestation
O24.414 + Z3A.30	30-weeks-pregnant female seen in physician's office with gestational diabetes; blood sugar reveals her diabetes is under good control with both diet and insulin

HIV Infection

During pregnancy, childbirth, or the puerperium, a patient admitted because of an HIV-related illness should receive a principal diagnosis from subcategory O98.7-, Human immunodeficiency [HIV] disease complicating pregnancy, childbirth and the puerperium, followed by the code(s) for the HIV-related illness(es). Patients with asymptomatic HIV infection status admitted during pregnancy, childbirth, or the puerperium should receive codes O98.7- and **Z21, Asymptomatic human immunodeficiency virus [HIV] infection status.** For example:

O98.711 + B20 + Z3A.00	First-trimester pregnant female with AIDS
O98.713 + Z21 + Z3A.30	30-weeks-pregnant female with complicating asymptomatic HIV status

Alcohol, Tobacco, and Drug Use

The Centers for Disease Control and Prevention (CDC) urge pregnant women not to drink alcohol any time during pregnancy. According to the CDC, there is no known safe amount of alcohol to drink while pregnant. Drinking alcohol during pregnancy can cause miscarriage, stillbirth, and a range of lifelong disorders known as fetal alcohol spectrum disorders. According to the U.S.

335

CHAPTER 23

*Complications
of Pregnancy,
Childbirth, and
the Puerperium*

Surgeon General, alcohol consumed during pregnancy increases the risk of alcohol-related birth defects, including growth deficiencies, facial abnormalities, central nervous system impairment, behavioral disorders, and impaired intellectual development. For any pregnancy case in which the mother uses alcohol during the pregnancy or postpartum, codes from subcategory O99.31-, Alcohol use complicating pregnancy, childbirth and the puerperium, should be assigned. A secondary code from category F10, Alcohol related disorders, should also be assigned to identify manifestations of the alcohol use.

Tobacco use also complicates pregnancy. Women who smoke prior to and during pregnancy are at risk for several adverse outcomes, such as premature rupture of membranes, placental abruption, and placenta previa during pregnancy. Babies born to women who smoke during pregnancy also have a higher risk of premature birth and low birth weight and are 1.4 to 3.0 times more likely to die of sudden infant death syndrome. Codes from subcategory O99.33-, Tobacco use disorder complicating pregnancy, childbirth, and the puerperium, should be assigned for any pregnancy case in which a mother uses any type of tobacco product during the pregnancy or postpartum. A secondary code from category F17, Nicotine dependence, should also be assigned to identify the type of nicotine dependence.

Drug use during pregnancy can have a direct impact on the fetus, including increased chances of birth defects, premature babies, underweight babies, and stillborn births. Codes under subcategory O99.32-, Drug use complicating pregnancy, childbirth, and the puerperium, should be assigned for any pregnancy case when a mother uses drugs during the pregnancy or postpartum. Secondary code(s) from categories F11–F16 and F18–F19 should also be assigned to identify manifestations of the drug use.

COMPLICATIONS OF LABOR AND DELIVERY

Complications of labor and delivery are classified to categories O60 through O77. This block of codes contains some of the most important codes for situations when code **O80, Encounter for full-term uncomplicated delivery,** cannot be used.

Category O60, Preterm labor, is defined in ICD-10-CM as "onset (spontaneous) of labor before 37 completed weeks of gestation." This category includes codes for cases with delivery as well as without delivery. Codes from category O60 should not be used with codes from subcategory O47.0- for false or threatened labor.

Failed induction of labor is classified to category O61. Fourth characters distinguish between medical (e.g., intravenous Oxytocin to stimulate contractions), instrumental (e.g., via mechanical or surgical induction, such as with transcervical Foley catheter balloon or laminaria), other, and unspecified methods of induction of labor.

Abnormalities of forces of labor are classified to category O62. Fourth characters specify primary inadequate contractions (O62.0); secondary uterine inertia (O62.1); other uterine inertia (O62.2); precipitate labor (O62.3); hypertonic, incoordinate, and prolonged uterine contractions (O62.4); other abnormalities of labor (O62.8); and unspecified abnormalities of labor (O62.9).

For patients with long labor, ICD-10-CM provides category O63, with the fourth character specifying the stages, such as prolonged first stage (O63.0); prolonged second stage (O63.1); delayed delivery of second twin, triplet, etc. (O63.2); and unspecified (O63.9).

Category O67 is used to classify intrapartum hemorrhage, not elsewhere classified. An Excludes1 note clarifies that antepartum hemorrhage, placenta previa, and premature separation of placenta are classified elsewhere.

Obstructed Labor

Obstructed labor occurs when the passage of the fetus through the pelvis is mechanically obstructed. The most common cause of obstructed labor is disproportion between the fetus's head

336

CHAPTER 23

*Complications
of Pregnancy,
Childbirth, and
the Puerperium*

and the mother's pelvis. Occasionally, however, obstruction is secondary to malpresentation, malposition, or fetal abnormalities. ICD-10-CM provides categories O64, O65, and O66 for obstructed labor due to different etiologies, as follows:

- Category O64, Obstructed labor due to malposition and malpresentation of fetus, is used to describe situations in which labor may be obstructed due to the position of the fetus. Fetal presentation refers to the part of the fetus that lies closest to or has entered the true pelvis at the time of delivery. Refer to figure 23.2 for examples of fetal presentations. Cephalic presentations are vertex, brow, face, and chin. Breech presentations include frank breech, complete breech, incomplete breech, and single or double footling breech. Shoulder presentations are rare and require cesarean delivery or turning before vaginal birth. Compound presentation involves the entry of more than one part into the true pelvis, most commonly a hand next to the head. Category O64 provides fourth characters to specify the varying fetal presentations causing the obstruction of labor, such as incomplete rotation of fetal head (O64.0), breech presentation (O64.1), face presentation (O64.2), brow presentation (O64.3), shoulder presentation (O64.4), compound presentation (O64.5), other malpresentation (O64.8), and unspecified malpresentation (O64.9).

FIGURE 23.2   Examples of Fetal Presentations

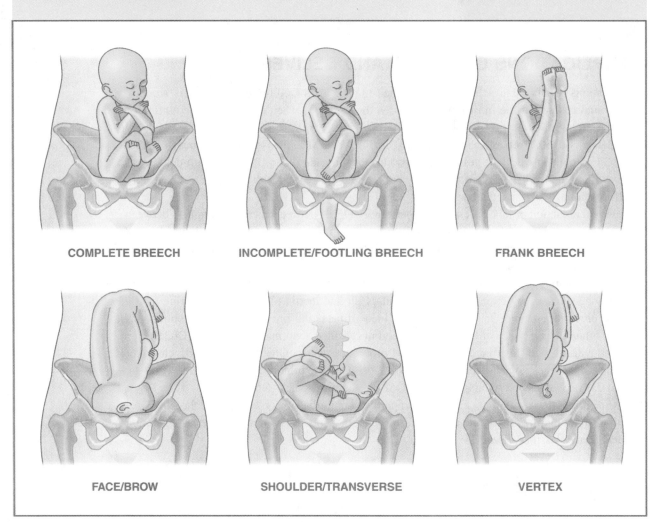

COMPLETE BREECH   INCOMPLETE/FOOTLING BREECH   FRANK BREECH

FACE/BROW   SHOULDER/TRANSVERSE   VERTEX

- Category O65, Obstructed labor due to maternal pelvic abnormality, is used to report obstructed labor caused by an abnormality in the mother's pelvis, such as deformity (O65.0), generally contracted pelvis (O65.1), pelvic inlet contraction (O65.2), pelvic outlet and mid-cavity contraction (O65.3), unspecified fetopelvic disproportion (O65.4), abnormality of maternal pelvic organs (O65.5), other maternal pelvic abnormalities (O65.8), and unspecified pelvic abnormality (O65.9).

- Category O66, Other obstructed labor, is used to classify other reasons for obstructed labor, such as shoulder dystocia (when the baby's shoulder gets stuck behind the mother's pubic bone) (O66.0), locked twins (a form of malpresentation in which a breech twin and a vertex twin become locked at the chin during labor and attempted delivery) (O66.1), unusually large fetus (O66.2), other abnormalities of fetus (including dystocia due to different etiologies) (O66.3), failed trial of labor (O66.4-), attempted application of vacuum extractor and forceps (O66.5), multiple fetuses (O66.6), other specified obstructed labor (O66.8 with an additional code to identify the cause of obstruction), and unspecified obstructed labor (O66.9).

Fetal Stress

Fetal stress is an uncommon complication of labor in which signs in a pregnant woman suggest that the fetus may not be well. It typically occurs when the fetus has not been receiving enough oxygen. Fetal stress may occur when the pregnancy lasts too long (postmaturity) or when complications of pregnancy or labor occur.

ICD-10-CM provides different codes related to fetal problems complicating labor and delivery, such as the following:

- **O68, Labor and delivery complicated by abnormality of fetal acid-base balance.** This code is used to describe fetal acidemia, fetal acidosis, fetal alkalosis, or fetal metabolic acidemia when these conditions complicate labor and delivery.

- Category O69, Labor and delivery complicated by umbilical cord complications. This category includes complications due to prolapse of cord; cord around neck, with compression; other cord entanglement, with compression; short cord; vasa previa; vascular lesion of cord; and other cord complications.

- **O76, Abnormality in fetal heart rate and rhythm complicating labor and delivery.** This code includes fetal problems such as bradycardia, heart rate decelerations, heart rate irregularity, tachycardia, and non-reassuring fetal heart rate or rhythm.

- Category O77, Other fetal stress complicating labor and delivery. This category includes codes for meconium in amniotic fluid (O77.0), fetal stress due to drug administration (O77.1), and other evidence of fetal stress (such as electrocardiographic or ultrasonic evidence) (O77.8). Unspecified fetal stress is classified to code O77.9.

It is important to remember that these codes should only be reported when the above conditions affect the management of the mother.

POSTPARTUM COMPLICATIONS

The postpartum period, clinically termed the "puerperium," begins immediately after delivery and includes the subsequent six weeks. A postpartum complication is defined as any complication that occurs during that six-week period. Postpartum complications are classified to categories O85 through O92.

One type of postpartum complication is a puerperal infection—a bacterial infection following childbirth. An estimated 2 percent to 4 percent of mothers who deliver vaginally may experience some

338

CHAPTER 23

*Complications
of Pregnancy,
Childbirth, and
the Puerperium*

form of puerperal infection. For cesarean delivery, the figure is five to 10 times higher. The genital tract is commonly the site of infection (e.g., endometritis: O86.12). Other types of infections include obstetric surgical wound infection (O86.00–O86.03, O86.09); sepsis following an obstetric procedure (O86.04); cervicitis (O86.11); vaginitis (O86.13); other infection of genital tract (O86.19); urinary tract infection (O86.20); infection of kidney (O86.21); infection of bladder (O86.22); other urinary infection (O86.29); pyrexia of unknown origin (O86.4); puerperal septic thrombophlebitis (O86.81); and other specified puerperal infections (O86.89). Assign an additional code to identify the causal organism with codes in category O86.

Puerperal sepsis refers to a postpartum infection involving the genital tract. Code **O85, Puerperal sepsis,** requires a secondary code to identify the causal organism. For example, for a bacterial infection, a code from categories B95 through B97 should be assigned. Codes from category A40, Streptococcal sepsis, or A41, Other sepsis, should not be used for puerperal sepsis. If the sepsis is documented to be severe sepsis, a code from subcategory R65.2, Severe sepsis, should be assigned as an additional code, along with the appropriate code for any associated acute organ dysfunction.

For sepsis following an obstetrical procedure, such as cesarean delivery, assign first a code from O86.00 to O86.03, Infection of obstetric surgical wound, that identifies the site of the infection (e.g. deep incisional site), if known. Assign an additional code for sepsis following an obstetrical procedure (O86.04). Use an additional code to identify the infectious agent, such as methicillin-resistant *Staphylococcus aureus* (MRSA), and assign a code from subcategory R65.2 if the sepsis is severe, with an additional code for any acute organ dysfunction.

Examples of code assignments for postpartum complications include the following:

- A patient who delivered a single healthy baby at 40 weeks develops endometritis two days following cesarean delivery while still in the hospital. Code **O86.12, Endometritis following delivery,** is assigned. This condition is considered a complication of childbirth and not a complication of pregnancy. In ICD-10-CM, there is an Index entry for "endometritis, puerperal, postpartum, childbirth." Additional codes are assigned to identify the reason for the C-section, the outcome of delivery, and weeks of gestation of pregnancy.

- A patient is admitted three weeks postpartum and treated for acute pyelonephritis due to *Escherichia coli* infection. Code **O86.21, Infection of kidney following delivery,** is assigned as the principal diagnosis. Code **B96.20, Unspecified Escherichia coli [E. coli] as the cause of diseases classified elsewhere,** is assigned as an additional code to provide specificity regarding the infection.

- A patient who delivered via low cervical C-section six days prior is readmitted with severe sepsis with acute kidney failure due to a MRSA infection deep within the C-section wound. Code **O86.02, Infection of obstetric surgical wound, deep incisional site,** is assigned for the postsurgical wound infection. For the MRSA sepsis with acute kidney failure, also assign codes **B95.62, Methicillin resistant Staphylococcus aureus as the cause of diseases classified elsewhere; O86.04, Sepsis following an obstetrical procedure; R65.20, Severe sepsis without septic shock;** and **N17.9, Acute kidney failure, unspecified.**

Uterine atony is a condition that can complicate delivery and refers to failure of the uterine muscle to contract adequately after the delivery. Uterine atony can occur with or without bleeding. Code **O62.2, Other uterine inertia,** is the default code for atony of the uterus without hemorrhage that is not otherwise specified or when the provider has documented that the uterine atony occurred during labor. Code **O72.1, Other immediate postpartum hemorrhage,** is assigned for postpartum uterine atony with hemorrhage when it occurs immediately following delivery of the baby and placenta. Code **O75.89, Other specified complications of labor and delivery,** is assigned for postpartum uterine atony without hemorrhage. For example:

- A patient develops postpartum hemorrhage due to uterine atony immediately after spontaneous vaginal delivery of twins at 38 weeks' gestation. The B-Lynch suture is performed

339

CHAPTER 23

*Complications
of Pregnancy,
Childbirth, and
the Puerperium*

to control the bleeding. The B-Lynch suture is a brace suture used to compress the uterus without compromising major vessels in cases of postpartum hemorrhage. Code **O72.1, Other immediate postpartum hemorrhage,** is assigned for postpartum uterine atony with hemorrhage. Also assign codes **O30.003, Twin pregnancy, unspecified number of placenta and unspecified number of amniotic sacs, third trimester; Z3A.38, 38 weeks gestation of pregnancy;** and **Z37.2, Twins, both liveborn.** Code **0UQ97ZZ, Repair uterus, via natural or artificial opening,** is assigned for the B-Lynch procedure.

- A nulliparous patient had a normal vaginal delivery at 40 weeks' gestation. After placental separation, uterine atony was noted, and the patient started to hemorrhage. The atony was unresponsive to bimanual massage, intravenous oxytocin, and intramuscular methylergonovine. The provider evacuated a 50-ml clot from the lower uterine segment, fundus firm with cessation of bleeding. The appropriate ICD-10-PCS procedure code for evacuation of clot is **0UC97ZZ, Extirpation of matter from uterus, via natural or artificial opening.** The correct root operation is "Extirpation," which is defined as taking or cutting out solid matter from a body part.

Pregnancy-associated cardiomyopathy is also referred to as peripartum cardiomyopathy because it may be diagnosed in the third trimester of pregnancy but may continue to progress months after delivery. Code **O90.3, Peripartum cardiomyopathy,** should be used only when the cardiomyopathy develops as a result of pregnancy in women who did not have pre-existing heart disease. For example:

- A patient is admitted due to peripartum cardiomyopathy with ejection fraction of 21 percent and heart failure. The patient is approximately two to three months postpartum. Code **O90.3, Peripartum cardiomyopathy,** is assigned as the principal diagnosis. The peripartum period is defined as the last month of pregnancy to five months postpartum.

For pre-existing heart disease complicating pregnancy and the puerperium, codes from subcategory O99.4, Diseases of the circulatory system complicating pregnancy, childbirth and the puerperium, should be used instead of the pregnancy-associated cardiomyopathy code.

OTHER MATERNAL DISEASES

ICD-10-CM provides category O99 to describe other maternal diseases classifiable elsewhere but complicating pregnancy, childbirth, and the puerperium. This category includes conditions that complicate the pregnant state, are aggravated by the pregnancy, or are a main reason for obstetric care. Examples include:

O99.0-	Anemia
O99.1-	Other diseases of the blood and blood-forming organs and certain disorders involving the immune mechanism
O99.2-	Endocrine, nutritional, and metabolic diseases
O99.3-	Mental disorders and diseases of the nervous system
O99.4-	Diseases of the circulatory system
O99.5-	Diseases of the respiratory system
O99.6-	Diseases of the digestive system
O99.7-	Diseases of the skin and subcutaneous tissue
O99.8-	Other specified diseases and conditions

An additional code is used to identify the specific condition. For example:

- A patient is admitted five weeks postpartum with acute cholecystitis and cholelithiasis. Code **O99.63, Diseases of the digestive system complicating the puerperium,** and code

K80.00, Calculus of gallbladder with acute cholecystitis without obstruction, are assigned.

- A patient, who is four weeks postpartum, is admitted secondary to postpartum depression. Code **O99.345, Other mental disorders complicating the puerperium,** and code **F53.0, Postpartum depression,** are assigned.

Malignant neoplasms complicating pregnancy, childbirth, and the puerperium are classified to subcategory O9A.1, with additional code(s) to identify the specific neoplasm. This subcategory is for conditions classified to C00 through C96. Maternal care for benign tumor of corpus uteri is coded to O34.1-, while maternal care for benign tumor of cervix is classified to O34.4-.

Coding of injury, poisoning, physical abuse, sexual abuse, and psychological abuse complicating pregnancy, childbirth, and the puerperium is discussed in chapter 29 of this handbook.

SEQUELAE OF COMPLICATION OF PREGNANCY, CHILDBIRTH, OR THE PUERPERIUM

Code **O94, Sequelae of complication of pregnancy, childbirth, and the puerperium,** is assigned when an initial complication of the obstetric experience develops a sequela that requires care or treatment at a later date. The sequelae include conditions specified as such, or as late effects, which may occur at any time after the postpartum period. Like all late effect codes, code O94 is sequenced after the code describing the residual condition. Examples include the following:

- A patient is admitted for repair of postpartal perineum prolapse secondary to traumatic laceration sustained during childbirth two years earlier. Code **N81.89, Other female genital prolapse,** is assigned first, with code **O94, Sequelae of complication of pregnancy, childbirth, and the puerperium,** assigned as an additional code.

- A patient presents with fatigue and cold intolerance. Her history indicates that she had experienced a severe hemorrhage during delivery of a normal liveborn seven months earlier. She was diagnosed with Sheehan's syndrome and treated with replacement hormones. Code **E23.0, Hypopituitarism,** is assigned for Sheehan's syndrome, followed by code **O94, Sequelae of complication of pregnancy, childbirth, and the puerperium.**

EXERCISE 23.4

Code the following diagnoses. Do not code procedures. Assign Z codes where applicable.

1. Intrauterine pregnancy, spontaneous
   delivery, single liveborn

2. Intrauterine pregnancy, 12 weeks' gestation,
   undelivered, with mild hyperemesis gravidarum

3. Intrauterine pregnancy, 39 weeks,
   delivered, left occipitoanterior, single liveborn
   Primary uterine inertia

4. Cesarean delivery of stillborn at 38 weeks'
    gestation owing to placental infarction

    _____

5. Intrauterine pregnancy, with pernicious
    anemia, second trimester

    _____

6. Intrauterine pregnancy, term, 40 weeks' gestation
    Spontaneous delivery, left occipitoanterior
    Single liveborn

7. Intrauterine pregnancy, twins, 33 weeks
    Premature rupture of membranes, onset of
    labor three hours later. Spontaneous delivery of
    premature twins, vertex presentation, both liveborn
    Postpartum pulmonary embolism

    _____

8. Premature delivery, third trimester, frank breech
    presentation, single female liveborn
    First-degree tear, vaginal wall

    _____

9. Term pregnancy, 39 weeks, delivered, single stillborn,
    left occipitoanterior
    Terminal abruptio placentae
    Cord wrapped tightly around neck with compression

    _____

10. Intrauterine pregnancy, 12 weeks;
    long-standing essential hypertension
    being monitored closely

    _____

OBSTETRIC PROCEDURES

When coding obstetric procedures using ICD-10-PCS, it is important to distinguish whether the
procedure is performed on the fetus or on the pregnant female. Procedures performed on the fetus

342

CHAPTER 23

*Complications
of Pregnancy,
Childbirth, and
the Puerperium*

FIGURE 23.3 Structure of Codes in the Obstetrics Section

Character 1	Character 2	Character 3	Character 4	Character 5	Character 6	Character 7
Section	Body System	Root Operation	Body Part	Approach	Device	Qualifier

(products of conception) are classified to the Obstetrics Section. Procedures performed on the pregnant female, on body parts other than the products of conception, are coded to the appropriate root operation in the Medical and Surgical Section. For example, amniocentesis is coded to the "products of conception" body part in the Obstetrics Section. However, repair of obstetric urethral laceration is coded to the "urethra" body part in the Medical and Surgical Section.

The ICD-10-PCS Obstetrics Section follows the same conventions found in the Medical and Surgical Section, with all seven characters retaining the same meaning, as shown in figure 23.3. The body system (character 2) in the Obstetrics Section is always "pregnancy." There are only three values used for body part in this section: "products of conception" (0); "products of conception, retained" (1); and "products of conception, ectopic" (2).

There are 12 root operations (as shown in figure 23.4) in the Obstetrics Section, 10 of which are also found in the Medical and Surgical Section. The two root operations unique to the Obstetrics Section are defined below:

- Abortion: Artificially terminating a pregnancy
- Delivery: Assisting the passage of the products of conception from the genital tract (This root operation applies only to manually assisted, vaginal delivery.)

FIGURE 23.4 Root Operations in the Obstetrics Section

Value	Root Operation	Definition
2	Change	Taking out or off a device from a body part and putting back an identical or similar device in or on the same body part without cutting or puncturing the skin or a mucous membrane
9	Drainage	Taking or letting out fluids and/or gases from a body part
A	Abortion	Artificially terminating a pregnancy
D	Extraction	Pulling or stripping out or off all or a portion of a body part
E	Delivery	Assisting the passage of the products of conception from the genital canal
H	Insertion	Putting in a nonbiological appliance that monitors, assists, performs, or prevents a physiological function but does not physically take the place of a body part
J	Inspection	Visually and/or manually exploring a body part
P	Removal	Taking out or off a device from a body part, region, or orifice
Q	Repair	Restoring, to the extent possible, a body part to its normal anatomic structure and function
S	Reposition	Moving to its normal location or other suitable location all or a portion of a body part
T	Resection	Cutting out or off, without replacement, all of a body part
Y	Transplantation	Putting in or on all or a portion of a living body part taken from another individual or animal to physically take the place and/or function of all or a portion of a similar body part

Cesarean deliveries are coded to the Obstetrics Section to the root operation "Extraction" rather than to the root operation "Delivery." The root operation "Extraction" is also used for vaginal deliveries requiring assistance with forceps, vacuum, or internal version. Occasionally, vacuum assistance is used with cesarean delivery. However, the use of the vacuum is not separately coded. Assign only the ICD-10-PCS code for the cesarean delivery.

Procedures performed following a delivery or an abortion for curettage of the endometrium or evacuation of retained products of conception are all coded in the Obstetrics Section to the root operation "Extraction" and the body part "products of conception, retained." Diagnostic or therapeutic dilation and curettage performed during times other than the postpartum or post-abortion period are all coded in the Medical and Surgical Section to the root operation "Extraction" and the body part "endometrium."

PROCEDURES ASSISTING DELIVERY

Delivery can be assisted in a number of ways. Manually assisted vaginal delivery is coded as follows:

Character 1 Section	Character 2 Body System	Character 3 Root Operation	Character 4 Body Part	Character 5 Approach	Character 6 Device	Character 7 Qualifier
1	0	E	0	X	Z	Z
Obstetrics	Pregnancy	Delivery	Products of conception	External	None	None

Labor may be induced by artificial rupture of the fetal membranes (AROM, which is classified to the Obstetrics Section, body system "Pregnancy," root operation "Drainage," body part "products of conception" and qualifier "amniotic fluid") or by other surgical induction, such as cervical dilatation (0U7C7ZZ). Cervidil (prostaglandin gel insert) can be inserted to soften and ripen the cervix before labor is induced. For cervical ripening with Cervidil, assign code **3E0P7VZ, Introduction of hormone into female reproductive, via natural or artificial opening.** Artificial rupture of membranes (10907ZC) may also be performed after labor has begun. Pitocin (oxytocin) can be used to either induce labor contractions or augment active labor by increasing the strength and frequency of ongoing labor contractions. When Pitocin is administered to augment active labor, it is not coded separately. If Pitocin is given intravenously to induce labor, assign code **3E033VJ, Introduction of other hormone into peripheral vein, percutaneous approach.** For example:

- A patient presents to the hospital at 40 weeks' gestation for induction of labor. Pitocin is administered intravenously in the peripheral vein, and AROM is carried out. The patient has a normal spontaneous vaginal delivery without complication. Assign code **O80, Encounter for full-term uncomplicated delivery.** Codes Z37.0 and Z3A.40 are also assigned for the outcome of delivery and completed weeks of gestation. For the assisted delivery, AROM, and induction of labor, the following ICD-10-PCS codes are assigned: **10E0XZZ, Delivery of products of conception, external approach; 10907ZC, Drainage of amniotic fluid, therapeutic from products of conception, via natural or artificial opening; and 3E033VJ, Introduction of other hormone into peripheral vein, percutaneous approach.**

Amnioinfusion (Administration Section, root operation "Introduction") is typically performed during labor via a transcervical approach after rupture of the fetal membranes. An intrauterine pressure catheter is used to infuse a lactated Ringer's or normal saline solution into the amniotic cavity. Alternatively, fluid can be infused through a needle transabdominally. Amnioinfusion is performed

344

CHAPTER 23 :

Complications
of Pregnancy,
Childbirth, and
the Puerperium :

as prophylactic treatment of oligohydramnios, for reduction of variable decelerations of the fetal heart rate because of cord compression during labor, or as treatment of preterm premature rupture of membranes.

For example, amnioinfusion of normal saline solution is coded as follows:

Character 1 Section	Character 2 Body System	Character 3 Root Operation	Character 4 Body System	Character 5 Approach	Character 6 Substance	Character 7 Qualifier
3	E	0	E	7	7	Z
Administration	Physiological systems and anatomical regions	Introduction	Products of conception	Via natural or artificial opening	Electrolytic and water balance substance	None

If rotation during delivery is carried out, this procedure is coded to the Obstetrics Section, root operation "Reposition," code **10S07ZZ, Reposition products of conception, via natural or artificial opening.** Whenever there is an assisted routine delivery, code **10E0XZZ, Delivery of products of conception, external approach,** is assigned. If, however, instrumentation such as forceps or vacuum extraction is used to assist delivery, assign a code describing forceps or vacuum delivery rather than code 10E0XZZ.

Forceps Delivery and Vacuum Extraction

Forceps, vacuum extraction, or internal and combined version may also assist delivery. These procedures are coded to the Obstetrics Section, root operation "Extraction." Codes are provided for low-forceps, mid-forceps, or high-forceps delivery. In a low-forceps delivery (seventh-character qualifier value 3), forceps are applied to a visible fetal head after it has entered the pelvic floor. Mid-forceps (seventh-character qualifier value 4) are applied to the head during its entry into the pelvic floor, and high forceps (seventh-character qualifier value 5) are applied to the head before it enters the pelvic brim. Breech presentations may require partial or total breech extraction, with or without forceps to the aftercoming head. Vacuum extraction (seventh-character qualifier value 6) applies a traction device, rather than forceps, to the fetal head for extraction of the fetus. When a vacuum is used to assist in the labor to bring the fetus down to a lower station, and forceps are used in the actual extraction procedure to deliver the baby, assign only code **10D07Z3, Extraction of products of conception, low forceps, via natural or artificial opening.** Because the same root operation was performed on the same body part, the process does not meet the definition of multiple procedures.

Episiotomy

An episiotomy is a surgical incision in the perineum made just before delivery to enlarge the vaginal opening and assist delivery. Code **0W8NXZZ, Division of female perineum, external approach,** is assigned for a routine episiotomy. The repair (episiorrhaphy) is not coded separately because the repair is integral to the procedure. When an episiotomy is performed in connection with a forceps delivery, two codes are assigned: a code for the delivery and code 0W8NXZZ for the episiotomy.

Duhrssen Incision

Occasionally during delivery, a Duhrssen cervical incision is performed to facilitate delivery of the infant's entrapped head. The purpose of the procedure is to widen the opening of an incompletely dilated cervix. The coding of a Duhrssen incision is similar to coding an episiotomy. Assign a code for the cervical dilation procedure (0U7C7ZZ). The repair of the incision is integral to the total procedure and is therefore not coded separately.

Perineal Lacerations

Perineal lacerations are classified as first, second, third, or fourth degree in category O70, Perineal laceration during delivery:

- First-degree tears (O70.0) involve damage to the fourchette and vaginal mucosa, and underlying muscles are exposed but not torn.

- Second-degree tears (O70.1) include the posterior vaginal walls and perineal muscles, but the anal sphincter is intact.

- Third-degree tears (O70.2-) extend to the anal sphincter, but the rectal mucosa is intact.

- Fourth-degree tears (O70.3) involve the rectal and anal mucosa.

Codes in subcategory O70.2, Third degree perineal laceration during delivery, are further subdivided according to type as follows:

Type IIIa	Less than 50% of external anal sphincter thickness torn
Type IIIb	More than 50% of external anal sphincter thickness torn
Type IIIc	Both external anal sphincter and internal anal sphincter torn

Code O70.4 describes an anal sphincter tear complicating delivery that is not associated with a third-degree perineal laceration. Code **O70.9, Perineal laceration during delivery, unspecified,** is used when there is no additional information on the degree of the perineal laceration.

Inclusion notes for these diagnosis codes indicate what is involved in each degree. When more than one degree is mentioned, only the code for the highest degree is assigned.

The repair of an obstetric perineal laceration is coded based on the degree of the tear and the tissue repaired. The body part is selected based on the furthest anatomical extent of the obstetric tear repaired. Coding of obstetric lacerations in this manner will help to standardize the data by maintaining the convention of assigning one code for each laceration when documented by degree (first through fourth). The *ICD-10-PCS Official Coding Guidelines* states the following about overlapping body layers (B3.5): "If the root operations Excision, Repair or Inspection are performed on overlapping layers of the musculoskeletal system, the body part specifying the deepest layer is coded." For example, repair of a second-degree laceration requires repair of the perineal muscle, vaginal mucosa, and skin; therefore, it is coded to the body part "perineum muscle." Because a second-degree perineal laceration equates to muscle injury, documentation of repair of a second-degree perineal laceration is sufficient to code the surgery as repair of perineal muscle. Assign the following ICD-10-PCS codes based on the degree of the perineal tear:

- **0HQ9XZZ, Repair perineum skin, external approach,** for repair of a first-degree perineal laceration

- **0KQM0ZZ, Repair perineum muscle, open approach,** for repair of a second-degree perineal laceration

- **0DQR0ZZ, Repair anal sphincter, open approach,** for repair of a third-degree perineal laceration

- **0DQP0ZZ, Repair rectum, open approach,** for the repair of the fourth-degree tear

Category O71, Other obstetric trauma, is used for other obstetric trauma, including trauma from instrument for the following injuries: rupture of uterus (spontaneous) before onset of labor (O71.0-) or during labor (O71.1), postpartum inversion of uterus (O71.2), obstetric laceration of cervix (O71.3), obstetric high vaginal laceration alone (O71.4), other obstetric injury to pelvic organs (O71.5), obstetric damage to pelvic joints and ligaments (O71.6), obstetric hematoma of pelvis (O71.7), other obstetric trauma (O71.8-), and unspecified obstetric trauma (O71.9).

Periurethral lacerations are tears that occur during delivery, which involve the vulva and tissues around the vaginal opening or the outermost layer of the vagina. Neither muscle nor the

346

CHAPTER 23

*Complications
of Pregnancy,
Childbirth, and
the Puerperium*

urethra are involved in the injury. Code **O71.82, Other specified trauma to perineum and vulva,** is assigned to describe a periurethral tear. Code **0UQMXZZ, Repair vulva, external approach,** is assigned for the repair of an obstetric periurethral laceration.

Occasionally, an episiotomy extends spontaneously to become a perineal laceration or tear. When an episiotomy extends to become a perineal laceration, ICD-10-PCS codes are assigned for the episiotomy, the assisted delivery, and the laceration repair. All of these codes are needed to completely describe this situation. For example:

- A patient had a normal vaginal delivery at 40 weeks' gestation. She had an assisted delivery and episiotomy, which extended to a third-degree perineal laceration. The laceration was repaired with sutures. Code **O70.20, Third degree perineal laceration during delivery, unspecified,** should be assigned as the principal diagnosis. Codes **Z3A.40, 40 weeks gestation of pregnancy,** and **Z37.0, Single live birth,** should also be assigned to indicate the weeks of gestation and the outcome of delivery. For the procedures, assign codes **0W8NXZZ, Division of female perineum, external approach,** for the episiotomy; **10E0XZZ, Delivery of products of conception, external approach,** for the assisted delivery; and **0DQR0ZZ, Repair anal sphincter, open approach,** for the repair of the third-degree laceration.

Fetal Monitoring

Continuous fetal heart rate monitoring is commonly done during labor. Monitoring sensors can either be placed externally or internally. In external fetal monitoring, sensors are placed on the abdomen and connected to a machine that records fetal heart rate as well as uterine contractions. Assign code **4A1HXCZ, Monitoring of products of conception, cardiac rate, external approach.** Internal (transvaginal) monitoring involves inserting an electrode through the vagina and attaching it to the fetal scalp, along with a tube to monitor contractions. The electrode and tube are attached to a device that continuously records fetal heart rate. Code **4A1H7CZ, Monitoring of products of conception, cardiac rate, via natural or artificial opening,** is assigned for this type of fetal monitoring.

Fetal oxygen monitoring provides the physician with a direct measure of fetal oxygen status when an irregular fetal heart rate is present. The intrapartum fetal oxygen monitor uses a single-use, disposable sensor that is inserted through the birth canal when one of the amniotic membranes has ruptured and the cervix is dilated more than 2 centimeters. The oxygen saturation is displayed on a monitor screen as a percentage. Assign code **10H073Z, Insertion of monitoring electrode into products of conception, via natural or artificial opening,** for this type of fetal monitoring.

Another type of monitoring can be done by using the intrauterine pressure monitoring device, which is a pressure gauge rather than a monitoring electrode. A pressure catheter is inserted into the uterus during labor to evaluate contractions. The device provides exact measurements of contractions, unlike external monitors. Code **10H07YZ, Insertion, products of conception, via natural or artificial opening, other device,** is assigned to describe the placement of an intrauterine pressure monitor.

Cesarean Delivery

Cesarean delivery is an operative delivery that is carried out when, for some reason, spontaneous delivery is impossible or seems inadvisable. C-sections are classified to the root operation "Extraction," body part "products of conception," and open approach. A classic C-section, which removes the fetus through an incision into the upper part of the uterus using an abdominal peritoneal approach, is assigned code **10D00Z0, Extraction of products of conception, high, open approach.** A low cervical C-section uses an incision into the lower portion of the uterus, with a pelvic cavity or an abdominal peritoneal incision, and is assigned code **10D00Z1, Extraction of products of conception, low, open approach.** There is also an extraperitoneal C-section (seventh-character qualifier value 2).

EXERCISE 23.5

Code the following procedures.

1. Induction of labor by cervical dilation

2. Assisted spontaneous delivery

3. Vaginal delivery using low forceps

4. Extraperitoneal C-section, low transverse incision

5. Mid-forceps vaginal delivery with routine episiotomy

SERVICES RELATED TO CONTRACEPTIVE MANAGEMENT

Category Z30, Encounter for contraceptive management, is assigned as the principal diagnosis for admissions or outpatient encounters for contraceptive management. Codes in this category cover services such as initiation of oral contraceptive measures (Z30.011); initiation of vaginal ring hormonal contraceptive device (Z30.015); initiation of transdermal patch hormonal contraceptive device (Z30.016); counseling in natural family planning to avoid pregnancy (Z30.02); insertion of intrauterine contraceptive device (Z30.430); removal of intrauterine contraceptive device (Z30.432); removal and reinsertion of intrauterine contraceptive device (Z30.433); sterilization (Z30.2); surveillance of injectable contraceptive (Z30.42); surveillance of vaginal ring hormonal contraceptive device (Z30.44); surveillance of transdermal patch hormonal contraceptive device (Z30.45); and surveillance of implantable subdermal contraceptive (Z30.46). Procedure codes must also be assigned when appropriate.

EXERCISE 23.6

Code the following diagnoses and procedures.

1. Family planning counseling

2. Encounter for insertion of intrauterine contraceptive device
    Insertion of intrauterine contraceptive device

3. Encounter for removal of intrauterine contraceptive device
    Removal of intrauterine contraceptive device

4. Encounter for lactation counseling

STERILIZATION

When a patient seeks health care for the purpose of contraceptive sterilization, code **Z30.2, Encounter for sterilization,** is assigned as the principal diagnosis. If there are underlying medical or psychological conditions that led to the decision to undergo sterilization, codes for these conditions may be assigned as additional diagnoses. Because sterilization may be performed as an elective procedure without any predisposing medical or psychological reasons, code Z30.2 can be used as a solo diagnosis code.

When an elective sterilization procedure is performed during a hospital episode in which an obstetric delivery has occurred, Z30.2 is assigned as a secondary code, with a code from chapter 15 of ICD-10-CM assigned as the principal diagnosis.

Note that code Z30.2 is assigned for both female and male patients for whom a contraceptive sterilization procedure is performed. Sterilization procedures for females are sometimes generically referred to as "tubal ligation." ICD-10-PCS classifies sterilization procedures for females to the female reproductive system and to different root operations ("Excision," "Occlusion," or "Destruction") depending on the technique used. For example:

- Partial salpingectomy, whereby a portion of the fallopian tubes are cut and tied with suture material: root operation "Excision"

- Clips or external rings, whereby the fallopian tubes are clipped (e.g., Filshie clip, Wolf clip) or blocked with an external ring (e.g., Falope ring, Yoon ring): root operation "Occlusion"

- Electrocoagulation, whereby a small portion of each fallopian tube is burnt or cauterized: root operation "Destruction"

Sterilization procedures for males are classified to the male reproductive system, root operation "Destruction" or "Excision."

Code Z30.2 is not assigned as either a principal or a secondary diagnosis when sterilization results from other treatment or when a sterilization procedure is performed as part of the treatment for another condition. In such cases, the original condition, any complications or comorbidities, and the procedures performed are coded. For example, when a hysterectomy is performed because of injury or damage to the uterus during delivery, only the obstetric diagnoses and procedures are coded, even though the procedure results in sterility. Code Z30.2 is used only for a sterilization performed specifically for contraception; assigning it when a sterilization is incidental to other treatment is inappropriate.

Other examples of appropriate coding of situations involving sterilization follow.

Z30.2 + F32.9 + Z64.1 + 0UL74ZZ	A patient with multiparity (five children) and reactive depression is admitted for elective sterilization; bilateral endoscopic ligation and division (root operation "Occlusion") of the fallopian tubes are carried out for sterilization
O32.1xx0 + Z30.2 + Z37.0 + Z3A.38 + 10D07Z6 + 0UL74CZ	Term pregnancy, liveborn delivered; breech presentation; 38 weeks' gestation; delivery by partial breech vacuum extraction; endoscopic bilateral tubal ligation with extraluminal device for sterilization

Sterilization procedures are intended to be permanent. However, there may be situations in which a patient may desire a reversal of the sterilization procedure. Admission for a tuboplasty or vasoplasty to reverse a previous sterilization procedure is coded to **Z31.0, Encounter for reversal of previous sterilization.**

EXERCISE 23.7

Code the following diagnostic statements and procedures.

1. Essential hypertension

   Admitted for sterilization

   Laparoscopy with bilateral partial salpingectomy

2. Endometriosis of uterus

   Admitted for sterilization

   Bilateral laparoscopic tubal ligation

   via electrocautery for sterilization

3. Pregnancy, 40 weeks' gestation, with breech delivery,

   female infant, followed by sterilization

   Vacuum breech extraction

   Laparoscopic occlusion of bilateral fallopian tubes

   with Falope (external) rings

4. Elective sterilization, patient request

   Vasectomy, bilateral (open)

5. Elective reversal of previous tubal ligation

   Laparoscopic salpingoplasty

PROCREATIVE MANAGEMENT

A code from category Z31, Encounter for procreative management, is assigned when a patient who is having difficulty becoming pregnant is seen for help in correcting this problem.

Code Z31.61 is assigned as the first-listed diagnosis for an encounter/visit for procreative counseling and advice using natural family planning. Couples seeking natural methods of family planning require training/counseling by a medical professional or a qualified counselor. There are five methods of natural family planning:

- Basal body temperature method

- Ovulation/cervical mucus method

- Symptothermal method

- Calendar method

- Lactational amenorrhea

Therapy for malignant neoplasms or other serious conditions can affect reproductive health and the ability to conceive. Antineoplastic drugs (e.g., alkylating agents) and radiotherapy to the pelvic area may impair ovarian and testicular function, leading to infertility. Depending on the

350

CHAPTER 23

*Complications
of Pregnancy,
Childbirth, and
the Puerperium*

dosage delivered and the length of treatment, healthy sperm cells and ovarian follicles can be destroyed along with cancer cells.

Code **Z31.62, Encounter for fertility preservation counseling,** is assigned for encounters for advice and counseling on available options to conceive a child or maintain pregnancy before the start of cancer treatment or the surgical removal of gonads. The discussion may include whether to conceive before cancer treatment; banking of sperm, eggs, ovarian tissue, or embryos; and/or modification of surgery to spare the uterus.

Code **Z31.84, Encounter for fertility preservation procedure,** is assigned for the fertility preservation encounter. Codes Z31.62 and Z31.84 are not limited to those seeking advice prior to cancer treatment or gonad removal. They may be assigned for patients having any treatment (not only cancer treatment) that may affect fertility.

Code **Z31.83, Encounter for assisted reproductive fertility procedure cycle,** is assigned for patients undergoing in vitro fertilization. An additional code should be assigned to identify the type of infertility. Code Z31.83 is not used for encounters for diagnostic testing prior to starting in vitro fertilization. Assign the reason for the encounter when the patient presents for diagnostic testing.

Code **Z31.7, Encounter for procreative management and counseling for gestational carrier,** is assigned for visits involving procreative management and counseling of a patient who is a gestational carrier. A gestational carrier gives birth for an individual who is unable to have children naturally. A gestational carrier is different from a surrogate. A surrogate provides the egg as well as giving birth, whereas a gestational carrier uses a fertilized egg that is provided from another woman, usually the intended mother. If a gestational carrier presents for care and the pregnancy is incidental to the encounter, assign code **Z33.3, Pregnant state, gestational carrier.**

When in vitro fertilization has been successful, a code from subcategory O09.81-, Supervision of pregnancy resulting from assisted reproductive technology, is assigned for subsequent encounters involving antenatal supervision and/or prenatal care.

Encounters for investigations such as sperm counts or fallopian tube insufflation are coded to **Z31.41, Encounter for fertility testing.** For encounters for sperm count following sterilization reversal, assign code **Z31.42, Aftercare following sterilization reversal,** instead of Z31.41.

ICD-10-CM provides the following codes to describe encounters for testing and counseling for genetic disease:

Z31.430	Encounter of female for testing for genetic disease carrier status for procreative management
Z31.438	Encounter for other genetic testing of female for procreative management
Z31.440	Encounter of male for testing for genetic disease carrier status for procreative management
Z31.441	Encounter for testing of male partner of patient with recurrent pregnancy loss
Z31.448	Encounter for other genetic testing of male for procreative management
Z31.5	Encounter for genetic counseling

If the encounter is for genetic screening not associated with procreative management, assign a code from subcategory Z13.7, Encounter for screening for genetic and chromosomal anomalies, rather than the Z31.4- series.

SUSPECTED MATERNAL AND FETAL CONDITIONS NOT FOUND

Codes from subcategory Z03.7, Encounter for suspected maternal and fetal conditions ruled out, are to be used in very limited circumstances on a maternal record when an encounter is for a suspected maternal or fetal condition that is ruled out during that encounter (for example, a maternal or fetal condition may be suspected due to an abnormal test result). These codes should not be used when

351

CHAPTER 23

Complications
of Pregnancy,
Childbirth, and
the Puerperium

the condition is confirmed. In those cases, the confirmed condition should be coded. These codes also should not be used if an illness or any signs or symptoms related to the suspected condition or problem are present. In those cases, the appropriate codes for the diagnosis and signs and symptoms should be reported instead.

Codes from subcategory Z03.7 can be used with other codes, but only if the conditions specified with the other codes are unrelated to the suspected condition being evaluated. Codes from subcategory Z03.7 may not be used for encounters for antenatal screening of the mother. For encounters for suspected fetal conditions that are inconclusive following testing and evaluation, assign the appropriate code from category O35, O36, O40, or O41.

Codes in subcategory Z03.7 describe suspected fetal/maternal problems not found, as follows:

Z03.71   Encounter for suspected problem with amniotic cavity and membrane ruled out
Z03.72   Encounter for suspected placental problem ruled out
Z03.73   Encounter for suspected fetal anomaly ruled out
Z03.74   Encounter for suspected problem with fetal growth ruled out
Z03.75   Encounter for suspected cervical shortening ruled out

---

EXERCISE 23.8

Code the following diagnostic statements and procedures. Assign Z codes where applicable.

1. Gestational diabetes treated with both diet and oral anti-diabetic medication; 40 weeks' gestation, spontaneous delivery of living female infant

   Manually assisted delivery
   Episiotomy and repair

2. Term pregnancy, 39 weeks' gestation, living dichorionic twins (diamniotic sacs), cesarean delivery performed because fetal stress noted prior to labor

   Low cervical cesarean delivery

3. Delivery, 38 weeks' gestation, living child, ROA presentation

   Manually assisted delivery
   Transvaginal fetal cardiac rate monitoring during labor
   Episiotomy and episiorrhaphy

352

CHAPTER 23

*Complications
of Pregnancy,
Childbirth, and
the Puerperium*

4. Uterine pregnancy, 39 weeks' gestation, delivered with
   obstructed labor due to transverse lie presentation
   Pre-existing hypertension with mild preeclampsia,
   single liveborn

   Classic high cesarean delivery

---

5. Intrauterine pregnancy, 37 weeks' gestation, delivered,
   spontaneous
   Third-stage hemorrhage with anemia
   secondary to acute blood loss
   Monochorionic twins, both liveborn, diamniotic placenta

---

6. Pregnancy, 38 weeks' gestation, delivered, frank breech
   presentation with liveborn male infant

   Partial breech extraction with mid-forceps to aftercoming head

---

7. Pregnancy, 40 weeks' gestation, delivered, spontaneous
   Liveborn, male infant

   Assisted spontaneous delivery
   Elective sterilization following delivery
   Bilateral endoscopic ligation and crushing of fallopian tubes

---

8. Intrauterine pregnancy, 26 weeks' gestation, with complicating
   incompetent cervix, undelivered
   Shirodkar cervical cerclage operation

---

9. Gestational hypertension
   Pregnancy, third trimester, 29 weeks' gestation, undelivered

---

10. Intrauterine pregnancy, 38 weeks' gestation, delivered,
    right occipitoanterior, liveborn male infant
    Episiotomy that extended to second-degree
    lacerations, perineum

    Amniotomy for induction of labor
    Low-forceps delivery with episiotomy
    Repair of perineal laceration

---

11. Delivery, stillborn, male infant, 40 weeks' gestation
brow presentation; obstructed labor

Extraction with internal version
Episiotomy and repair

___

12. Twin pregnancy, 38 weeks' gestation, with malposition fetus 2
One liveborn twin, one stillborn (fetus 2), two placentas
and two amniotic sacs

Classical cesarean section

___

13. Postpartum uterine atony without hemorrhage
occurring two weeks after delivery

___

14. Encounter for testing of female for genetic disease
carrier status (patient planning on pregnancy)

___

15. Encounter for in vitro fertilization (IVF);
infertility due to obstructed fallopian tube

___

16. Visit for procreative counseling using natural family planning

___

17. 32-year-old gravida 2, para 0, admitted at 39 weeks' gestation
for an elective primary low cesarean section.
The patient had a completely normal prenatal course,
a normal pregnancy, and an unremarkable postoperative
course. She elected to have a cesarean section
because of fear of vaginal delivery. She had a normal
single liveborn without complications.

___

18. Woman is admitted to the hospital and delivers a healthy
baby. Four years ago, the woman used heroin and cocaine
and currently is receiving prescribed methadone as a result
of past dependence. She had a normal single liveborn without
complications. The final diagnoses are "Term, 40 weeks' gestation,
manually assisted delivery, and methadone use."

___

CHAPTER 24

Abortion and Ectopic Pregnancy

CHAPTER OVERVIEW

- Codes for pregnancy with an abortive outcome are found in categories O00 through O08 in chapter 15 of ICD-10-CM.

- The primary axis for coding abortion is the type of abortion (spontaneous, induced, or failed).

- Category Z3A codes (weeks of gestation) should not be assigned for pregnancies with abortive outcomes (categories O00–O08) nor for postpartum conditions because category Z3A is not applicable to these conditions.

- Subcategories further specify if the abortion is complete, incomplete, or unspecified and whether a complication is present.

- An encounter for an elective abortion without complication is coded Z33.2.

- If the attempted termination of pregnancy results in a liveborn infant, code **Z33.2, Encounter for elective termination of pregnancy,** is used along with a code from category Z37, Outcome of delivery.

- Molar pregnancies and other abnormal products of conception are coded to categories O01 and O02.

- Codes for ectopic pregnancies have a fourth character to indicate the location, and a fifth character to identify with or without intrauterine pregnancy (O00.0–O00.9).

LEARNING OUTCOMES

After studying this chapter, you should be able to:

- Classify abortive outcomes by type of abortion.

- Select the appropriate code to indicate whether the abortion is complete, incomplete, or unspecified.

- Code complications of abortion.

- Understand how to code different types and occurrences of abortions.

- Classify abnormal products of conception (such as molar and ectopic pregnancies).

INTRODUCTION

The expulsion or extraction of all or part of the placenta or membrane with an estimated gestation of less than 20 completed weeks is considered an abortive outcome (abortion). Although requirements for fetal death reporting vary from state to state, these requirements should not be confused with ICD-10-CM rules for classifying abortions; they are entirely separate.

Pregnancy with abortive outcome is classified in categories O00 through O08. Note that the term "abortion" in the disease classification of ICD-10-CM refers to a fetal death. It is important to distinguish between an encounter for the purpose of performing an elective abortion versus one for dealing with a spontaneous abortion or a complication of an abortion. Encounters for the purpose of performing an elective abortion are classified to **Z33.2, Encounter for elective termination of pregnancy.** If a procedure to terminate the pregnancy is performed in the hospital, the procedure code is also required.

TYPES OF ABORTION

The primary axis for coding abortion is the type of abortion. Abortive outcome is classified by type in ICD-10-CM as follows:

- *Spontaneous abortion (category O03):* One that occurs without any instrumentation or chemical intervention.

- *Complications following (induced) termination of pregnancy (O04):* Complications after an abortion performed for either therapeutic or elective termination of pregnancy (terms such as "elective abortion," "induced abortion," "artificial abortion," and "termination of pregnancy" are used when this type of abortion is performed).

- *Failed attempted termination of pregnancy (Category O07):* One in which an induction of termination of pregnancy has failed to evacuate or expel the fetus and the patient is still pregnant. It includes incomplete elective abortion.

COMPLETE VERSUS INCOMPLETE SPONTANEOUS ABORTION

Codes in subcategories O03.0 through O03.4 indicate that the abortion is incomplete, while codes in subcategories O03.5 through O03.9 indicate that the abortion is complete or unspecified. Incomplete abortion refers to retained products of conception—whether from a spontaneous abortion or an elective termination of pregnancy. When the provider documentation does not specify whether the spontaneous abortion is complete or incomplete, ICD-10-CM classifies it to "complete or unspecified." The fact that a follow-up dilatation and curettage (D & C) is performed is not evidence in itself that an abortion is incomplete; the physician makes this determination.

COMPLICATIONS ASSOCIATED WITH ABORTION

Codes in categories O03, O04, and O07 indicate whether a complication is present and the general type of complication, such as a genital or pelvic infection; delayed or excessive hemorrhage; embolism; or other complications, including shock, renal failure, venous complications, cardiac arrest, sepsis, or urinary tract infection.

For subsequent encounters when there are retained products of conception following either a spontaneous abortion or an elective termination of pregnancy without complications, assign code **O03.4, Incomplete spontaneous abortion without complication,** or code **O07.4, Failed**

attempted termination of pregnancy without complication. This advice applies even when the patient was discharged previously with a discharge diagnosis of complete abortion. If the patient has a specific complication associated with the spontaneous abortion or elective termination of pregnancy in addition to retained products of conception, assign the appropriate complication code (e.g., O03.-, O04.-, O07.-) instead of code O03.4 or O07.4.

In ICD-10-CM's Tabular List, Chapter 15, Pregnancy, Childbirth and the Puerperium (O00–O9A), there is an instructional note that states: "Use additional code from category Z3A, Weeks of gestation, to identify the specific week of the pregnancy, if known." This note applies to all codes in the obstetric chapter. However, the weeks of gestation may not be documented or may not be relevant in cases of nonviable pregnancies. The *ICD-10-CM Official Guidelines for Coding and Reporting* have been revised to state "Category Z3A codes should not be assigned for pregnancies with abortive outcomes (categories O00–O08), elective termination of pregnancy (code Z33.2), nor for postpartum conditions, as category Z3A is not applicable to these conditions." The Centers for Disease Control and Prevention National Center for Health Statistics will be considering a future Coordination and Maintenance Committee proposal to revise the conflicting note in the Tabular List. In the interim, this handbook follows the Official Coding Guidelines regarding category Z3A.

For sepsis related to abortion, additional codes may be assigned to identify the infectious organism, and a code from R65.2- to identify severe sepsis, if applicable. Examples follow.

- A patient is admitted with incomplete spontaneous abortion, and a D & C is performed to remove any retained products of conception. There is evidence of pelvic infection. The patient is discharged on the fourth hospital day with the infection cleared. The principal diagnosis is **O03.0, Genital tract and pelvic infection following incomplete spontaneous abortion.**

- One week following discharge after a termination of pregnancy, a patient is readmitted because she has developed endometritis. Code **O04.5, Genital tract and pelvic infection following (induced) termination of pregnancy,** is assigned as the principal diagnosis, with an additional code for the endometritis.

- A patient is admitted in renal failure one week after discharge following a complete spontaneous abortion. Code **O03.82, Renal failure following complete or unspecified spontaneous abortion,** is assigned as the principal diagnosis.

- A patient who underwent an elective abortion one week earlier is admitted because of continued bleeding. A D & C is performed, and the pathology report shows retained products of conception. Code **O04.6, Delayed or excessive hemorrhage following (induced) termination of pregnancy,** is assigned.

- Five days following discharge for spontaneous abortion, a patient is admitted with a diagnosis of infection due to retained fetal tissue. The retention of fetal tissue indicates that the abortion was not complete; therefore, code **O03.0, Genital tract and pelvic infection following incomplete spontaneous abortion,** is assigned even though the patient was hospitalized for the abortion previously.

EXERCISE 24.1

Code the following diagnoses. Consider the diagnostic statements given below as the only information available in the medical record. Do not assign procedure codes.

1. Failed attempted abortion complicated by hemorrhage

2. Incomplete early abortion (spontaneous)

3. Therapeutic abortion, complete, with electrolyte imbalance

4. Electively induced abortion, complete, with amniotic
   fluid embolism

5. Patient readmitted with bleeding due to retained
   placenta one week following previous hospital
   admission for spontaneous abortion

6. Discharge #1: Electively induced abortion, complete
   Discharge #2 (same patient): Sepsis following induced
   abortion during previous admission

MATERNAL CONDITION AS REASON FOR ABORTION

Codes from categories O20 through O29 and O30 through O77 can be assigned as an additional code to indicate a maternal condition that influenced the decision to proceed with an elective abortion. Pregnancy can be terminated on a purely elective basis, however, and it is not necessary to assign a code to indicate a reason for the abortion. For example:

- A patient who is 12 completed weeks' gestation is admitted for elective abortion, based on her physician's advice that her severe heart disease indicates that an abortion might be advisable to prevent cardiac complications. In this case, the principal diagnosis code is **Z33.2, Encounter for elective termination of pregnancy.** Code **O99.411, Diseases of the circulatory system complicating pregnancy, first trimester,** is also assigned, along with an additional code to identify the particular heart disease.

- A patient who had rubella at six weeks' gestation requests abortion because of the possibility of fetal abnormality. Code **Z33.2, Encounter for elective termination of pregnancy,** is designated as the principal diagnosis, with code **O35.3xx0, Maternal care for (suspected) damage to fetus from viral disease in mother,** as a secondary diagnosis.

- A patient who is 26 weeks' pregnant presents for elective termination of pregnancy due to fetal anomalies. Assign code **Z33.2, Encounter for elective termination of pregnancy,** as the principal diagnosis. Code **O35.9xx0, Maternal care for (suspected) fetal abnormality and damage, unspecified,** is assigned as an additional diagnosis.

- A first-trimester pregnant patient is admitted with placenta previa. She does not request abortion, but after evaluating various treatment possibilities, her physician concludes that an abortion is necessary. The patient consents, and the abortion is carried out. In this case, the code for placenta previa (O44.01) is sequenced first, followed by the abortion code.

INADVERTENT ABORTION

When an inadvertent abortion occurs because of surgery or as the result of trauma or other condition unrelated to the pregnancy, the obstetric codes (O00–O9A) are sequenced first. Codes from other chapters may be assigned along with the obstetric codes to further specify the condition. A code from category O03, Spontaneous abortion, is assigned to indicate that an abortion occurred. For example:

- A woman was admitted to the hospital at 12 weeks' gestation with acute cholecystitis. The surgeon performed a laparoscopic cholecystectomy. During the stay, the patient had an inadvertent spontaneous abortion.

Principal diagnosis:	O99.611	Diseases of the digestive system complicating pregnancy, first trimester
Additional diagnoses:	O03.9	Spontaneous abortion
	K81.0	Acute cholecystitis
Principal procedure:	0FT44ZZ	Resection of gallbladder, percutaneous endoscopic approach

- Open appendectomy was performed because of acute appendicitis with peritonitis. On the second postoperative day, the patient experienced an inadvertent abortion (complete) at 12 weeks' gestation.

Principal diagnosis:	O99.611	Diseases of the digestive system complicating pregnancy, first trimester
Additional diagnoses:	K35.2	Appendicitis with peritonitis
	O03.9	Spontaneous abortion
Principal procedure:	0DTJ0ZZ	Resection of appendix, open approach

ABORTION PROCEDURE RESULTING IN LIVEBORN INFANT

Occasionally, an attempt to terminate a pregnancy results in a liveborn infant. Note that a fetus that has any heartbeat, respiration, or involuntary muscle movement after expulsion is considered to be a live birth, no matter how short a time it survives. In this situation, code Z33.2, Encounter for elective termination of pregnancy, and a code from category Z37, Outcome of delivery, are assigned. A code for the procedure used in the attempt to terminate the pregnancy should also be assigned. For example:

- A patient delivers a liveborn infant with extreme immaturity following attempted abortion by insertion of laminaria. Code Z33.2, Encounter for elective termination of pregnancy, is assigned, along with code Z37.0 (for the single liveborn). Assign also the procedure code for the insertion of the laminaria.

LOSS OF FETUS WITH REMAINING FETUS

Occasionally, a patient with multiple gestation is admitted for what appears to be a spontaneous abortion during which one or more fetuses are expelled but one or more live fetuses remain in utero. In such cases, no code from category O00–O08 is assigned; instead, a code from either subcategory O31.1, Continuing pregnancy after spontaneous abortion of one fetus or more, or subcategory O31.2, Continuing pregnancy after intrauterine death of one fetus or more, is assigned.

CONTINUING PREGNANCY FOLLOWING ELECTIVE FETAL REDUCTION

Subcategory code O31.3 identifies continuing pregnancy after elective fetal reduction during the current pregnancy. These pregnancies are considered high risk, and there is a need to identify them, even if the pregnancy is reduced to a single fetus. For example, when the woman delivers the single newborn, these codes make it possible to document that this case was originally a multiple gestation that underwent fetal reduction. Note that subcategory O31.3 refers to fetal reduction, whereas subcategories O31.1 and O31.2, described in the preceding section, are for spontaneous abortion or involuntary fetal loss.

The subcategories for multiple gestation following fetal reduction are as follows:

O31.30   Continuing pregnancy after elective fetal reduction of one fetus or more, unspecified trimester

O31.31   Continuing pregnancy after elective fetal reduction of one fetus or more, first trimester

O31.32   Continuing pregnancy after elective fetal reduction of one fetus or more, second trimester

O31.33   Continuing pregnancy after elective fetal reduction of one fetus or more, third trimester

Codes in category O31 require a seventh character. Seventh character 0 is for single gestations and multiple gestations where the fetus (e.g., fetus 1 or fetus A) is unspecified. Seventh characters 1–9 are for cases of multiple gestations to identify the fetus for which the code applies. If more than one fetus is affected by a condition, a separate code with the appropriate seventh character is assigned to identify each fetus. For example, if fetus 2 and fetus 4 are affected by papyraceous fetus, codes O31.00x2 and O31.00x4 are both assigned. The appropriate code from category O30, Multiple gestation, must also be assigned when assigning a code from category O31 that has a seventh character of 1–9.

For example:

- A patient in her 24th week of pregnancy presents with monochorionic (monoamniotic) twin gestation complicated by inter-twin vascular communication. She undergoes elective reduction of the fetus because of inter-twin vascular communication. One fetus had developed polyhydramnios. Code **O31.32x1, Continuing pregnancy after elective fetal reduction of one fetus or more, second trimester, fetus 1,** is assigned as the principal diagnosis. As additional diagnoses, assign codes **O35.8xx1, Maternal care for other (suspected) fetal abnormality and damage, fetus 1; O40.2xx1, Polyhydramnios, second trimester, fetus 1; O30.012, Twin pregnancy, monoamniotic/monochorionic, second trimester;** and **Z3A.24, 24 weeks of gestation of pregnancy.**

- A patient with an initial twin pregnancy had previously undergone fetal reduction of one fetus because of suspected chromosomal anomalies. The patient is now in her 38th week and is admitted and delivers a normal single liveborn infant. Code **O31.33x2, Continuing pregnancy after elective fetal reduction of one fetus or more, third trimester,** is assigned as the principal diagnosis. As additional diagnoses, assign codes **Z37.0, Single live birth; Z3A.38, 38 weeks of gestation of pregnancy;** and **O30.003, Twin pregnancy, unspecified, third trimester.**

PROCEDURES FOR TERMINATION OF PREGNANCY

ICD-10-PCS classifies procedures performed on the products of conception to the Obstetrics Section. Abortion procedures are coded to the Obstetrics Section, root operation "Abortion," which is defined as "artificially terminating a pregnancy," as shown in the excerpt from the ICD-10-PCS Tables in figure 24.1.

The root operation "Abortion" is subdivided according to whether an additional device, such as a laminaria (a medical product used to dilate the cervix and to induce labor in abortions) or an abortifacient (a substance that causes an abortion), is used, or whether the abortion was performed

FIGURE 24.1 Excerpt from ICD-10-PCS Table for Abortion Procedures

Section	1	Obstetrics
Body System	0	Pregnancy
Operation	A	Abortion: Artificially terminating a pregnancy

Body Part	Approach	Device	Qualifier
0 Products of Conception	0 Open 2 Open Endoscopic 3 Percutaneous 4 Percutaneous Endoscopic 8 Via Natural or Artificial Opening Endoscopic	Z No Device	Z No Qualifier
0 Products of Conception	7 Via Natural or Artificial Opening	Z No Device	6 Vacuum W Laminaria X Abortifacient Z No Qualifier

by mechanical means. If either a laminaria, an abortifacient, or a vacuum is used, then the approach is via natural or artificial opening. All other abortion procedures are those performed by mechanical means (the products of conception are physically removed with the aid of instrumentation), and the device value is Z, no device.

Coding examples follow.

10A07ZZ	Abortion induced by dilatation and curettage
10A07ZW	Transvaginal insertion of laminaria
10A07ZX	Abortion by insertion of prostaglandin suppository

Procedures performed following an abortion for curettage of the endometrium or evacuation of retained products of conception are all coded in the Obstetrics Section to the root operation "Extraction" and the body part "products of conception, retained." For example, dilatation and curettage for an incomplete spontaneous abortion is coded to **10D17ZZ, Extraction of products of conception, retained, via natural or artificial opening.**

EXERCISE 24.2

Code the following diagnoses and procedures.

1. Therapeutic abortion, complete (10 weeks' gestation),

   performed because of severe reactive psychosis

   Vaginal vacuum abortion

   _____

2. Inadvertent spontaneous abortion (complete)

   prompted by radiation treatment damage to fetus

   (single fetus)

   _____

3. Elective abortion (complete) performed because
    of chromosomal abnormality of fetus (single fetus)

    Abortion using laminaria

ECTOPIC AND MOLAR PREGNANCIES

Ectopic and molar pregnancies and other abnormal products of conception are classified to the following categories, with an additional code from category O08 when any complication occurs:

O00   Ectopic pregnancy
O01   Hydatidiform mole
O02   Other abnormal product of conception

A molar pregnancy occurs when a blighted ovum within the uterus develops into a mole or benign tumor. A blighted ovum typically occurs within the first trimester when a fertilized egg attaches itself to the uterine wall but the embryo does not develop. Cells develop to form the pregnancy sac but not the embryo itself. A high level of chromosome abnormalities can cause a blighted ovum. The hydatidiform mole is a particular type of molar pregnancy and is classified separately (O01.-) in ICD-10-CM. All other molar pregnancies are included in code **O02.0, Blighted ovum and nonhydatidiform mole.**

Human chorionic gonadotropin (hCG) is a hormone produced in the body during pregnancy. An hCG blood test measures the level of hCG detectable in the blood. The test can be qualitative or quantitative. In early pregnancy, the hCG level should double approximately every two to three days. A decrease in the hCG doubling time may be an indication of a miscarriage or ectopic pregnancy. Although the hCG blood level and pregnancy tests will be positive, the gestational sac will not be visible on ultrasound. An ectopic pregnancy must be ruled out when the ultrasound does not demonstrate an intrauterine pregnancy; if it is ruled out, the miscarriage is confirmed. Assign code **O02.81, Inappropriate change in quantitative human chorionic gonadotropin (hCG) in early pregnancy.**

A biochemical pregnancy is the earliest form of miscarriage. The term "biochemical" refers to a situation in which the pregnancy is too early to confirm except through biochemical means. In a biochemical pregnancy, the fertilized egg will not implant properly in the uterus, resulting in an early miscarriage. Biochemical pregnancy is included under code O02.81.

Utilization of assisted technologies has resulted in an increase in multiple gestational pregnancies in which an intrauterine pregnancy may coexist with an ectopic pregnancy. An ectopic pregnancy (O00.0-; O00.1-; O00.2-; O00.8-; and O00.9-) occurs when a fertilized ovum is implanted and develops anywhere outside the uterus. The fourth character indicates the extrauterine location of the ectopic pregnancy, and the fifth character indicates with or without intrauterine pregnancy. The sixth character for subcategories O00.1, Tubal pregnancy, and O00.2, Ovarian pregnancy, describes right, left, or unspecified tubal or ovarian pregnancy. The codes are as follows:

O00.00   Abdominal pregnancy without intrauterine pregnancy
O00.01   Abdominal pregnancy with intrauterine pregnancy
O00.101   Right tubal pregnancy without intrauterine pregnancy
O00.102   Left tubal pregnancy without intrauterine pregnancy
O00.109   Unspecified tubal pregnancy without intrauterine pregnancy
O00.111   Right tubal pregnancy with intrauterine pregnancy

O00.112	Left tubal pregnancy with intrauterine pregnancy
O00.119	Unspecified tubal pregnancy with intrauterine pregnancy
O00.201	Right ovarian pregnancy without intrauterine pregnancy
O00.202	Left ovarian pregnancy without intrauterine pregnancy
O00.209	Unspecified ovarian pregnancy without intrauterine pregnancy
O00.211	Right ovarian pregnancy with intrauterine pregnancy
O00.212	Left ovarian pregnancy with intrauterine pregnancy
O00.219	Unspecified ovarian pregnancy with intrauterine pregnancy
O00.80	Other ectopic pregnancy without intrauterine pregnancy
O00.81	Other ectopic pregnancy with intrauterine pregnancy
O00.90	Unspecified ectopic pregnancy without intrauterine pregnancy
O00.91	Unspecified ectopic pregnancy with intrauterine pregnancy

Patients with a history of an ectopic or molar pregnancy have an increased risk of having the same complication in another pregnancy. Assign code O09.1- for an encounter involving supervision of an obstetric patient with a previous history of ectopic pregnancy. Codes from subcategory O09.A are assigned during the prenatal period for pregnant women who are high risk because of a previous history of molar pregnancy.

As previously noted, the *ICD-10-CM Official Guidelines for Coding and Reporting* have been revised to state "Category Z3A codes should not be assigned for pregnancies with abortive outcomes (categories O00-O08), elective termination of pregnancy (code Z33.2), nor for postpartum conditions, as category Z3A is not applicable to these conditions."

Tubal Pregnancy

Tubal pregnancy is the most common type of ectopic pregnancy. Surgical procedures for removing a tubal ectopic pregnancy include salpingotomy and salpingostomy; in both procedures, the ectopic pregnancy is removed from the fallopian tube by means of an incision into the tube. An ectopic pregnancy can also be removed by salpingectomy (excision of the tube) with the ectopic pregnancy intact. Removal of ectopic pregnancy is classified to the Obstetrics Section, body system "pregnancy," and body part "product of conception, ectopic." If the removal of the ectopic pregnancy is performed via salpingotomy or salpingostomy, the root operation is "Extraction"; if the procedure is performed via salpingectomy, the root operation is "Resection."

Coding examples follow.

O00.102	Left tubal pregnancy	
	10T24ZZ	Laparoscopy with resection of ectopic tubal pregnancy
O00.101	Right tubal pregnancy	
	10T20ZZ+0UB50ZZ	Laparotomy, salpingectomy with removal of right tubal pregnancy and excision of portion of right fallopian tube
O00.00	Abdominal pregnancy	
	10T20ZZ	Removal of abdominal pregnancy (open approach)
O00.80	Cornual pregnancy	
	10T24ZZ	Laparoscopic removal of cornual pregnancy

Complications of Molar and Ectopic Pregnancies

Unlike complications of abortions, complications of ectopic and molar pregnancies are classified in category O08, whether they occur during the initial episode of care or during a later episode. When the complication occurs during an episode of care for the purpose of treating the ectopic or molar pregnancy, a code from the O00 through O02 series is sequenced first, followed by a code from category O08. When the patient is readmitted for a complication following treatment of an ectopic or molar pregnancy, assign a code from category O08 as the principal diagnosis. An additional code that describes the complication more specifically can be assigned as needed. Sample codes include the following:

O00.101 + O08.0   Pelvic peritonitis following right ectopic tubal pregnancy
                            (this admission)

O08.1   Hemorrhage following ruptured ectopic tubal pregnancy removed on
                            previous admission

MISSED ABORTION

The term "missed abortion" refers to fetal death that occurs prior to the completion of 20 weeks of gestation, with the dead fetus retained for a period of time in the uterus. This condition may be indicated by a cessation of growth, hardening of the uterus, or actual diminution in size of the uterus. Absence of fetal heart tones after they had been previously heard is also indicative of a missed abortion. The retained fetus may be expelled spontaneously, or surgical or chemical intervention may be required. For example:

- A patient in the 19th week of gestation reports that she is no longer feeling any fetal movement. The physician cannot hear any fetal heart tones, although they were present one month ago. On examination, the uterus is hard and possibly smaller than on the last visit. Code **O02.1, Missed abortion,** is assigned.

- A patient presents at 19 weeks gestation for induction of labor due to intrauterine fetal demise. The patient experiences a retained placenta with hemorrhage resulting in an acute blood loss anemia. Codes **O02.1, Missed abortion; O04.6, Delayed or excessive hemorrhage, following (induced) termination of pregnancy;** and **D62, Acute posthemorrhagic anemia,** are assigned. The acute blood loss anemia resulted from the hemorrhage and was not a complication of the pregnancy.

When the period of gestation is longer than 20 weeks, retention of a dead fetus is considered a missed intrauterine death (O36.4-).

Code O02.1 is not assigned for blighted ovum, nonhydatidiform mole, or hydatidiform mole. Instead, assign code **O02.0, Blighted ovum and nonhydatidiform mole,** or a code from category O01, Hydatidiform mole, instead. For example:

- A patient is diagnosed with a blighted ovum and has a vacuum dilatation and curettage (D&C) performed. Code **O02.0, Blighted ovum and nonhydatidiform mole,** is assigned for the blighted ovum. For the procedure, code **10D07Z6, Extraction of products of conception, vacuum, via natural or artificial opening,** is assigned.

EXERCISE 24.3

Code the following diagnoses. Do not assign procedure codes.

1. Therapeutic abortion, complete, with embolism

2. Failed attempted induction of abortion

3. Ruptured right tubal pregnancy with peritonitis due to
   group A *Streptococcus*

   _____

4. Incomplete early abortion at 8 weeks' gestation
   (spontaneous)

   _____

5. Eighteen-week spontaneous abortion, complete,
   with excessive hemorrhage

   _____

6. Electively induced abortion with liveborn, 21 weeks

   _____

7. Electively induced abortion, complete,
   complicated by shock

   _____

8. Ectopic pregnancy, right fallopian tube
   with intrauterine pregnancy

   _____

9. Carneous mole

   _____

10. Hydatidiform mole

    _____

11. Missed abortion, 19 weeks' gestation

    _____

12. Ten-week pregnancy with electively induced abortion,
    complete
    Family problems due to multiparity

    _____

CHAPTER 25 — Congenital Anomalies

CHAPTER OVERVIEW

- Congenital anomalies are classified in chapter 17 of ICD-10-CM.

- Congenital and acquired conditions are often distinguished with a parenthetical note in the main term or subterm of a condition in the Alphabetic Index.

- In a few specific cases, separate codes are provided for the congenital and acquired versions of a condition.

- Congenital anomalies are classified first by the body system involved.

- Although congenital anomalies are present at birth, they may not be recognized until later in life.

- Patient age plays no role in assigning chapter 17 codes. They can be used at any age.

- In the case of newborns, congenital conditions that may have future implications are reported even though they may not be treated during the current episode of care.

- Conditions caused by mechanical factors during gestation are coded to categories Q65–Q79, Congenital malformations and deformations of the musculoskeletal system.

- Conditions due to birth injury are considered perinatal and are not part of the congenital classifications.

LEARNING OUTCOMES

After studying this chapter, you should be able to:

Distinguish between congenital and acquired conditions in the Alphabetic Index.

Code for a congenital anomaly even if the classification does not provide a specific code for it.

Explain the relationship of patient age to codes for congenital anomalies.

Explain the difference between congenital and perinatal deformities.

TERM TO KNOW

Congenital anomaly
abnormal condition present at birth, which may not be recognized until later in life

REMEMBER . . .

There are about 4,000 congenital anomalies. Not all have been classified with a specific code.

INTRODUCTION

Congenital anomalies are classified in categories Q00 through Q99 in chapter 17 of ICD-10-CM. Congenital anomalies are abnormal conditions that are present at birth, although they may not be recognized until later. Codes from chapter 17 may be used throughout the life of the patient.

Many congenital conditions can now be repaired because of medical advances, and patients are left with no residual condition. If a congenital anomaly has been corrected, a personal history code should be used to identify the history of the anomaly. Codes in subcategory Z87.7, Personal history of (corrected) congenital malformations, are assigned for history of congenital anomalies that have been surgically corrected. If the congenital malformation has been partially corrected or repaired but still requires medical treatment, assign a code for the congenital malformation, rather than a personal history code.

LOCATION OF TERMS IN THE ALPHABETIC INDEX

A distinction between acquired and congenital conditions is often noted in the Alphabetic Index by a nonessential modifier associated with the main term or a subterm. When either "acquired" or "congenital" appears in parentheses with the main term, the alternative term can ordinarily be located as a subterm.

Note that some conditions are congenital by definition and have no acquired version; others are always considered to be acquired. For many conditions, of course, no distinction is made. When the diagnostic statement does not describe a condition as being either acquired or congenital, ICD-10-CM often makes a presumption that it is one or the other.

The following example from the Alphabetic Index demonstrates this usage:

Deformity . . .

-breast (acquired) N64.89

--congenital Q83.9

--reconstructed N65.0

-bronchus (congenital) Q32.4

--acquired NEC J98.09

In this example, the Alphabetic Index assumes that deformity of the breast without other qualification is classified as acquired, whereas deformity of the bronchus is classified as congenital if not otherwise specified. The Tabular List may offer additional guidance by means of an exclusion note. For example, the entry under category K57, Diverticular disease of intestine, refers the user elsewhere for congenital diverticulum of intestine, coded **Q43.8, Other specified congenital malformations of intestine.** For code Q43.8, the inclusion note indicates that congenital diverticulum of the colon is appropriately classified here.

Congenital anomalies are classified first by the body system involved. Many congenital anomalies have specific codes in ICD-10-CM; others are located under such general terms as "anomaly" and "deformity" rather than under the name of the specific condition. For example:

Q45.8   Congenital malposition of gastrointestinal tract

Q22.5   Ebstein's anomaly

Q40.1   Congenital hiatus hernia

Q82.5   Strawberry nevus

Q03.9   Congenital hydrocephalus

Because approximately 4,000 congenital anomalies have been identified, it is impossible for the classification to provide a specific code for each. When the type of anomaly is specified in the medical record but no specific code is provided, the code for other specified anomaly of that type and site should be assigned. Often, only the code for unspecified anomaly of that general type or site can be assigned. When a specific code is not available, additional codes for manifestations of the anomaly should be assigned to the extent possible. Use additional secondary codes from other chapters to specify conditions associated with the anomaly. For example:

- A 10-month-old infant is diagnosed with cardiofaciocutaneous (CFC) syndrome. CFC syndrome is a genetic condition associated with mutation in four known genes: BRAF, MEK1, MEK2, and KRAS. Assign code **Q87.89, Other specified congenital malformation syndromes, not elsewhere classified,** for CFC syndrome. Additional codes may be assigned for any manifestations of the condition as instructed by the guideline on congenital anomalies.

RELATIONSHIP OF AGE TO CODES

Codes from chapter 17 can be reported for a patient of any age. Many congenital anomalies, although actually present at birth, do not manifest themselves until later in life. In addition, many cannot be corrected and persist throughout life, and these conditions may be reported for an adult patient. Patient age is not the determining factor in assigning these codes. Following are examples:

- A patient, 30 years of age, with Marfan's syndrome was admitted for a heart valve replacement and repair of an abdominal aortic aneurysm. In this case, the code **Q87.40, Marfan's syndrome,** is assigned in spite of the patient's age because the condition is an inherited disorder of the connective tissue that is transmitted as an autosomal dominant trait.
- A patient, age 25 years, was admitted for brain surgery, which revealed a colloid cyst of the right third ventricle. In this case, code **Q04.6, Congenital cerebral cysts,** is assigned because a colloid cyst of the third ventricle is always congenital and the patient's age does not influence code assignment.

NEWBORN WITH CONGENITAL CONDITIONS

When a diagnosis of a congenital condition is made during the hospital episode in which an infant is born, the appropriate code from chapter 17 of ICD-10-CM should be assigned as an additional code, with the appropriate code from category Z38, Liveborn infants, according to place of birth and type of delivery, used as the principal diagnosis. (See chapter 26 of this handbook.) Examples follow:

Z38.00 + Q36.9   Term birth, single male, vaginal delivery; incomplete cleft lip on right side

Z38.00 + Q54.9   Term birth, single male, vaginal delivery; hypospadias

Note that the following is an exception to the guidelines for reporting other conditions: Congenital conditions that may have future health care implications are reported for newborns even if they are not further evaluated or treated during the current episode of care. Therefore, it is appropriate to assign congenital anomalies codes (Q00–Q99) whenever a congenital condition is diagnosed by the physician.

CONGENITAL DEFORMITIES VERSUS PERINATAL DEFORMITIES

Certain musculoskeletal deformities that result from a mechanical factor during gestation, such as intrauterine malposition or pressure, are classified in categories Q65–Q79, Congenital malformations and deformations of the musculoskeletal system. Conditions due to birth injury are classified as perinatal conditions in categories P10–P15, Birth trauma, in chapter 16 of ICD-10-CM, with an additional code assigned to identify the specific condition whenever possible. Examples of congenital and perinatal deformities include the following:

Q65.1   Bilateral congenital dislocation of hip

Q68.2   Congenital dislocation of knee

P13.4   Fracture of clavicle due to birth trauma

HYDROCEPHALUS AND SPINA BIFIDA

ICD-10-CM provides separate codes for congenital hydrocephalus (Q03.-), spina bifida with hydrocephalus (Q05.-), acquired secondary normal pressure hydrocephalus (G91.0), obstructive hydrocephalus (G91.1), and acquired idiopathic normal pressure hydrocephalus (G91.2).

Congenital hydrocephalus is defined as an excessive accumulation of cerebrospinal fluid (CSF) in the brain that is present at birth. The excessive fluid leads to increased intracranial pressure and possibly brain damage. A code from category Q03, Congenital hydrocephalus, is assigned for this birth defect. ICD-10-CM provides fourth characters to further specify malformation of aqueduct of Sylvius (Q03.0), atresia of foramina of Magendie and Luschka (Q03.1), and other congenital hydrocephalus (Q03.8); when this information is not available, the condition is coded to **Q03.9, Congenital hydrocephalus, unspecified.** If the medical record documentation does not specify whether the hydrocephalus is congenital or acquired, the classification defaults to acquired, and code **G91.9, Hydrocephalus, unspecified,** is assigned.

Spina bifida is a congenital anomaly involving incomplete closure of the embryonic neural tube, resulting in a spinal cord defect. Many individuals with spina bifida have an associated abnormality of the cerebellum, referred to as Chiari II malformation. In affected individuals, the back portion of the brain is displaced from the skull into the upper neck. Hydrocephalus develops in approximately 90 percent of individuals with myelomeningocele/spina bifida because the displaced cerebellum obstructs the flow of CSF. For spina bifida without hydrocephalus, assign a code from Q05.5 through Q05.8, depending on the portion of the spine affected. If spina bifida is present with hydrocephalus, assign a code from Q05.0 through Q05.4 for this type of congenital anomaly, depending on the portion of the spine affected, as follows:

Q05.0   Cervical spina bifida with hydrocephalus

Q05.1   Thoracic spina bifida with hydrocephalus

Q05.2   Lumbar spina bifida with hydrocephalus

Q05.3   Sacral spina bifida with hydrocephalus

Q05.4   Unspecified spina bifida with hydrocephalus

For a diagnostic statement of spina bifida without further specification, assign code **Q05.9, Spina bifida, unspecified.** Use an additional code for any paraplegia or paraparesis (G82.2-) associated with spina bifida.

CONGENITAL MALFORMATIONS OF THE GREAT ARTERIES

Congenital malformations of the great arteries (category Q25) include congenital malformations of the aorta, pulmonary artery, and other great arteries.

Congenital Malformations of the Aorta

Congenital malformations of the aorta are very common. The aorta is divided into segments according to its anatomical course. It starts from the left ventricle as the ascending aorta, which travels superiorly from the aortic valve and then makes a hairpin turn known as the aortic arch. Coarctation of the aorta is a discrete narrowing of the aorta, which typically involves a thoracic location distal to the left subclavian artery but proximal to the patent ductus arteriosus. The most extreme form of coarctation is an interrupted aortic arch, which may also be called "atresia of the aortic arch." In aortic atresia, there is no opening from the left ventricle into the aorta. Due to the missing heart structure, blood cannot move from the left ventricle to the body, and the only source of blood flow is through the ductus arteriosus. Congenital aortic atresia and hypoplasia of aorta are usually associated with hypoplastic left heart and involve the aortic valvular orifice and the ascending aorta. Other aortic malformations include congenital aneurysm, congenital dilatation, persistence of the right aortic arch, persistence of the fetal double aortic arch, and anomalies of the origin of the left or right subclavian artery.

ICD-10-CM codes for congenital malformations of the aorta include coarctation of aorta (Q25.1), interruption of aortic arch (Q25.21), and other atresia of aorta (Q25.29). Most of these defects are found at birth, but they may also be identified later in life.

Other congenital malformations of the aorta are classified in subcategory Q25.4 as follows: congenital malformation of aorta NOS (Q25.40); absence and aplasia of aorta (Q25.41); hypoplasia of aorta (Q25.42); congenital aneurysm of aorta (Q25.43); congenital dilation of aorta (Q25.44); double aortic arch (Q25.45); tortuous aortic arch (Q25.46); right aortic arch (Q25.47); anomalous origin of subclavian artery (Q25.48); and other congenital malformations of aorta (Q25.49).

Pulmonary Artery Anomalies

Pulmonary artery atresia (Q25.5) is the incomplete formation of the pulmonary valve (located between the right ventricle and the pulmonary artery), which obstructs the flow of blood through the leaflets and into the lungs. In a newborn, the deoxygenated blood can flow through the patent ductus arteriosus into the pulmonary artery and get to the lungs. However, when the ductus arteriosus closes shortly after birth, the baby will increasingly become cyanotic and will have difficulty breathing because of the defective pulmonary valve.

Pulmonary artery coarctation (Q25.71) refers to narrowing or stenosis of the pulmonary artery. Narrowing of the main pulmonary artery or its branches makes it difficult for blood that is deficient in oxygen to pass from the right ventricle to the lungs to get the oxygen necessary for the body. The heart becomes overworked when it has to pump harder to get the blood into the lungs. A moderate or severe degree of pulmonary artery stenosis can lead to pulmonary hypertension at rest or during exercise. Pulmonary artery stenosis is usually associated with congenital cardiovascular anomalies such as pulmonary valve stenosis and tetralogy of Fallot.

A pulmonary arteriovenous malformation (AVM), referred to as pulmonary arteriovenous aneurysm or pulmonary arteriovenous fistula (Q25.72), is an abnormal communication between the pulmonary artery and the pulmonary vein. The abnormally direct connection between high-pressure arteries and low-pressure veins may be detected via stethoscope as a rhythmic whooshing sound caused by excessively rapid blood flow through the arteries and veins. While pulmonary AVMs are most commonly congenital, they may be acquired through conditions such as hepatic cirrhosis, mitral stenosis, trauma, and metastatic thyroid carcinoma.

NEUROFIBROMATOSIS

Neurofibromatosis (subcategory Q85.0) refers to a group of autosomal dominant genetic disorders that cause tumors to grow along the nerves. Schwannomas (Q85.03) may occur along any nerve of the body, including spinal, cranial, and peripheral nerves, except on the vestibular nerve. As the tumors grow they compress nerves and cause pain, numbness, tingling, weakness, and other neurological symptoms.

CYSTIC KIDNEY DISEASE

There are major differences in the clinical characteristics, pathophysiology, and prognosis of the various types of congenital cystic kidney disease. This fact augments the importance of being as specific as possible about the type when assigning a code. For example, symptoms and problems for polycystic kidney disease, infantile type (Q61.19), progress slowly as more and more cysts develop over the years; this disease is relatively common. Medullary cystic kidney (Q61.5) is a hereditary disorder in which cysts in the center of each kidney cause the kidneys to gradually lose their ability to work; late in the disease, symptoms of chronic kidney disease may develop. When the diagnostic statement does not indicate whether a renal cyst is congenital or acquired, ICD-10-CM presumes that the cyst is acquired.

CONGENITAL MALFORMATIONS OF GENITAL ORGANS

The development of the female reproductive tract is a complex process that involves a highly orchestrated series of events, including cellular differentiation, migration, fusion, and canalization. Failure of any part of the process results in congenital anomalies. Mullerian anomalies refer to all congenital anomalies of the uterus, cervix, and vagina. ICD-10-CM provides unique codes for the spectrum of congenital uterine, cervical, and vaginal anomalies in categories Q50 through Q52:

Q50   Congenital malformations of ovaries, fallopian tubes and broad ligaments
Q51   Congenital malformations of uterus and cervix
Q52   Other congenital malformations of female genitalia

A vaginal septum (subcategory Q52.12) occurs when the female reproductive tract does not develop properly, creating a dividing wall of tissue within the vagina. When lateral fusion defects occur during organogenesis of the reproductive tract, complete duplication of the reproductive tract may occur, leading to uterus didelphys with a longitudinal vaginal septum that creates two vaginas. Another presentation includes an oblique orientation of the longitudinal vaginal septum that leads to obstruction of one of the vaginas, while the other vagina is patent. The obstructing longitudinal vaginal septum may be right or left sided, or may also be microperforate.

Codes in subcategory Q52.12 classify nonobstructing and obstructing longitudinal vaginal septum as follows: longitudinal vaginal septum, nonobstructing (Q52.120); longitudinal vaginal septum, obstructing, right side (Q52.121); longitudinal vaginal septum, obstructing, left side (Q52.122); longitudinal vaginal septum, microperforate, right side (Q52.123); longitudinal vaginal septum, microperforate, left side (Q52.124); and longitudinal vaginal septum, unspecified (Q52.129).

Codes in subcategory Q51.2 classify "other doubling of the uterus" and include septate uterus. The septate uterus occurs in two versions: partial septate uterus and complete septate uterus. The following codes specifically identify these congenital malformations: complete doubling of uterus (Q51.21), partial doubling of uterus (Q51.22), and other and unspecified doubling of uterus (Q51.28).

Congenital malformations of male genital organs are classified to categories Q53 through Q55. These categories include conditions such as undescended and ectopic testes, hypospadias, and other congenital malformations of male genital organs.

Cryptorchidism refers to incomplete testicular descent; the condition may be unilateral or bilateral. The term encompasses palpable, nonpalpable, and ectopic testicles. The position of the testis can be abdominal, inguinal, prescrotal, or gliding. ICD-10-CM classifies undescended and ectopic testicle to category Q53. Code Q53.0- describes ectopic testis, and codes Q53.1- and Q53.2- describe undescended testis. The fifth character in subcategories Q53.1 and Q53.2 indicates the location of the undescended testicle (abdominal, ectopic perineal, high scrotal, inguinal, or unspecified). For example, the undescended testicle may be unilateral intraabdominal (Q53.111), unilateral inguinal (Q53.112), unilateral high scrotal (Q53.13), bilateral intraabdominal (Q53.211), bilateral inguinal (Q53.212), or bilateral high scrotal (Q53.23).

Hypospadias is a somewhat common congenital anomaly whereby the opening of the urethra is on the underside, rather than at the end, of the penis. ICD-10-CM classifies hypospadias to category Q54, Hypospadias, with additional fourth characters to specify balanic (Q54.0), penile (Q54.1), penoscrotal (Q54.2), perineal (Q54.3), congenital chordee (ventral curvature of the penis, caused by presence of a fibrous band of tissue instead of normal skin along the corpus spongiosum) (Q54.4), other (Q54.8), or unspecified (Q54.9). Procedures to repair hypospadias are classified to the root operation "Reposition," body part "urethra."

In addition to the above female and male genital malformations, ICD-10-CM provides category Q56, Indeterminate sex and pseudohermaphroditism, which distinguishes among hermaphroditism, not elsewhere classified (Q56.0); male pseudohermaphroditism (Q56.1); female pseudohermaphroditism (Q56.2); pseudohermaphroditism, unspecified (Q56.3); and indeterminate sex, unspecified (Q56.4).

OMPHALOCELE AND GASTROSCHISIS

An omphalocele is a distinct ventral wall defect. The intestines are usually covered by a membranous sac, with the intestine being exposed only if the sac ruptures. An omphalocele is commonly associated with other structural and chromosomal anomalies. Code **Q79.2, Exomphalos,** is assigned for a congenital omphalocele.

Gastroschisis is an anomaly involving a defect of the ventral body wall to the right of the umbilical cord insertion. This anomaly is caused by failure of the developing abdominal wall to completely close, allowing the intestines to protrude from the defect. The exposed intestines are not covered by a membranous sac. Assign code **Q79.3, Gastroschisis,** for congenital gastroschisis.

EXERCISE 25.1

Code the following diagnoses and procedures. Do not assign External cause of morbidity codes.

---

1. Polycystic kidneys, adult type

---

2. Congenital chordee

   Repair of hypospadias and release of chordee

   (open approach)

---

3. Congenital pyloric stenosis

   Endoscopic dilation of the pylorus

---

4. Congenital dislocation of both hips

   Closed reduction of dislocation of both hips with

   immobilization in plaster casts

---

5. Congestive heart failure in patient with congenital

   interatrial septal defect

---

6. Posterior subcapsular cataract, left eye, congenital

7. Accessory fifth digit, right foot

8. Esophageal web with esophageal spasm and reflux
    esophagitis

9. Left trigger thumb, congenital
    Open tenolysis of flexor sheath of left thumb

10. Urachal cyst and patent urachus

11. Thoracoabdominal coarctation of aorta

12. Hallux rigidus, left

13. Down syndrome

14. Bilateral talipes equinovarus, congenital

15. Unilateral cleft lip and cleft palate, soft and hard
    Correction of cleft hard and soft palate via incisions on both sides
    of the cleft, and repositioning of the tissue and muscles
    Repair of cleft upper lip, open

16. Cystic lung, congenital

17. Congenital nevus flammeus

18. Large congenital atrial septal defect (ASD)
    and patent foramen ovale (PFO)
    Repair of ASD/PFO with insertion of synthetic prosthesis across
    atrial septum via cardiac catheter to reinforce atrial septum

19. A two-month-old infant with polydactyly and a supernumerary digit
    of the right fifth finger underwent complete surgical removal,
    involving excision of bone and other tissues

CHAPTER 26

Perinatal Conditions

CHAPTER OVERVIEW

- Perinatal conditions other than congenital anomalies are classified in chapter 16 of ICD-10-CM.
- These conditions can be found under the main term **Birth** or as a subterm under the condition's main term.
- Perinatal conditions are sequenced as the principal diagnosis but follow the appropriate Z38 code for the birth episode.
- Codes for perinatal conditions can be used throughout the patient's life. There is no prohibition due to age.
- Conditions are coded if they meet the definition of reportable conditions or if they have an implication for the newborn's future care.
- Newborn immaturity and prematurity are classified by birth weight. Codes for these conditions are never assigned without a physician's clinical evaluation as indicated in the diagnostic statement.
- Newborn postmaturity is classified by length of gestation.
- The perinatal conditions in chapter 16 cover fetal distress, metabolic abnormalities, difficulties due to aspiration, and more.
- Codes in categories P00–P04 are assigned only when a maternal condition is the cause of confirmed morbidity or potential mortality in the newborn.
- A code from category Z05 is assigned when a healthy infant is evaluated for a suspected condition that is not found.
- Infections specific to the perinatal period are considered congenital.
- Infections that occur after birth but within the perinatal period may or may not be classified in chapter 16.
- Z codes are used for routine newborn vaccination and health supervision.

LEARNING OUTCOMES

After studying this chapter, you should be able to:

- Locate codes and follow general guidelines with regard to perinatal conditions.
- Use Z codes to classify the birth, and use them with other codes for perinatal conditions.
- Code situations involving newborn immaturity, prematurity, and postmaturity.
- Code for evaluation and observation of newborns and infants.
- Determine what chapter to use to classify a newborn or infant infection.
- Know how and when to assign codes for maternal condition on the newborn record.

TERMS TO KNOW

Newborn immaturity
implies a birth of less than 37 completed weeks' gestation

Newborn postmaturity
a gestational period of more than 42 weeks

Newborn low birth weight
implies a birth weight of 1,000–2,499 grams

Newborn extremely low birth weight
implies a birth weight of 500–999 grams

REMEMBER . . .

Codes from chapter 16 are never found on a maternal record, and codes from chapter 15 are never found on a newborn's record.

INTRODUCTION

With the exception of congenital anomalies, conditions that originate in the perinatal period are classified in chapter 16 of ICD-10-CM and categories P00 through P96. The perinatal period is defined as before birth through the first 28 days after birth. The perinatal period ends on the 29th day of life because the World Health Organization considers the day of birth as "day zero" for international comparisons.

LOCATING CODES FOR PERINATAL CONDITIONS IN THE ALPHABETIC INDEX

Codes for perinatal conditions are located in the Alphabetic Index by referring to the main term **Birth** or to the main term for the condition and then to such subterms as "newborn," "neonatal," "fetal," "infants," and "infantile." If the Alphabetic Index does not provide a specific code for a perinatal condition, assign code **P96.89, Other specified conditions originating in the perinatal period,** followed by the code from another chapter that specifies the condition.

GENERAL PERINATAL GUIDELINES

Codes from chapter 16 are never used on maternal records. By the same token, codes from chapter 15, Pregnancy, Childbirth and the Puerperium, should never be reported on the newborn record.

Generally, chapter 16 codes are sequenced as the principal or first-listed diagnosis on the newborn record, except for the appropriate code from the Z38 series for the birth episode. Codes from other chapters may be assigned as secondary diagnoses to provide additional detail.

The perinatal guidelines for secondary diagnoses are the same as the general coding guidelines for "additional diagnoses" (refer to chapter 3 of this handbook). In addition, assign codes for any conditions that have been specified by the provider as having implications for future health care needs. Assign codes from chapter 16 only for definitive diagnoses established by the provider. If a definitive diagnosis has not been established, codes for signs and symptoms may be assigned.

Sometimes, a newborn may have a condition that may be either due to the birth process or community acquired. If the documentation does not specify which it is, the default code selected should be due to the birth process, and a chapter 16 code should be selected. When the condition is community acquired, do not report a chapter 16 code.

RELATIONSHIP OF AGE TO CODES

Most conditions originating during the perinatal period are transitory in nature. However, some conditions that originate during the perinatal period persist, and some do not manifest themselves until later in life. Such conditions are classified in chapter 16, no matter how old the patient is, and may be reported throughout the life of the patient if the condition is still present. For example:

- A 53-year-old woman is admitted for treatment of vaginal carcinoma due to intrauterine exposure to prescribed DES (diethylstilbestrol) taken by her mother during pregnancy. Code **C52, Malignant neoplasm of vagina,** and code **P04.18, Newborn affected by other maternal medication,** are assigned because the intrauterine exposure remains an important element in the patient's condition, even though the problem did not present itself until later in the patient's life.

- An 18-year-old man was admitted for workup because he had begun experiencing respiratory problems. A diagnosis of bronchopulmonary dysplasia was made, and the patient was discharged to be seen in the physician's office in two weeks. Code **P27.1, Broncho-**

pulmonary dysplasia originating in the perinatal period, is assigned because broncho-pulmonary dysplasia is a congenital condition even though it may not become a problem until later in the patient's life.

CLASSIFICATION OF BIRTHS

A code from category Z38 is assigned as the principal diagnosis for any newborn. The first axis for coding is whether the birth is single, twin, or multiple. The codes further specify whether the birth occurred in the hospital, outside the hospital, or unspecified as to place of birth. If the birth occurred in the hospital, additional characters indicate the type of delivery (vaginal or cesarean). The medical record will provide sufficient information regarding the type of delivery to permit selection of the code.

A code from this series is assigned only on the newborn record and is assigned only for the episode in which the birth occurred. If a newborn is discharged and readmitted or transferred to another facility, the code for the condition responsible for the transfer or readmission is designated as the principal diagnosis. For example:

- A single liveborn vaginally delivered in the hospital with an associated diagnosis of sub-dural hemorrhage due to birth trauma is coded as **Z38.00, Single liveborn infant, delivered vaginally,** and **P10.0, Subdural hemorrhage due to birth injury,** with the Z code sequenced first.

- If the infant is discharged and readmitted or transferred to another facility for treatment of the hemorrhage, the principal diagnosis for that admission is P10.0; no code from category Z38 is assigned.

- If the admission of an infant born outside the hospital is delayed and the newborn is admitted later because of a complication, the complication code is assigned as the principal diagnosis; no code from category Z38 is assigned.

OTHER DIAGNOSES FOR NEWBORNS

A code from category Z38 indicates only that a birth occurred. Additional codes are assigned for all clinically significant conditions noted on the examination of the newborn. A newborn condition is clinically significant when it has implications for the newborn's future health care. This is an exception to the Uniform Hospital Discharge Data Set guidelines.

Insignificant or transient conditions that resolve without treatment are not coded. Medical records of newborns sometimes mention conditions such as fine rashes, molding of the scalp, and minor jaundice. Because these conditions usually resolve without treatment and require no additional workup, they are not coded. For example:

- The physician documents diagnoses of syndactyly and hydrocele on the newborn's diagnostic statement. Even though no treatment is given and no further evaluation is performed during the infant's hospital stay, both of these conditions will require treatment at some time in the future, and so they are reported.

- The physician mentions on the newborn delivery record that the infant has slight jaundice. No further evaluation is performed, and the jaundice clears by the following day. No code for jaundice is assigned.

- The pediatrician documents in the newborn medical record that the baby's heart murmur is benign and most likely due to a patent ductus arteriosus/patent foramen ovale (PDA/PFO). He orders a cardiac consult and an echocardiogram to evaluate the PDA/PFO. Assign code **Q21.1, Atrial septal defect,** for the PFO and code **Q25.0, Patent ductus**

arteriosus, for the PDA. These conditions are being evaluated further; therefore, they can be reported.

- During a routine physical examination of a newborn, the pediatrician notes a possible systolic ejection murmur and recommends further workup post discharge. Assign code **P29.89, Other cardiovascular disorders originating in the perinatal period.** At this point, the underlying cause of the murmur has not been identified.

PREMATURITY, LOW BIRTH WEIGHT, AND POSTMATURITY

Newborns delivered before full term are defined as either immature or premature by both birth weight and gestational age and are classified in category P07 as follows:

- Extremely low birth weight (P07.0-) implies a birth weight of 500–999 grams.
- Low birth weight (P07.1-) implies a birth weight of 1,000–2,499 grams.
- Extreme immaturity (P07.2-) implies less than 28 completed weeks (less than 196 completed days) of gestation.
- Preterm (P07.3-) implies 28 completed weeks (196 completed days) or more, but less than 37 completed weeks (259 completed days) of gestation.

When both birth weight and gestational age of the newborn are available, both should be coded, with birth weight (P07.0-, P07.1-) sequenced before gestational age (P07.2-, P07.3-). Providers use different criteria in determining prematurity. A code for prematurity should not be assigned unless a diagnosis of prematurity is documented.

Even when a newborn is not premature, it may be appropriate to assign a code from category P05, Disorders of newborn related to slow fetal growth and fetal malnutrition. The assigned code does not imply prematurity but indicates that the newborn is smaller than expected for the length of gestation.

Occasionally, the obstetrician will document the gestational age in the mother's record, and the pediatrician will document a different gestational age in the infant's chart. The discrepancy reflects the fact that different providers (e.g., obstetrician and pediatrician) may use different criteria in determining weeks of gestation for the mother versus the gestational age of the infant. For the newborn, assign the appropriate codes for gestational age based on the documentation of the attending provider for the infant (e.g., the pediatrician).

To indicate the birth weight, fifth characters are assigned to codes for low birth weight newborns (P07.0- to P07.1-), newborn light for gestational age (P05.0-), and newborn small for gestational age (P05.1-). Note that the weight expressed by the fifth character should be reasonably consistent with the four-character code to which it is applied. Although most preterm births (liveborn infant less than 37 completed weeks of gestation) are associated with low birth weight, at least 10 percent of newborns in their 37th week of gestation weigh more than 2,500 grams. Code **P05.09, Newborn light for gestational age, 2500 grams and over,** is assigned for a newborn who is light for gestational age but weighs more than 2,500 grams. Code **P05.19, Newborn small for gestational age, other,** should be assigned for an infant who is small for gestational age but weighs 2,500 grams or more.

When a diagnosis of prematurity has been established by the provider, assignment of codes in categories P05, Disorders of newborn related to slow fetal growth and fetal malnutrition, and P07, Disorders of newborn related to short gestation and low birth weight, not elsewhere classified, are based on the recorded birth weight and estimated gestational age at the time of birth. For example, an infant born at hospital A at 34 weeks' gestation and transferred to hospital B after 14 days for further evaluation of a congenital anomaly could still have a code for prematurity assigned at hospital B as an additional diagnosis. The fifth character for these codes is always based on birth weight, not the infant's weight at the time of transfer or readmission.

For example, a 12-month-old child who was born preterm is being seen for acute bronchiolitis due to respiratory syncytial virus (RSV). The physician lists "acute bronchiolitis due to RSV, ex-26 week preemie" in the diagnostic statement. Code **J21.0, Acute bronchiolitis due to respiratory syncytial virus,** is assigned as the first-listed diagnosis. Code **P07.25, Extreme immaturity of newborn, gestational age 26 completed weeks,** is assigned to indicate that the child was born at 26 weeks of gestation.

As noted earlier, chapter 16 codes may be used regardless of the patient's age if the condition originates in the perinatal period and continues through the life of the patient. Moreover, codes from category P07, Disorders of newborn related to short gestation and low birth weight, not elsewhere classified, may be assigned for a child or an adult if the provider indicates the patient's prematurity and gestational age are contributing conditions affecting the patient's current health status.

Post-term is defined as a gestational period of more than 40 completed weeks to 42 completed weeks. Prolonged gestation or postmaturity is defined as a gestational period of more than 42 completed weeks. Category P08 classifies a long gestation and/or high birth weight as follows:

P08.0   Exceptionally large newborn baby (usually implies weight of 4,500 grams or more)
P08.1   Other heavy for gestational age newborn (heavy- or large-for-dates newborns, regardless of period of gestation)
P08.21 Post-term newborn
P08.22 Prolonged gestation of newborn

Codes **P08.21, Post-term newborn,** and **P08.22, Prolonged gestation of newborn,** may be assigned based only on the gestational age of the newborn as documented in the infant's record by the pediatrician. A specific condition or disorder does not have to be associated with the longer gestational period for these codes to be assigned.

FETAL DISTRESS AND ASPHYXIA

Fetal distress may be defined as signs that indicate a critical response to stress. It implies metabolic abnormalities such as hypoxia and acidosis that affect the functions of vital organs to the point of temporary or permanent injury or even death. ICD-10-CM provides different codes for fetal distress, depending on the specific condition, as follows:

P19.0   Metabolic acidemia in newborn first noted before onset of labor
P19.1   Metabolic acidemia in newborn first noted during labor
P19.2   Metabolic acidemia noted at birth
P19.9   Metabolic acidemia, unspecified
P84   Other problems with newborn

Category P84 includes the following conditions in newborns without further specification: acidemia, acidosis, anoxia, asphyxia, hypercapnia, hypoxemia, hypoxia, and mixed metabolic and respiratory acidosis.

Asphyxia refers to a decreased level of oxygen delivered to the body or an organ with a buildup of carbon dioxide. Birth asphyxia occurs when an infant does not receive enough oxygen before, during, or just after birth, and it can cause decreased heart rate, decreased blood flow, and low blood pressure leading to cellular and organ damage. When the duration of the asphyxia is brief, the infant can recover without any long-lasting injury. If the time period is longer, it may lead to reversible damage, and when prolonged, irreversible injury. Birth asphyxia is classified to code P84.

Hypoxic-ischemic encephalopathy (HIE) is a life-threatening condition that usually results from damage to the cells of the brain and spinal cord secondary to inadequate oxygen during the birth process. HIE is evidence of acute or subacute brain injury due to asphyxia. It is the most common cause of neurological disease during the neonatal period and is associated with significant mortality and morbidity. Infants with the mild form of HIE are hyperalert and overreact to the slightest stimulus. This stage usually lasts 24 hours or less. Infants can recover with normal neurological function. Moderate HIE is associated with lethargy, clinical seizures, suppressed tendon reflexes, bradycardia, and periodic breathing. This stage may last from 2 to 14 days. A good neurological prognosis is seen in infants who can recover within five days. Severe HIE is characterized by stupor to coma, primitive to no reflexes, variable heart rate, and apnea. Half of infants with severe HIE die. Eighty percent of those who survive have intellectual disabilities, epilepsy, cerebral palsy, and learning disabilities. Only 10 percent survive with no neurological disability. The codes for HIE distinguish among mild (P91.61), moderate (P91.62), severe (P91.63), and unspecified (P91.60).

Neonatal encephalopathy is a clinically defined syndrome of neurological dysfunction in the newborn infant, manifested by difficulty initiating and maintaining respiration, depression of tone and reflexes, subnormal level of consciousness, and seizures. A newborn may meet the diagnostic criteria for HIE but can also have an underlying condition not associated with HIE. Code **P91.811, Neonatal encephalopathy in diseases classified elsewhere,** is assigned for neonatal encephalopathy that is caused by a condition other than HIE. When assigning code P91.811, code first the underlying cause, if known. If neonatal encephalopathy is caused by a hypoxic ischemic brain injury, assign the appropriate code from subcategory P91.6, Hypoxic ischemic encephalopathy [HIE], rather than code P91.811. Assign code P91.819 for unspecified neonatal encephalopathy.

Codes for fetal distress or abnormality of heart rate and rhythm are assigned to the newborn record only when the condition is specifically identified by the physician. These codes are never assigned on the basis of other information in the newborn record.

NEONATAL CEREBRAL INFARCTION

Neonatal cerebral infarction (or stroke) is a cerebrovascular condition that occurs between 20 weeks of fetal life through the 28th postnatal day. The condition involves severe disorganization or complete disruption of the gray matter of the developing brain caused by embolic, thrombotic, or ischemic events. ICD-10-CM codes for neonatal cerebral infarction are assigned based on the affected side, as follows:

P91.821 Neonatal cerebral infarction, right side
P91.822 Neonatal cerebral infarction, left side
P91.823 Neonatal cerebral infarction, bilateral
P91.829 Neonatal cerebral infarction, unspecified side

FETAL AND NEWBORN ASPIRATION

Category P24, Neonatal aspiration, describes meconium aspiration and other types of fetal aspiration in the following subcategories/codes:

P24.0- Meconium aspiration
P24.1- Neonatal aspiration of (clear) amniotic fluid and mucus
P24.2- Neonatal aspiration of blood
P24.3- Neonatal aspiration of milk and regurgitated food
P24.8- Other neonatal aspiration
P24.9 Neonatal aspiration, unspecified

Subcategories P24.0- through P24.8- provide an additional fifth character to identify the presence or absence of respiratory symptoms. If applicable, an additional code, I27.2, should be assigned to identify any secondary pulmonary hypertension.

Meconium aspiration in newborns occurs when the fetus gasps while still in the birth canal and inhales meconium-stained amniotic, vaginal, or oropharyngeal fluids. Tachypnea, wheezing, and apnea are sometimes present in meconium aspiration; these conditions may resolve over a short period or may take a more prolonged course. In the milder forms of this condition, dyspnea occurs soon after birth, lasts two or three days, and is followed by rapid recovery. Therapy includes bronchoscopic suction of meconium, oxygen administration, humidity control, and prophylactic antibiotics. Massive aspiration syndrome is synonymous with massive fetal aspiration. Although meconium aspiration syndrome and massive meconium aspiration are somewhat different conditions, they have similar clinical presentation and course, and code **P24.01, Meconium aspiration with respiratory symptoms,** is assigned for both. Code P96.83 is assigned for meconium staining.

Meconium ileus and meconium plug syndrome (a transient disorder of the newborn's colon with delayed passage of meconium and intestinal dilatation) are coded to **P76.0, Meconium plug syndrome,** except when specified as meconium ileus in cystic fibrosis, which is coded to E84.11 instead. Code P03.82 is assigned for meconium passage (without aspiration) during delivery.

HEMOLYTIC DISEASE OF THE NEWBORN

Rh-positive infants born to Rh-negative mothers often develop hemolytic disease owing to fetal-maternal blood group incompatibility. These conditions are classified in category P55, Hemolytic disease of newborn. Note that an indication of incompatibility on a routine cord blood test is not conclusive. Do not assign a code from category P55 on the basis of this finding alone; a diagnosis of isoimmunization or hemolytic disease requires provider confirmation.

NECROTIZING ENTEROCOLITIS

Necrotizing enterocolitis (NEC) is a severe gastrointestinal condition that involves injury to the bowel, intestinal mucosal disruption associated with enteric feedings, infectious pathogens, and immature immune response. It is a major cause of morbidity and mortality in premature infants. Although NEC commonly affects premature infants with a birth weight of less than 1,500 grams, it can also occur in infants with low risk factors. The exact etiology of NEC is unknown; however, it is thought that the intestine of the premature infant is weakened by too little oxygen and blood flow. The infant then has an increased risk of developing NEC because of difficulty with blood and oxygen circulation, digestion, and fighting infection. When feedings are started and the food moves into the weakened area of the intestinal tract, bacteria from the food can damage the intestinal tissues. These tissues can develop necrosis and perforation, leading to acute abdominal infection. ICD-10-CM classifies necrotizing enterocolitis according to the following stages:

P77.1   Stage 1 necrotizing enterocolitis in newborn
P77.2   Stage 2 necrotizing enterocolitis in newborn
P77.3   Stage 3 necrotizing enterocolitis in newborn
P77.9   Necrotizing enterocolitis in newborn, unspecified

NEONATAL CEREBRAL LEUKOMALACIA

Periventricular leukomalacia, also known as neonatal cerebral leukomalacia (P91.2), refers to necrosis of white matter adjacent to lateral ventricles with formation of cyst. It is a major risk factor for cerebral palsy and other neurological disorders. Risk for leukomalacia is greatest in infants with very low birth weight. Although the cause of this condition is still obscure, recent studies have associated it with intrauterine growth retardation, intrauterine infections, and pregnancies involving monozygotic twins. The condition is frequently associated with severe intraventricular hemorrhage, but the leukomalacia is not necessarily the cause of the problem. An additional code is reported when intraventricular hemorrhage (P52.0, P52.1, P52.21, P52.22, P52.3) is associated with periventricular leukomalacia.

DISORDERS OF STOMACH FUNCTION AND FEEDING PROBLEMS

Persistent vomiting in a newborn may be a sign of a very serious condition. ICD-10-CM separately classifies vomiting, bilious emesis, failure to thrive, and other feeding problems in newborns. These codes are used for newborns up to the 28th day of life who are experiencing feeding problems (P92.9), bilious vomiting (P92.01), other vomiting (P92.09), regurgitation and rumination (P92.1), slow feeding (P92.2), underfeeding (P92.3), overfeeding (P92.4), neonatal difficulty in feeding at breast (P92.5), failure to thrive (P92.6), and other feeding problems (P92.8). For example, a 10-day-old baby presents for weight recheck and feeding problems. Code **Z00.111, Health examination for newborn 8 to 28 days old,** is assigned, along with code **P92.9, Feeding problems of newborn, unspecified.** Codes in the main classification are used for infants and children older than 28 days.

OBSERVATION AND EVALUATION OF NEWBORNS AND INFANTS

Codes in category Z05, Encounter for observation and evaluation of newborn for suspected diseases and conditions ruled out, are assigned when an infant within the perinatal period is evaluated for a suspected condition that is found not to be present when the study is complete. A code from category Z05 is not assigned when a definite condition is diagnosed or when the patient presents with signs or symptoms of a suspected problem that is not ruled out. Instead, assign a code for the diagnosed condition or the appropriate codes for the signs and symptoms.

During the birth episode, first assign a code from category Z38. A code from category Z05 may also be assigned as the principal diagnosis for a later readmission or encounter during the perinatal period of 28 days when a code from Z38 no longer applies. For example:

- The physician is concerned that a vaginally delivered newborn with a drug-dependent mother may have been adversely affected by exposure to drugs in utero. Drug screens are carried out on the newborn, and the newborn is temporarily placed in the intensive care nursery for closer observation of potential withdrawal symptoms. No withdrawal symptoms are noted and drug screens are negative. Codes **Z38.00, Single liveborn infant, delivered vaginally,** and **Z05.8, Observation and evaluation of newborn for other specified suspected condition ruled out,** are assigned.

- A newborn infant is readmitted two days after discharge because of slight cyanosis and the possibility of a perinatal respiratory problem. A complete workup discloses no problem, including no observable cyanosis, and the patient is discharged without any diagnosis having been established. Code **Z05.3, Observation and evaluation of newborn for suspected respiratory condition ruled out,** is assigned as the principal diagnosis.

- A newborn infant is readmitted two days after discharge because of cyanosis and the possibility of a perinatal respiratory problem. The infant is diagnosed as having respiratory distress syndrome. Code **P22.0, Respiratory distress syndrome,** is assigned. No code from category Z05 is assigned.

- The mother of a newborn tested positive for group B *Streptococcus* (GBS) at delivery. After clinical evaluation and workup, GBS infection in the newborn is ruled out. Code **Z05.1, Observation and evaluation of newborn for suspected infectious condition ruled out,** is assigned.

- The mother of a newborn tested positive for GBS at delivery. After clinical evaluation and workup, the provider states, "Newborn affected by maternal group B *Streptococcus;* unable to completely rule out active GBS infection," and the infant is treated for GBS. In this case, assign codes **P00.89, Newborn affected by other maternal conditions,** and **B95.1, Streptococcus, group B,** as the cause of diseases classified elsewhere. Unlike the previous example, the provider has not completely ruled out an active GBS infection. In the inpatient setting, an uncertain diagnosis documented at the time of discharge is coded as if the condition exists.

Ordinarily, no additional code is assigned when codes in category Z05 are sequenced as the principal diagnosis. However, additional codes can be assigned for a perinatal or congenital condition that requires continuing therapy or monitoring during the stay. Codes for congenital conditions that do not receive further evaluation or therapeutic treatment are not assigned when a newborn is admitted for observation.

It is inappropriate to assign codes in subcategory Z03.7, Encounter for suspected maternal and fetal conditions ruled out, for the newborn. This code subcategory is only reported on the maternal record.

INFECTIONS ORIGINATING DURING THE PERINATAL PERIOD

Many infections specific to the perinatal period are considered to be congenital and may be classified in chapter 16 of ICD-10-CM when they are acquired before birth via the umbilicus (for example, rubella) or during birth (for example, herpes simplex). Codes are located by referring to the main term for the infection and then identifying subterms, such as "neonatal," "newborn," "congenital," "perinatal," or "maternal, affecting fetus or newborn." However, certain perinatal infections (for example, congenital syphilis) appear in chapter 1 of ICD-10-CM, Certain Infectious and Parasitic Diseases.

Infections that occur after birth but appear during the 28-day perinatal period may or may not be classified in chapter 16. When none of the subterms mentioned above is listed, the usual infection code is assigned. If an infection does not appear for a week or more after birth, the record should be reviewed to see whether there is any indication that it may be due to exposure to the infection rather than being congenital. Clarification should be sought from the physician when the record is not completely clear.

If a newborn has sepsis, assign a code from category P36, Bacterial sepsis of newborn. If the P36 code includes the causal organism, do not assign an additional code from category B95, Streptococcus, Staphylococcus, and Enterococcus as the cause of diseases classified elsewhere, or category B96, Other bacterial agents as the cause of diseases classified elsewhere. If the P36 code does not include the causal organism, assign an additional code from category B95 or B96. If applicable, use additional codes to identify severe sepsis (R65.2-) and any associated acute organ dysfunction, such as acute respiratory failure (P28.5).

As mentioned in chapter 13 of this handbook, ELISA or Western blot tests of newborns with HIV-positive mothers are often positive. This result usually indicates the antibody status of the mother rather than that of the newborn. Code **R75, Inconclusive laboratory evidence of human immunodeficiency virus (HIV),** is assigned to the newborn chart because the HIV antibodies can cross the placenta into the newborn and may persist for as long as 18 months, producing a false positive test result in the newborn. The newborn may later lose these antibodies, which means that there was never any actual HIV infection.

If a newborn tests positive for COVID-19 during the birth admission, assign first the appropriate code from category Z38, Liveborn infants according to place of birth and type of delivery, as the principal diagnosis. Additional codes for the COVID-19 infection will depend on the provider's documentation of the type of transmission. If the provider explicitly documents the COVID-19 as being contracted in utero or during the birth process, assign codes **P35.8, Other congenital viral diseases,** and **U07.1, COVID-19.** If the provider's documentation does not indicate a specific type of transmission, assign code U07.1 and the appropriate codes for any associated manifestation(s) in neonates/newborns. According to the Centers for Disease Control and Prevention, transmission of the virus responsible for COVID-19 to neonates is thought to occur primarily through respiratory droplets during the postnatal period when neonates are exposed to mothers, other caregivers, visitors, or healthcare personnel with COVID-19.

MATERNAL CONDITIONS AFFECTING THE FETUS OR NEWBORN

Codes from categories P00 through P04 are assigned only on the newborn's record and only when the maternal condition is the cause of morbidity or mortality in the newborn. The fact that the mother has a related medical condition or has experienced a complication of pregnancy, labor, or delivery does not warrant assignment of a code from these categories on the newborn's record. For example:

- A living child born to a diabetic mother in a term birth and delivered by cesarean section is coded as Z38.01. No code from the series P00 through P04 is assigned because the medical record does not document a problem affecting the newborn.

Many drugs that are taken by the mother during pregnancy can cross over the placenta to the fetus. These medications or substances may be prescribed, available over the counter, or obtained illicitly (e.g., drugs of addiction) and can adversely affect the newborn. ICD-10-CM classifies newborns affected by noxious substances transmitted via placenta or breast milk to the following codes and subcategories:

P04.0	Newborn affected by maternal anesthesia and analgesia in pregnancy, labor and delivery
P04.1-	Newborn affected by other maternal medication
P04.2	Newborn affected by maternal use of tobacco
P04.3	Newborn affected by maternal use of alcohol
P04.4-	Newborn affected by maternal use of drugs of addiction
P04.5	Newborn affected by maternal use of nutritional chemical substances
P04.6	Newborn affected by maternal exposure to environmental chemical substances
P04.8-	Newborn affected by other maternal noxious substances
P04.9	Newborn affected by maternal noxious substance, unspecified

When the newborn experiences drug withdrawal due to maternal illicit drug use, assign the appropriate code from subcategory P04.4, along with code **P96.1, Neonatal withdrawal symptoms from maternal use of drugs of addiction.** Both codes are assigned to capture the infant's withdrawal symptoms and the specific drug causing the withdrawal. Examples follow.

- A newborn delivered of a mother addicted to cocaine shows signs of withdrawal. The infant's drug screen is positive for cocaine. Assign codes **P04.41, Newborn affected by maternal use of cocaine,** and **P96.1, Neonatal withdrawal symptoms from maternal use of drugs of addiction,** on the newborn's record.

- A newborn is diagnosed with hypermagnesemia. The provider documents that the infant had developed hypermagnesemia due to the mother's treatment with magnesium sulfate for pregnancy-related eclampsia prior to delivery. Assign codes **P71.8, Other transitory neonatal disorders of calcium and magnesium metabolism,** and **P04.18, Newborn affected by other maternal medication,** on the newborn's record.

When a specific condition in the infant that resulted from the mother's condition is identified, a code for that condition is assigned rather than a code from categories P00 through P04. For example, infants born to diabetic mothers sometimes experience a transient abnormally low blood glucose level (hypoglycemia), classified as **P70.1, Syndrome of infant of a diabetic mother,** or they may have a transient diabetic state (hyperglycemia), sometimes referred to as pseudodiabetes, which is coded as **P70.2, Neonatal diabetes mellitus.** When fetal or newborn conditions result in hospitalization or other obstetric care of the mother, code assignment on the maternal record is from category O35, Maternal care for known or suspected fetal abnormality and damage, or category O36, Maternal care for other fetal problems (see chapter 23 of this handbook).

SURGICAL OPERATION ON MOTHER AND FETUS

ICD-10-CM provides several codes to capture newborns affected by amniocentesis, in utero procedures, surgery performed on the mother during pregnancy, and other maternal factors unrelated to the current pregnancy (i.e., mother's history of surgery not associated with pregnancy). These codes are only assigned on the newborn's record. If the management of the pregnancy is affected because of complications of in utero surgery, assign the appropriate code from subcategory O35.7xx-, Maternal care for (suspected) damage to fetus by other medical procedures, on the mother's record. Obstetric codes from chapter 11 of ICD-10-CM should not be used on the newborn's record.

Specific codes for a newborn affected by the mother's surgery or medical procedure unrelated to the pregnancy are as follows:

P00.6   Newborn affected by surgical procedure on mother
P00.7   Newborn affected by other medical procedures on mother, not elsewhere classified

ENDOCRINE AND METABOLIC DISTURBANCES SPECIFIC TO THE FETUS AND NEWBORN

ICD-10-CM classifies transitory endocrine and metabolic disorders specific to the newborn to categories P70 through P74. This code range includes transitory endocrine and metabolic disturbances caused by the infant's response to maternal endocrine and metabolic factors or its adjustment to the extrauterine environment.

Metabolic acidosis may be caused by renal failure, septicemia, hypoxia, hypothermia, hypotension, cardiac failure, dehydration, electrolyte disturbances, hyperglycemia, anemia, intraventricular hemorrhage, and/or metabolic disorders. The underlying cause of the acidosis must be treated to correct the problem. Late metabolic acidosis of newborn is coded to P74.0.

Transitory metabolic disturbances in the major serum electrolytes (sodium, potassium, chloride, and bicarbonate) may occur during birth or shortly thereafter. ICD-10-CM provides specific codes to differentiate between hyper- and hyponatremia and hyper- and hypokalemia as well as abnormal serum concentrations of chloride or bicarbonate as follows: hypernatremia of newborn (P74.21); hyponatremia of newborn (P74.22); hyperkalemia of newborn (P74.31); hypokalemia of newborn (P74.32); alkalosis of newborn (P74.41); hyperchloremia of newborn (P74.421); and hypochloremia of newborn (P74.422).

INFANTILE COLIC

A colicky baby is a healthy, well-fed baby who cries more than three hours a day, three days a week, for more than three weeks. The crying usually occurs at about the same time every day for no apparent reason and may be intense, with the baby having clenched fists and tensed abdominal muscles. The baby may be inconsolable. There is no known cause for colic. It may last from the first few weeks of birth through four months of age. Code **R10.83, Colic,** is assigned for infantile colic. Assign code **R10.84, Generalized abdominal pain,** for colic in an adult or a child more than 12 months old.

APPARENT LIFE-THREATENING EVENT

Apparent life-threatening event (ALTE) refers to an episode that may be characterized by any of the following signs: apnea, cyanosis, changes in muscle tone, and/or choking or gagging. It was previously referred to as near-miss sudden infant death syndrome (SIDS) or aborted crib death, but these terms should not be used because they imply an association between ALTE and SIDS. Code **R68.13, Apparent life threatening event in infant,** is assigned for ALTE in a newborn or an infant.

Because of the wide variety of presentations of the ALTE episode, signs and symptoms may be coded as additional diagnoses in any of the following circumstances:

- When no confirmed diagnosis or identifiable cause of the ALTE is established

- When signs and symptoms are not associated routinely with the confirmed cause of the ALTE

- When the reporting of signs and symptoms provides additional information about the cause of the ALTE

ROUTINE VACCINATION OF NEWBORNS

Newborns are vaccinated shortly after birth against hepatitis B and varicella. When the need for vaccination is indicated during the newborn stay, code **Z23, Encounter for immunization,** may be assigned. ICD-10-CM provides several codes in category Z28, Immunization not carried out and underimmunization status, to identify a variety of reasons why a vaccine is not administered. For example, if the newborn's vaccination is not administered because of parental refusal, assign code **Z28.82, Immunization not carried out because of caregiver refusal.** Procedure codes are required to identify the type of immunization given. In the inpatient setting, the following ICD-10-PCS codes are available to report vaccinations (although most hospitals generally do not code them):

3E0134Z	Introduction of serum, toxoid and vaccine into subcutaneous tissue, percutaneous approach
3E0234Z	Introduction of serum, toxoid and vaccine into muscle, percutaneous approach

HEALTH SUPERVISION OF INFANT OR CHILD

A code from subcategory Z00.1, Encounter for newborn, infant and child health examinations, is assigned for routine encounters of infants and children when no problem has been identified. Codes from subcategory Z00.1 are not assigned for a hospital admission.

Codes from subcategory Z00.11, Newborn health examination, are assigned for a routine examination or health check for children less than 29 days old, with an additional code to identify any abnormal findings. Code Z00.110 is used for newborns less than 8 days old, and code Z00.111 is for newborns 8 to 28 days old. Code Z00.111 includes newborn weight check.

Codes Z00.121 and Z00.129 are used for routine child health examinations for children over 28 days old and include developmental testing. Code Z00.129 is assigned when no abnormal findings are documented during the routine exam. Code Z00.121 is assigned for a routine health examination with abnormal findings. The abnormal finding can be either a condition/diagnosis that is newly found or a change in the severity of a chronic condition (e.g., uncontrolled diabetes or an acute exacerbation of a chronic condition). In this context, chronic conditions or previously diagnosed problems are not considered abnormal findings unless they are documented as either exacerbated or uncontrolled during a current well-child exam.

If any vaccinations are administered during a routine examination, also assign code **Z23, Encounter for immunization.**

EXERCISE 26.1

Code the following diagnoses and procedures as they would be assigned to a newborn's or child's record. Presume that all births were delivered in the hospital and were vaginally delivered unless stated otherwise.

1. Term birth, living male, cesarean delivery,

   with hemolytic disease due to ABO isoimmunization

2. Term birth, living child, vaginal delivery

   Physiological neonatal jaundice

3. Normal, full-term female, spontaneous vaginal delivery

   Congenital left hip subluxation

4. Newborn, male, premature (33 weeks' gestation, 1,400 grams)

   Hyaline membrane disease

5. Term birth, living male

   Ophthalmitis of newborn due to

   maternal gonococcal infection

6. Near-term birth, living male, delivered by

   cesarean section with neonatal hypoglycemia

7. Term birth, living child
   Intrauterine growth retardation

   _____

8. Premature birth, living female infant (27 weeks'
   gestation, 1,850 grams)
   Withdrawal syndrome in infant due to maternal
   heroin addiction

   _____

9. Term birth, twin, with fracture of right
   clavicle during birth

   _____

10. Five-year-old child with Erb's palsy secondary to
    birth trauma

    _____

11. Infant with hemolytic disease due to Rh isoimmunization
    (patient received by transfer from other facility)
    Skin phototherapy, single

    _____

12. Patient born in Community Hospital, with erythroblastosis
    fetalis due to ABO incompatibility; transferred immediately
    after birth to intensive care nursery at University Hospital
    for further care

    a. Codes for Community Hospital stay

    b. Code for University Hospital stay

    _____

13. Normal, male infant, delivered by cesarean section
    when fetal acidemia was noted early in labor
    Fetal distress due to cord compression

    _____

14. Newborn born on the way to hospital
    and admitted directly to newborn nursery
    Anemia due to acute blood loss from umbilical stump

    _____

15. Term birth with severe sepsis due to *E. coli* caused by
    amnionitis

---

16. Term birth, delivered with meconium
    aspiration syndrome due to prolonged labor,
    first stage
    Cord around neck of infant two times

---

17. Term birth, living male, with partial facial paralysis

---

18. Premature infant (25 weeks, 1,300 grams) transferred
    from University Hospital's intensive care
    nursery to Community Hospital for supervision
    of weight gain with diagnosis of "slow feeding"

---

19. Newborn twins, spontaneous vaginal delivery,   #1:
    twin #1 delivered in parking lot of hospital,   #2:
    twin #2 delivered after admission of mother

---

20. Term birth, living child; mother known to be a
    chronic alcoholic; newborn placed in intensive care
    nursing for observation for possible alcohol-related
    problems; none found

---

21. Routine visit to well-baby clinic for checkup;
    healthy 14-day-old infant

---

22. Term infant with sickle-cell trait born in hospital

Coding OF Circulatory System Diseases AND Neoplastic Diseases

CHAPTER 27

Diseases of the Circulatory System

CHAPTER OVERVIEW

- Circulatory disorders are classified in chapter 9 of ICD-10-CM.

- Rheumatic fever is classified with and without rheumatic heart disease.

- Ischemic heart disease is a general term for conditions affecting the myocardium.

  — Type 1 myocardial infarctions are classified with a fourth character to indicate the wall involved. They are also classified as to whether there is an ST-segment elevation.

  — The code for intermediate coronary syndrome includes a range of anginas.

  — Atherosclerosis is one of the conditions included in the category "other forms of heart disease."

- If a patient is admitted with stable angina (currently a rare practice), the underlying cause is the principal diagnosis.

- There are two main categories of heart failure—systolic and diastolic. Heart failure is further classified by left- and right-sided failure.

- The assignment and sequencing of cardiac arrest depends on the circumstances of the hospitalization. It does not matter whether the patient is resuscitated or not.

- An aneurysm is diagnosed and then classified according to its location.

  — Sometimes, a term is used to describe its appearance.

  — A term may also describe its etiology.

- Nontraumatic conditions affecting the cerebral arteries are coded together. These conditions include strokes.

- Hypertension is classified by type (primary or secondary).

- Hypertensive crisis can involve hypertensive urgency or emergency.

- Hypertension can be paired with heart disease, chronic kidney disease, or both.

- Procedures for treating circulatory disorders are varied and appear throughout this chapter of the handbook.

LEARNING OUTCOMES

After studying this chapter, you should be able to:

Classify the disorders related to the heart and the rest of the circulatory system.

Distinguish between the different conditions regarded as ischemic heart disease.

Classify heart failure by category and location.

Code for a variety of procedures involving the circulatory system and the heart.

TERMS TO KNOW

Diastolic heart failure
occurs when the heart has a problem relaxing between contractions to allow enough blood into the ventricles

Systolic heart failure
occurs when the ability of the heart to contract decreases

Thrombophlebitis of a vein
a condition indicated by a clot that has become inflamed

Thrombosis of a vein
a condition indicated by the forming of a clot

REMEMBER . . .

The range of circulatory disorders is broad and complex, requiring close attention to instructional terms.

INTRODUCTION

Chapter 9 of ICD-10-CM classifies circulatory disorders except for those that have been reclassified to chapter 15 (obstetric conditions) or to chapter 17 (congenital anomalies). This chapter covers a broad range of conditions, many of which are commonly seen for patients admitted to acute care hospitals. Because these are complex disorders and many are interrelated, it is particularly important for coding professionals to be alert to all instructional terms.

RHEUMATIC HEART DISEASE

Rheumatic heart disease occurs as the result of an infection with group A hemolytic *Streptococcus*. ICD-10-CM classifies rheumatic fever with and without rheumatic heart disease. The first axis distinguishes whether the fever is acute (I00–I02) or inactive (quiescent) (I05–I09), and the second axis determines whether there is heart involvement.

FIGURE 27.1   Major Vessels of the Arterial System

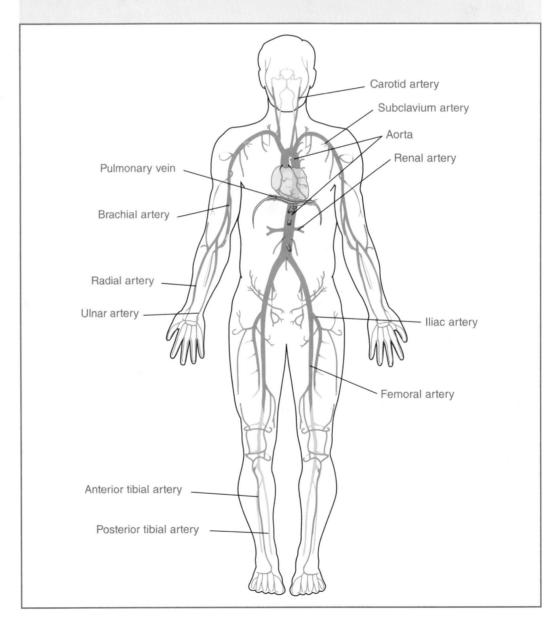

Chronic rheumatic heart disease includes heart disease that has resulted from a previously active rheumatic infection. The heart valves are most often involved. ICD-10-CM presumes that certain mitral valve disorders of unspecified etiology are rheumatic in origin. When the diagnostic statement includes more than one condition affecting the mitral valves, one of which is presumed to be rheumatic, all are classified as rheumatic. For example:

I05.0   Mitral valve stenosis
I34.0   Mitral valve insufficiency
I05.2   Mitral valve stenosis and insufficiency

In these examples, the mitral valve stenosis is presumed to be of rheumatic origin, but the mitral valve insufficiency is not. In the third example, the combination code presumes both disorders to be rheumatic because the stenosis is presumed to be rheumatic.

FIGURE 27.2   Major Vessels of the Venous System

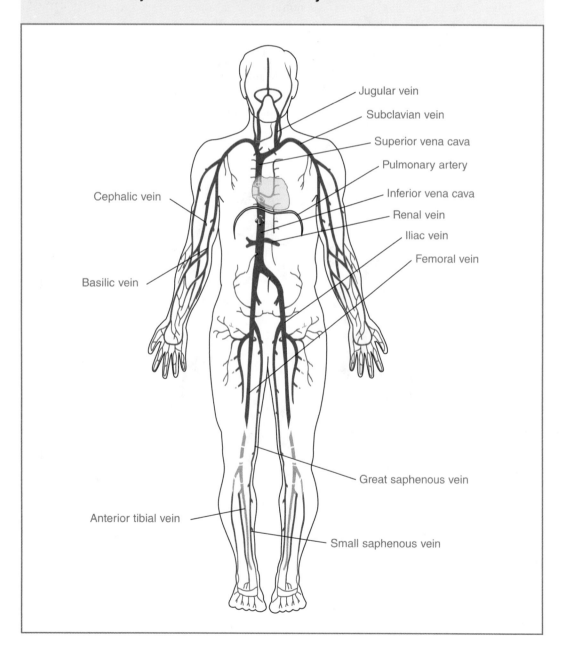

ICD-10-CM presumes that a disorder affecting both the mitral and aortic valves is rheumatic in origin. Otherwise, the aortic condition is classified as rheumatic only when specifically stated as such. For example:

I35.1   Aortic valve insufficiency
I08.0   Mitral valve insufficiency with aortic valve insufficiency
I35.0   Aortic valve stenosis
I06.0   Rheumatic aortic stenosis
I08.0   Mitral stenosis and aortic stenosis

ICD-10-CM presumes that valve insufficiency and stenosis affecting multiple valves is rheumatic in origin. For example:

I08.3   Mitral valve stenosis, aortic insufficiency and tricuspid insufficiency
I08.8   Mitral valve insufficiency, aortic insufficiency, tricuspid insufficiency and pulmonary insufficiency

When both aortic valve stenosis and mitral valve insufficiency are present, ICD-10-CM presumes the condition has a rheumatic origin. Code **I08.0, Rheumatic disorders of both mitral and aortic valves,** is assigned when the provider does not specify the cause of the valve disease. ICD-10-CM assumes rheumatic origin when valve disease affects multiple valves and the cause is not documented as nonrheumatic. Category I08, Multiple valve disease, includes multiple valve diseases specified as rheumatic or unspecified. This is a World Health Organization international default, and coding professionals must follow the conventions in the classification.

FIGURE 27.3   The Interior of the Heart

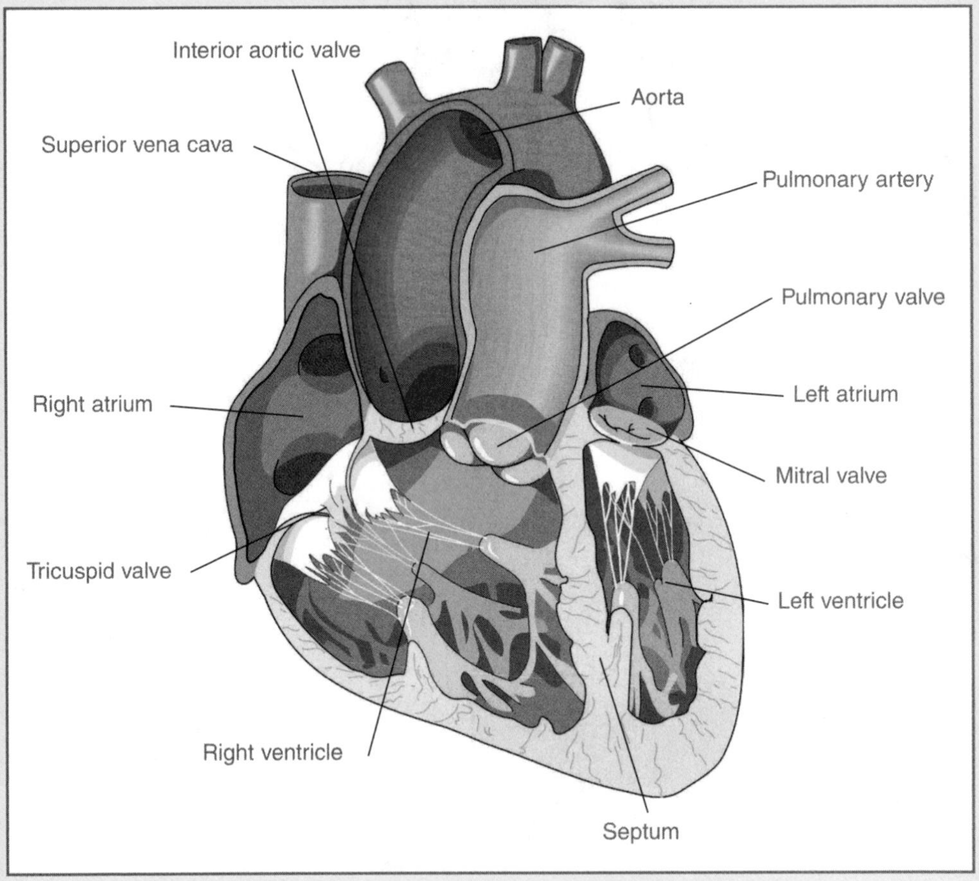

A diagnosis of heart failure in a patient who has rheumatic heart disease is classified as **I09.81, Rheumatic heart failure,** unless the physician specifies a different cause. An additional code from category I50, Heart failure, is assigned to identify the type of heart failure. However, do not assume that congestive heart failure is rheumatic in nature. Unless ICD-10-CM directs coding professionals to assign the code for "rheumatic," it is inappropriate to assign a code for rheumatic congestive heart failure. For example:

I09.81 + I50.9 + I42.0 + I05.1	End-stage congestive heart failure due to rheumatic heart disease and dilated cardiomyopathy with mitral valve insufficiency
I50.9 + I08.1 + Z95.2	Congestive heart failure, severe mitral valve regurgitation, tricuspid valve regurgitation, and a history of aortic valve stenosis status post valve replacement

EXERCISE 27.1

Code the following diagnoses.

1. Mitral regurgitation

2. Mitral valve stenosis with congestive heart failure

3. Severe mitral stenosis and mild aortic insufficiency

4. Aortic and mitral insufficiency with long-standing, persistent atrial fibrillation

5. Mitral insufficiency, congenital

6. Mitral valve insufficiency with aortic regurgitation

7. Chronic aortic and mitral valve insufficiency, rheumatic, with acute congestive heart failure due to rheumatic heart disease

ISCHEMIC HEART DISEASE

Ischemic heart disease is the general term for a number of disorders affecting the myocardium that are caused by a decrease in the blood supply to the heart due to coronary insufficiency. The insufficiency is usually caused by deposits of atheromatous material in the epicardial portions of the coronary artery that progressively obstruct its branches so that the lumen of the arteries become either partially or completely occluded. Other common terms for ischemic heart disease are arteriosclerotic heart disease, coronary ischemia, coronary artery disease, and coronary arteriosclerosis (atherosclerosis).

Ischemic heart disease is classified in categories I20 through I25 as follows:

I20   Angina pectoris

I21   Acute myocardial infarction

I22   Subsequent myocardial infarction

I23   Current complications following myocardial infarction

I24   Other acute ischemic heart disease

I25   Chronic ischemic heart disease

An additional code is used to identify hypertension (I10–I16) when present.

Angina Pectoris

Angina pectoris (category I20) is an early manifestation of ischemic heart disease; however, in rare instances, it occurs as a result of congenital abnormalities of the coronary arteries or such conditions as aortic stenosis, valvular insufficiency, aortic syphilis, or Raynaud's phenomenon. It is characterized by chest pain (usually perceived by the patient as a sensation of tightness, squeezing, pressing, choking, or burning), heartburn or gas, or an ill-defined discomfort. The pain is similar to that of unstable angina, but it is less severe, more easily controlled, and usually relieved in a predictable manner by either rest or the administration of nitroglycerin.

Angina pectoris can be produced by any activity or situation that increases the oxygen requirements of the myocardium, such as exercise, walking into the wind, cold weather, consumption of a large meal, emotional stress, or elevation of blood pressure. Angina pectoris may also occur even when the patient is at rest and without apparent stimulation, such as during the night. This condition is referred to as nocturnal or decubitus angina and is classified as I20.8. A variant type that also occurs at rest is known as Prinzmetal angina. Angina described as angiospastic, Prinzmetal, spasm induced, or variant is coded to **I20.1, Angina pectoris with documented spasm.** Code **I20.8, Other forms of angina pectoris,** includes stable angina, angina equivalent, angina of effort, and stenocardia. Symptoms associated with angina equivalent are assigned additional codes.

In today's health care environment, it is unlikely that a patient would be admitted to the hospital for treatment of stable angina except for the purpose of undergoing diagnostic studies to determine its underlying cause. In this case, sequence the combination code (I25.1-) for angina with atherosclerotic heart disease (ASHD) as the principal diagnosis when the ASHD is the underlying cause.

Code **I20.0, Unstable angina,** includes conditions described as accelerated angina, crescendo angina, de novo effort angina, intermediate coronary syndrome, preinfarction angina, or worsening effort angina. These conditions occur after less exertion has been expended than in angina pectoris; the pain is more severe and less easily relieved by nitroglycerin. Without treatment, unstable angina often progresses to acute myocardial infarction.

Code I20.0 is designated as the principal diagnosis only when the underlying condition is not identified and there is no surgical intervention. Patients with severe coronary arteriosclerosis and unstable angina may be admitted for cardiac bypass surgery or a percutaneous transluminal coronary angioplasty to prevent further progression to infarction. In such cases, the combination code for coronary arteriosclerosis with unstable angina (I25.110) is assigned as the principal diagnosis. Examples of appropriate coding follow.

- A patient is admitted with unstable angina and undergoes right and left heart catheterization, which shows coronary arteriosclerosis. A coronary bypass procedure is recommended, but the patient feels he needs some time to think it over and discuss it with his family. For this admission, the coronary arteriosclerosis with unstable angina (I25.110) is the principal diagnosis.

- A patient is admitted with unstable angina and a history of myocardial infarction five years ago. She is treated with intravenous nitroglycerin, and the angina subsides by the end of the first hospital day. No other complications are noted, and no additional diagnostic studies are carried out. In this case, the unstable angina (I20.0) is the principal diagnosis. Assign also code I25.2 to describe the old myocardial infarction.

EXERCISE 27.2

Code the following diagnoses and procedures.

---

1. Crescendo angina due to coronary arteriosclerosis

    Right and left cardiac catheterization, percutaneous

---

2. Angina pectoris with essential

    hypertension

Myocardial Infarction

The American College of Cardiology and the American Heart Association classify acute myocardial infarction (MI) into five types. When there is no information regarding the type of MI, type 1 is the default.

A spontaneous type 1 myocardial infarction (T1MI) is an acute ischemic condition that ordinarily appears following prolonged myocardial ischemia. It is usually precipitated by an occlusive coronary thrombosis at the site of an existing arteriosclerotic stenosis. Although ischemic heart disease is a progressive disorder, it is often silent for long periods with no clinical manifestations, and then it can appear suddenly in an acute form without any intervening symptoms having been experienced.

An MI described as acute or with a duration of four weeks or less is classified in category I21, ST elevation (STEMI) and non-ST elevation (NSTEMI) myocardial infarction, with a fourth character indicating the wall involved (such as anterolateral wall or inferior wall). Codes from I21.0- through I21.2- also have a fifth character to indicate the coronary artery involved (e.g., left main coronary artery). Codes I21.0- through I21.3 identify type 1 transmural infarctions; code I21.4 identifies type 1 subendocardial infarctions that do not extend through the full thickness of the myocardial wall. Diagnostic statements do not always mention the affected wall, but this information can almost always be found in the electrocardiographic report. Code **I21.3, ST elevation (STEMI) myocardial infarction of unspecified site,** includes a type 1 ST elevation myocardial infarction of unspecified site. Code I21.3 should not be assigned unless no information regarding the site is documented in the medical record. If only STEMI or transmural MI without the site is documented, query the provider as to the site, or assign code I21.3.

Type 1 MIs can also be classified according to whether there is ST-segment elevation (codes I21.0- through I21.3) or non-ST-segment elevation (code I21.4). STEMI and NSTEMI share the same pathophysiology, and both are considered type 1 MIs. If there is no information regarding whether there is ST elevation or non-ST elevation, or information regarding the site of the MI, assign code **I21.9, Acute myocardial infarction, unspecified.** If an MI is documented as nontransmural or subendocardial, but the site is provided, it is still coded as a subendocardial MI. Acute MIs specified by site (except subendocardial or nontransmural MIs), and not described as either STEMI or NSTEMI, are coded as acute STEMI by site.

If a type 1 NSTEMI evolves to an STEMI, assign the code for the STEMI. If an STEMI converts to an NSTEMI due to thrombolytic therapy, assign the code for STEMI. Be careful to note that these codes are used for documented acute MIs and should not be confused with abnormal findings on electrocardiograms (EKGs) of ST-segment elevation.

An acute type 2 MI (T2MI) can occur secondary to cardiac stress due to other causes (i.e., demand ischemia or ischemic imbalance, resulting from a supply-and-demand mismatch), without atherosclerotic plaque rupture, but with myocardial necrosis. Code **I21.A1, Myocardial infarction type 2,** is assigned for a T2MI. Code first the underlying cause, such as anemia, chronic obstructive pulmonary disease, paroxysmal tachycardia, and so forth.

In a type 3 MI (T3MI), the patient expires from a presumed cardiac etiology without confirmatory cardiac biomarkers. Myocardial infarctions associated with revascularization procedures are classified as type 4 and type 5 MIs. Type 4 MI (T4MI) occurs in the context of percutaneous coronary intervention (PCI) and/or stent implantation. There are subclassifications of T4MIs (e.g., 4a, 4b, and 4c) reflecting the different contexts in which biomarkers can turn positive in percutaneous coronary intervention (PCI) procedures. Type 5 MI (T5MI) is related to coronary artery bypass graft surgery. Code **I21.A9, Other myocardial infarction type,** is assigned for types 3, 4a, 4b, 4c, and 5 MIs. If the T4MI or T5MI is postprocedural following cardiac surgery, assign first, if applicable, code **I97.190, Other postprocedural cardiac functional disturbances following cardiac surgery.**

When the MI meets the definition of a reportable diagnosis, codes from category I21 may continue to be reported for the duration of four weeks (28 days) or fewer from onset, regardless of the health care setting. This includes patients who are transferred from the acute care setting to the post–acute care setting within the four-week time frame. For encounters after the four-week time frame in which the patient requires continued care related to the MI, assign the appropriate aftercare code, rather than a code from category I21. Otherwise, code **I25.2, Old myocardial infarction,** may be assigned for an old or healed MI not requiring further care.

Troponins are proteins found in skeletal and cardiac muscle fibers that regulate muscular contraction. Troponin tests measure the level of cardiac-specific troponin in the blood to evaluate whether a patient has experienced an acute MI. **Assign code R79.89, Other specified abnormal findings of blood chemistry,** for an abnormal troponin test without a diagnosis of acute myocardial infarction.

When a patient has a new type 1 MI within four weeks of an acute type 1 MI, a code from category I22, Subsequent ST elevation (STEMI) and non-ST elevation (NSTEMI) myocardial infarction, should be used in conjunction with a code from category I21. The sequencing of the I21 and I22 codes depends on the circumstances of admission.

If a subsequent myocardial infarction of one type occurs within four weeks of a myocardial infarction of a different type, assign the appropriate codes from category I21 to identify each type. Do not assign a code from category I22. Codes from category I22 should only be assigned if both the initial and subsequent myocardial infarctions are type 1 or unspecified. Subsequent type 2, 4, or 5 MIs are coded by type rather than by using codes from category I22.

Figure 27.4 illustrates a process for sequencing an acute type 1 MI and a subsequent type 1 MI. Part A shows a decision tree for a patient admitted for acute MI. Part B shows a decision tree for a patient admitted due to conditions other than acute MI who has an acute MI during this admission.

Examples illustrating the sequencing of acute type 1 MI codes are as follows:

- A patient is admitted to the hospital due to an acute MI and has a subsequent acute MI within four weeks while still in the hospital. Code I21.- is sequenced first as the reason for the admission, with code I22.- sequenced as a secondary code.

- A patient suffers a subsequent acute MI after discharge for care of an initial acute MI that occurred 18 days earlier. The I22 code should be sequenced first, followed by the I21 code. An I21 code must accompany an I22 code to identify the site of the initial acute MI and to indicate that the patient is still within the four-week time frame of healing from the initial acute MI.

The guidelines for assigning the correct code from category I22 are the same as for the initial MI.

FIGURE 27.4 Decision Tree for Coding Acute Type 1 Myocardial Infarction

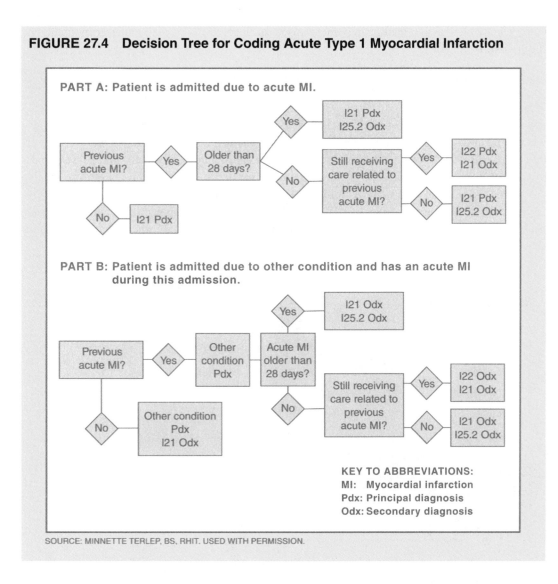

Patients with acute MI sometimes experience an associated postinfarction hypotension. In this situation, the code for the acute MI is sequenced first, with an additional code of **I95.89, Other hypotension.**

For both acute MIs and subsequent MIs, additional codes may be assigned to identify risk factors, such as the following:

Z77.22	Exposure to environmental tobacco smoke
Z87.891	History of nicotine dependence
Z57.31	Occupational exposure to environmental tobacco smoke
F17.-	Nicotine dependence
Z72.0	Tobacco use

Evolving Myocardial Infarction

An evolving myocardial infarction sometimes precipitates right ventricular failure that progresses to congestive heart failure. The patient may then be admitted because of this precursor condition, which then progresses to an acute myocardial infarction. After study, the principal diagnosis in this situation is the infarction, with an additional code assigned for the heart failure. Additional codes should also be assigned for any mention of cardiogenic shock, ventricular arrhythmia, and fibrillation. For example:

I21.09 + I50.9 + I49.01   Congestive heart failure with acute myocardial infarction of anterolateral wall with ventricular fibrillation

If the infarction is described as old or healed, review the medical record to determine whether the infarction is actually old and/or healed or whether the diagnosis refers to a more recent infarction still under care. A diagnosis of old myocardial infarction is usually made on the basis of electrocardiographic findings or some other investigation in a patient who is not experiencing symptoms. Code **I25.2, Old myocardial infarction,** is essentially a history code, even though it is not included in the Z-code chapter of ICD-10-CM. It should not be assigned when current ischemic heart disease is present and should be assigned as an additional code only when it has some significance for the current episode of care.

EXERCISE 27.3

Code the following diagnoses; do not code procedures.

---

1. A patient felt well until around 10:00 p.m., when he began having severe chest pain, which continued to increase in severity. He was brought to the emergency department by ambulance. There was no previous history of cardiac disease, but the EKG showed an acute posterolateral myocardial infarction, and the patient was admitted immediately for further care.

---

2. A patient with compensated congestive heart failure on Lasix began to have extreme difficulty in breathing and was brought to the emergency department, where she was found to be in congestive failure. Because it was thought that an impending infarction was possible, a percutaneous transluminal coronary angioplasty was performed, but the patient went on to have an acute inferolateral infarction.

---

3. A patient was admitted with acute myocardial infarction involving the left main coronary artery with no history of previous infarction or previous care for this episode. A week later during the hospital stay, he also experienced an acute anterolateral infarction.

---

4. A patient was admitted to Community Hospital with severe chest pain, which was identified as an acute anterolateral wall infarction (no history of earlier care). Patient was transferred to University Hospital two days later for angioplasty, returned to

Community Hospital after three days at University to continue

recovery, and stayed for four days.

Code for first admission to Community Hospital

Code for transfer to University Hospital

Code for transfer back to Community Hospital

---

5. The patient in the situation described in item 4 above

    was readmitted to Community Hospital a week later

    because she was having severe chest pains and was

    diagnosed with a new inferior wall MI.

Current Complications Following Myocardial Infarction

ICD-10-CM provides codes within category I23 to identify current complications following acute myocardial infarctions when those complications occur within the 28-day period, as follows:

I23.0   Hemopericardium

I23.1   Atrial septal defect

I23.2   Ventricular septal defect

I23.3   Rupture of cardiac wall without hemopericardium

I23.4   Rupture of chordae tendineae

I23.5   Rupture of papillary muscle

I23.6   Thrombosis of atrium, auricular appendage, and ventricle

I23.7   Postinfarction angina

I23.8   Other complications

A code from category I23 must be used in conjunction with a code from category I21 or category I22. Sequencing of the code from category I23 will depend on the circumstances of admission, as follows:

- If the complication of the MI is the reason for the encounter, the I23 code should be sequenced first.

- If the complication of the MI occurs during the encounter for the MI, the I23 code should be sequenced after the I21 or I22 code.

Other Acute Ischemic Heart Disease

A diagnosis of acute ischemic heart disease or acute myocardial ischemia does not always indicate an infarction. It is often possible to prevent infarction by means of surgery and/or the use of thrombolytic agents if the patient is treated promptly. If there is occlusion or thrombosis of the artery without infarction, code **I24.0, Acute coronary thrombosis not resulting in myocardial infarction,** is assigned. Code **I24.8, Other forms of acute ischemic heart disease,** includes coronary insufficiency and subendocardial ischemia. If the patient presents for treatment of an acute type 2 myocardial infarction caused by demand ischemia, assign code **I21.A1, Myocardial infarction type 2,** rather than code I24.8.

Assign code **I51.89, Other ill-defined heart diseases,** for nontraumatic myocardial injury not specified as an acute myocardial infarction.

Postmyocardial Infarction Syndrome and Postmyocardial Angina

Patients with acute myocardial infarction sometimes experience postmyocardial infarction syndrome (I24.1). Postmyocardial infarction, also called Dressler's syndrome, is a pericarditis characterized by fever, leukocytosis, pleurisy, pleural effusion, joint pains, and occasionally pneumonia. No codes from category I20, Angina pectoris, nor from category I30, Acute pericarditis, can be used with codes from category I24.

Patients with acute myocardial infarction may also experience angina described as postinfarction angina (I23.7). Codes from category I20, Angina pectoris, cannot be used with code **I23.7, Postinfarction angina.** Codes from category I23 must be used in conjunction with a code from category I21 or category I22 to identify the acute or subsequent myocardial infarction. Sequencing depends on the circumstances of admission.

Postinfarction angina together with atherosclerosis is another form of angina and is coded to I25.118. It is not appropriate to use code **I25.10, Atherosclerotic heart disease of native coronary artery without angina pectoris,** because the postinfarction angina is present. For example:

- A patient with known atherosclerotic coronary artery disease who presents with an acute non-ST elevation myocardial infarction subsequently develops postinfarction angina. Code **I21.4, Non-ST elevation (NSTEMI) myocardial infarction,** is assigned as the principal diagnosis. Code **I23.7, Postinfarction angina,** and code **I25.118, Atherosclerotic heart disease of native coronary artery with other forms of angina pectoris,** are assigned as secondary diagnoses.

EXERCISE 27.4

Code the following diagnoses.

---

1. Acute myocardial infarction, transmural inferolateral wall
   Third-degree atrioventricular block

---

2. Acute myocardial infarction of inferoposterior wall
   Congestive heart failure
   Hypertension

---

3. Impending myocardial infarction (crescendo angina)
   resulting in occlusion of coronary artery

---

4. Acute coronary insufficiency

---

5. Hemopericardium as a complication of acute
   myocardial infarction of the inferior wall, which
   occurred three weeks ago; patient had been
   discharged a week before

Chronic Ischemic Heart Disease

Category I25, Chronic ischemic heart disease, includes such conditions as coronary atherosclerosis, old myocardial infarction, coronary artery dissection, chronic coronary insufficiency, myocardial ischemia, and aneurysm of heart. Diagnoses of coronary artery disease or coronary heart disease without any further qualification are too vague to be coded accurately; the physician should be asked to provide a more specific diagnosis. Code **I25.9, Chronic ischemic heart disease, unspecified,** should rarely be assigned in an acute care hospital setting.

Subcategory I25.1-, Atherosclerotic heart disease of native coronary artery, includes conditions described as atherosclerotic cardiovascular disease, coronary (artery) atheroma, coronary artery disease, and coronary artery sclerosis. The fifth character indicates the presence or absence of angina pectoris, with a sixth character specifying the type of angina (unstable, with documented spasm, other, or unspecified).

ICD-10-CM has combination codes for atherosclerotic heart disease with angina pectoris, which are included in subcategories I25.11 and I25.7. It is not necessary to use an additional code for angina pectoris when these combination codes are used. A causal relationship can be assumed in a patient with both atherosclerosis and angina pectoris, unless the documentation indicates that the angina is due to a condition other than atherosclerosis. If a patient with coronary artery disease is admitted due to an acute myocardial infarction, the acute MI should be sequenced before the coronary artery disease.

Subcategory I25.7, Atherosclerosis of coronary artery bypass graft(s) and coronary artery of transplanted heart with angina pectoris, includes a fifth character to provide additional information on the type of bypass graft (unspecified, autologous vein, autologous artery, nonautologous biological coronary artery bypass graft, native artery of transplanted heart, bypass graft of coronary artery of transplanted heart). A sixth character specifies the type of angina pectoris (unstable, with documented spasm, other, or unspecified). For atherosclerosis of other coronary vessels without angina pectoris, codes from I25.81-, Atherosclerosis of other coronary vessels without angina pectoris, are reported. The sixth character indicates the type of coronary artery (bypass graft, native artery of transplanted heart, or bypass graft of transplanted heart).

Atherosclerosis of the native coronary arteries and bypass grafts is classified as follows:

I25.10	Native coronary artery without angina pectoris
	Unspecified type of vessel, native or graft
I25.710	Autologous vein bypass graft with unstable angina
I25.810	Nonautologous biological bypass graft without angina
	Artery bypass graft, including internal mammary artery
	Unspecified type of bypass graft
I25.750	Native coronary artery of transplanted heart with unstable angina
I25.812	Bypass graft (artery) (vein) of transplanted heart

Physicians rarely include information regarding the type of graft in the diagnostic statement, but it is almost always available in the medical record. If the medical record makes it clear that there has been no previous bypass surgery, a code from subcategory I25.1, Atherosclerotic heart disease of native coronary artery, can be assigned. If there is atherosclerosis of a previous bypass graft and information indicating the material used in the bypass is available, a code from I25.70- through I25.73-, I25.79-, or I25.810 should be assigned. Note that arteriosclerosis of a bypass vessel is not classified as a postoperative complication.

When atherosclerosis of a native coronary artery in a transplanted heart is identified in the diagnostic statement, code I25.75- or I25.811 is assigned. Code I25.76- or code **I25.812, Atherosclerosis of bypass graft of coronary artery of transplanted heart,** is assigned to identify atherosclerosis of a bypass graft in a transplanted heart.

Chronic Total Occlusion

A chronic total occlusion of a coronary artery (I25.82) involves complete blockage of a coronary artery that has been present for an extended period (e.g., months or years). The chronic total occlusion develops when plaque accumulates in the artery, leading to a substantial reduction in blood flow and the development of bypass collateral blood flow. Although well-developed collaterals do not completely compensate for diminished blood flow, they help to preserve the viability of the myocardium and prevent resting ischemia. Patients with chronic total occlusion who present with a change in anginal status that is directly related to physical activity have an increased risk of myocardial infarction or death. Chronic total occlusion of a coronary artery may be treated with angioplasty (root operation "Dilation") or stent placement, usually a drug-eluting stent. These types of obstructions are more resistant to guide wire crossing and are more difficult to treat than other types of coronary stenosis. Advanced methods in treatment have been developed to specifically handle chronic total coronary occlusions.

Code I25.82 should be used as an additional code assignment if coronary atherosclerosis (code series I25.1-, I25.7-, I25.81-) is present with a chronic total occlusion of a coronary artery. An excludes1 note explains that code I25.82 should not be assigned if the patient is also diagnosed with acute coronary occlusion or an acute myocardial infarction. However, both conditions can be coded when the culprit lesion responsible for the myocardial infarction (I21.-, I22.-) is in a different vessel than the chronic total occlusion. This is an exception to the excludes1 instruction.

Code **I25.83, Coronary atherosclerosis due to lipid rich plaque,** describes coronary atherosclerosis with the exact composition of the atherosclerotic plaque. The presence of lipid rich atherosclerotic plaque can precipitate an acute coronary event. The identification of plaque as lipid rich or non–lipid rich is clinically significant because this information can assist interventional cardiologists in determining the correct treatment (i.e., drug-eluting stent or non-drug-eluting stent). Near infrared spectroscopy (8E023DZ) is a new intravascular diagnostic tool that can detect and differentiate lipid rich atherosclerotic plaque. When the provider documents lipid rich plaque, the appropriate code for the coronary atherosclerosis (I25.1-, I25.7-, I25.81-) should be sequenced first, followed by code I25.83 as an additional code assignment.

Code **I25.84, Coronary atherosclerosis due to calcified coronary lesion,** is used to differentiate calcified coronary lesions from other ischemic coronary lesions. The calcium deposits in these types of lesions present a rigid obstacle that can result in an increased risk for complications, such as inadequate stent expansion, acute stent thrombosis, and restenosis, when treated by angioplasty with stent placement. When coding a calcified coronary lesion, sequence first the appropriate coronary atherosclerosis code (I25.1-, I25.7-, I25.81-), followed by code I25.84.

HEART FAILURE

Heart failure occurs when an abnormality of cardiac function results in the inability of the heart to pump blood at a rate commensurate with the body's needs or the ability to do so only from an abnormal filling pressure. This decrease in blood supply to body tissue results in unmet needs for oxygen as well as in a failure to meet other metabolic requirements. This in turn results in pulmonary and/or systemic circulatory congestion and reduced cardiac output. Precipitating causes of heart failure include cardiac arrhythmias, pulmonary embolism, infections, anemia, thyrotoxicosis, myocarditis, endocarditis, hypertension, and myocardial infarction.

All codes for heart failure include any associated pulmonary edema; therefore, no additional code for this edema is assigned. A diagnosis of acute pulmonary edema in the absence of underlying heart disease is classified with conditions affecting the respiratory system. (See chapter 18 of this handbook for more information on the respiratory system.)

There are two main categories of heart failure: systolic and diastolic. Systolic heart failure (I50.2-) occurs when the ability of the heart to contract decreases. Diastolic heart failure (I50.3-)

occurs when the heart has a problem relaxing between contractions (diastole) to allow enough blood to enter the ventricles. Heart failure with combined systolic (congestive) and diastolic (congestive) heart failure is assigned code I50.4-. Fifth characters further specify whether the heart failure is unspecified, acute, chronic, or acute on chronic. Other classifications of heart failure include right heart failure, unspecified (I50.810); acute right heart failure (I50.811); chronic right heart failure (I50.812); acute on chronic right heart failure (I50.813); right heart failure due to left heart failure (I50.814); biventricular heart failure (I50.82); high output heart failure (I50.83); end stage heart failure (I50.84); other heart failure (I50.89); and heart failure, unspecified (I50.9).

A more contemporary term for diastolic heart failure is heart failure with preserved ejection fraction (HFpEF). Contemporary terms for systolic heart failure include heart failure with reduced ejection fraction (HFrEF), heart failure with low ejection fraction, and heart failure with reduced systolic function. HFpEF and HFrEF can be further described as acute or chronic. When the provider has documented HFpEF, HFrEF, or other similar terms, coding professionals may interpret the diagnosis to be "diastolic heart failure" or "systolic heart failure," respectively (or a combination of both diastolic and systolic heart failure, if indicated), and assign the appropriate ICD-10-CM codes. These new terms have now been incorporated as inclusion terms under the respective ICD-10-CM codes.

The term "congestive heart failure" is often mistakenly used interchangeably with "heart failure." Congestion—pulmonary or systemic fluid buildup—is one feature of heart failure, but it does not occur in all patients. Congestive heart failure is included in the codes for systolic and diastolic heart failure. Therefore, when the diagnostic statement lists congestive heart failure along with either systolic or diastolic heart failure, only the code for the type of heart failure is assigned: diastolic and/or systolic. If congestive heart failure is documented without further specification, it is classified to **I50.9, Heart failure, unspecified.**

Heart dysfunction without mention of heart failure is indexed to **I51.89, Other ill-defined heart diseases.** It is not appropriate to assume that a patient is in heart failure when only "diastolic dysfunction" or "systolic dysfunction" is documented. When the provider has linked either diastolic or systolic dysfunction with acute or chronic heart failure, it should be coded as "acute/chronic diastolic or systolic heart failure." For example, assign code **I50.31, Acute diastolic (congestive) heart failure,** when the provider links acute heart failure with diastolic dysfunction. If there is no provider documentation linking the two conditions, assign code **I50.9, Heart failure, unspecified.**

Heart failure is differentiated clinically by whether the right or left ventricle is primarily affected. Left-sided heart failure (left ventricular failure) is due to the accumulation of excess fluid behind the left ventricle. Code **I50.1, Left ventricular failure,** includes associated conditions such as dyspnea, orthopnea, bronchospasm, cardiac asthma, edema of lung with heart disease, edema of lung with heart failure, left heart failure, pulmonary edema with heart disease, and pulmonary edema with heart failure; therefore, no additional codes are assigned for these conditions. Heart failure, unspecified, is coded to I50.9. However, because I50.9 is a vague code, an effort should be made to determine whether a code from the series I50.1 through I50.8- is more appropriate.

Right-sided failure ordinarily follows left-sided failure, and right heart failure due to left heart failure is assigned code I50.814. This code includes any left-sided failure that is present; therefore, only code I50.814 is required. Code also the type of left ventricular failure, if known (I50.2–I50.43).

Providers may occasionally document "stage A heart failure." The American Heart Association defines "stage A heart failure" as the presence of heart failure risk factors—but no heart disease and no symptoms. (Although at risk for developing the condition, these patients do not have heart failure.) Code **Z91.89, Other specified personal risk factors, not elsewhere classified,** is assigned to capture the increased risk. If other conditions and/or factors influence risk—such as hypertension, coronary artery disease, valvular disease, and so forth—assign additional codes for those conditions.

Compensated, Decompensated, and Exacerbated Heart Failure

When heart failure occurs, the heart muscle commonly develops compensatory mechanisms such as cardiac hypertrophy, raised arterial pressure, ventricular dilation, or increased force of contraction. When compensatory mechanisms develop, the heart failure may be described as *compensated,* permitting near-normal function. When these compensatory mechanisms can no longer meet the increased workload, decompensation of the heart function results; this situation is often described as decompensated heart failure. Code assignment is not affected by the use of these terms; the code for the type of heart failure is assigned. An exacerbation is an increase in the severity of a disease or any of its symptoms. The terms "exacerbated" and "decompensated" indicate that there has been a flare-up (acute phase) of a chronic condition. An acute exacerbation of a chronic condition (such as heart failure) is coded as acute on chronic. For example:

- A patient with a known history of congestive heart failure is admitted with an exacerbation of diastolic congestive heart failure. Code **I50.33, Acute on chronic diastolic (congestive) heart failure,** is assigned.

Hypertensive Heart Disease and Heart Failure

Hypertensive heart disease (with or without heart failure) is classified in category I11, with a code from category I50 to identify the type of heart failure (if present) as an additional diagnosis. If chronic kidney disease (N18.-) or unspecified contracted kidney (N26.-) due to hypertension or arteriosclerosis of kidney, arteriosclerotic nephritis, hypertensive nephropathy, or nephrosclerosis is present, a code from category I12 is assigned. The appropriate code from N18.1–N18.6 or N18.9 is assigned as an additional diagnosis to identify the stage of chronic kidney disease. If hypertensive heart disease and hypertensive chronic kidney disease are present, a code from category I13 is used. Category I13 provides different codes to indicate hypertensive heart and chronic kidney disease with or without heart failure as well as the stage of the chronic kidney disease. When using a code from category I13, also assign a code from category I50 to identify the type of heart failure (if present) and a code from N18.1–N18.6 or N18.9 to identify the stage of chronic kidney disease. When a hypertensive crisis such as hypertensive urgency or emergency is documented along with hypertensive heart or chronic kidney disease or a combination of both diseases, a code from category I16, Hypertensive crisis, is assigned along with a code from categories I11, I12, or I13. Further information in classifying hypertension and other associated conditions is provided later in this chapter.

CARDIAC TAMPONADE

Cardiac tamponade (I31.4), also referred to as pericardial tamponade or tamponade, is the compression of the heart caused by the accumulation of fluid inside the pericardium. Cardiac tamponade is often associated with viral or bacterial pericarditis. This condition typically occurs as a result of chest trauma, heart rupture, dissecting aortic aneurysm, cancer, cardiac surgery, renal failure, and/ or acute myocardial infarction. The underlying cause of the tamponade should be sequenced first, followed by code I31.4.

Cardiac tamponade can be life threatening if left untreated. The goals of therapy are to improve heart function, relieve symptoms, and treat the tamponade. This can be accomplished with pericardiocentesis (root operation "Drainage," body part "pericardial cavity") or creation of a pericardial window (root operation "Drainage," body part "pericardium").

For example, a patient develops increased pericardial effusion and undergoes pericardiocentesis (percutaneous approach) due to rapid pericardial tamponade. Assign code **I31.4, Cardiac tamponade.** For the procedure, assign code **0W9D3ZZ, Drainage of pericardial cavity, percutaneous approach.**

CARDIOMYOPATHY

Cardiomyopathy (I42.-) presents a clinical picture of a dilated heart, flabby heart muscles, and normal coronary arteries. Hypertrophic cardiomyopathy (HCM) is a condition, usually inherited, in which the heart muscle becomes thickened without any obvious cause. It is a known cause of sudden cardiac death in younger athletes, and young people are more likely to develop a more severe form of hypertrophic cardiomyopathy than older adults. HCM can be either obstructive (I42.1) or nonobstructive (I42.2) and is frequently asymptomatic until sudden cardiac death. Common types of cardiomyopathy are the following:

I42.0   Dilated cardiomyopathy, which includes congestive cardiomyopathy

I42.1   Obstructive hypertrophic cardiomyopathy, including idiopathic hypertrophic subaortic stenosis

I42.2   Other hypertrophic cardiomyopathy, including nonobstructive hypertrophic cardiomyopathy

I42.3   Endomyocardial (eosinophilic) disease, including endomyocardial (tropical) fibrosis and Löffler's endocarditis

I42.4   Endocardial fibroelastosis, including congenital cardiomyopathy and elastomyofibrosis

I42.5   Other restrictive cardiomyopathy, including constrictive cardiomyopathy not otherwise specified

I42.6   Alcoholic cardiomyopathy due to alcohol consumption: a code for alcoholism (F10.-) is also assigned if present

I42.7   Cardiomyopathy due to drug and external agent: code first the poisoning due to drug or toxin, if applicable (T36–T65 with fifth or sixth character 1–4 or 6); if the condition is caused by an adverse effect, use an additional code, if applicable, to identify the drug (T36–T50 with fifth or sixth character 5)

I42.8   Other cardiomyopathies

I42.9   Unspecified cardiomyopathy

Congestive cardiomyopathy (I42.0) has essentially the same symptoms as congestive heart failure, and the condition is often associated with congestive heart failure. Treatment ordinarily revolves around management of the congestive heart failure. Therefore, heart failure (I50.-) is designated as the principal diagnosis, with an additional code assigned for the cardiomyopathy.

Two codes may be required for cardiomyopathy due to other underlying conditions; for example, cardiomyopathy due to amyloidosis is coded **E85.4, Organ-limited amyloidosis,** and **I43, Cardiomyopathy in diseases classified elsewhere.** The underlying disease, amyloidosis, is sequenced first. Hypertensive cardiomyopathy should be coded to category I11, Hypertensive heart disease, with I43 assigned as an additional code. Assign first code **G71.11, Myotonic muscular dystrophy,** with I43 as an additional code assignment for cardiomyopathy due to myotonia atrophica.

The term "ischemic cardiomyopathy" is sometimes used to designate a condition in which ischemic heart disease causes diffuse fibrosis or multiple infarction, leading to heart failure with left ventricular dilation. This is not a true cardiomyopathy and is coded to **I25.5, Ischemic cardiomyopathy,** when no further clarification is provided by the attending physician.

CARDIAC ARREST

Code **I46.9, Cardiac arrest, cause unspecified,** may be assigned as a principal or first-listed diagnosis if the underlying condition is unknown. It does not matter whether the patient is resuscitated. The assignment and sequencing of code I46.9 is dependent on the circumstances of the hospitalization. If the patient is admitted due to cardiac arrest and an underlying cause is not established before the patient is discharged or expires, it is appropriate to assign code I46.9 as the principal or first-listed diagnosis.

I46.9 may be assigned as a secondary code when cardiac arrest occurs during the hospital episode and the cause of the arrest is unknown. If the provider indicates a cardiac cause for the arrest, the underlying cardiac condition is designated as the principal diagnosis, with code **I46.2, Cardiac arrest due to underlying cardiac condition,** as an additional code. If the provider indicates a noncardiac cause, code **I46.8, Cardiac arrest due to other underlying condition,** is assigned as an additional code.

Some providers may document pulseless electrical activity (PEA) rather than cardiac arrest. PEA refers to electrical activity on a monitor without a detectable pulse. It is one of the rhythms that cause a pulseless cardiac arrest. PEA usually has some underlying cause that can be treated; the most common cause in emergency situations is hypovolemia. PEA can be caused by respiratory failure with hypoxia, as the cardiac muscle in this case is unable to generate a sufficient force despite an electrical depolarization. True PEA is the absence of myocardial contraction despite coordinated electrical activity. Code **I46.9, Cardiac arrest, cause unspecified,** may be assigned as a principal or first-listed diagnosis if the underlying condition causing the PEA is unknown. Note that codes are not assigned for symptoms integral to the condition, such as bradycardia and hypotension.

Asystole is a medical term used to describe a cardiac arrest rhythm, in which there is no discernible electrical activity on electrocardiogram (EKG). In the Alphabetic Index of Diseases and Injuries, the entry for the term **Asystole (heart)** instructs users to see **Arrest, cardiac.** However, asystole is not coded as cardiac arrest when a brief pause of electrical activity with spontaneous recovery of sinus rhythm is noted on an EKG. For example, a patient was admitted due to syncopal episodes and was diagnosed with a complete heart block. He underwent implantation of a dual chamber permanent pacemaker. The cardiologist noted that the EKG showed a complete atrioventricular block with periods of asystole over six seconds with conversion to sinus bradycardia. There was no mention of cardiac arrest. Assign only code **I44.2, Atrioventricular block, complete.** In this case, the brief pause noted on EKG was due to the complete heart block.

Cardiac arrest that occurs as a complication of surgery is coded as **I97.710, Intraoperative cardiac arrest during cardiac surgery,** or **I97.711, Intraoperative cardiac arrest during other surgery,** depending on the type of surgery. Code **O75.4, Other complications of obstetric surgery and procedures,** is assigned for cardiac arrest complicating obstetric surgery or procedures.

Note that none of these cardiac arrest codes is assigned to indicate that a patient has died. Therefore, do not code cardiac arrest to indicate a patient's death.

ANEURYSM

An aneurysm is a localized abnormal dilation of blood vessels. A dissecting aneurysm is one in which blood enters the wall of the artery and separates the layers of the vessel wall. As the aneurysm progresses, tension increases and the aneurysm is likely to rupture, which usually results in death.

Aneurysms are diagnosed primarily according to their location, such as the following:

I25.41	Coronary artery aneurysm
I71.02	Dissecting aneurysm of abdominal aorta
I71.3	Aneurysm of abdominal aorta with rupture
I71.2	Aneurysm of thoracic artery
I71.1	Ruptured aneurysm of thoracic artery
I71.6	Thoracoabdominal aneurysm
I72.5	Aneurysm of other precerebral arteries
I72.6	Aneurysm of vertebral artery
I77.70	Dissection of unspecified artery
I77.74	Dissection of vertebral artery
I77.75	Dissection of other precerebral arteries
I77.76	Dissection of artery of upper extremity

I77.77   Dissection of artery of lower extremity

I77.79   Dissection of other specified artery

Occasionally, a term describing the aneurysm's appearance is used, such as "berry aneurysm" (I67.1), or a term may describe its etiology, such as "syphilitic aneurysm of aorta" (A52.01) or "traumatic aneurysm" (S25.00-, S25.20-).

CEREBROVASCULAR DISORDERS

Acute organic (nontraumatic) conditions affecting the cerebral arteries include hemorrhage, infarction, occlusion, and thrombosis and are coded in the I60–I68 series. Category I63, Cerebral infarction, is used to describe occlusion and stenosis of cerebral and precerebral arteries resulting in cerebral infarction. Please refer to figure 27.5 for an illustration of the types of cerebral infarction. Category I63 is subdivided on the basis of whether the cerebral infarction is due to thrombosis, embolism, occlusion, or stenosis and whether it is a precerebral or cerebral artery, with sixth characters identifying the artery and laterality (e.g., right carotid artery, right middle cerebral artery, or bilateral carotid arteries). A cerebral infarction may occasionally be caused by a bilateral arterial lesion.

Codes from category I63 should not be assigned unless cerebral infarction is clearly documented in the medical record and the physician has indicated a relationship between the infarction and the cerebral artery thrombosis, embolism, occlusion, or stenosis. Never assume that infarction has occurred. These codes apply to the current episode of care only; they do not indicate that the patient has had a cerebral infarction in the past.

FIGURE 27.5   Types of Cerebral Infarction

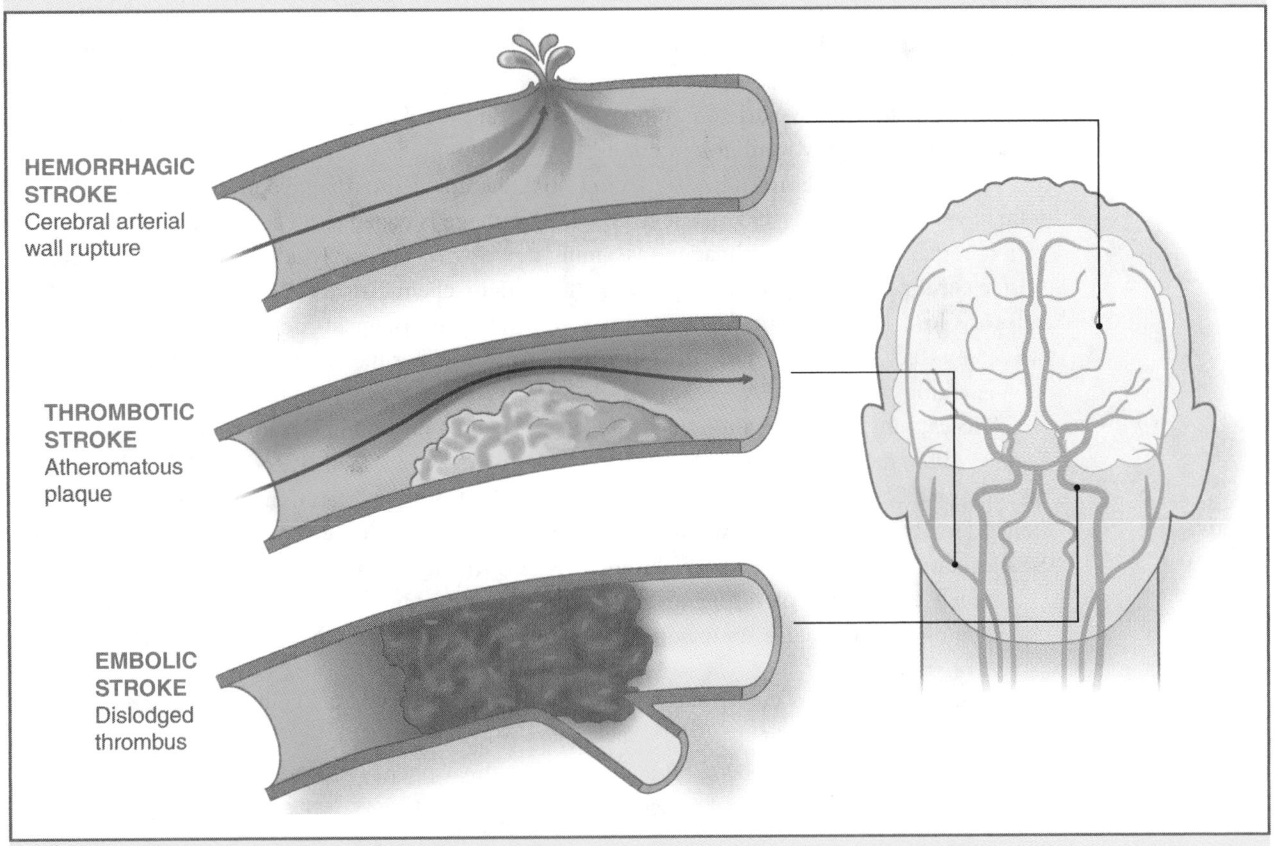

HEMORRHAGIC STROKE
Cerebral arterial wall rupture

THROMBOTIC STROKE
Atheromatous plaque

EMBOLIC STROKE
Dislodged thrombus

When occlusion and stenosis of precerebral or cerebral arteries are documented without mention of cerebral infarction, codes from category I65, Occlusion and stenosis of precerebral arteries, not resulting in cerebral infarction, or category I66, Occlusion and stenosis of cerebral arteries, not resulting in cerebral infarction, should be used. Other terms classified to these categories are "embolism," "narrowing," "obstruction" (complete) (partial), and "thrombosis." Fifth characters are provided in subcategories I65.0, I65.2, I66.0, I66.1, and I66.2 to indicate whether the condition is present on the right, left, bilateral, or unspecified arteries.

Diagnostic statements often are not specific regarding the site or type of the cerebrovascular condition. When the diagnosis is stated as cerebrovascular accident (CVA) or stroke without any further qualification, it is important to review the medical record for more definitive information or to consult with the physician. When no further information is available, code **I63.9, Cerebral infarction, unspecified,** is assigned for the diagnosis of stroke or CVA to allow for improved uniformity in coding and statistical data.

Although the Alphabetic Index of Diseases and Injuries references code I63.9 for a chronic cerebral infarction, this code assignment is not appropriate when a chronic stroke is documented. Typically, a chronic stroke is seen six months to years after a stroke's acute onset. If a patient with a diagnosis of chronic stroke presents with neurological deficits, assign a code from category I69, Sequelae of cerebrovascular disease. When the post-stroke patient presents without neurological deficits or residual conditions, assign code **Z86.73, Personal history of transient ischemic attack (TIA), and cerebral infarction without residual deficits.** More information on code assignment from category I69 is provided in the next section of this chapter.

Code I63.9 is assigned for an aborted CVA when there is no further specification as to the type of CVA. Patients who present with symptoms of an acute cerebrovascular infarction and are treated with tissue plasminogen activator (tPA) have actually had a cerebral infarction. Although brain damage may not be demonstrated by computerized tomography scan, brain damage would be visible microscopically. The administration of tPA is coded to "other thrombolytic." For example, code **3E03317, Introduction of other thrombolytic into peripheral vein, percutaneous approach,** is assigned when tPA is administered into peripheral vein. Administration of tPA is effective in treating ischemic stroke caused by blood clots that are blocking blood flow to the brain. It is also effective in treating myocardial infarctions.

Occasionally after the administration of tPA therapy, hemorrhagic conversion of an ischemic infarction can occur. The subsequent cerebral hemorrhage is coded as an adverse effect of the medication, rather than as a complication (assuming that tPA was properly administered). Code **I63.89, Other cerebral infarction,** is assigned for the initial ischemic stroke. The appropriate code from category I61, Nontraumatic intracerebral hemorrhage, is assigned along with code **T45.615A, Adverse effect of thrombolytic drugs, initial encounter,** for the hemorrhagic transformation following administration of tPA.

To capture the information that the patient is status post administration of tPA at a different facility within the past 24 hours prior to admission to the current facility, code Z92.82 is assigned as an additional code along with codes from category I63, Cerebral infarction; category I21, ST elevation (STEMI) and non-ST elevation (NSTEMI) myocardial infarction, or category I22, Subsequent ST elevation (STEMI) and non-ST elevation (NSTEMI) myocardial infarction.

Each component of a diagnostic statement identifying cerebrovascular disease should be coded unless the Alphabetic Index or the Tabular List instructs otherwise. For example:

I60.7 + I67.2	Cerebrovascular arteriosclerosis with subarachnoid hemorrhage due to ruptured berry aneurysm
I61.9 + G93.6	Intracerebral hemorrhage with vasogenic edema
E85.4 + I68.0	Cerebral amyloid angiopathy

ICD-10-CM provides codes to report a postoperative stroke. However, medical record documentation must clearly specify the cause-and-effect relationship between the medical intervention and the cerebrovascular accident in order to assign a code for intraoperative or postprocedural cerebrovascular accident. Proper code assignment depends on whether the cerebrovascular accident was an infarction or a hemorrhage and whether it occurred intraoperatively or postoperatively. If it were a cerebral hemorrhage, code assignment depends on the type of procedure performed. For example:

G97.31   Intraoperative hemorrhage and hematoma of a nervous system organ or structure complicating a nervous system procedure

G97.32   Intraoperative hemorrhage and hematoma of a nervous system organ or structure complicating other procedure

I97.810 Intraoperative cerebrovascular infarction during cardiac surgery

I97.811 Intraoperative cerebrovascular infarction during other surgery

I97.820 Postprocedural cerebrovascular infarction following cardiac surgery

I97.821 Postprocedural cerebrovascular infarction following other surgery

For codes from subcategory I97.8, assign an additional code to identify the specific type of stroke/cerebrovascular accident. The general coding rule for postoperative complications is that when the complication code does not specifically identify the condition, an additional code should be assigned to more fully explain it.

When conditions classifiable in categories I00 through I99 occur during pregnancy, childbirth, or the puerperium, they are reclassified in subcategory O99.4, Diseases of the circulatory system complicating pregnancy, childbirth and the puerperium. Because code O99.4- does not indicate the nature of the circulatory system condition, it is appropriate to assign an additional code from chapter 9 of ICD-10-CM for greater specificity.

Sequelae of Cerebrovascular Disease

Codes from category I69, Sequelae of cerebrovascular disease, allow for greater specificity in reporting the residual effects of cerebrovascular diseases. These "late effects" include neurological deficits that persist after initial onset of cerebrovascular conditions classifiable to categories I60 through I67. The neurological deficits caused by cerebrovascular disease may be present from the onset or may arise at any time after the onset of the condition classifiable to categories I60 through I67. Fourth-character subclassifications indicate the causal condition (e.g., nontraumatic subarachnoid hemorrhage, cerebral infarction), as follows:

I69.0-   Sequelae of nontraumatic subarachnoid hemorrhage

I69.1-   Sequelae of nontraumatic intracerebral hemorrhage

I69.2-   Sequelae of other nontraumatic intracranial hemorrhage

I69.3-   Sequelae of cerebral infarction

I69.8-   Sequelae of other cerebrovascular diseases

I69.9-   Sequelae of unspecified cerebrovascular diseases

Fifth and sixth characters provide information regarding the neurological deficits. The corresponding neurological deficits are as follows:

- Cognitive deficits
- Speech and language deficits
- Monoplegia of upper limb
- Monoplegia of lower limb
- Hemiplegia/hemiparesis
- Other paralytic syndrome
- Other sequelae (includes apraxia, dysphagia, facial weakness, ataxias, and other sequelae)

Providers may occasionally document unilateral weakness due to cerebral infarction. When unilateral weakness is clearly documented as following a stroke, it is considered synonymous with hemiparesis/hemiplegia (I69.35-). Unilateral weakness outside of this clear association cannot be assumed to be hemiparesis/hemiplegia unless it is associated with some other brain disorder or injury.

Codes for other paralytic syndrome following cerebrovascular disease (I69.06-, I69.16-, I69.26-, I69.36-, I69.86-, and I69.96-) provide an instructional note to assign additional codes to indicate the type of paralytic syndrome, such as locked in state (G83.5) or quadriplegia (G82.5-). Also, an additional code should be added to codes I69.091, I69.191, I69.291, I69.391, I69.891, and I69.991 to identify the type of dysphagia, if known. For "other sequelae of cerebrovascular disease" (codes I69.098, I69.198, I69.298, I69.398, I69.898, and I69.998), assign additional codes to identify the specific sequelae.

Codes from category I69 are assigned for any remaining deficits when the patient is admitted at a later date. Like other late effect codes, codes from category I69 are assigned only when they are significant for the current episode of care. Code **Z86.73, Personal history of transient ischemic attack (TIA), and cerebral infarction without residual deficits,** should be assigned rather than a code from category I69 when the patient has a history of a cerebrovascular infarction or CVA with no residual conditions, a history of TIA, a history of prolonged reversible ischemic neurological deficit (PRIND), or a history of reversible ischemic neurological deficit (RIND). Codes from category I69 differ from other late effect codes in two ways:

- These codes can be assigned as the principal diagnosis when the purpose of the admission is to deal with the late effect.

- Codes from category I69 may be assigned on a medical record with codes from categories I60–I67 when a patient presents with a new cerebral infarction, or when intracerebral hemorrhage and deficits from an earlier episode remain.

Unlike other late effects, neurological deficits such as hemiplegia and aphasia due to cerebrovascular accidents are often present from the onset of the disease rather than arising after the original condition itself has cleared. Report any neurological deficits caused by a CVA even if they have resolved at the time of discharge from the hospital. For example, a patient is admitted because of subarachnoid hemorrhage with associated aphasia and hemiplegia, which clear by the time of discharge. Even though these deficits have cleared at discharge, the following codes are assigned:

I60.9   Nontraumatic subarachnoid hemorrhage, unspecified
R47.01   Aphasia
G81.90   Hemiplegia

Note that codes from category I69 are not assigned for sequelae of traumatic intracranial injuries. Instead, assign codes from category S06, Intracranial injury, with the seventh-character value "S" for sequelae.

EXERCISE 27.5

Code the following diagnoses.

1. Occlusion of right internal carotid artery with cerebral infarction
   with mild hemiplegia resolved before discharge

2. Hemiplegia on right (dominant) side
   due to old cerebral thrombosis with infarction

3. Admission for treatment of new cerebral embolism with

    cerebral infarction and with aphasia remaining at discharge

    (patient had a cerebral embolism with infarction

    one year ago, with residual apraxia and dysphagia)

    _____

4. Cerebral infarction due to thrombosis

    with right hemiparesis (dominant) and aphasia

    _____

5. Cerebral embolism right anterior cerebral artery

    _____

6. Insufficiency of vertebrobasilar arteries

    _____

7. Admission for rehabilitation because of monoplegia of the right

    arm and right leg, each affecting dominant side (patient had a

    nontraumatic extradural [intracranial] hemorrhage one month ago)

    _____

8. Quadriplegia due to ruptured berry aneurysm five years ago

    _____

HYPERTENSION

ICD-10-CM classifies hypertension by type as essential or primary (categories I10–I13) and secondary (category I15). Categories I10 through I13 classify primary hypertension according to a hierarchy of the disease from its vascular origin (I10) to the end-organ involvement of the heart (I11), chronic kidney disease (I12), or heart and chronic kidney disease combined (I13). Essential hypertension is also described as high blood pressure, primary hypertension, hypertensive vascular disease, or systemic hypertension.

The classification presumes a causal relationship between hypertension and heart involvement and hypertension and kidney involvement, as the two conditions are linked by the term "with" in the Alphabetic Index. These conditions should be coded as related even in the absence of provider documentation explicitly linking them, unless the documentation clearly states the conditions are unrelated. If the documentation states that the heart disease or chronic kidney disease is unrelated to the hypertension, code the conditions separately. Sequence the diagnoses according to the circumstances of the admission/encounter.

Primary, Transient, and Secondary Hypertension

Malignant hypertension is a sudden and rapid development of extremely high blood pressure. The lower (diastolic) blood pressure reading, which is normally around 80 mm Hg, is often above 130 mm Hg. Without effective treatment, malignant hypertension can lead to congestive heart failure, hypertensive encephalopathy, intracerebral hemorrhage, uremia, and even death. Codes in category I16, Hypertensive crisis, classify hypertensive urgency (I16.0), hypertensive emergency

(I16.1), and hypertensive crisis, unspecified (I16.9). Assign a code from category I16 for any documented hypertensive urgency, hypertensive emergency, or unspecified hypertensive crisis. Also assign a code for any identified hypertensive disease (I10–I15). The sequencing is based on the reason for the encounter.

The term "benign hypertension" refers to a relatively mild degree of hypertension of prolonged or chronic duration. Although malignant hypertension is almost always identified in the diagnostic statement, benign hypertension is rarely specified as a diagnosis. From an ICD-10-CM coding perspective, hypertension described as accelerated, benign, essential, idiopathic, malignant, or systemic is assigned to code **I10, Essential (primary) hypertension.**

Occasionally, the hypertension may be described as controlled or uncontrolled. Controlled hypertension or hypertension documented as "history of" usually refers to an existing state of hypertension that is under control by therapy. Uncontrolled hypertension may refer to untreated hypertension or hypertension that does not respond to the current therapeutic regimen. However, whether the hypertension is controlled or not does not affect code selection. Assign the appropriate code from categories I10 through I15, Hypertensive disease.

When the hypertension is documented as "history of," review the medical record to determine whether the hypertension is still under treatment. If so, the appropriate code from categories I10 through I15 should be assigned.

When the hypertension is described as transient, assign code **R03.0, Elevated blood pressure reading without diagnosis of hypertension,** unless the patient has an established diagnosis of hypertension. For transient hypertension of pregnancy, assign a code from category O13, Gestational [pregnancy-induced] hypertension without significant proteinuria, or O14, Pre-eclampsia.

Secondary hypertension (category I15) is the result of some other primary disease or underlying condition. When the condition causing the hypertension can be cured or brought under reasonable control, the secondary hypertension may stabilize or disappear entirely. Two codes are required to report secondary hypertension: one for the underlying cause and one from category I15 to identify the secondary hypertension. The sequencing of these codes depends on the circumstances of admission or encounter. For example:

M32.10 + I15.8	Hypertension due to systemic lupus erythematosus
I15.2 + E22.0	Acromegaly with secondary hypertension; patient seen for hypertension management

HYPERTENSIVE HEART DISEASE

ICD-10-CM presumes a causal relationship between hypertension and heart involvement and classifies hypertension and heart conditions to category I11, Hypertensive heart disease, as the two conditions are linked by the term "with" in the Alphabetic Index. These conditions should be coded as related even in the absence of provider documentation explicitly linking them. Code first **I11.0, Hypertensive heart disease with heart failure,** as instructed by the note at category I50, Heart failure. However, if the provider has specifically documented different causes for the hypertension and the heart condition, code the heart condition (I50.-, I51.4–I51.7, I51.89, I51.9) and hypertension separately. Sequencing of these conditions depends on the circumstances of the admission/encounter.

Category I11 is subdivided to indicate whether heart failure is present. An additional code from category I50 is required to specify the type of heart failure, if known. For example:

I11.0 + I50.9	Congestive heart failure due to hypertension
I11.0 + I50.9	Hypertensive heart disease with congestive heart failure
I11.0 + I50.9	Congestive heart failure with hypertension

A causal relationship is presumed to exist for a cardiac condition when it is associated with another condition classified as hypertensive heart disease. For example:

I11.0+I50.9   Hypertensive myocarditis with congestive heart failure
I11.0+I50.9   Hypertensive cardiovascular disease with congestive heart failure

Review the medical record for any reference to the presence of conditions such as coronary arteriosclerosis or chronic coronary insufficiency that could merit additional code assignments.

HYPERTENSION AND CHRONIC KIDNEY DISEASE

When the diagnostic statement includes both hypertension and chronic kidney disease, ICD-10-CM assumes that there is a cause-and-effect relationship; a code from category I12, Hypertensive chronic kidney disease, is assigned, as the two conditions are linked by the term "with" in the Alphabetic Index. These conditions should be coded as related even in the absence of provider documentation explicitly linking them, unless the documentation clearly states the conditions are unrelated. A fourth character is used with category I12 to indicate the stage of the chronic kidney disease. The appropriate code from category N18 should be used as a secondary code to identify the stage of chronic kidney disease.

Kidney conditions that are not indexed to hypertensive chronic kidney disease may or may not be hypertensive; if the physician indicates a causal relationship, only the code for hypertensive chronic kidney disease is assigned. Sample codes for cases of hypertensive chronic kidney disease include the following:

I12.9   Hypertensive nephropathy, benign
I12.9   Hypertensive nephrosclerosis
I12.9+N18.30   Accelerated hypertension with chronic kidney disease stage 3

When the diagnostic statement indicates hypertension and diabetes mellitus are both responsible for chronic kidney disease, assign the appropriate code from category I12, along with the code from categories E08 through E13, for diabetes with chronic kidney disease. Sequencing is optional. An additional code is assigned for the stage of chronic kidney disease (N18.-).

Note that acute kidney failure is an entirely different condition from chronic kidney disease and is not caused by hypertension. Therefore, codes from category I12 are not assigned for acute kidney failure and hypertension. If a patient has hypertensive chronic kidney disease and acute renal failure, the acute renal failure should also be coded. Sequence according to the circumstances of the admission or encounter. If a patient has acute kidney failure with renal papillary necrosis and hypertension, assign codes N17.2 and I10. Sequencing depends on the circumstances of the admission or encounter.

HYPERTENSIVE HEART AND CHRONIC KIDNEY DISEASE

The codes in category I13, Hypertensive heart and chronic kidney disease, are combination codes that include hypertension, heart disease, and chronic kidney disease. The inclusion note at category I13 specifies that the conditions classified to categories I11 and I12 are included together in I13. Therefore, if a patient has hypertension, heart disease, and chronic kidney disease, then a code from I13 should be used rather than individual codes for hypertension, heart disease, and chronic kidney disease, or codes from I11 or I12.

Fourth and fifth characters indicate with or without heart failure, as well as the stage of the chronic kidney disease. Assume a relationship between the hypertension and the chronic kidney disease and heart disease, whether or not the condition is so designated. If heart failure is present, assign an additional code from category I50 to identify the type of heart failure. When a code from category I13 is assigned, the appropriate code from category N18, Chronic kidney disease, should be used as a secondary code to identify the stage of chronic kidney disease. For patients with both acute renal failure and chronic kidney disease, the acute renal failure should also be coded. Sequence the codes according to the circumstances of the admission or encounter.

HYPERTENSION WITH OTHER CONDITIONS

Although hypertension is often associated with other conditions and may accelerate their development, ICD-10-CM does not provide combination codes to describe these associated conditions. Codes for each condition must be assigned to fully describe the patient's condition. For example:

I70.0+I10	Atherosclerosis of aorta with essential hypertension
I25.10+I10	Coronary atherosclerosis and systemic hypertension
I25.10+I10	Arteriosclerotic heart disease with essential hypertension

Hypertensive Cerebrovascular Disease

For hypertensive cerebrovascular disease, first assign the appropriate code from categories I60 through I69, followed by the appropriate hypertension code (I10–I15).

Hypertensive Retinopathy

For hypertensive retinopathy, a code from subcategory H35.0, Background retinopathy and retinal vascular changes, should be used with a code from categories I10–I15, Hypertensive diseases, to include the systemic hypertension. The sequencing is based on the reason for the admission or encounter.

EXERCISE 27.6

Code the following diagnoses.

1. Left heart failure with hypertension

2. Hypertensive cardiomegaly

3. Congestive heart failure with hypertension
   and cardiomegaly

4. Acute congestive diastolic heart failure due to
   hypertension

5. Hypertensive heart disease
   Myocardial degeneration

6. Acute cerebrovascular insufficiency

7. Cerebral thrombosis
   Moderate arterial hypertension

8. Arteriosclerotic cerebrovascular disease

    Hypertension, primary

---

9. Chronic coronary insufficiency

    Essential hypertension

---

10. Acute coronary insufficiency

    Hypertensive heart disease

HYPERTENSION COMPLICATING PREGNANCY, CHILDBIRTH, AND THE PUERPERIUM

Hypertension associated with pregnancy, childbirth, or the puerperium is considered a complication unless the physician specifically indicates that it is not. This condition includes pre-existing hypertension as well as transient hypertension of pregnancy or hypertension arising during pregnancy. Hypertension complicating pregnancy, childbirth, and the puerperium is reclassified in categories O10 through O11 and O13 through O16. (See chapter 23 of this handbook.)

ELEVATED BLOOD PRESSURE VERSUS HYPERTENSION

Blood pressure readings vary from time to time and tend to increase with age. Because of these variables, a diagnosis of hypertension must be made on the basis of a series of blood pressure readings rather than a single reading. A diagnosis of elevated blood pressure reading, without a diagnosis of hypertension, is assigned code R03.0. This code is never assigned on the basis of a blood pressure reading documented in the medical record; the physician must have specifically documented a diagnosis of elevated blood pressure.

True postoperative hypertension is classified as a complication of surgery, and code **I97.3, Postprocedural hypertension,** is assigned. However, a diagnosis of postoperative hypertension often refers only to an elevated blood pressure that reflects the patient's agitation or inadequate pain control and would be coded to R03.0.

When the surgical patient has a pre-existing hypertension, only a code from categories I10 through I13 is assigned; neither pre-existing hypertension nor simple elevated blood pressure is classified as a postoperative complication. Any other diagnosis of transient hypertension except that occurring in pregnancy, childbirth, and the puerperium, or a diagnosis of postoperative hypertension not clearly documented in the medical record should be discussed with the physician to determine whether it represents an elevated blood pressure reading or a true hypertension.

ATHEROSCLEROSIS OF EXTREMITIES

Atherosclerosis of the native arteries of the extremities is classified into subcategory I70.2. Fifth characters used with subcategory I70.2 indicate the progression of the disease, as follows:

*   Code I70.21- indicates atherosclerosis of the extremities with intermittent claudication.

*   Code I70.22- indicates the presence of rest pain; it includes any intermittent claudication.

- Codes I70.23-, I70.24-, and I70.25- indicate a condition that has progressed to ulceration; each code includes any rest pain and/or intermittent claudication. Code L97.- is used with I70.23- and I70.24-, and code L98.49- is used with I70.25-, to identify the severity of the ulcer.

- Code I70.26- indicates the presence of gangrene; it includes any or all of the preceding conditions. Code L98.49- is assigned as an additional code to identify the severity of any ulcer, if applicable.

Codes in subcategory 170.2, Atherosclerosis of native arteries of the extremities, provide inclusion terms identifying critical limb ischemia and chronic limb-threatening ischemia, with rest pain, with ulceration, and with gangrene. Critical limb ischemia is a severe blockage in the arteries of the lower extremities.

Atherosclerosis of extremities involving a graft is coded to subcategories I70.3 through I70.7, as follows:

I70.3-	Unspecified graft
I70.4-	Autologous vein bypass graft
I70.5-	Nonautologous biological bypass graft
I70.6-	Nonbiological bypass graft
I70.7-	Other type of bypass graft

Codes from subcategories I70.3 through I70.7 provide inclusion terms describing critical limb ischemia and chronic limb-threatening ischemia, as well as additional characters to indicate the same progression of disease previously discussed under subcategory I70.2, Atherosclerosis of native arteries of the extremities (namely, intermittent claudication, rest pain, ulceration, and gangrene).

A chronic total occlusion of an artery of the extremities (I70.92) develops when hard, calcified plaque accumulates in an artery over an extended period of time, resulting in a clinically significant decrease in blood flow. Approximately 40 percent of patients with peripheral vascular disease present initially with partial occlusion, which progresses to a chronic total occlusion. Intervention with angioplasty and stenting is more complex because passing a guide wire through a total occlusion is extremely difficult.

Code I70.92 should be used as an additional code assignment with subcategories I70.2 through I70.7 when a chronic total occlusion is present with atherosclerosis of the extremities. An acute occlusion of arteries of the extremity is assigned to code series I70.2-, I70.3-, or I70.4-.

SECONDARY PULMONARY HYPERTENSION

Secondary pulmonary hypertension (PH) is defined as "increased pressure in the pulmonary arteries" and is usually caused by other conditions. Subcategory I27.2, Other secondary pulmonary hypertension, differentiates the various types of secondary PH. They are clinically classified into five groups:

- Group 1, *Secondary pulmonary arterial hypertension* (I27.21): Secondary pulmonary arterial hypertension (PAH) is the most widely recognized category of PH. It includes primary pulmonary hypertension as well as idiopathic and inheritable PAH. Other secondary causes of PH in this group are drug- and toxin-induced PH, pulmonary hypertension associated with congenital heart disease, and HIV infection.

- Group 2, *Pulmonary hypertension due to left heart disease* (I27.22): Pulmonary hypertension in group 2 occurs secondary to left heart failure (systolic or diastolic) or secondary to left heart valvular disease.

- Group 3, *Pulmonary hypertension due to lung disease and hypoxia* (I27.23): The major causes of PH in group 3 are alveolar hypoxia due to lung disease, impaired control of breathing, and high altitudes.

- Group 4, *Chronic thromboembolic pulmonary hypertension* (I27.24): Pulmonary hypertension in group 4 can develop due to obstruction of the pulmonary arterial vessels caused by thromboemboli, tumors, or foreign bodies.
- Group 5, *Other secondary pulmonary hypertension* (I27.29): In this group, the mechanism for the development of PH is either unclear or multifactorial. Group 5 includes hematologic disorders; systemic disorders (i.e., sarcoidosis and pulmonary Langerhans cell histiocytosis); metabolic disorders, such as glycogen storage disease; Gaucher disease; thyroid disorders; and other conditions.

Code I27.20 is assigned for unspecified pulmonary hypertension. When assigning codes from subcategory I27.2, code also any associated conditions, if applicable, such as lung disease, HIV disease, heart disease, thromboemboli, and so forth. The sequencing is based on the reason for the encounter, except in cases involving adverse effects of drugs. See chapter 31 of this handbook for guidance on the sequencing of adverse effect codes.

PULMONARY EMBOLISM

An embolus is a blood clot that usually occurs in the veins of the legs (deep vein thrombosis, or DVT). Emboli can dislodge and travel to other organs in the body. A pulmonary embolism is a clot that lodges in the lungs, blocking the pulmonary arteries and reducing blood flow to the lungs and heart. Pulmonary embolic disease may be acute or chronic (long-standing, having occurred over many weeks, months, or years). In most cases, acute pulmonary emboli do not cause chronic disease because the body's mechanisms will generally break down the blood clot.

An acute embolus is usually treated with anticoagulants, such as intravenous (IV) heparin and warfarin or oral Coumadin, to dissolve the clot and prevent new ones. For acute pulmonary embolism, anticoagulant therapy may be carried out for three to six months. Therapy is discontinued when the embolus dissolves. A filter to interrupt the vena cava is another treatment option. The device filters the blood returning to the heart and lungs until the pulmonary embolism dissolves.

The tulip filter device is indicated in cases of recent pulmonary embolism and proximal DVT with a contraindication to anticoagulation, and as prophylaxis following trauma. When the tulip filter is used on a temporary basis, complications of permanent filters (i.e., thrombosis, migration of the filter, inferior vena cava occlusion or perforation, filter fragmentation, and increased risk for DVT) can be avoided. The tulip filter device consists of four legs that form the shape of a cone. A small hook at the base of each leg is used for fixation of the device. Filter wires form the shape of tulip petals, giving the device its name. A hook at the apex of the cone allows the filter to be retrieved, although it may be used as a permanent fixture to manage thromboembolic disease. For example:

- A patient with pulmonary embolism underwent placement of a tulip filter into the interior vena cava. Code **06H03DZ, Insertion of intraluminal device into inferior vena cava, percutaneous approach,** is assigned for insertion of the tulip filter.

Acute pulmonary embolisms are classified to category I26, Pulmonary embolism, with fourth characters to indicate whether there is acute cor pulmonale, and fifth characters to indicate subsegmental pulmonary emboli, saddle embolus, or septic pulmonary embolism. For example:

- I26.01   Septic pulmonary embolism with acute cor pulmonale
- I26.90   Septic pulmonary embolism without acute cor pulmonale
- I26.93   Single subsegmental pulmonary embolism without acute cor pulmonale
- I26.94   Multiple subsegmental pulmonary emboli without acute cor pulmonale

Code **I26.99, Other pulmonary embolism without acute cor pulmonale,** is used for an acute pulmonary embolism not otherwise specified. Code **I27.82, Chronic pulmonary embolism,** is assigned for a chronic or recurrent pulmonary embolism. In addition to code I27.82, assign code

Z79.01, Long-term (current) use of anticoagulants, to describe any associated long-term use of anticoagulant therapy. If the pulmonary embolism has completely resolved and the provider indicates history of pulmonary embolism, assign code **Z86.711, Personal history of pulmonary embolism.**

SADDLE EMBOLISM

Saddle emboli are among the most severe and life-threatening forms of embolism. Patient survival depends on early diagnosis and treatment. The aorta is the most common site for a saddle embolus, but saddle emboli can occur at other sites, such as the pulmonary artery at the level of the bifurcation of the pulmonary trunk and extending into the main right and left pulmonary arteries. The following codes are assigned for saddle embolism: saddle embolus of pulmonary artery with acute cor pulmonale (I26.02), saddle embolus of pulmonary artery without acute cor pulmonale (I26.92), saddle embolus of abdominal aorta (I74.01), and other arterial embolism and thrombosis of abdominal aorta (I74.09). Treatment can involve various methods, including IV heparin, IV tPA, and/or thrombectomy.

THROMBOSIS AND THROMBOPHLEBITIS OF VEINS OF EXTREMITIES

Deep vein thrombosis and thrombophlebitis are two distinct processes that can coexist. A patient can develop a thrombus with or without inflammation. A diagnosis of thrombosis of a vein indicates that a clot has formed; a diagnosis of thrombophlebitis indicates that the clot has become inflamed. When both thrombosis and thrombophlebitis of the lower extremities are documented, assign only a code from subcategory I82.4-, Acute embolism and thrombosis of deep veins of lower extremity; I82.5-, Chronic embolism and thrombosis of deep veins of lower extremity; or I82.81-, Embolism and thrombosis of superficial veins of lower extremities. A separate code for the thrombophlebitis is not assigned.

Thrombophlebitis of the extremities is classified according to the veins involved, as follows:

I80.0-	Superficial vessels of lower extremities
I80.1-	Femoral vein
I80.20-	Unspecified deep vessels of lower extremities
I80.21-	Iliac vein
I80.22-	Popliteal vein
I80.23-	Tibial vein
I80.24-	Peroneal vein
I80.25-	Calf muscular vein
I80.29-	Other deep vessels of lower extremities
I80.3-	Lower extremities, unspecified
I80.8	Other sites
I80.9	Unspecified site

Deep vein thrombosis, also referred to as venous thromboembolism, is a blood clot in a major vein. DVT generally involves the veins of the lower extremity, but it can also occur in the veins of the upper extremity. With the use of catheters for venous access and cardiac devices, there is increased risk of developing DVT in the upper extremities, such as the axillary, subclavian, or brachiocephalic veins. DVT can occur following orthopedic surgery, pelvic/abdominal surgery, or prolonged inactivity (e.g., long-distance travel, bed rest due to injury or illness, paralysis). Some individuals have a predisposition for developing blood clots due to an abnormality in their blood clotting system (e.g., factor V mutation, protein C or S deficiency, lupus).

Treatment involves anticoagulants to inhibit further development of blood clots or clot-dissolving drugs. In the hospital, heparin is usually administered intravenously. In some cases, a filter is placed in the vena cava to prevent emboli or clots from traveling to the heart and lungs. Following discharge, anticoagulant therapy is recommended for three to six months (or longer). High-risk patients may be maintained on anticoagulant therapy for an indefinite period.

Venous embolism and thrombosis can be of deep vessels or superficial vessels, and the condition can be acute or chronic, with recurrent episodes. Recurrent DVT can be prevented through prophylactic anticoagulant therapy, venous stasis prevention with gradient elastic stockings, and intermittent pneumatic compression of the legs. Clinical studies have not been done to determine when DVT becomes chronic. In ICD-10-CM, the default is acute and the inclusion terms at category I82.4- affirm that this code category is used for DVT not otherwise specified.

When DVT has completely resolved and the provider documentation indicates past history of DVT, assign code **Z86.718, Personal history of other venous thrombosis and embolism.**

ICD-10-CM classifies venous embolism and thrombosis to category I82, Other venous embolism and thrombosis, according to the veins involved, with the codes for veins of the extremities being further specified as acute or chronic, as follows:

I82.0	Budd-Chiari syndrome
I82.1	Thrombophlebitis migrans
I82.2-	Vena cava and other thoracic veins
I82.3	Renal vein
I82.4-	Deep veins of lower extremity (acute)
I82.5-	Deep veins of lower extremity (chronic)
I82.6-	Veins of upper extremity (acute)
I82.7-	Veins of upper extremity (chronic)
I82.A-	Axillary vein (acute and chronic)
I82.B-	Subclavian vein (acute and chronic)
I82.C-	Internal jugular vein (acute and chronic)
I82.81-	Superficial veins of lower extremities
I82.89-	Other specified veins (acute and chronic)
I82.9-	Unspecified veins

Code **Z79.01, Long-term (current) use of anticoagulants,** is reported along with codes in subcategories I82.5 and I82.7 to describe any associated long-term use of anticoagulant therapy.

Atheroembolism is separate and distinct from atherosclerosis, thrombosis, or embolism. Thrombosis and embolism involve true clots, whereas atheroembolism involves cholesterol crystals from atheromatous plaques from vessels such as the aorta or the renal artery. Atheroembolism is most commonly associated with the extremities. Category I75 is used to report atheroembolism.

OTHER CIRCULATORY CONDITIONS

In general, the coding principles applicable throughout ICD-10-CM apply to other sections of the ICD-10-CM chapter on circulatory diseases, which are not discussed specifically in this handbook.

EXERCISE 27.7

Code the following diagnoses and procedures.

---

1. Stasis ulcer, left lower extremity

   Left lesser saphenous vein stripping

   (percutaneous)

---

2. Chronic venous embolism and thrombosis
   of subclavian veins on long-term Coumadin therapy
   Chronic orthostatic hypotension

3. Arteriosclerosis of legs with intermittent claudication

4. Septic embolism pulmonary artery due to *Staphylococcus Aureus* sepsis
   Saphenous phlebitis, right leg

5. Pulmonary hypertension

6. Raynaud's syndrome with gangrene

7. Esophageal varices, hemorrhagic

8. Bleeding esophageal varices due to portal hypertension
   Ligation of esophageal varices (transorifice endoscopic)

9. Arteriosclerotic ulcer and gangrene of left lower leg

10. Patient was admitted with acute headache and problems with
    vision; condition deteriorated rapidly, and patient died within
    four hours of admission; final diagnosis: ruptured berry aneurysm

11. Dissecting aneurysm of thoracic aorta
    Excision of the aneurysm with anastomosis (open approach)

STATUS Z CODES

ICD-10-CM provides several Z codes to indicate that the patient has a health status related to the circulatory system, such as the following:

Z94.1	Heart transplant status
Z95.0	Presence of cardiac pacemaker
Z95.1	Presence of aortocoronary bypass graft
Z95.2	Presence of prosthetic heart valve
Z95.3	Presence of xenogenic heart valve
Z95.4	Presence of other heart-valve replacement
Z95.5	Presence of coronary angioplasty implant and graft

Z95.810	Presence of automatic (implantable) cardiac defibrillator
Z95.811	Presence of heart assist device
Z95.812	Presence of fully implantable artificial heart
Z95.818	Presence of other cardiac implants and grafts
Z95.820	Peripheral vascular angioplasty status with implants and grafts
Z95.828	Presence of other vascular implants and grafts

These codes are assigned only as additional codes and are reportable only when the status affects the patient's care for a given episode. When the physician evaluates the patient's cardiac condition in any care setting, assign first a code for the specific cardiac condition along with a code describing the presence of a cardiac device (i.e., pacemaker, automatic cardioverter/defibrillator [AICD], cardiac resynchronization pacemaker [CRT-P], or biventricular defibrillator [CRT-D]). For example, when a patient presents with sick sinus syndrome (SSS) and is status post pacemaker insertion, assign codes **I49.5, Sick sinus syndrome**, and **Z95.0, Presence of cardiac pacemaker.** The SSS is a reportable chronic condition. Although the pacemaker is controlling the heart rate, it does not cure SSS and the condition is still being managed/monitored.

PROCEDURES INVOLVING THE CIRCULATORY SYSTEM

Several complex diagnostic tests have been developed for evaluating a patient's circulatory status, and several intensive procedures are currently in use for treating diseases of the circulatory system. The coronary artery bypass, used for patients with severe blockage in the coronary arteries, has been augmented by less-invasive procedures, such as angioplasty. Some of these tests and procedures are described briefly in this section.

The majority of the *ICD-10-PCS Official Coding Guidelines* are covered in chapters 7 and 9 of this handbook. However, there are three specific guidelines for selection of the "body part" values of note for the procedures of the circulatory system:

- *Branches of body parts:* If a specific branch of a body part does not have its own body part value in ICD-10-PCS, the body part is typically coded to the closest proximal branch that has a specific body part value. In the cardiovascular body systems, if a general body part is available in the correct root operation table and coding to a proximal branch would require assigning a code in a different body system, the procedure is coded using the general body part value. For example, occlusion of the bronchial artery is coded to the body part value "upper artery" in the body system "upper arteries," not to the body part value "thoracic aorta, descending" in the body system "heart and great vessels."

- *Continuous section of tubular body part:* If a procedure is performed on a continuous section of a tubular body part, code the body part value corresponding to the furthest anatomical site from the point of entry. For example, a procedure performed on a continuous section of artery from the femoral artery to the external iliac artery with the point of entry at the femoral artery is coded to the external iliac artery body part.

- *Coronary arteries:* The coronary arteries are classified as a single body part that is further specified by the number of arteries treated. One procedure code specifying multiple arteries is used when the same procedure is performed, including the same device and qualifier values. For example, angioplasty of two distinct coronary arteries with placement of two stents is coded as "dilation of coronary artery, two arteries with two intraluminal devices," whereas angioplasty of two distinct coronary arteries, one with stent placed and one without, is coded as two separate procedures: "dilation of coronary artery, one artery with intraluminal device" and "dilation of coronary artery, one artery with no device."

Coding Clinic has provided the following guidance in relation to selection of body part values for vessels. In sections of ICD-10-PCS containing values that distinguish central vessels from peripheral vessels, a coding convention can be applied to determine whether the procedure site is a central vessel or a peripheral vessel for coding purposes. The following vessels are coded to the "central artery/vein" body part value(s):

- Coronary artery
- Coronary vein
- Pulmonary trunk
- Pulmonary artery
- Pulmonary vein
- Inferior vena cava
- Superior vena cava
- Thoracic aorta

All other vessels are coded to the "peripheral artery/vein" body part value(s).

Diagnostic Cardiac Catheterization

Cardiac catheterization is an invasive diagnostic procedure performed for diagnosing and assessing the severity of cardiovascular disease. The procedure includes recording intracardiac and intravascular pressures, recording tracings, obtaining blood for blood-gas testing, and measuring cardiac output. A number of other tests involve the insertion of cardiac catheters, but they are not classified as diagnostic catheterization unless a separate procedure with a report including the measurements listed in the preceding sentence has been documented.

ICD-10-PCS classifies cardiac catheterizations to the Measurement and Monitoring Section; "physiological systems" body system; and function/device (character 6) "sampling and pressure"; a qualifier (character 7) specifies whether the procedure is a left heart, right heart, or bilateral catheterization, as shown below.

Character 1 Section	Character 2 Body System	Character 3 Root Type	Character 4 Body Part	Character 5 Approach	Character 6 Function/Device	Character 7 Qualifier
4	A	0	2	3	N	7
Measurement and monitoring	Physiological systems	Measurement	Cardiac	Percutaneous	Sampling and pressure	Left heart

Other examples of cardiac catheterization codes include:

4A023N8   Measurement of cardiac sampling and pressure, bilateral, percutaneous approach

4A023N6   Measurement of cardiac sampling and pressure, right heart, percutaneous approach

4A020N7   Measurement of cardiac sampling and pressure, left heart, open approach

Angiocardiography

Cardiac angiography is a diagnostic test ordinarily performed in conjunction with diagnostic cardiac catheterization. Ergonovine provocation testing is often performed in association with coronary arteriograms to diagnose coronary spasm and is included in the code for the coronary arteriogram. Angiographies and arteriographies are classified in ICD-10-PCS in the Imaging Section, root operation "Fluoroscopy," with the body part character identifying the vessel imaged and whether the contrast material used was high osmolar, low osmolar, or other contrast. Coding professionals should work together with their radiologists to determine which contrast media is being used for imaging and then develop internal facility-specific guidelines identifying the type of contrast to code these procedures. For example, a facility may use only low osmolar contrast for imaging studies. For cardiac angiographies, ICD-10-PCS distinguishes in the body part character whether the procedure involves single or multiple coronary arteries and whether the procedure is performed on a bypass graft. For example:

B2120ZZ   Fluoroscopy of single coronary artery bypass graft using high osmolar contrast

B211YZZ   Fluoroscopy of multiple coronary arteries using other contrast

Intraoperative Fluorescence Vascular Angiography

Intraoperative fluorescence vascular angiography (IFVA) is a new imaging technology that allows real-time evaluation of the coronary vasculature and cardiac chambers during coronary artery bypass graft (CABG) procedures. IFVA is used to assess the quality of the vascular anastomoses and patency of the graft, with results that are similar to selective coronary arteriography and cardiac catheterization. This new imaging technique is accomplished in less time and without the use of potentially harmful contrast material. Codes for IFVA procedures in ICD-10-PCS are similar to codes for conventional angiographies with fluoroscopy, but they are distinguished by the use of the qualifier "laser" in character 6 and the qualifier "intraoperative" in character 7. For example, compare these codes for coronary IFVA procedures with the two fluoroscopy examples previously listed under angiocardiography:

B212010   Fluoroscopy of single coronary artery bypass graft using high osmolar contrast, laser intraoperative

B211Y10   Fluoroscopy of multiple coronary arteries using other contrast, laser intraoperative

Intraoperative fluorescence vascular angiography can also be used in noncoronary applications, such as breast cancer surgery, pediatric microsurgery, reconstructive surgery, and other types of tissue reconstruction. In addition, IFVA not only visualizes the coronary vasculature but also enables intraoperative visualization of blood perfusion to the heart muscle, allowing surgeons to successfully perform transmyocardial revascularization (TMR).

Electrophysiological Stimulation and Recording Studies

Electrophysiological stimulation and recording studies, commonly referred to as EP studies, are performed as part of the diagnosis and therapeutic management of patients with ventricular tachycardia or ventricular fibrillation, both forms of cardiac arrhythmia that carry a high risk of sudden death. EP studies are also performed for patients who have unexplained syncope and palpitation or supraventricular tachycardia. Sometimes, a bundle of His electrocardiography will be done as part of an EP study. The bundle of His electrocardiography is a test that measures electrical activity in a part of the heart that carries the signals that control the time between heartbeats (contractions).

The EP study involves inserting a catheter—a narrow, flexible tube—attached to electricity monitoring electrodes, into a blood vessel, often through a site in the groin or neck, and winding the catheter wire up into the heart. After cardiac access is obtained either percutaneously or via cutdown, specialized electrophysiological catheter electrodes are inserted and guided into position under fluoroscopy. Once the catheter reaches the heart, electrodes at its tip gather data and a variety of electrical measurements are made. These data pinpoint the location of the faulty electrical site. During this "electrical mapping," the cardiac arrhythmia specialist, an electrophysiologist, may instigate, through pacing (the use of tiny electrical impulses), arrhythmias that are the crux of the problem.

Invasive EP studies are assigned code **4A0234Z, Measurement of cardiac electrical activity, percutaneous approach.** Code **3E063KZ, Introduction of other diagnostic substance into central artery, percutaneous approach,** may also be assigned.

For noninvasive programmed electrical stimulation, assign code **4A02X4Z, Measurement of cardiac electrical activity, external approach.** This noninvasive study can also be done using a transesophageal approach. ICD-10-PCS does not provide a specific transesophageal approach value for measurement of cardiac rhythm. The external approach (4A02X4Z) is the closest available equivalent.

An ablative procedure can also be performed. The cardiac conduction system includes the sinoatrial node, the atrioventricular node, the bundle of HIS, and all other specialized pathways in the atria and ventricles that govern the stimulation of the heart's pumping action. The cardiac conduction system is the site of any arrhythmogenic focus treated by an ablation procedure, and such procedures are coded to the body part value "conduction mechanism." For example:

- A patient diagnosed with ventricular tachycardia undergoes percutaneous ablation of ventricular tachycardia. Assign code **02583ZZ, Destruction of conduction mechanism, percutaneous approach.**

A newer hybrid ablation convergent procedure is a catheter-based endocardial ablation performed in the electrophysiology laboratory, along with epicardial ablation performed via a minimally invasive approach by a cardiothoracic surgeon. This procedure is effective in blocking conduction mechanisms for the treatment of persistent and longstanding persistent atrial fibrillation.

Implant of Automatic Cardioverter Defibrillator

The automatic implantable cardioverter defibrillator (AICD) is an electronic device designed to detect and treat life-threatening tachyarrhythmias by means of countershocks. Patients receiving this therapy have usually had one or more episodes of life-threatening arrhythmias that cannot be controlled by other therapy.

A total cardioverter defibrillator system implant is usually performed as a single procedure. It includes the formation of a subcutaneous tissue pocket or an abdominal fascia pocket, implantation or replacement of the defibrillator with epicardial patches and any transvenous leads, intraoperative procedures for evaluation of the lead signal, defibrillator threshold measurements, and tests of the implanted device with induction of arrhythmia. During the surgery to implant the AICD, the device is tested by inducing ventricular fibrillation (VF). Shocks are delivered by use of a defibrillator and normal sinus rhythm is restored. A diagnosis of ventricular fibrillation is not coded when it is induced by the use of a defibrillator (shocking) to make sure the AICD recognizes the VF because the arrhythmia is being induced to check the functioning of the device.

Although a single procedure is more typical, the AICD implant is sometimes performed in two stages. The leads are implanted first, and the generator is implanted on a subsequent day during the same hospital admission.

Coding of the insertion of an AICD requires multiple codes, as follows:

1. A code for the insertion of the defibrillator generator into the subcutaneous pocket in either the chest or the abdomen, using either an open approach or a percutaneous approach. For example:

   0JH608Z   Insertion of defibrillator generator into chest subcutaneous tissue and fascia, open approach

   0JH838Z   Insertion of defibrillator generator into abdomen subcutaneous tissue and fascia, percutaneous approach

2. A code for the insertion of the defibrillator lead(s). There are multiple possible codes depending on whether the lead is inserted into the right atrium, left atrium, right ventricle, or left ventricle. There are also different codes based on whether the leads were inserted using the open, percutaneous, or percutaneous endoscopic approach. Conventional defibrillators rely on transvenous leads for cardiac sensing and defibrillation. For example:

02H60KZ   Insertion of defibrillator lead into right atrium, open approach

02H73KZ   Insertion of defibrillator lead into left atrium, percutaneous approach

02HK4KZ   Insertion of defibrillator lead into right ventricle, percutaneous endoscopic approach

The newer, totally subcutaneous implantable cardioverter defibrillators use subcutaneous rather than transvenous leads. For example:

0JH60FZ   Insertion of subcutaneous defibrillator lead into chest subcutaneous tissue and fascia, open approach

0JH63FZ   Insertion of subcutaneous defibrillator lead into chest subcutaneous tissue and fascia, percutaneous approach

3. Any extracorporeal circulation (continuous cardiac output) (5A1221Z) or any other concomitant surgical procedure should also be coded.

There are two codes for the revision or relocation of a cardiac device pocket, one for open approach and the other for percutaneous approach, as follows:

0JWT0PZ   Revision of cardiac rhythm related device in trunk subcutaneous tissue and fascia, open approach

0JWT3PZ   Revision of cardiac rhythm related device in trunk subcutaneous tissue and fascia, percutaneous approach

These codes may be used for the creation of a pocket for a loop recorder or pocket for an implantable, patient-activated cardiac event recorder. Insertion and relocation of both devices are included in these codes.

There are two codes for removal of subcutaneous defibrillator leads and three codes for their revision, as follows:

0JPT0FZ   Removal of subcutaneous defibrillator lead from trunk subcutaneous tissue and fascia, open approach

0JPT3FZ   Removal of subcutaneous defibrillator lead from trunk subcutaneous tissue and fascia, percutaneous approach

0JWT0FZ   Revision of subcutaneous defibrillator lead in trunk subcutaneous tissue and fascia, open approach

0JWT3FZ   Revision of subcutaneous defibrillator lead in trunk subcutaneous tissue and fascia, percutaneous approach

0JWTXFZ   Revision of subcutaneous defibrillator lead in trunk subcutaneous tissue and fascia, external approach

When a patient is admitted for replacement or adjustment of an AICD, code **Z45.02, Encounter for adjustment and management of automatic implantable cardiac defibrillator,** is assigned as the principal diagnosis unless the procedure is being performed because of a mechanical complication, in which case a code from subcategory T82.1, Mechanical complication of cardiac electronic device, is assigned. When only the leads are replaced, code the removal of the old lead and then the insertion of the new lead. When only the pulse generator is replaced, code the removal of the old generator as well as the insertion of the new generator. For example, if the pulse generator is removed from the chest and replaced with a new one, code both procedures using the open approach:

0JPT0PZ   Removal of cardiac rhythm related device from trunk subcutaneous tissue and fascia, open approach

0JH608Z   Insertion of defibrillator generator into chest subcutaneous tissue and fascia, open approach

Automatic implantable cardioverter/defibrillators sometimes require checking of the pacing thresholds or interrogation without arrhythmia induction. This procedure is coded to **4B02XTZ, Measurement of cardiac defibrillator, external approach.** For example, a bedside check or interrogation of an AICD device is assigned to code 4B02XTZ.

Cardiac Pacemaker Therapy

Cardiac pacemaker therapy (figure 27.6) involves electrical control of the heart rate. ICD-10-PCS codes differentiate between the insertion of temporary pacemakers and the insertion of permanent pacemakers. In a temporary pacemaker insertion, transvenous pacing wires are placed via a catheter and attached to an external pulse generator. This type of pacemaker is generally used for an acutely ill patient until a permanent pacemaker can be inserted. Another type of temporary pacemaker is used intraoperatively or immediately following surgery, with the pacing wires placed into the myocardium in an already-opened chest. Temporary pacemaker procedures are classified to **5A1213Z, Performance of cardiac pacing, intermittent,** or **5A1223Z, Performance of cardiac pacing, continuous.** In ICD-10-PCS, devices used during a procedure are not coded unless the device remains after the procedure is completed. Therefore, a temporary pacemaker used only during surgery is not coded.

A temporary transmyocardial pacemaker, in which a needle is inserted into the chest and into the myocardium with leads fed through the needle directly into the heart muscle and attached to an

FIGURE 27.6   Pacemaker Insertion

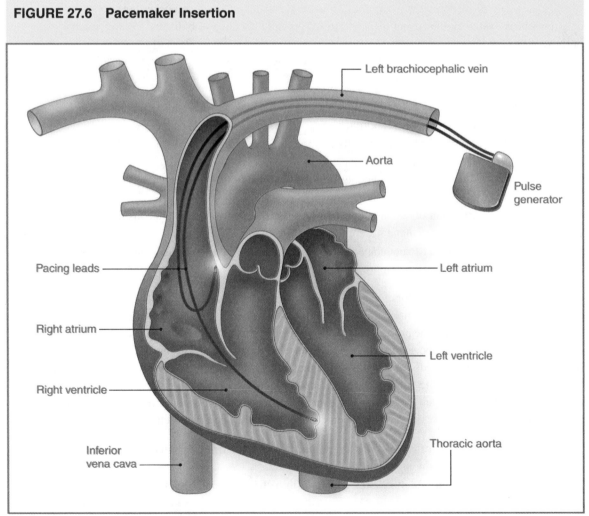

external pacing device, is sometimes used in an effort at cardiopulmonary resuscitation. This procedure is considered an integral part of cardiopulmonary resuscitation (5A2204Z), and no additional code is assigned.

At least two codes are required for the initial insertion of a permanent pacemaker. One code indicates the type of device, commonly called a pulse generator, which is coded to the Medical and Surgical Section; "subcutaneous tissue and fascia" body system; and root operation "Insertion"; with character 6, device, providing information regarding the type of pacemaker (single chamber, single chamber rate responsive, or dual chamber). Additional codes are used to report the insertion of the leads.

Pacemaker leads (electrodes) can be placed either transvenously into the inside of the heart or epicardially onto the outside of the heart. To insert a transvenous lead into the ventricle, an incision is made in the skin and the lead is passed into the subclavian vein, down the superior vena cava, across the right atrium, and into the right ventricle. When transvenous leads are used, the pacemaker device is ordinarily placed in a subcutaneous pocket in the upper chest wall. Code 0JWT0PZ or 0JWT3PZ is assigned for the revision or relocation of a pocket for a pacemaker, defibrillator, or other implanted cardiac device.

No incision into the chest cavity is needed for the insertion of an epicardial lead. When epicardial leads are used, the most common site for the pacemaker pocket is the abdominal wall.

There are three types of pacemaker devices on the market—single chamber, single chamber rate responsive, and dual chamber—each of which has a unique ICD-10-PCS sixth-character value for its insertion. For example, for a single chamber pacemaker inserted into a chest pocket using an open approach, code **0JH604Z, Insertion of single chamber pacemaker into chest subcutaneous tissue and fascia, open approach,** is assigned.

A single chamber device uses a single lead; a dual chamber device requires two leads, one in the atrium and one in the ventricle. It is important to be sure that the code for the lead insertion and the code for the pacemaker device are compatible.

For example, insertion of a dual chamber permanent pacemaker with electrodes into the right atrium and right ventricle is coded as follows:

0JH606Z	Insertion of pacemaker, dual chamber into chest subcutaneous tissue and fascia, open approach
02H63JZ	Insertion of pacemaker lead into right atrium, percutaneous approach
02HK3JZ	Insertion of pacemaker lead into right ventricle, percutaneous approach

A rate-responsive device is one in which the pacing rate is determined by physiological variables other than the atrial rate. This type of pacemaker permits patients to lead a more normal life and is strongly preferred for a potentially active patient. Physicians use various terms for this ability to respond, and, in many cases, they mention only the device number in documenting an insertion. The coding department should work with the hospital operating room staff and/or physicians to identify the devices commonly used in the facility and how those devices might be consistently identified in the operative report.

Sometimes, the pulse generator in a pacemaker must be replaced, or there may be a need to upgrade from a single chamber pacemaker to a dual chamber pacemaker. ICD-10-PCS provides individual codes for each component of these procedures. For example, a replacement of the pulse generator alone requires codes for the removal of the old generator and insertion of the new generator. Similarly, if replacement of the existing leads is required, codes will be required for the removal of the old leads, as well as codes for the insertion of the new leads.

For example, if a single chamber pacemaker is removed from the chest and replaced with a new one, code both procedures using the open approach:

0JPT0PZ	Removal of cardiac rhythm related device from trunk subcutaneous tissue and fascia, open approach
0JH604Z	Insertion of pacemaker, single chamber into chest subcutaneous tissue and fascia, open approach

When an existing pacemaker device is replaced with a new device, the type of device removed does not affect the removal code. ICD-10-PCS provides a single code (0JPT0PZ) for removal of a cardiac rhythm–related device from the chest or abdomen—whether pacemaker or cardiac defibrillator. However, the codes for device insertion do provide information regarding the type of cardiac rhythm device.

When a patient is admitted for routine removal, replacement, or reprogramming of a cardiac pacemaker, code **Z45.010, Encounter for checking and testing of cardiac pacemaker pulse generator [battery],** or code **Z45.018, Encounter for adjustment and management of other part of cardiac pacemaker,** is assigned as the principal diagnosis. Reprogramming is a simple nonoperative procedure that does not require a procedure code. Physicians sometimes indicate that a patient is being admitted for battery replacement. This is something of a misnomer because pacemakers no longer use batteries and the whole device is actually replaced. When the pacemaker device is being replaced only because it is nearing the end of its expected life, code Z45.010 or Z45.018 is assigned as the principal diagnosis. When the pacemaker is being replaced because of a mechanical complication of the device, a code from subcategory T82.1, Mechanical complication of cardiac electronic device, is assigned.

Intracardiac pacemakers are also known as "leadless" pacemakers and "transcatheter" pacemakers. Conventional pacemaker devices require two components: a generator in a subcutaneous pocket on the chest plus a lead or leads tunneled below the skin and advanced into one or more heart chambers. The components of an intracardiac pacemaker are combined into a single device implanted within a heart chamber. This type of pacemaker does not require either a subcutaneous pocket or a tunneled lead. All components are miniaturized into a capsule-like device that is inserted into a peripheral vessel, typically the femoral vein, and then advanced into the heart chamber, fixed to the chamber wall, and released. Although intracardiac pacemakers are also referred to as "leadless" pacemakers, a tiny electrode at the end of the battery capsule actually delivers the pacing pulse to the heart tissue.

Intracardiac pacemakers are currently placed within the right ventricle for single chamber pacing. An intracardiac pacemaker can be placed via a percutaneous endoscopic approach, an open approach, or a percutaneous approach. The device must be programmed when placed and then periodically interrogated and reprogrammed. When the device eventually reaches its end-of-battery-life, a new device must be placed. The old device can be removed percutaneously, or it can be turned off and abandoned in place. The following are examples of intracardiac pacemaker codes:

02H43NZ	Insertion of intracardiac pacemaker into coronary vein, percutaneous approach
02H44NZ	Insertion of intracardiac pacemaker into coronary vein, percutaneous endoscopic approach
02H60NZ	Insertion of intracardiac pacemaker into right atrium, open approach
02H63NZ	Insertion of intracardiac pacemaker into right atrium, percutaneous approach
02H64NZ	Insertion of intracardiac pacemaker into right atrium, percutaneous endoscopic approach
02H70NZ	Insertion of intracardiac pacemaker into left atrium, open approach
02H73NZ	Insertion of intracardiac pacemaker into left atrium, percutaneous approach
02H74NZ	Insertion of intracardiac pacemaker into left atrium, percutaneous endoscopic approach
02HK0NZ	Insertion of intracardiac pacemaker into right ventricle, open approach
02HK3NZ	Insertion of intracardiac pacemaker into right ventricle, percutaneous approach
02HK4NZ	Insertion of intracardiac pacemaker into right ventricle, percutaneous endoscopic approach
02HL0NZ	Insertion of intracardiac pacemaker into left ventricle, open approach
02HL3NZ	Insertion of intracardiac pacemaker into left ventricle, percutaneous approach
02HL4NZ	Insertion of intracardiac pacemaker into left ventricle, percutaneous endoscopic approach

Cardiac Resynchronization Therapy

Cardiac resynchronization therapy (CRT) is a newer technology similar to conventional pacemaker therapy and implantable cardioverter defibrillators. In CRT, leads are placed in the right atrium and right ventricle with a third lead that is positioned in a vein on the outer surface of the left ventricle. CRT treats heart failure by providing strategic electrical stimulation to the right atrium, right ventricle, and left ventricle of the heart to recoordinate ventricular contractions and improve cardiac output. CRT is also sometimes referred to as biventricular pacing because both ventricles are electrically stimulated at the same time.

ICD-10-PCS codes distinguish between the insertion of cardiac resynchronization pacemaker without internal cardiac defibrillator (CRT-P) and the insertion of cardiac resynchronization defibrillator (CRT-D). The codes differ in the values for the seventh-character qualifier, which distinguish between "cardiac resynchronization pacemaker pulse generator" and "cardiac resynchronization defibrillator pulse generator," as shown in the following examples of codes for the insertion of a pulse generator using a percutaneous approach:

0JH637Z   Insertion of cardiac resynchronization pacemaker pulse generator into chest subcutaneous tissue and fascia, percutaneous approach

0JH639Z   Insertion of cardiac resynchronization defibrillator pulse generator into chest subcutaneous tissue and fascia, percutaneous approach

No additional codes are assigned for the creation of the pocket to hold the device, implantation of the device, or intraoperative procedures to evaluate lead signals. However, separate codes are required for the insertion of the transvenous leads.

For the CRT-P, codes are needed for the insertion of pacemaker leads into the right or left ventricle (e.g., **02HK3JZ, Insertion of pacemaker lead into right ventricle, percutaneous approach**). For the CRT-D, codes are needed for the insertion of defibrillator leads based on the documentation of where the leads are placed (e.g., **02H63KZ, Insertion of defibrillator lead into right atrium, percutaneous approach; 02HK3KZ, Insertion of defibrillator lead into right ventricle, percutaneous approach; 02HL3KZ, Insertion of defibrillator lead into left ventricle, percutaneous approach; or 02H43KZ, Insertion of defibrillator lead into coronary vein, percutaneous approach**).

Over time, there may be a need to replace the lead into the left ventricular coronary venous system, replace the pacemaker pulse generator on a CRT-P, or replace the defibrillator pulse generator on a CRT-D. In all of these situations, code the device removal and the insertion of the replacement device separately. When the leads are repositioned only (not replaced), the code for the root operation "Revision" is assigned. For example, code **02WA3MZ, Revision of cardiac lead in heart, percutaneous approach,** is assigned for repositioning of the CRT-D or CRT-P lead only via a percutaneous approach.

Percutaneous Mitral Valve Repair

The MitraClip® implant is a minimally invasive, closed chest, catheter-based approach for intracardiac repair of mitral regurgitation caused by valve pathology and/or left ventricular dysfunction. The procedure is performed on a beating heart and is an alternative to the open heart surgical approach. Interventional cardiologists can perform the procedure in the cardiac catheterization laboratory or in a hybrid operating suite under general anesthesia. The procedure does not require cardiopulmonary bypass. Insertion of the MitraClip® implant is coded to **02UG3JZ, Supplement mitral valve with synthetic substitute, percutaneous approach.**

Percutaneous Aortic and Pulmonary Valve Repair

Transcatheter aortic and pulmonary valve replacements are catheter-based procedures that allow for implantation of a prosthetic valve within the diseased native valve without invasive surgery or cardiopulmonary bypass. There are two approaches to transcatheter aortic and pulmonary valve replacement: endovascular and transapical. A bioprosthetic valve is delivered by catheter across the diseased native valve through the femoral artery or vein (endovascular approach) or through the apex of the heart by means of a thoracotomy incision (transapical approach). In both approaches, a balloon valvuloplasty catheter is advanced through the aorta and placed over the diseased native aortic or pulmonary valve. A balloon valvuloplasty is then performed. The delivery catheter is placed over the native valve, and the new bioprosthetic valve is put in place, destroying the native valve underneath it. Endovascular or transapical replacement of the aortic or pulmonary valves is coded to the root operation "Replacement." For example:

02RF3JZ	Replacement of aortic valve with synthetic substitute, percutaneous approach
02RH3JH	Replacement of pulmonary valve with synthetic substitute, transapical, percutaneous approach

When a procedure is performed to correct a portion of a malfunctioning or displaced device, the procedure is coded to the root operation "Revision." However, the "aortic valve" body part is not currently available in the ICD-10-PCS tables for a percutaneous Revision procedure; therefore, the procedure is coded to the body part "heart." For example:

- A patient had previously undergone aortic valve replacement. The valve is now leaking along the perimeter where the bioprosthetic valve is attached. The surgeon performs percutaneous closure of the paravalvular leak. Code **02WA3JZ, Revision of synthetic substitute in heart, percutaneous approach,** is assigned.

Percutaneous Balloon Valvuloplasty

Percutaneous balloon valvuloplasty (027H3ZZ) is a noninvasive treatment for pulmonary valve stenosis. It involves a balloon wedge catheter that is advanced via the femoral vein into the heart and across the stenotic valve. The balloon is then inflated by hand pressure. There is no need for general anesthesia, the hospital stay is short, and no scarring results from the procedure.

Percutaneous Transluminal Coronary Angioplasty

Percutaneous transluminal coronary angioplasty (PTCA) procedures are classified in the Medical and Surgical Section to the root operation "Dilation," percutaneous approach. Code selection is based on the number of coronary arteries treated, with the fourth-character body part value used to indicate one, two, three, or four or more arteries. The code assignment reflects the number of coronary arteries treated as well as the number of stents that are inserted. The codes also indicate a sixth-character device value for the type of stent used (drug-eluting or non-drug-eluting), if applicable. Assign a code for each coronary artery (lesion) treated, unless a single lesion extends into more than one artery.

When a thrombolytic agent is also administered, assign a separate code (e.g., code **3E03317, Introduction of other thrombolytic into peripheral vein, percutaneous approach**).

Because reclosure often occurs following angioplasty, a stent is frequently inserted to prevent reclosure. Please refer to figure 27.7 for an illustration of angioplasty with stent insertion. In this procedure, a small, stainless steel mesh stent is inserted during angioplasty to prop open the blocked coronary arteries. After the balloon has been threaded into the coronary artery and inflated to squash plaque deposits against the vessel wall, the process is repeated with a second balloon carrying the stent. Expansion of the balloon pushes the stent against the artery wall, where it remains to maintain patency.

ICD-10-PCS provides different values for character 6, device, to identify whether a "drug-eluting intraluminal device (stent)," "intraluminal device (stent)," "radioactive intraluminal device," or no device was used. Note that a separate procedure code is assigned for each artery dilated when the device value differs for each artery. For example, when PTCA procedures are performed on two coronary arteries, one with a drug-eluting stent and the other with a non-drug-eluting stent, assign

FIGURE 27.7   Angioplasty with Stent Insertion

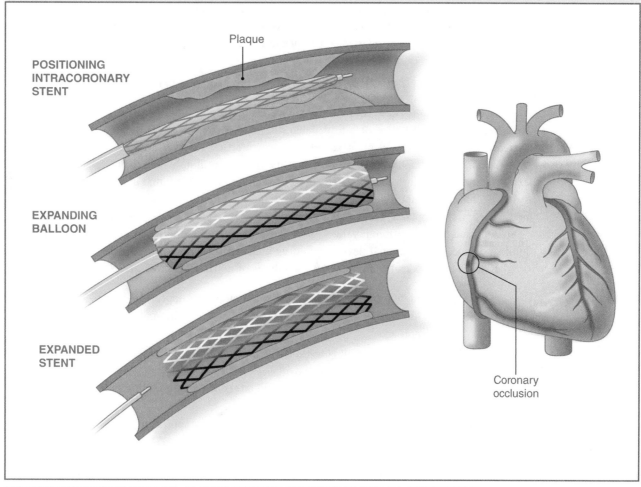

Plaque

POSITIONING
INTRACORONARY
STENT

EXPANDING
BALLOON

EXPANDED
STENT

Coronary
occlusion

codes **027034Z, Dilation of coronary artery, one artery with drug-eluting intraluminal device, percutaneous approach,** and **02703DZ, Dilation of coronary artery, one artery with intraluminal device, percutaneous approach.**

Minor intimal tears often occur during angioplasty or the newer rotational atherectomy procedures. These minor tears are considered to be an unavoidable part of the procedure and are not classified as complications.

Transluminal Coronary Atherectomy

Transluminal coronary atherectomy is a minimally invasive catheter-based procedure that removes plaque from coronary arteries. This procedure is effective in removing calcification due to plaque buildup and removing blockages, allowing blood to circulate unobstructed to the heart muscle. The types of mechanical atherectomy are rotational, directional, and transluminal extraction. Transluminal extraction atherectomy, which uses a device that cuts plaque off the vessel walls, is used to clear bypass grafts.

Coronary atherectomy procedures are classified in the Medical and Surgical Section to the root operation "Extirpation," percutaneous approach. Code selection is based on the number of coronary artery sites treated. The fourth-character body part value indicates coronary artery at one site, two sites, three sites, or four or more sites. For example, when two sites are treated, assign code **02C13ZZ, Extirpation of matter from coronary artery, two arteries, percutaneous approach.**

Coronary atherectomy procedures can be used instead of, or along with, angioplasty with or without stent insertion. When an atherectomy is performed along with a PTCA and infusion of a thrombolytic agent, assign separate codes for the PTCA, atherectomy, and thrombolytic infusion.

Angioplasty and Atherectomy of Noncoronary Vessels

ICD-10-PCS provides myriad unique codes to report angioplasty of noncoronary vessels. Because of the level of detail available, the circulatory system is divided into several body systems, such as "heart and great vessels," "upper arteries," "lower arteries," "upper veins," and "lower veins." The diaphragm is the dividing line for determining where the code is classified. For example, the subclavian vein is located above the diaphragm and is found in the "upper veins" body system, while the femoral vein is located below the diaphragm and is found in the "lower veins" body system. Angioplasty procedures of noncoronary vessels are classified to the root operation "Dilation" and include different values for the device character 6 to distinguish "drug-eluting intraluminal device," "intraluminal device (non-drug eluting)," or no device.

Examples of codes for angioplasty procedures of noncoronary vessels include:

027V3ZZ	Dilation of superior vena cava, percutaneous approach
047H3DZ	Dilation of right external iliac artery with intraluminal device, percutaneous approach
047P34Z	Dilation of right anterior tibial artery with drug-eluting intraluminal device, percutaneous approach
037J34Z	Dilation of left common carotid artery with drug-eluting intraluminal device, percutaneous approach
037G3ZZ	Dilation of intracranial artery, percutaneous approach

Atherectomy is a minimally invasive catheter-based procedure to remove plaque that can be performed on noncoronary vessels. To treat a blockage, a guide wire is advanced across the area of stenosis/occlusion, and an atherectomy catheter is advanced into the diseased arterial segment. On the tip of the catheter is either a high-speed rotating device (burr) or a sharp blade. The burr grinds the plaque into minute particles, whereas the blade shaves the plaque away. The plaque is ground up or suctioned out. ICD-10-PCS provides procedure codes for atherectomy of noncoronary vessels, such as the common carotid arteries, the internal and external carotid arteries, the vertebral arteries, and the other extracranial arteries. It classifies atherectomy to the root operation "Extirpation." Extirpation is defined as taking or cutting out solid matter from a body part. When an atherectomy is done along with an angioplasty, assign codes for both procedures. Examples of codes describing noncoronary atherectomy procedures include:

03CG3ZZ	Extirpation of matter from intracranial artery, percutaneous approach
03CH3ZZ	Extirpation of matter from right common carotid artery, percutaneous approach

If a thrombolytic agent is used, it should be assigned as an additional code, with the appropriate code from the Administration Section, root operation "Introduction." For example:

3E03317	Introduction of other thrombolytic into peripheral vein, percutaneous approach
3E04317	Introduction of other thrombolytic into central vein, percutaneous approach
3E05317	Introduction of other thrombolytic into peripheral artery, percutaneous approach

FIGURE 27.8   Coronary Artery Bypass Graft

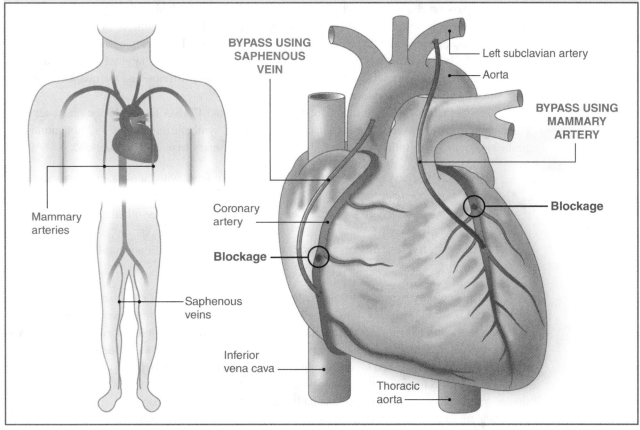

BYPASS USING
SAPHENOUS
VEIN

Left subclavian artery

Aorta

BYPASS USING
MAMMARY
ARTERY

Mammary
arteries

Coronary
artery

Blockage

Blockage

Blockage

Saphenous
veins

Inferior
vena cava

Thoracic
aorta

Coronary Artery Bypass Graft

CABGs are performed to revascularize the myocardium when a blockage in a coronary artery limits the blood supply to the heart. The grafts bypass the obstructions in the coronary arteries. (See figure 27.8.)

Coronary circulation consists of two main arteries, right and left, each with several branches:

- Right coronary artery (RCA)
  —Right marginal
  —Right posterior descending (PDA)

- Left main coronary artery (LMCA)
  —Left anterior descending branch (LAD)
  —Diagonal
  —Septal
  —Circumflex (LCX)
  —Obtuse marginal (OM)
  —Posterior descending
  —Posterolateral

The aortocoronary artery bypass is the most commonly used type of CABG. It brings blood from the aorta into the obstructed coronary artery, bypassing the obstruction by means of a segment of the patient's own saphenous vein, nonautologous biological material, or, occasionally, a segment of the internal mammary artery (IMA).

Coronary artery bypass graft procedures are coded differently from other bypass procedures. In other bypass procedure codes, the body part axis identifies the body part bypassed from. However, the body part value in a CABG procedure code identifies the number of coronary arteries bypassed to, and the qualifier specifies the vessel bypassed from. For example, aortocoronary artery bypass of the left anterior descending coronary artery and the obtuse marginal coronary artery is classified in the body part axis of classification as two coronary arteries, and the qualifier specifies the aorta as the body part bypassed from.

ICD-10-PCS identifies the type of tissue used in the CABG in the device character 6 as "autologous venous tissue," "autologous arterial tissue," "synthetic substitute," or "nonautologous tissue substitute." The following are examples of aortocoronary bypass procedure codes:

021009W   Bypass coronary artery, one artery from aorta with autologous venous tissue, open approach

02100JW   Bypass coronary artery, one artery from aorta with synthetic substitute, open approach

02110KW   Bypass coronary artery, two arteries from aorta with nonautologous tissue substitute, open approach

Not all coronary bypass procedures involve the aorta. The internal mammary–coronary artery bypass graft is accomplished by loosening the internal mammary artery from its normal position and using it as a conduit to bring blood from the subclavian artery to the occluded coronary artery. When coding internal mammary–coronary artery bypass grafts, the body part value identifies the number of coronary arteries bypassed to, and the qualifier specifies the vessel bypassed from—namely, the IMA. ICD-10-PCS identifies the type of tissue used in the device character 6 as "autologous venous tissue," "autologous arterial tissue," "synthetic substitute," or "nonautologous tissue substitute." The following are examples of internal mammary–coronary artery bypass procedure codes:

02100Z8   Bypass coronary artery, one artery from right internal mammary, open approach

02110J9   Bypass coronary artery, two arteries from left internal mammary with synthetic substitute, open approach

The internal mammary artery is traditionally used as a pedicle (in situ) graft in coronary artery bypass surgery. This is reflected in ICD-10-PCS by the seventh-character qualifier. However, occasionally the length of the right IMA is not sufficient to reach the desired position on the target artery. In these situations, length can be compensated for by excising the right IMA and using it as a free graft or by adding an additional conduit (graft extension).

Other arteries are also used to bypass an obstruction in the coronary artery. ICD-10-PCS distinguishes these procedures by the use of different values for character 7, qualifier, such as thoracic artery and abdominal artery. For example:

02130ZC   Bypass coronary artery, four or more arteries from thoracic artery, open approach
02130ZF   Bypass coronary artery, four or more arteries from abdominal artery, open approach

It is rare for only one coronary artery to be bypassed. When multiple coronary arteries are bypassed, a separate procedure is coded for each coronary artery that uses a different device and/ or qualifier. For example, it is fairly common to perform both an internal mammary–coronary artery bypass and an aortocoronary bypass at the same operative episode. When this occurs, the aortocoronary artery bypass and internal mammary–coronary artery bypass are coded separately. The surgeon's brief statement of the operation performed does not always distinguish the types of bypasses involved. Refer to the body of the operative report when the brief statement is not clear.

If an autograft is obtained from a different procedure site to complete the objective of the procedure, a separate procedure is coded. For example, when a coronary bypass with excision of saphenous vein graft is done, the excision of the saphenous vein is coded separately.

An additional code should also be assigned for any use of extracorporeal circulation (continuous cardiac output) (5A1221Z) during the coronary artery bypass procedure. However, procedures such as hypothermia, cardioplegia, intraoperative pacing, and chest tube insertions are considered to be integral to bypass surgery; no separate codes are assigned for them.

In coding coronary artery bypass procedures, it is important to keep the following points in mind:

- The use of a detached segment of the IMA as graft material for an aortocoronary bypass does not make the procedure an internal mammary–coronary artery bypass. The internal mammary–coronary artery bypass involves the use of the IMA itself as a still-vascularized conduit for the blood supply and does not involve the aorta.

- When more than one coronary artery is involved in either type of graft (an internal mammary–coronary artery bypass or an aortocoronary artery bypass graft), the anastomosis is sometimes carried out in a sequential manner, bypassing more than one artery. The mention of sequential anastomoses does not affect the code in any way.

The following examples may provide further assistance in coding coronary bypass grafts:

- Coronary artery vascularization (via thoracotomy) is carried out with four grafts: the aorta to the diagonal branch of the left coronary and, in sequential fashion, to the obtuse marginal branch of the circumflex, the right coronary artery, and the left anterior descending coronary artery. This procedure involves only the aorta and the coronary arteries. Because four coronary arteries were bypassed, assign code **02130AW, Bypass coronary artery, four or more arteries from aorta with autologous arterial tissue, open approach.**

- During an open procedure, grafts from the aorta to the coronary arteries are carried out by grafting the bifurcated left anterior descending system with a 1.5-millimeter excised section of the left internal mammary artery as a free graft. The first diagonal artery is then grafted side-to-side with a 4-millimeter section of the saphenous vein. Next, the obtuse marginal branch is grafted with a 4-millimeter section of the saphenous vein. Finally, the posterior descending artery, which was diffusely diseased, is grafted with a 4-millimeter section of the right saphenous vein. All four grafts bring blood from the aorta to the coronary arteries. Sections of both the right saphenous vein and the left internal mammary artery are used for this purpose. Because four arteries (LAD, diagonal, obtuse marginal, and posterior descending) have been bypassed, the following codes are assigned: **02100AW, Bypass coronary artery, one artery from aorta with autologous arterial tissue, open approach,** for the bypass from the aorta to the left anterior descending artery with left internal mammary artery as free graft; **021209W, Bypass coronary artery, three arteries from aorta with autologous venous tissue, open approach,** for the bypass from the aorta to the first diagonal, obtuse marginal, and posterior descending arteries with saphenous vein; and **06BP0ZZ, Excision of right saphenous vein, open approach.**

- Bypass grafts are performed (via thoracotomy) by bringing the left internal mammary artery to the left anterior ascending artery; a right saphenous vein graft is then used to bring blood from the aorta to the obtuse marginal branch of the circumflex artery, to the diagonal artery, and to the proximal PDA. In this case, a single internal mammary–coronary artery bypass and three aortocoronary bypass grafts are placed (OM, diagonal, PDA). The codes assigned are **02100Z9, Bypass coronary artery, one artery from left internal mammary, open approach; 06BP0ZZ, Excision of right saphenous vein, open approach;** and **021209W, Bypass coronary artery, three arteries from aorta with autologous venous tissue, open approach.** The sequence of the codes is optional.

• The left internal mammary artery is loosened and used to bypass the left anterior descending artery; grafts of the right saphenous vein are bypassed to the posterior descending artery and to the obtuse marginal branch of the circumflex. In this case, three coronary arteries are bypassed, one by an internal mammary–coronary artery bypass and two by aortocoronary bypasses. The codes assigned are **02100Z9, Bypass coronary artery, one artery from left internal mammary, open approach; 06BP0ZZ, Excision of right saphenous vein, open approach; and 021109W, Bypass coronary artery, two arteries from aorta with autologous venous tissue, open approach.**

Heart revascularization is also performed by other techniques. Transmyocardial revascularization is a procedure that uses a laser to bore holes through the myocardium to restore perfusion to areas of the heart where blood flow may be impaired due to diseased or clogged arteries. TMR is coded to the root operation "Repair" (restoring, to the extent possible, a body part to its normal anatomical structure and function). Although TMR does not restore the heart's anatomical structure, the procedure is performed to restore function to the heart. The procedure can be performed by open approach (02QA0ZZ, 02QB0ZZ, or 02QC0ZZ), percutaneous endoscopic approach (02QA4ZZ, 02QB4ZZ, or 02QC4ZZ), and percutaneous or endovascular procedures (02QA3ZZ, 02QB3ZZ, or 02QC3ZZ).

EXERCISE 27.8

Code the following diagnoses and procedures.

---

1. A patient was admitted through the emergency department complaining of chest pain with radiation down the left arm increasing in severity over the past three hours. Initial impression was impending myocardial infarction, and the patient was taken directly to the surgical suite, where percutaneous transluminal angioplasty with insertion of coronary stent was carried out on the right coronary artery. Infarction was aborted, and the diagnosis was listed as acute coronary insufficiency.

---

2. Atherosclerosis of previous coronary artery bypass graft with unstable angina
   Right saphenous vein graft was used to bring blood from the aorta to the right coronary artery, the left coronary artery, and the left anterior descending artery. Intraoperative continuous pacing pacemaker was used during the procedure as well as extracorporeal circulatory assistance. Temporary pacemaker leads were inserted in left atria and ventricle.

---

3. Occlusion of the right coronary artery
   Right and left diagnostic cardiac catheterization

---

4. A patient with known native vessel coronary atherosclerosis
   and unstable angina underwent percutaneous balloon angioplasty
   carried out on three coronary arteries
   Insertion of two stents

5. A patient with sick sinus syndrome was admitted
   for initial insertion of dual chamber pacemaker
   device into chest, open approach
   Pacemaker leads were placed percutaneously
   in the right ventricle and right atrium

6. A patient was admitted for replacement of single
   chamber pacemaker device because the battery was
   expected to fail within a short time; device was replaced
   with single chamber, rate-responsive pacemaker device.
   No leads needed to be replaced.

7. A patient was admitted for open revision of
   displaced and protruding pacemaker device
   with single chamber, rate-responsive device

8. A patient with ventricular tachycardia underwent
   catheter-based invasive electrophysiological
   cardiac study (via femoral artery)

Exclusion or Excision of the Left Atrial Appendage

Exclusion or excision of the left atrial appendage (LAA) is a component of most operations to treat atrial fibrillation (AF) and reduces late thromboemboli in patients with AF undergoing mitral valve surgery. Code **I51.3, Intracardiac thrombosis, not elsewhere classified,** is assigned for an atrial appendage thrombus. The clot occurs in the heart, not the coronary vessels. There are several surgical strategies to manage the LAA, such as clipping, suture ligation, excision and suture closure, or stapling exclusion with or without excision. Some of these procedures use a permanently implanted device at the LAA site. For example, the following code is assigned for left-sided thoracoscopic stapling of the left atrial appendage to occlude the LAA:

02L74ZK   Occlusion left atrium, percutaneous endoscopic approach

Ablation of Heart Tissue (Maze Procedure)

The maze procedure is a surgical treatment used for atrial fibrillation that creates lines of conduction block in the heart itself. The maze procedure and other types of ablative procedures performed in the electrophysiological laboratory relate to the conduction mechanism (electrical pathway), which involves various parts of the heart, including the atria. The focus of the procedure is ablation of the conduction mechanism (to correct aberrant arrhythmia), not ablation of the atrial muscle. Because the conduction mechanism is the part of the heart being treated, it is the correct body part, rather than the atrium or atrial appendage, to use for code assignment for this procedure.

The classic maze procedure is performed through an open chest approach (02580ZZ) via a median sternotomy or thoracotomy, with the surgeon using a scalpel to make a carefully placed pattern of incisions in the atrial tissue. Scar tissue (lesions) forms as the incisions heal, which creates the conduction block. There are variations called maze 1, maze 2, and maze 3, which represent different patterns of incisions.

Making multiple atrial incisions is difficult and risky. Therefore, other open approach techniques have been developed that use a series of linear ablations instead of incisions. A variety of energy sources are used for ablation (e.g., radiofrequency, cryothermy, microwave, laser, ultrasound). The energy source is delivered via a probe or a clamp instrument and can be applied at strategic locations within the heart or on the heart's surface. The creation of the incisions/ablation lines can be directly visualized with the open approach.

Endovascular (percutaneous) approaches (02583ZZ) through peripherally inserted cardiac catheters have also been developed. Endovascular ablations have been very effective in the treatment of arrhythmias, including atrial fibrillation and atrial flutter, resulting from a single abnormal source (i.e., ectopic focus) of electrical stimulation on the right side of the heart.

The thoracoscopic approach (02584ZZ) is the newest technique. Notably, what is commonly referred to as the thoracoscopic approach should more accurately be referred to as "thoracoscopically assisted" because the thoracoscope is used for illumination and visualization only, while the actual surgical ablation instruments are inserted via a (mini) thoracotomy or a subxiphoid incision rather than through the scope itself. However, a total thoracoscopic approach has recently been established. As with the open approach, the thoracoscopically assisted and total thoracoscopic techniques require opening up the pericardium. Significant dissection of the pericardial sinuses and other vital structures is required to gain access to target areas of the heart. Additionally, as with the open technique, incisions can be made into the atria thoracoscopically, but linear ablations are most often done. For example:

- A patient with chronic persistent atrial fibrillation undergoes a minimally invasive epicardial radiofrequency maze procedure via pericardioscopic assistance (convergent procedure). During surgery, the thorax is entered and a full-thickness ablation of right atrial tissue is accomplished. Code **02584ZZ, Destruction of conduction mechanism, percutaneous endoscopic approach,** is assigned for the minimally invasive epicardial radiofrequency maze procedure.

Implantable Heart Assist Devices

Heart circulatory support systems can provide temporary left, right, or biventricular support for patients whose hearts have failed but have the potential for recovery. A heart circulatory support system can also be used as a bridge for patients who are awaiting a heart transplant. It involves an electromechanically driven pump the size of a human heart implanted within the abdominal wall. This system provides circulatory support by taking over most of the workload of the left ventricle. Blood enters the pump through an inflow conduit connected to the left ventricle and is ejected through an outflow conduit into the body's arterial system.

The system is monitored by an electronic controller and powered by primary and reserve battery packs worn on a belt around the waist or carried in a shoulder bag. There is also a stationary system that consists of a small bedside monitor. The controller is connected to the implanted pump by a percutaneous lead (a small tube containing control and power wires) through the patient's skin.

The implantation of a total internal biventricular heart replacement system (02RK0JZ and 02RL0JZ) involves substantial removal of part or all of the biological heart. Both ventricles are resected, and the native heart is no longer intact. A ventriculectomy is included in this procedure, so it should not be coded separately. However, any associated procedures performed in conjunction with the placement of the total internal biventricular system, such as combined heart-lung transplantation or heart transplantation, should be reported.

ICD-10-PCS provides the following codes for the implantation, repair, and removal of implantable heart assist systems:

Synthetic substitute heart/ventricle

02RK0JZ	Replacement of right ventricle with synthetic substitute, open approach
02RL0JZ	Replacement of left ventricle with synthetic substitute, open approach
02WA0JZ	Revision of synthetic substitute in heart, open approach

Implantable heart assist system

02HA0QZ	Insertion of implantable heart assist system into heart, open approach
02HA3QZ	Insertion of implantable heart assist system into heart, percutaneous approach
02HA4QZ	Insertion of implantable heart assist system into heart, percutaneous endoscopic approach
02WA0QZ	Revision of implantable heart assist system in heart, open approach
02WA3QZ	Revision of implantable heart assist system in heart, percutaneous approach
02WA4QZ	Revision of implantable heart assist system in heart, percutaneous endoscopic approach
02PA0QZ	Removal of implantable heart assist system from heart, open approach
02PA3QZ	Removal of implantable heart assist system from heart, percutaneous approach
02PA4QZ	Removal of implantable heart assist system from heart, percutaneous endoscopic approach

Short-Term External Heart Assist Devices

Short-term external heart assist devices are generally classified as hemodynamic support devices that unload the left ventricle, mini heart pumps/ventricular assist devices (VAD), and temporary circulatory support and recovery devices. Generally, these heart assist devices include an inflow cannula, a pump, an outflow graft, and an external controller component.

ICD-10-PCS provides the following codes for the insertion, revision, and removal of short-term external heart assist systems:

02HA0RS	Insertion of biventricular short-term external heart assist system into heart, open approach
02HA3RS	Insertion of biventricular short-term external heart assist system into heart, percutaneous approach
02HA4RS	Insertion of biventricular short-term external heart assist system into heart, percutaneous endoscopic approach
02WA0RZ	Revision of short-term external heart assist system in heart, open approach
02WA3RZ	Revision of short-term external heart assist system in heart, percutaneous approach
02WA4RZ	Revision of short-term external heart assist system in heart, percutaneous endoscopic approach
02PA0RZ	Removal of short-term external heart assist system from heart, open approach
02PA3RZ	Removal of short-term external heart assist system from heart, percutaneous approach
02PA4RZ	Removal of short-term external heart assist system from heart, percutaneous endoscopic approach

One example of a temporary heart assist device is the Impella®. When a patient is admitted and has an Impella® device inserted, two ICD-10-PCS codes should be reported: a code from Table 02H that describes the insertion of the device, and a code from Table 5A0 that describes assistance with an impeller pump. For example:

- A patient underwent insertion of a biventricular Impella® CP left ventricular assist device, which was introduced via the femoral artery, using a combination of fluoroscopic and transesophageal echo guidance. The patient's hemodynamics were stabilized and pressure requirements reduced. Assign **code 02HA3RS, Insertion of biventricular short-term heart assist system into heart, percutaneous approach,** to identify the insertion of a biventricular external heart assist device, and code **5A0221D, Assistance with cardiac output using impeller pump, continuous,** to identify the assistance with the impeller pump.

If a patient is subsequently transferred with the Impella® still in place, the only procedure code reported by the second facility is a code for the removal of the device if the device is removed.

Insertion of external heart assist devices is an example of the ICD-10-PCS guideline B6.1a, which describes limited root operations in which the classification provides the qualifier value "intraoperative" for specific procedures involving clinically significant devices. The device will be utilized for a brief duration during the procedure or current inpatient stay. When an external heart assist device such as the Impella® is inserted intraoperatively and removed at the completion of the procedure, assign code **02HA3RJ, Insertion of short-term external heart assist system into heart, intraoperative, percutaneous approach,** and code **5A0221D, Assistance with cardiac output using impeller pump, continuous.**

INTRA-AORTIC BALLOON PUMP

An intra-aortic balloon pump (IABP) helps the heart pump blood. Specifically, it is a polyethylene balloon mounted on a catheter that is typically inserted into the descending aorta through the femoral artery. The other end of the catheter attaches to a computer console containing a pump that inflates the balloon. As the balloon at the end of the catheter inflates and deflates with the rhythm of the heart, it helps the heart to pump blood into the body. At the start of diastole, the balloon inflates augmenting coronary perfusion. At the beginning of systole, the balloon deflates and blood is ejected from the left ventricle, increasing cardiac output. These actions decrease the workload on the heart and allow the heart to pump more blood. IABP therapy was first used for surgical patients but is now being used with interventional cardiology procedures and medical therapy. An IABP may be used pre-, intra-, or postoperatively to support the patient for a few hours or up to several days.

An IABP differs from an external heart assist device and is not classified as a device in ICD-10-PCS. Because an IABP is not considered a device under ICD-10-PCS, it is not appropriate to use the root operations "Insertion" or "Removal" for the placement or removal, respectively, of the intra-aortic balloon. Typically, auxiliary procedures done solely to support the performance of a surgical procedure are not coded separately. However, cardiopulmonary bypass and IABP are exceptions. When a surgical procedure is performed using IABP, the use of IABP (root operation "Assistance") should be assigned the separate code: **5A02210, Assistance with cardiac output using balloon pump, continuous.**

Totally Implantable and Tunneled Vascular Access Devices

A totally implantable vascular access device (VAD), often referred to as an implantable port or port-a-cath, consists of an injection port and a catheter system. A totally implantable VAD is used for multiple purposes, such as infusion of total parenteral nutrition and bolus injections of medication. It is designed to provide repeated access to the vascular system without the trauma or complications of multiple venipunctures. The devices can be left in place for weeks or months, as opposed to days, and are generally placed in patients who require long-term intermittent access, such as for chemotherapy. The "port" is inserted subcutaneously into the chest area without any portion of it exiting the skin. The catheter is inserted into one of the main veins of the upper chest (subclavian, internal jugular, or superior vena cava) and tunneled through the subcutaneous tissue. The tip of the catheter is advanced into a point in the superior vena cava just outside the right atrium; the other end of the catheter is then connected to the port, which can be accessed percutaneously using a needle.

A totally implantable VAD is a two-part device; two ICD-10-PCS codes are required to capture insertion of the device. Assign the following ICD-10-PCS codes for placement of the catheter and placement of the subcutaneous port:

02HV33Z   Insertion of infusion device into superior vena cava, percutaneous approach

0JH60WZ   Insertion of totally implantable vascular access device into chest subcutaneous tissue and fascia

A tunneled VAD is placed through a small incision at the neck into the internal jugular vein, where the catheter tip is advanced into the superior vena cava or right atrium. The opposite end of the catheter is tunneled through subcutaneous tissue and exits the body through a small incision at the chest wall. Tunneled VADs are used for long-term needs such as chemotherapy, hemodialysis, or total parenteral nutrition. For example, a patient underwent placement of a tunneled catheter in the right atrium. Codes **02H633Z, Insertion of infusion device into right atrium, percutaneous approach,** and **0JH63XZ, Insertion of tunneled vascular access device into chest subcutaneous tissue and fascia, percutaneous approach,** are assigned, respectively, for insertion of the catheter and the VAD.

When a tunneled catheter is exchanged by placing a new access catheter through the existing tunnel and into the right atrium using fluoroscopic guidance, the root operation "Change" is assigned for placing the catheter into the same exact position as the previous catheter. "Change" is defined as taking out or off a device from a body part and putting back an identical or similar device in or on the same body part without cutting or puncturing the skin or a mucous membrane. All "Change" procedures are coded by using the approach "external."

The use of an infusion pump that remains outside the body and infuses medication through a subcutaneous or venous needle is not coded. Only the procedure for placing a venous needle or catheter is coded. The application of this device includes the insertion of a permanent catheter.

Simple venous catheters (also called heparin locks) are sterile catheter systems that provide repeated access to the vascular system for procedures such as blood withdrawal and medication or fluid administration. The catheter is inserted into a peripheral vein, such as the cephalic vein, by puncturing the skin and then taping the catheter in place. These catheters remain in place for a much shorter period of time than totally implantable or tunneled VADs. Examples of simple venous catheters include Angiocaths, Abbott catheters, and Jelco catheters. For example, code **05HB03Z, Insertion of infusion device into right basilic vein, open approach,** is assigned for insertion of a simple catheter system into the basilic vein in the right arm.

A peripherally inserted central catheter (PICC) can be removed at bedside by simply removing sutures and pulling out the line. This bedside procedure is considered a nonoperative removal. Nonoperative removal of a PICC line is not typically coded. However, if facilities wish to capture this information, assign the following ICD-10-PCS code:

02PYX3Z Removal of infusion device from great vessel, external approach

Refer to figure 27.9 for a central venous catheter and figure 27.10 for a PICC.

Selection of the body part value for insertion of VADs as well as simple venous catheters is based on the site in which the catheter resides after the insertion procedure is completed, meaning the end placement of the device rather than the point of entry. For example, a PICC inserted in the

FIGURE 27.9 Central Venous Catheter (CVC)

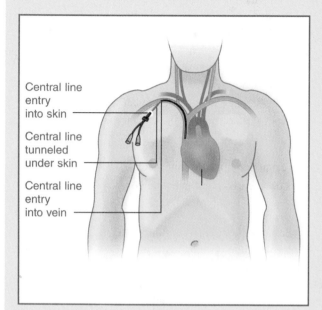

Central line entry into skin

Central line tunneled under skin

Central line entry into vein

FIGURE 27.10 Peripherally Inserted Central Catheter (PICC)

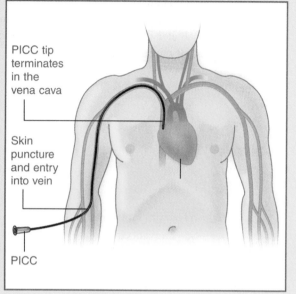

PICC tip terminates in the vena cava

Skin puncture and entry into vein

PICC

right arm with the tip ending in the superior vena cava is coded to **02HV33Z, Insertion of infusion device into superior vena cava, percutaneous approach.**

Implantable Hemodynamic Monitor

The implantable hemodynamic monitoring system allows clinicians to identify early signs of volume overload before signs and symptoms of heart failure become apparent. Clinicians can then adjust treatment to prevent acute decompensated heart failure and the need for hospital admission. The device consists of two key components. A lead with a pressure sensor is placed within the right ventricle at the right ventricular outflow tract. The other component is the monitoring device, which includes pressure-sensing circuitry with memory to process and collect the data obtained by the sensor. For example:

02HK30Z   Insertion of pressure sensor monitoring device into right ventricle, percutaneous approach

0JH600Z   Insertion of hemodynamic monitoring device into chest subcutaneous tissue and fascia, open approach

0JH800Z   Insertion of hemodynamic monitoring device into abdomen subcutaneous tissue and fascia, open approach

Intravascular and Intra-Aneurysm Pressure Measurement

Measurement of intra-aneurysm sac pressure during endovascular repair of an abdominal or thoracic aortic aneurysm can help to detect and treat endoleaks (blood flow within the aneurysm sac but outside the endoluminal graft). This procedure is classified by ICD-10-PCS to the Medical and Surgical Section, root operation "Insertion," body part either "abdominal aorta" or "thoracic aorta," and pressure sensor device. An example is **02HW30Z, Insertion of pressure sensor monitoring device into thoracic aorta, descending, percutaneous approach:**

Character 1 Section	Character 2 Body System	Character 3 Root Operation	Character 4 Body Part	Character 5 Approach	Character 6 Device	Character 7 Qualifier
0	2	H	W	3	0	Z
Medical and surgical	Heart and great vessels	Insertion	Thoracic aorta, descending	Percutaneous	Monitoring device, pressure sensor	No qualifier

Intravascular pressure measurement of coronary arteries provides physiological assessment of intravascular lesions. The specialized guide wire–mounted pressure sensor measures pressure and flow and can be used during diagnostic cardiac catheterization to determine the significance of a blockage in a coronary artery. Pressure wire measurement can confirm therapeutic results in coronary vessel stenting, identify culprit vessels, assist in developing an individual therapeutic strategy, and provide step-by-step guidance during complex interventional procedures. This procedure is classified to the Measurement and Monitoring Section, "physiological systems" body system, root operation "Measurement," pressure function, coronary qualifier. A code example is **4A033BC, Measurement of arterial pressure, coronary, percutaneous approach:**

Character 1 Section	Character 2 Body System	Character 3 Operation	Character 4 Body System	Character 5 Approach	Character 6 Function/Device	Character 7 Qualifier
4	A	0	3	3	B	C
Measurement and monitoring	Physiological systems	Measurement	Arterial	Percutaneous	Pressure	Coronary

Any other diagnostic or therapeutic procedures performed in conjunction with intravascular pressure measurement of coronary arteries are coded separately.

Intravascular pressure measurement can be performed on other vessels, such as intrathoracic arteries (i.e., assessment of the aorta, aortic arch, and carotid arteries), pulmonary arteries, and peripheral arteries, including assessment of vessels of the arms and legs. Assign additional codes for any synchronous diagnostic or therapeutic procedures performed.

Implantation of Carotid Sinus Stimulation System

The baroreflex system helps to regulate function of the heart, kidneys, and peripheral vasculature to maintain an appropriate blood pressure. The carotid sinus baroreflex activation device is currently the only medical device used to treat refractory hypertension. It consists of an implantable pulse generator, bilateral carotid sinus leads, and a computer programming system. The pulse generator is placed in a subcutaneous pocket in the pectoral region below the collar bone. Electrodes are placed bilaterally on the carotid arteries, which are two main blood pressure control points, and the leads run under the skin and connect to the pulse generator. Placement of the leads is determined by intraoperative blood pressure responses to test activations. The programming system regulates the activation energy from the device to the leads and can be adjusted based on the needs of the patient.

When the device is activated, the programming system delivers activation energy through the leads to the carotid sinus. The baroreceptors of the carotid arteries send signals through neural pathways to the brain that there is a rise in blood pressure that needs to be corrected. The brain sends signals to other parts of the body to counteract the rise in blood pressure by modulating the nervous system and hormones to dilate blood vessels and allow blood to flow more freely, reduce the heart rate, and influence fluid handling by the kidneys. This results in reduced blood pressure, reduced workload by the heart, improved circulation, and a more optimal neurohormonal balance.

Insertion of a complete system is coded by assigning separate codes for each of the following components of the surgery:

0JH60MZ	Insertion of stimulator generator into chest subcutaneous tissue and fascia, open approach
03HK3MZ	Insertion of stimulator lead into right internal carotid artery via percutaneous approach
03HL3MZ	Insertion of stimulator lead into left internal carotid artery via percutaneous approach

In the event that it becomes necessary to revise the leads or the pulse generator, ICD-10-PCS provides separate codes for these procedures as well. For example:

- A patient who is status post implantation of a carotid sinus baroreflex activation device due to refractory hypertension is admitted to have the lead adjusted and repositioned (via percutaneous approach) within the left carotid sinus for better signal activation. Assign code **Z45.09, Encounter for adjustment and management of other cardiac device,** as the principal diagnosis. Assign code **I10, Essential (primary) hypertension,** as an additional diagnosis. Assign code **03WY3MZ, Revision of stimulator lead in upper artery, percutaneous approach,** for repositioning of the lead.

Implantation of Cardiomyostimulation System

Dynamic cardiomyoplasty is a fairly complicated, new surgical technique performed using a two-step open procedure that involves elevating the latissimus dorsi muscle and then wrapping it around the heart. A stimulator similar to a pacemaker is implanted and connected to both the heart and the wrapped muscle. There are a number of components to the procedure, which are all coded separately, as follows:

- Transfer of the trunk muscle, either left (0KXG0ZZ) or right (0KXF0ZZ)
- Resection of the rib, either left (0PT20ZZ) or right (0PT10ZZ)
- Insertion of cardiac lead into pericardium, open approach (02HN0MZ)

Heart Transplantation

Heart transplantation is carried out when the heart is failing and does not respond to therapies. The main reasons for heart transplants are cardiomyopathy, severe coronary artery disease, and congenital defects of the heart. The number of organs available for transplantation is insufficient to meet the need. A patient may wait months for a transplant, and many patients do not live long enough to receive the organ. Code **02YA0Z0, Transplantation of heart, allogeneic, open approach,** or **02YA0Z1, Transplantation of heart, syngeneic, open approach,** is used to report the transplantation of a heart from a donor. "Allogeneic" refers to transplant from a genetically similar, but not identical, donor; "syngeneic" refers to a transplant from a genetically identical or closely related donor. For example:

- A patient underwent an orthostatic cardiac allograft transplantation utilizing total cardiopulmonary bypass along with an open sternotomy. Because excessive transfusions were required, a Mahurkar catheter was inserted percutaneously through the left common femoral vein and the end tip placed in the inferior vena cava. The patient also had an IABP for counterpulsation, which was left in place after the procedure. The pacemaker was also left in place at the end of the procedure due to coagulopathy. The following codes are assigned:

02YA0Z0	Transplantation of heart, allogeneic, open approach
5A02210	Assistance with cardiac output using balloon pump, continuous
5A1223Z	Performance of cardiac pacing, continuous

5A1221Z   Performance of cardiac output, continuous

06H033Z   Insertion of infusion device into inferior vena cava, percutaneous approach

Typically, auxiliary procedures done solely to support the performance of a surgical procedure are not coded separately. Cardiopulmonary bypass and IABP are exceptions. When a surgical procedure is performed with cardiopulmonary bypass and IABP, they are coded separately in ICD-10-PCS. In this case, the transfusion catheter and the temporary pacing were required to be continued beyond the operative episode of the heart transplant. In that sense, these procedures are more than just temporary auxiliary support of the surgical procedure and therefore are coded separately.

Procedures on Aneurysms

An aneurysm of a vessel is an abnormal dilatation, causing the vessel to become enlarged and weakened, which can lead to rupture. In ICD-10-PCS, the selection of the appropriate root operation for aneurysm repair depends on the primary physical action performed to correct the aneurysm.

The open aneurysmectomy (see figure 27.11) is the gold standard for abdominal aortic aneurysm repair. In this surgery, the aneurysm sac is cut open and repaired by the use of a long tubular (e.g., Dacron® or polytetrafluoroethylene) graft. The graft is sutured to the aorta, connecting one end of the aorta at the site of the aneurysm to the other end of the aorta. If the aneurysm is repaired by cutting open the aneurysm and removing the affected section of artery and replacing it with a graft, the root operation is "Replacement." ICD-10-PCS provides distinct values for different types of grafts, such as autologous and nonautologous tissue substitutes, synthetic substitutes, and zooplastic tissue. If graft material is derived from an animal, and the "zooplastic" device value is not available, it is appropriate to use "nonautologous tissue substitute" as the device value. ICD-10-PCS provides clinical detail on the specific segment of the thoracic aorta that is being treated. The body part value "X" is used for the ascending and arch segments of the thoracic aorta; the body part value "W" is used for procedures performed on the descending segment of the thoracic aorta. The following codes are examples of open repair of abdominal aortic aneurysms:

04R007Z   Replacement of abdominal aorta with autologous tissue substitute, open approach

04R00JZ   Replacement of abdominal aorta with synthetic substitute, open approach

04R00KZ   Replacement of abdominal aorta with nonautologous tissue substitute, open approach

02RW08Z   Replacement of thoracic aorta, descending, with zooplastic tissue, open approach

Abdominal aortic aneurysm repair can also be performed using an interposition tube graft without removing the aneurysm (see figure 27.12). During surgery, the aneurysm sac is opened; an interposition tube graft (Dacron® or GORE-TEX®) is sutured into place; and the vessel is closed over the graft. Although this type of aneurysm repair is not performed via an endovascular approach, the root operation "Restriction" still applies. The intraluminal device is placed to narrow the lumen of the vessel using an open approach; it is not replacing the vessel because the aneurysm is not resected. The following code is an example of open repair of abdominal aortic aneurysm using an interposition graft:

04V00DZ   Restriction of abdominal aorta with intraluminal device, open approach

Endovascular aneurysm repair (EVAR) (see figure 27.13) is a minimally invasive procedure used to treat an aneurysm. In this type of repair, a stent graft is deployed under radiological guidance using a catheter via the femoral artery into the site of the aneurysm. After deployment, the stent graft expands, relieving pressure on the aneurysm. The stent graft restricts the aneurysm from circulating blood, thus preventing its expansion and rupture. If the aneurysm is repaired by putting

FIGURE 27.11 Open Aneurysmectomy

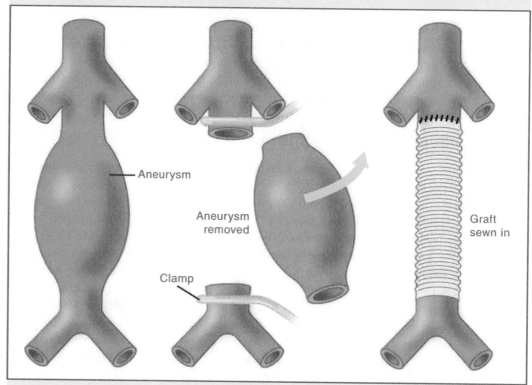

COPYRIGHT ©2018 BY HEALTH FORUM, INC., AN AMERICAN HOSPITAL ASSOCIATION COMPANY. ALL RIGHTS RESERVED.

FIGURE 27.12 Open Surgical Aneurysm Repair via Tube Graft

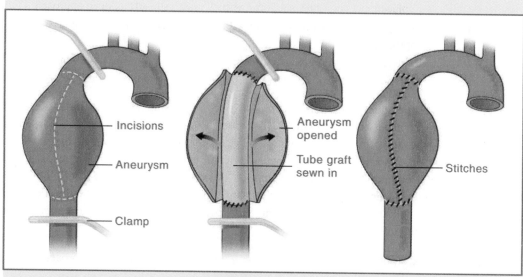

COPYRIGHT ©2018 BY HEALTH FORUM, INC., AN AMERICAN HOSPITAL ASSOCIATION COMPANY. ALL RIGHTS RESERVED.

in a stent graft or other device into the lumen of the artery, the root operation is "Restriction" and the device is "intraluminal." If the aneurysm is repaired by wrapping or otherwise deploying material or a device (e.g., clip, sleeve, and so forth) on or around the outside of the artery, the root operation is "Restriction" and the device is "extraluminal." The simplest aortic endografts are essentially straight tubes that reline a segment of the aorta to exclude the aneurysm from circulation. However, these tubes cannot be used to treat aneurysms close to or involving major branches of the aorta because the tube could cover the origins of the branches and cut off blood flow to the organs supplied by the branches. Branched and fenestrated endografts were developed to address this issue.

The following codes are examples of procedures for endovascular repair of aneurysms:

04V03DZ	Restriction of abdominal aorta with intraluminal device, percutaneous approach
04V93CZ	Restriction of right renal artery with extraluminal device, percutaneous approach
04V53DZ	Restriction of superior mesenteric artery with intraluminal device, percutaneous approach

Bifurcated endografts may be used for treating aneurysms located at or just above the distal bifurcation of the abdominal aorta into the left and right common iliac arteries (e.g., aorto-iliac aneurysm). In such cases, no separate codes are assigned for additional endograft limbs or extensions placed in the common iliac arteries unless the aneurysm continues distally into the internal iliac artery, external iliac artery, or external femoral artery, necessitating another endograft.

Endograft procedures always involve a "landing zone," also called a "seal zone." This is a segment of healthy tissue into which the endograft extends so it can form a proper seal and reduce the risk of endoleaks. Finding a landing zone for an aneurysm may involve crossing anatomical boundaries into another body part. For example, an abdominal aortic endograft may have a proximal

FIGURE 27.13 Endovascular Aneurysm Repair

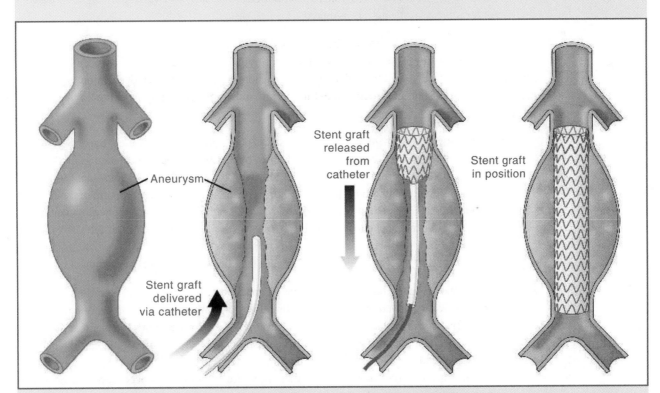

Aneurysm

Stent graft delivered via catheter

Stent graft released from catheter

Stent graft in position

landing zone in the thoracic aorta or a distal landing zone in the common iliac artery. That is, the aneurysm itself is entirely within the abdominal aorta, but the endograft extends up into the thoracic aorta or down into the common iliac artery simply to achieve a proper seal. A separate code is not assigned for the landing zone, even if it is in a different body part.

Endovascular aneurysm repair involves restriction of the aneurysmal sac from the systemic circulation. If restriction is inadequate, patients can develop an endoleak, resulting in aneurysm expansion with an increased risk of rupture. For example:

- A patient status post endovascular aneurysm repair develops a type 1 endoleak and undergoes another EVAR, in which the surgeon uses an endostaple device to attach the stent graft. Code **04WY3DZ, Revision of intraluminal device in lower artery, percutaneous approach,** is assigned.

In the above case, the type 1 endoleak involved leaking at the graft attachment site. Endostaples were used to secure the position of the endograft. The objective of the surgery is to correct the leak. The appropriate root operation is "Revision" because the endostaple device was used to reattach the stent graft (endograft). In ICD-10-PCS, stent grafts are considered intraluminal devices; however, staples are considered supplies integral to the procedure, and they are not coded as a device.

A pseudoaneurysm, also referred to as a false aneurysm, is a hematoma adjacent to a puncture or other disruption of the arterial wall. It is caused by the slow leaking of blood into the surrounding tissues, which gives the hematoma the appearance of a sac, even though the collection of blood is outside the arterial wall. A pseudoaneurysm is distinct from a true aneurysm. The latter is an abnormal widening of the arterial wall itself and, unless it is a dissecting aneurysm, involves all three layers of the arterial wall. If untreated, the pseudoaneurysm can lead to thrombosis, rupture, or distal embolization. The following is an example of code assignment for a procedure to treat pseudoaneurysm:

- A patient presents for repair of right femoral artery pseudoaneurysm. At surgery, dissection is undertaken down to the inguinal ligament, and the common femoral artery is identified. The pseudoaneurysm site is sutured. Code **04QK0ZZ, Repair right femoral artery, open approach,** is assigned.

In the above example, the cut down and suturing of the pseudoaneurysm are coded as a "Repair."

Pseudoaneurysm following femoral-popliteal bypass is uncommon but can occur as a complication of the surgery. Endovascular repair of pseudoaneurysm can include balloon angioplasty and self-expanding stent graft deployment in the previously placed femoral-popliteal bypass graft. For example:

- A patient with peripheral artery disease, status post right femoral popliteal bypass grafting, using saphenous vein, presented one year post bypass with a totally occluded graft. At that time, he underwent recanalization of the graft with balloon angioplasty and stent placement. He now presents with a right lower extremity pseudoaneurysm due to rupture of the femoral popliteal graft. The patient undergoes endovascular repair with stent graft deployment at the site of the existing saphenous vein graft. Codes **04WY37Z, Revision of autologous tissue substitute in lower artery, percutaneous approach,** and **04UK3JZ, Supplement right femoral artery with synthetic substitute, percutaneous approach,** are assigned.

In the example above, the pseudoaneurysm was a complication of the previously placed graft. At surgery, a stent graft was deployed inside of the existing graft for reinforcement and to prevent recurrence of the rupture. Two codes are assigned. The root operation "Revision" captures the fact that the previously placed saphenous vein graft was repaired. The root operation "Supplement" captures the fact that a stent graft was placed inside the existing graft to reinforce the previous bypass site.

When an intraoperative intra-aneurysm sac pressure monitoring procedure is performed in conjunction with an endovascular repair, the procedure to insert the monitoring device may be coded separately along with the endovascular repair. For example:

02VW3DZ Restriction of thoracic aorta, descending, with intraluminal device, percutaneous approach

02HW30Z Insertion of pressure sensor monitoring device into thoracic aorta, descending, percutaneous approach

Endovascular implantation of a branching or fenestrated graft into the aorta is a new technology used as an endovascular repair option for patients who are not anatomical candidates for standard endovascular repair of abdominal aortic aneurysms. The branching or fenestrated endograft is a tubular fabric graft with supporting metal stents that feature custom-positioned holes (fenestrations) to ensure proper blood flow through the aorta and to the kidneys and nearby organs. Each

---

FIGURE 27.14   Aorta and Lower Side Branches

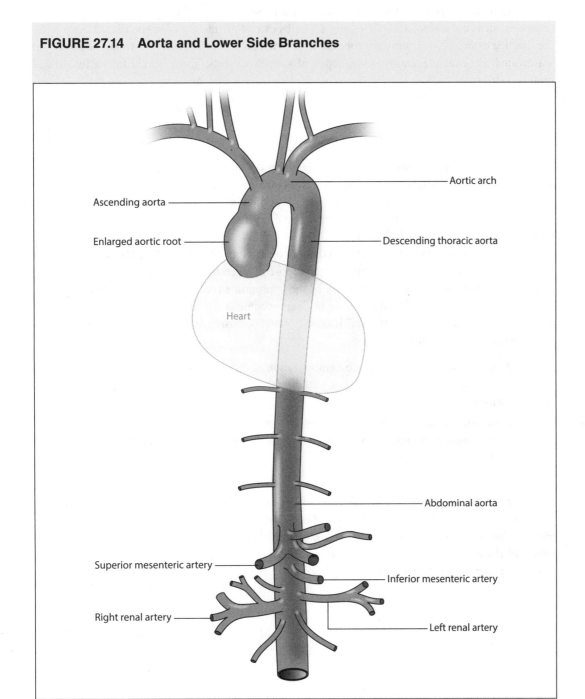

fenestrated graft is customized for the individual aneurysm. This type of graft is captured by the device value "E, Intraluminal device, branched or fenestrated, one or two arteries," or by the device value "F, Intraluminal device, branched or fenestrated, three or more arteries." In the abdominal aorta, four side branches must be kept open: the right renal artery, left renal artery, superior mesenteric artery, and celiac trunk—collectively referred to as the visceral arteries. In the thoracic aorta, specifically the aortic arch, three branches must be kept open: the left subclavian artery, left common carotid artery, and brachiocephalic (innominate) artery—collectively referred to as the precerebral arteries.

For both clinical and coding purposes, it is important to understand that stents placed through the nubs or fenestrations into the side branches are not equivalent to a regular stent procedure. In a regular stent procedure, the objective is to reopen an occluded vessel. In contrast, the objective of placing a stent during EVAR is to ensure that a vessel that was already open remains open. A separate code is not assigned for the endograft limbs extending into the common iliac arteries or for the iliac leg extension. It is only appropriate to assign a code for the vessel in which the aneurysm was treated. For example, endovascular repair of abdominal aortic aneurysms with one fenestrated graft is coded to **04V03EZ, Restriction of abdominal aorta with branched or fenestrated intraluminal device, one or two arteries, percutaneous approach.**

Other Endovascular Procedures

Endovascular embolization uses particulate agents (such as gelfoam, polyvinyl alcohol, and spherical embolics), coils, liquid sclerosing agents (such as alcohol and tissue adhesives), and other types of embolic materials (such as Onyx-18, a liquid embolic). Microcoils and microbeads are classified as intraluminal devices. The device key entry for "embolization coils" advises coding professionals to use intraluminal devices.

It is important to distinguish between the root operations "Restriction" and "Occlusion" when the documentation refers to embolization. The purpose of an embolization procedure is to terminate blood flow out of the vessel. The selection of the appropriate root operation depends on how the procedure is being defined. If the objective of the procedure is to obliterate the vessel (total occlusion), the root operation is "Occlusion." If only a partial occlusion is being done, the root operation is "Restriction." For example:

- A patient has a percutaneous coil embolization of the right uterine artery; code **04LE3DT, Occlusion of right uterine artery with intraluminal device, percutaneous approach,** is assigned.

- A patient with gastrointestinal bleeding undergoes microbead embolization of the inferior mesenteric artery. This procedure is performed to totally occlude the artery. Code **04LB3DZ, Occlusion of inferior mesenteric artery with intraluminal device, percutaneous approach,** is assigned.

Esophageal varices are enlarged veins in the esophagus, which can spontaneously rupture and cause severe bleeding. Transorifice endoscopic banding of esophageal varices involves complete occlusion of blood flow and meets the definition of the root operation "Occlusion." The lumen of the esophageal vein is being banded, not the esophagus. The Index entry for Ligation directs the user to see "Occlusion." Assign code **06L38CZ, Occlusion of esophageal vein with extraluminal device, via natural or artificial opening endoscopic,** for endoscopic banding of esophageal varices.

EXERCISE 27.9

Code the following diagnoses and procedures.

1. Second degree prolapsed hemorrhoids

    Hemorrhoidectomy by cryosurgery (open)

2. Painful varicose veins, right lower leg

    Right greater saphenous ligation and stripping for

    varicosities, open

3. Mitral stenosis and aortic insufficiency

    Permanent atrial fibrillation

    Hypertension

4. Abdominal aortic aneurysm

    Hypertensive cardiovascular disease essential

    Open repair of abdominal aortic aneurysm with

    interposition tube graft

5. Acute type 2 myocardial infarction, anterior wall

6. Renovascular hypertension secondary to

    fibromuscular hyperplasia, right renal artery

    Nuclear renal scan with Tc-99m

7. Congestive heart failure due to

    hypertensive heart disease

8. Acute systolic congestive heart failure

    End-stage dilated cardiomyopathy

    Permanent cardiac pacemaker in place

    Percutaneous revision of external heart assist

    device due to exposed wire and device malfunction

9. Cerebral occlusion, thrombotic with cerebral infarction

    Hypertensive cardiovascular disease

10. Hypertension

    Chronic kidney disease

11. Postoperative multiple subsegmental pulmonary emboli,
    initial encounter

---

12. Hypertensive encephalopathy due to
    hypertensive urgency

---

13. Percutaneous insertion of pacemaker leads (right
    ventricle and right atrium), insertion of dual chamber
    pacemaker device in chest pocket (open)

---

14. Arteriosclerosis of autologous vein bypass graft
    (four-vessel bypass graft with saphenous
    vein carried out two years ago)

---

15. Acute pulmonary edema with left ventricular failure

---

16. Cerebral infarction, acute, with thrombosis
    Residual hemiplegia, right, dominant side,
    and aphasia (at discharge)
    Essential hypertension

---

17. Severe stenosis of left main coronary arteries in patient
    with no previous history of bypass surgery
    Aortocoronary bypass, left diagonal and left circumflex
    arteries with right greater saphenous vein graft, open
    Cardiopulmonary bypass (extracorporeal cardiac)

CHAPTER 28

Neoplasms

CHAPTER OVERVIEW

- Neoplastic diseases are classified in chapter 2 of ICD-10-CM.
- Neoplasms are categorized by two axes.
  - The first axis for coding is by behavior (malignant, benign, carcinoma in situ, uncertain behavior, and unspecified behavior).
  - The second axis for coding is by anatomical site.
- The morphology of tumor cells is studied for classifying a neoplasm by its tissue origin.
- Neoplastic diseases are indexed by morphological type and common terms.
- The Neoplasm Table lists anatomical sites alphabetically. It uses behavior type to indicate the correct code.
- There are two types of malignant neoplasms.
  - Solid neoplasms have a localized point of origin and are considered to be the primary neoplasm of the site. They often metastasize to secondary sites.
    - The statement "metastatic to" indicates that the site of a metastatic tumor is secondary, while "metastatic from" indicates a primary site.
    - When coding, refer to the morphology type in the Alphabetic Index.
  - Lymphatic and hematopoietic tumors often circulate through the bloodstream and lymphatic system.
    - These tumors can spread to secondary sites. All sites to which they spread through circulation are considered secondary.
    - Special coding requirements are in place for Hodgkin disease and non-Hodgkin lymphomas.
- Sometimes, treatment can be a guide when selecting a principal diagnosis.
  - When the treatment is directed at the primary site, the malignancy of that site is often the principal diagnosis.
  - When the treatment is directed at a secondary site, the malignancy of the primary site is an additional code.
  - Admission solely for chemotherapy, immunotherapy, or external beam radiation therapy treatment requires a Z code as the principal diagnosis.

LEARNING OUTCOMES

After studying this chapter, you should be able to:

Explain the various classifications of neoplasms.

Locate codes for neoplastic diseases.

Code for malignant neoplasms (both solid and hematopoietic or lymphatic).

Code for the treatment of neoplastic diseases.

TERMS TO KNOW

Direct extension
the invasion of adjacent sites by a malignant neoplasm

Invasive
the extension of tumor cells to other adjacent sites

Metastasis
the resulting spread of invasive tumor cells

Neoplasm
a new or abnormal growth

REMEMBER . . .

Morphology codes are optional but are used in tumor registries and pathology indexes.

INTRODUCTION

A neoplasm is a new or abnormal growth. In the ICD-10-CM classification system, neoplastic disease is classified in categories C00 through D49. Certain benign neoplasms, such as prostatic adenomas, may be found in the specific body system chapters.

BEHAVIOR CLASSIFICATION

The first axis for coding neoplasms is behavior; the second axis is the anatomical site. ICD-10-CM classifies neoplasms into five behavior groups and a sixth for unspecified behavior:

C00–C96	Malignant
C7A, C7B, D3A	Neuroendocrine
D00–D09	Carcinoma in situ
D10–D36	Benign
D37–D48	Uncertain behavior
D49	Unspecified behavior

Malignant Neoplasms

Malignant neoplasms are tumor cells that extend beyond the primary site, attaching themselves to adjacent structures or spreading to distant sites. They are characterized by relentless growth and are difficult to cure. The term "invasive" is often used to describe the extension of the tumor cells to other adjacent sites. The resulting spread is called "metastasis."

Certain types of malignant neoplasms are noted for their invasive properties (for example, malignant melanoma of the skin) and usually require excision beyond the primary site because of their potential microinvasiveness. In such cases, a biopsy finding of malignancy on tissue removed during outpatient surgery may indicate the need for more extensive surgery on an inpatient basis. When such further surgery is performed, however, the pathology report may or may not indicate further malignancy. When no further malignancy is found, the physician ordinarily documents the diagnosis as a malignancy in accordance with the findings of the initial biopsy, because that condition is the reason for admission and the primary neoplasm may, in fact, require further treatment. In this situation, the diagnosis provided by the physician should be coded even though the current pathology report does not confirm the diagnosis. A copy of the original pathology report should be obtained and filed with the current medical record if at all possible.

Neuroendocrine Tumors

Neuroendocrine tumors (categories C7A, C7B, and D3A) arise from endocrine or neuroendocrine cells scattered throughout the body. The most common sites are the bronchi, stomach, small intestine, appendix, and rectum. These tumors are commonly classified according to the presumed embryonic site of origin, such as the foregut (bronchi and stomach), midgut (small intestine and appendix), and hindgut (colon and rectum).

A carcinoid tumor is a tumor that develops from enterochromaffin cells. These cells produce hormones that normally are found in the small intestine, appendix, colon, rectum, bronchi, pancreas, ovaries, testes, bile ducts, liver, and other organs. Carcinoid tumors are capable of producing these same hormones, often in large quantities, and can cause carcinoid syndrome (E34.0). Carcinoid tumors can be found throughout the body, but the majority are found in the gastrointestinal tract. Approximately 25 percent of carcinoid tumors are found in the bronchial airways and the lung. In some cases, it may not be possible to locate the site of origin of the carcinoid tumors, although symptoms of carcinoid syndrome may be present. Carcinoid tumors can present as a primary malignancy (category C7A), as a secondary or metastatic tumor (category C7B), or as a benign tumor (category D3A). Codes Z85.020, Z85.030, Z85.040, Z85.060, Z85.110, Z85.230, and Z85.520 are used to describe the history of a malignant neuroendocrine tumor that has been previously excised or eradicated with no further treatment.

When multiple endocrine neoplasia (MEN) syndrome is associated with malignant or benign neuroendocrine tumors, code also the MEN syndrome (E31.2-). However, this code is not assigned when the health record documentation does not support the condition. If there is an associated endocrine syndrome, assign the appropriate additional code, such as carcinoid syndrome (E34.0). For example:

C7A.092 + E31.21 + E34.0   Malignant carcinoid tumor of the stomach, Wermer's
                             syndrome, and carcinoid syndrome

Merkel Cell Carcinoma

Merkel cell carcinoma, also called neuroendocrine carcinoma of the skin, arises from the uncontrolled growth of Merkel cells in the skin. It is a rare skin cancer and potentially life threatening; aggressive therapy may be needed. Merkel cell carcinoma does not have a distinctive appearance and usually develops on sun-exposed skin (e.g., head, neck, arms) as a painless, firm, flesh-colored to red or blue bump. It is diagnosed via skin biopsy. The following subcategories and codes are assigned for Merkel cell carcinoma:

C4A.0   Merkel cell carcinoma of lip
C4A.1-   Merkel cell carcinoma of eyelid, including canthus
C4A.2-   Merkel cell carcinoma of ear and external auricular canal
C4A.3-   Merkel cell carcinoma of other and unspecified parts of face
C4A.4   Merkel cell carcinoma of scalp and neck
C4A.5-   Merkel cell carcinoma of trunk
C4A.6-   Merkel cell carcinoma of upper limb, including shoulder
C4A.7-   Merkel cell carcinoma of lower limb, including hip
C4A.8   Merkel cell carcinoma of overlapping sites
C4A.9   Merkel cell carcinoma, unspecified

Malignant Neoplasms of Ectopic Tissue

Malignant neoplasms of ectopic tissue are coded to the site of origin mentioned in the documentation. For example, ectopic pancreatic malignant neoplasms involving the stomach are coded to **C25.9, Malignant neoplasm of pancreas, unspecified.**

Benign Neoplasms

Benign neoplasms are not invasive and do not spread to either adjacent or distant sites. They may, however, cause local effects such as displacement, pressure on an adjacent structure, impingement on a nerve, or compression of a vessel and therefore require surgery. Uterine myomas, for example, may cause pressure on the urinary bladder, which results in urinary symptoms. Most benign tumors can be cured by total excision.

Carcinoma in Situ

Tumor cells in carcinoma described as in situ are undergoing malignant changes but are still confined to the point of origin without invasion of the surrounding normal tissue. Other terms that describe carcinoma in situ include "intraepithelial," "noninfiltrating," "noninvasive," and "preinvasive" carcinoma. Severe cervical or vulvar dysplasia described as CIN III or VIN III is classified as carcinoma in situ. (See chapter 20 of this handbook for more information.)

Neoplasms of Uncertain Behavior

The ultimate behavior of certain neoplasms cannot be determined at the time they are discovered, and a firm distinction between benign and malignant tumor cells cannot be made. For example, certain benign tumors may be undergoing malignant transformation; as a result, continued study is necessary to arrive at a conclusive diagnosis.

Neurofibromatosis refers to a group of autosomal dominant genetic disorders that cause tumors to grow along the nerves. Code **Q85.00, Neurofibromatosis, unspecified,** is assigned for neurofibromatosis.

Schwannomas may occur along any nerve of the body, including spinal, cranial, and peripheral nerves, except on the vestibular nerve. As the tumors grow, they compress nerves and cause pain, numbness, tingling, weakness, and other neurological symptoms. Code **Q85.03, Schwannomatosis,** is assigned for this condition.

Neoplasms of Unspecified Behavior

It is important not to confuse neoplasms of unspecified behavior with those of uncertain behavior. Category D49 is provided for those situations in which neither the behavior nor the morphology of the neoplasm is specified in the diagnostic statement or elsewhere in the medical record. This usually occurs when a patient is transferred to another medical care facility for further diagnosis and possible treatment before diagnostic studies are completed, or when a patient is given a working diagnosis in an outpatient setting pending further study. Category D49 includes terms such as "growth," "neoplasm," "new growth," and "tumor" when the neoplasms are not otherwise specified. With one exception, a code from category D49 would not be used for a neoplasm treated in an acute care facility because more definitive information should always be available.

The exception for coding neoplasm of unspecified behavior in the acute care setting is when coding dark areas or spots of the retina, which are referred to as neoplasms or suspected melanoma. These spots are often difficult to biopsy and must be continually evaluated. Code **D49.81, Neoplasm of unspecified behavior, retina and choroid,** is assigned for this condition. Because a biopsy of the retina poses a risk to the eye and is only performed if the lesion extends, there is usually no tissue biopsy taken to confirm the diagnosis. Therefore, code D49.81 is appropriately assigned for this condition.

Unspecified Mass or Lesion

It is incorrect to select a code from category D49, Neoplasms of unspecified behavior, when only the term "mass" or "lesion" is used. When coding a diagnosis documented as mass or lesion of a particular site, first refer to the main term **Mass** or **Lesion.** If the site is not listed under the main term, follow the cross-references under the main term that represent the documented diagnosis. For example, under the main term **Mass,** the index subentry for "substernal thyroid" directs the user to see **Goiter.**

If the diagnosis is "mass" and there is no Index entry for the specific site under **Mass,** follow the instruction provided at **Mass,** specified organ NEC, to see **Disease,** by site. Similarly, if a final diagnosis is documented as "lesion," and there is no Index entry for the specified organ or site under the main term **Lesion,** look up the main term **Disease.** The Index directs the user to see **Disease,** by site, for **Lesion,** organ or site NEC. If a final diagnosis is documented as "lump" of any body site except breast, look up the main term **Mass,** as directed by the "see also" note under the main term **Lump.**

EXERCISE 28.1

By referring to the following subcategories in the Tabular List, match the codes in the left column with the descriptions listed in the right column.

1. C18.4   Transverse colon _____   a. Benign

2. D44.10   Adrenal gland   _____   b. Carcinoma in situ

3. C43.0   Lip   _____   c. Malignant

4. D02.1   Trachea   _____   d. Uncertain behavior

5. D49.4   Bladder   _____   e. Unspecified behavior

6. D10.6   Nasopharynx   _____

7. C7A.025 Sigmoid colon   _____

MORPHOLOGY CLASSIFICATION

Morphology of neoplasms refers to the form and structure of tumor cells. It is studied to classify a neoplasm by its tissue of origin. The tissue of origin and the type of cells that make up a malignant neoplasm often determine the expected rate of growth, the severity of illness, and the type of treatment given. Metastatic neoplasms are identified at the metastatic site by their morphology, which is different from the normal tissue at that site but the same as that at the primary site.

A tumor registry is a cancer data system that provides follow-up on all cancer patients. It documents and stores all major aspects of a patient's cancer history and treatment, and its database includes demographics, medical history, diagnostic findings, primary site, metastasis, histology, stage of disease, treatments, recurrence, subsequent treatment, and end results. Use the completed cancer staging form for coding purposes when it is authenticated by the attending physician. If staging classes are being documented in the hospital medical record, obtain copies of the current classifications for use in decoding the numerical/alphabetical designations.

EXERCISE 28.2

Mark the following statements either true or false.

1. Morphology of neoplasms refers to the study of the form and structure   _____
    of the tissue and cells from which the neoplasm arises.

2. Metastatic neoplasms can be identified by their morphology, which is   _____
    identical to the morphology of the surrounding normal tissue and
    cells at the metastatic site.

3. The completed cancer staging form may be used for coding   _____
    purposes when it is authenticated by the attending physician.

LOCATING CODES FOR NEOPLASTIC DISEASE

The first step in locating the code for a neoplasm is to refer to the main term for the morphological type in the Alphabetic Index of Diseases and Injuries and then to review the subentries. For some types, a specific diagnosis code is provided. For example, for a diagnosis of renal cell carcinoma, the Alphabetic Index lists the main term **Carcinoma** and the subterm "renal cell" as follows:

> **Carcinoma . . .**
>
> -renal cell C64.-

When the site is not listed as a subterm or when a specific code is not given in the Alphabetic Index, a cross-reference to the Neoplasm Table in volume 2 of the Index appears. Cross-references should be followed closely; the following entries indicate the help the coding professional can receive when the type of neoplasm is referenced in the Alphabetic Index:

> **Sarcoma . . .**
>
> -cerebellar C71.6 . . .
>
> -embryonal—*see* Neoplasm, connective tissue, malignant . . .
>
> -Ewing's—*see* Neoplasm, bone, malignant

The Neoplasm Table (part of which is reproduced as table 28.1) lists anatomical sites alphabetically on the far left. (The indention levels have the same significance as those used elsewhere in the Alphabetic Index.) Columns to the right indicate the code for each behavior type for that site.

To use the Table, first locate the anatomical site in the list, move across the page to the behavior type, and then select the appropriate code. For each site, there are six possible code numbers according to whether the neoplasm in question is malignant, benign, in situ, of uncertain behavior, or of unspecified nature. The description of the neoplasm will often indicate which of the six columns is appropriate (e.g., malignant melanoma of skin, benign fibroadenoma of breast, carcinoma in situ of cervix uteri). Where such descriptors are not present, the remainder of the Index should be consulted, where guidance is given to the appropriate column for each morphological (histological) variety listed, such as Mesonephroma—*see* Neoplasm, malignant, by site; Embryoma—*see also* Neoplasm, uncertain behavior, by site; Bowen's disease—*see* Neoplasm, skin, in situ. However, the guidance in the Index can be overridden if one of the descriptors mentioned above is present; for example, malignant adenoma of colon is coded to C18.9 and not to D12.6, as the adjective "malignant" overrides the Index entry "Adenoma—*see also* Neoplasm, benign, by site." Codes listed with a dash (-) following the code have a required fifth character for laterality. Codes from the Neoplasm Table should be verified in the Tabular List.

TABLE 28.1 Section of the Neoplasm Table in the Alphabetic Index of Diseases and Injuries

Neoplasm, neoplastic—*continued*	Malignant Primary	Malignant Secondary	Ca in Situ	Benign	Uncertain Behavior	Unspecified Behavior
-nostril	C30.0	C78.39	D02.3	D14.0	D38.5	D49.1
-nucleus pulposus	C41.2	C79.51	—	D16.6	D48.0	D49.2
-occipital						
--bone	C41.0	C79.51	—	D16.4-	D48.0	D49.2
--lobe or pole, brain	C71.4	C79.31	—	D33.0	D43.0	D49.6
-odontogenic—see Neoplasm, jaw bone						
-olfactory nerve or bulb	C72.2-	C79.49	—	D33.3	D43.3	D49.7
-olive (brain)	C71.7	C79.31	—	D33.1	D43.1	D49.6
-omentum	C48.1	C78.6	—	D20.1	D48.4	D49.0

EXERCISE 28.3

Code the following diagnoses.

1. Bronchial adenoma

2. Burkitt lymphoma of intrapelvic lymph nodes

3. Lipoma of head

4. Hairy cell leukemia in remission

5. Endometrial sarcoma

6. Hodgkin sarcoma

BASIC TYPES OF MALIGNANT NEOPLASMS

There are two basic types of malignant neoplasms:

C00–C75, C76–C80   Solid
C81–C96   Hematopoietic and lymphatic

Solid tumors have a single, localized point of origin and are considered to be primary neoplasms of that site. Solid tumors tend to spread to adjacent or remote sites, with such sites classified as secondary or metastatic neoplasms. For example, a diagnosis of carcinoma of the lung with metastasis to the brain indicates that a primary neoplasm of the lung has metastasized to a secondary site in the brain.

Lymphatic and hematopoietic neoplasms arise in the reticuloendothelial and lymphatic systems and the blood-forming tissues. These neoplasms differ from solid malignant neoplasms in several ways, including the following:

- They may arise in a single site or in several sites simultaneously.
- Tumor cells often circulate in large numbers in the bloodstream and the lymphatic system rather than remaining confined to a single site.

Because of the differences between solid and hematopoietic-lymphatic diseases, this handbook deals with the two types of malignant neoplasms separately. Solid tumors are covered first, and then the discussion moves on to tumors that arise in the hematopoietic and lymphatic systems.

CODING OF SOLID MALIGNANT NEOPLASMS

A solid malignant neoplasm may spread from its site of origin by either direct extension or metastasis. Direct extension is the invasion of adjacent sites; "metastasis" refers to the spread to distant sites and the establishment of a new center of malignancy. ICD-10-CM does not make a distinction between these two types of extension. The terms "metastatic" and "secondary" are generally used interchangeably.

Overlapping Sites

When a primary malignant neoplasm overlaps two or more contiguous (next to each other) sites, it is classified to the subcategory/code ".8," signifying "overlapping lesion," unless the combination is specifically indexed elsewhere. For example, ICD-10-CM provides the following codes for certain malignant neoplasms whose stated sites overlap two or more boundaries:

C00.8   Neoplasm of overlapping sites of the lip whose point of origin cannot be assigned to any other code within category C00

C16.8   Neoplasm of stomach whose point of origin cannot be assigned to any other code within category C16

C34.80   Neoplasm of overlapping sites of lung, bronchus, and trachea whose point of origin cannot be assigned to any other code within category C34

When there are multiple neoplasms of the same site that are not contiguous, such as tumors in different quadrants of the same breast, codes for each site should be assigned.

EXERCISE 28.4

Code the following diagnoses.

1. Carcinoma of upper and middle third of esophagus

2. Carcinoma of oral cavity and pharynx

3. Adenocarcinoma of rectum and anus

Malignancy in Two or More Noncontiguous Sites

A patient may have more than one malignant tumor in the same organ. These tumors may represent different primary cancers or metastatic disease, depending on the site. When the documentation is unclear, the provider should be queried regarding the status of each tumor in order to select the correct codes.

When more than one primary cancer occurs in the same organ system, these are called "synchronous primary cancers." This condition can occur in the lungs where the target organ, in this case the respiratory epithelium, is attacked/altered by the inciting agent (e.g., tobacco smoke). However, the physician must designate whether one of the tumors represents a second primary cancer or a metastasis. For example:

- A patient with stage IV non–small cell lung cancer of the left lower lobe is admitted with extensive peritoneal metastasis and liver metastasis. A CT scan of the lung shows a large tumor in the left lung base with diffuse extension to the right lung. When queried, the provider documents that the tumor had started in the left lung and metastasized to the right lung. Because the provider has clearly documented that the primary malignancy of the left lung had extended to the right lung, assign code **C34.32, Malignant neoplasm of lower lobe, left bronchus or lung,** as the principal diagnosis and code **C78.01, Secondary malignant neoplasm of right lung,** as a secondary diagnosis. In addition, assign codes **C78.6, Secondary malignant neoplasm of retroperitoneum and peritoneum,** and **C78.7, Secondary malignant neoplasm of liver and intrahepatic bile duct.**

Neoplasms Described as Metastatic

The terms "metastatic" and "metastasis" are often used ambiguously in describing neoplastic disease, sometimes meaning that the site named is primary and sometimes meaning that it is secondary. When the diagnostic statement is not clear in this regard, review the medical record for further information. When none is available, however, the following guidelines apply.

"Metastatic To"

The statement "metastatic to" indicates that the site mentioned is secondary. For example, a diagnosis of metastatic carcinoma to the lung is coded as secondary malignant neoplasm of the lung (C78.0-). A code for the primary neoplastic site should also be assigned when the primary neoplasm is still present.

When the primary neoplasm has been excised or eradicated and is no longer under any type of treatment, a history code from subcategories Z85.0–Z85.8 should be assigned. The fourth character of category Z85 indicates the body system where the prior neoplasm occurred, and the fifth and sixth characters indicate the specific organ or site involved.

Please note that history codes in subcategories Z85.0–Z85.85 are only assigned for the former site of a primary malignancy, not the former site of a secondary malignancy. However, code **Z85.89, Personal history of malignant neoplasm of other organs and systems,** may be assigned to the former site(s) of either a primary or secondary malignancy that has been excised or eradicated and is no longer under treatment.

Ordinarily, no history code is assigned when the patient has had a prior benign or in-situ neoplasm or neoplasm of uncertain behavior. The exceptions are a few neoplasms that are included in subcategory Z86.0, as follows:

Z86.000   Personal history of in-situ neoplasm of breast
Z86.001   Personal history of in-situ neoplasm of cervix uteri
Z86.002   Personal history of in-situ neoplasm of other and unspecified genital organs
Z86.003   Personal history of in-situ neoplasm of oral cavity, esophagus, and stomach
Z86.004   Personal history of in-situ neoplasm of other and unspecified digestive organs

Z86.005	Personal history of in-situ neoplasm of middle ear and respiratory system
Z86.006	Personal history of melanoma in-situ
Z86.007	Personal history of in-situ neoplasm of skin
Z86.008	Personal history of in-situ neoplasm of other site
Z86.010	Personal history of colonic polyps
Z86.011	Personal history of benign neoplasm of the brain
Z86.012	Personal history of benign carcinoid tumor
Z86.018	Personal history of other benign neoplasm
Z86.03	Personal history of neoplasm of uncertain behavior

"Metastatic From"

The statement "metastatic from" indicates that the site mentioned is the primary site. For example, a diagnosis of metastatic carcinoma from the breast indicates that the breast is the primary site (C50.9-). A code for the metastatic site should also be assigned.

Single Metastatic Site

When only one site is described as metastatic without any further qualification and no more definitive information can be obtained by reviewing the medical record, refer first to the morphology type in the Alphabetic Index and code to the primary condition of that site. For example, a diagnosis of metastatic renal cell carcinoma of the lung indicates that the primary site is the kidney and the secondary site is the lung. The correct coding for this is **C64.9, Malignant neoplasm of unspecified kidney, except renal pelvis,** and **C78.00, Secondary malignant neoplasm of unspecified lung.** When a specific site for the morphology type is not indicated in a code entry or is not indexed, assign the code for unspecified site within that anatomical site. For example, oat cell carcinoma of unspecified site is indexed to **C34.90, Malignant neoplasm of unspecified part of unspecified bronchus or lung,** when a more specific site is not stated in the medical record.

Multiple Metastatic Sites

When two or more sites are described as "metastatic" in the diagnostic statement, each of the stated sites should be coded as secondary or metastatic. A code should also be assigned for the primary site when this information is available; code **C80.1, Malignant (primary) neoplasm, unspecified,** should be assigned when it is not.

No Site Stated

Code **C80.0, Disseminated malignant neoplasm, unspecified,** is for use only in those cases where the patient has advanced metastatic disease and no known primary or secondary sites are specified. It should not be used in place of assigning codes for the primary site and all known secondary sites. Code **C80.1, Malignant (primary) neoplasm, unspecified,** equates to Cancer, unspecified. This code should only be used when no determination can be made as to the primary site of a malignancy. This code should rarely be used in the inpatient setting. Code **C79.9, Secondary malignant neoplasm of unspecified site,** is assigned when no site is identified for the secondary neoplasm.

When no site is indicated in the diagnostic statement but the morphology type is qualified as metastatic, the code provided for that morphological type is assigned for the primary diagnosis along with an additional code for secondary neoplasm of unspecified site. For example, a diagnosis of metastatic apocrine adenocarcinoma with no site specified is coded as a primary malignant neoplasm of the skin, site unspecified (C44.99). An additional code of C79.9 is assigned for the secondary neoplasm. Code C44.99 is obtained by referring to the following main term and subterms in the Alphabetic Index:

Adenocarcinoma . . .

-apocrine . . .

--unspecified site C44.99

EXERCISE 28.5

Code the following diagnoses.

1. Metastatic carcinoma of right lung

2. Metastatic carcinoma to brain

3. Metastatic carcinoma from prostate to pelvic bone
   Previous prostatectomy with no
   recurrence at primary site

4. Metastatic carcinoma to brain from lung
   Previous resection of lung with no
   recurrence at primary site

5. Metastatic carcinoma from prostate to
   pelvic bone

6. Metastatic carcinoma of brain and lung

7. Metastatic carcinoma of pancreas and
   omentum

8. Metastatic adenocarcinoma of transverse
   colon

9. Metastatic carcinoma of bronchus

10. Metastatic serous papillary adenocarcinoma
    of bone

_____

11. Metastatic infiltrating duct cell carcinoma, female

_____

12. Metastatic odontogenic fibrosarcoma

_____

13. Chondroblastic osteosarcoma of limb with metastasis

_____

CODING OF MALIGNANCIES OF HEMATOPOIETIC AND LYMPHATIC SYSTEMS

Neoplasms that arise in lymphatic and hematopoietic tissues can spread to secondary sites. The site to which the neoplasm spreads is considered a secondary malignant neoplasm. For example, in leukemic meningitis, cancer cells have spread from the primary tumor to the meninges; therefore, the meningitis is coded as a secondary malignant neoplasm. Figure 28.1 shows the location of the lymph nodes in the body.

Neoplasms of Lymph Nodes or Glands

Primary malignant neoplasms of lymph nodes or glands are classified in categories C81 through C88, with a fourth character providing more specificity about the particular type of neoplasm and a fifth character indicating the nodes involved (except for categories C86 and C88, which do not specify site). If the neoplasm involves lymph nodes or glands of additional sites, the fifth character 8 is assigned to indicate that the malignancy involves multiple sites. For example, code **C83.38, Diffuse large B-cell lymphoma, lymph nodes of multiple sites,** is assigned for a diagnosis of diffuse large B-cell lymphoma of intra-abdominal and intrathoracic lymph nodes; individual codes are not assigned for each type of lymph node affected.

When a solid tumor has spread to the lymph nodes, a code from category C77 is assigned. For example, adenocarcinoma of right female breast with metastasis to lymph nodes of the axilla is coded to **C50.911, Malignant neoplasm of unspecified site of right female breast,** and **C77.3, Secondary and unspecified malignant neoplasm of axilla and upper limb lymph nodes.** No code from categories C81 through C88 is assigned.

Lymphomas can be malignant or benign. Benign lymphomas are classified to code **D36.0, Benign neoplasm of lymph nodes.** Malignant lymphomas are located by referencing the subterms for the site under the main term **Lymphoma.** When a diagnostic statement of lymphoma does not match any subentry under **Lymphoma** in the Index, the user may find that the pathology report indicates the neoplasm's behavior. However, the physician should be queried for confirmation before code selection.

Hodgkin Lymphoma

Hodgkin lymphoma (category C81) is a type of cancer originating from lymphocytes. It is characterized by the orderly spread of disease from one lymph node group to another and by the development of systemic symptoms with advanced disease. Hodgkin lymphoma may be treated with

FIGURE 28.1   The Lymphatic System

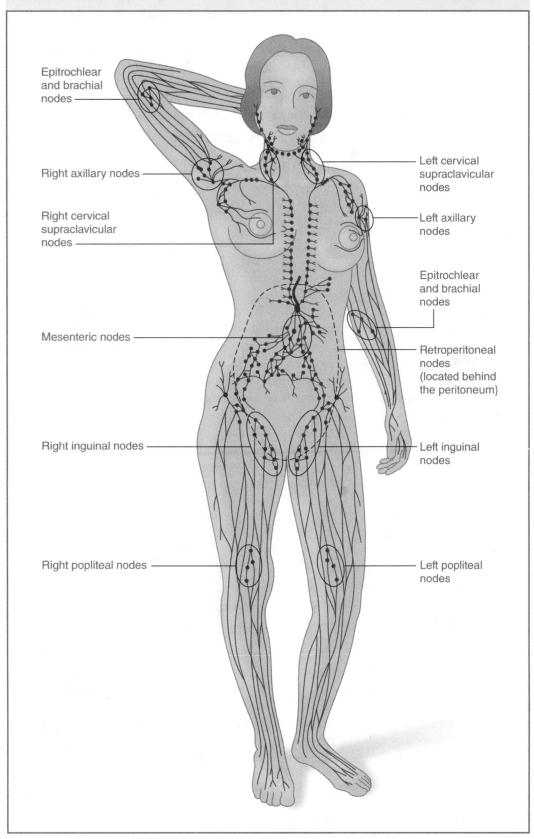

Epitrochlear and brachial nodes

Right axillary nodes

Right cervical supraclavicular nodes

Mesenteric nodes

Right inguinal nodes

Right popliteal nodes

Left cervical supraclavicular nodes

Left axillary nodes

Epitrochlear and brachial nodes

Retroperitoneal nodes (located behind the peritoneum}

Left inguinal nodes

Left popliteal nodes

radiation therapy, chemotherapy, or hematopoietic stem cell transplantation. The choice of treatment depends on the age and sex of the patient and the stage, bulk, and histological subtype of the disease.

Category C81 provides a fourth-character subclassification to identify the pathological subtype of Hodgkin lymphoma and fifth characters to identify the lymph nodes affected (e.g., unspecified site; head, face, and neck; intrathoracic; intra-abdominal; axilla and upper limb; inguinal region and lower limb; intrapelvic; spleen; multiple sites; extranodal and solid organ sites). The pathological subtype is identified in the following subcategories:

C81.0   Nodular lymphocyte predominant Hodgkin lymphoma (a rare subtype)

C81.1   Nodular sclerosis Hodgkin lymphoma (the most common subtype)

C81.2   Mixed cellularity Hodgkin lymphoma (a common subtype, most often associated with Epstein-Barr virus infection)

C81.3   Lymphocytic depletion Hodgkin lymphoma (a rare subtype)

C81.4   Lymphocyte-rich Hodgkin lymphoma

C81.7   Other Hodgkin lymphoma

C81.9   Hodgkin lymphoma, unspecified

Non-Hodgkin Lymphomas

Non-Hodgkin lymphomas are a heterogeneous group of malignant lymphomas that present a clinical picture that is broadly similar to Hodgkin disease but with the absence of the giant Reed-Sternberg cells that are characteristic of Hodgkin lymphoma. Lymphomas develop from the lymphoid components of the immune system. The main cell found in lymphoid tissue is the lymphocyte, an infection-fighting white blood cell, of which there are two main types: B lymphocytes (B-cells) and T lymphocytes (T-cells). Non-Hodgkin lymphomas can occur at any age and are often marked by lymph nodes that are larger than normal and by fever and weight loss. There are many different types of non-Hodgkin lymphoma. These types can be divided into aggressive (fast-growing) and indolent (slow-growing) types, and they can be formed from either B-cells or T-cells.

Throughout the years, the classification of lymphoma has changed considerably based on new insights provided by technological advances, as well as advances in the understanding of the clinical behavior of lymphoma. ICD-10-CM provides the following categories for non-Hodgkin lymphomas:

C82   Follicular lymphoma

C83   Non-follicular lymphoma

C84   Mature T/NK-cell lymphomas

C85   Other specified and unspecified types of non-Hodgkin lymphoma

C86   Other specified types of T/NK-cell lymphoma

C88   Malignant immunoproliferative diseases and certain other B-cell lymphomas

Follicular lymphoma (category C82) is the most common of the indolent non-Hodgkin lymphomas, and the second most common form of non-Hodgkin lymphoma overall. It is defined as a lymphoma of follicle center B-cells (centrocytes and centroblasts), which has at least a partially follicular pattern. Category C82 utilizes a dual-axis classification to allow the classification to accommodate the differences in terminology often encountered in medical records. Category C82 allows the classification of follicular lymphoma according to morphological grades (e.g., grade I) or the description of the follicle (e.g., diffuse follicle center), as follows:

C82.0-   Follicular lymphoma grade I

C82.1-   Follicular lymphoma grade II

C82.2-   Follicular lymphoma grade III, unspecified

C82.3-   Follicular lymphoma grade IIIa

C82.4-   Follicular lymphoma grade IIIb

C82.5-   Diffuse follicle center lymphoma

C82.6-   Cutaneous follicle center lymphoma

C82.8-   Other types of follicular lymphoma

C82.9-   Follicular lymphoma, unspecified

ICD-10-CM classifies non-follicular lymphoma to category C83, as follows:

C83.0   Small cell B-cell lymphoma

C83.1   Mantle cell lymphoma

C83.3   Diffuse large B-cell lymphoma

C83.5   Lymphoblastic (diffuse) lymphoma

C83.7   Burkitt lymphoma

C83.8   Other non-follicular lymphoma

C83.9   Non-follicular (diffuse) lymphoma, unspecified

Similar to category C81, Hodgkin lymphoma, categories C82 through C85 provide fifth characters to identify the lymph nodes affected (e.g., unspecified site; head, face, and neck; intrathoracic; intra-abdominal; axilla and upper limb; inguinal region and lower limb; intrapelvic; spleen; multiple sites; extranodal and solid organ sites).

Multiple Myeloma, Other Immunoproliferative Neoplasms, and Leukemias

Multiple myeloma and malignant plasma cell neoplasms are classified in category C90, with a fourth character indicating the particular type of neoplasm. Leukemias are classified in categories C91 through C95, with the fourth character indicating either the stage of the disease (acute or chronic) or the type of leukemia (e.g., adult T-cell, prolymophocytic leukemia of T-cell type). For all codes in categories C90 through C95, a fifth character is used to indicate the status of the patient, as follows:

0   Not having achieved remission (failed remission)

1   In remission

2   In relapse

Fifth character 0 is assigned if the health record documentation does not indicate that the patient has achieved remission. When the provider documents that the malignancy is in remission, assign fifth character 1. This character is only assigned when the physician specifically describes the neoplasm as being in remission. If the patient experiences a recurrence and the provider documents "relapse," assign fifth character 2. A relapse or recurrence can occur at any time during therapy or after completion of treatment, even months or years after remission.

It is important not to confuse "in remission" with personal history. The categories for leukemia, and category C90, Multiple myeloma and malignant plasma cell neoplasms, have codes indicating whether the condition has achieved remission. Additionally, the personal history codes **Z85.6, Personal history of leukemia,** and **Z85.79, Personal history of other malignant neoplasms of lymphoid, hematopoietic and related tissues,** are available. Personal history codes identify a patient's past medical condition that no longer exists and is not receiving treatment but has the potential for recurrence, and therefore may require continued monitoring. If the documentation is unclear as to whether the leukemia, myeloma, or other malignant plasma cell neoplasm should be coded as "in remission," the provider should be queried.

EXERCISE 28.6

Code the following diagnoses.

1. Aleukemic myeloid leukemia,
   in remission

2. Reticulum cell sarcoma of the spleen

3. Sarcoma, reticulum cell, intrathoracic

4. Intrapelvic Hodgkin granuloma

5. Chronic myeloid leukemia

6. Plasma cell leukemia

7. Carcinoma of lung with metastatic
   carcinoma of intrathoracic lymph nodes

8. Mycosis fungoides of intrathoracic and
   intra-abdominal lymph nodes

9. Chlamydial lymphogranuloma

10. Adenolymphoma of left female breast

11. Diffuse large B-cell lymphoma intra-abdominal

12. Peripheral T-cell lymphoma neck

SEQUENCING OF CODES FOR NEOPLASTIC DISEASES

The basic rule for designating principal diagnoses is the same for neoplasms as for any other condition; that is, the principal diagnosis is the condition found after study to have occasioned the current admission or encounter. There is no guideline that indicates a code for malignancy takes precedence. Because the principal diagnosis is sometimes difficult to determine in a patient with a malignant neoplasm, however, the thrust of treatment can often be used as a guide to select the principal diagnosis.

Some neoplasms are functionally active in that they may affect the activity of endocrine glands. All neoplasms are classified in chapter 2 of ICD-10-CM, whether they are functionally active or not. The code for these primary neoplasms is assigned first, followed by a code from chapter 4 to identify the endocrine dysfunction associated with any neoplasm. For example:

C56.1 + E28.0   Hyperestrogenism due to carcinoma of right ovary

C56.1 + L68.0   Carcinoma of right ovary with hirsutism

Treatment Directed at Primary Site

When treatment is directed toward the primary site, the malignancy of that site is designated as the principal diagnosis, in which case the primary malignancy is coded as the principal diagnosis, followed by any metastatic sites. The only exception to this guideline is if a patient admission/encounter is solely for the administration of chemotherapy, immunotherapy, or external beam radiation therapy, in which case the appropriate Z51.- code is assigned as the first-listed or principal diagnosis, and the diagnosis or problem for which the service is being performed is assigned as a secondary diagnosis. For example:

C18.7 + C78.7   Carcinoma of sigmoid colon with small metastatic nodules on the liver; sigmoid resection of the colon carried out

Z51.11 + C18.7   Carcinoma of sigmoid colon with prior resection; admitted for chemotherapy

Sometimes, two primary sites are present; in this case, each is coded as a primary neoplasm. When treatment is directed primarily toward one site, the neoplasm of that site should be designated as the principal diagnosis. When treatment is directed equally toward both, either may be designated as the principal diagnosis.

Occasionally, a patient admitted for surgery to correct a nonneoplastic condition has a pathology report indicating that a microscopic focus of malignancy is also present. In this situation, the condition that occasioned the admission remains the principal diagnosis, with an additional code assigned for the malignancy. For example:

- A patient with severe urinary retention due to hypertrophy of the prostate is admitted for prostatectomy. Transurethral resection of the prostate is carried out, and the patient is discharged with a diagnosis of benign hypertrophy of the prostate. When the pathology report is received, this diagnosis is confirmed, but a microscopic focus of adenocarcinoma is also identified. Code **N40.1, Benign prostatic hyperplasia with lower urinary tract symptoms,** is assigned as the principal diagnosis, with codes **C61, Malignant neoplasm of prostate,** and **R33.8, Other retention of urine,** as additional diagnoses.

- A patient is admitted for treatment of endometriosis of the uterus, and a total abdominal hysterectomy is carried out. The pathology report confirms the endometriosis but indicates that carcinoma in situ of the cervix is also present. In this case, the endometriosis is the reason for admission and remains the principal diagnosis. An additional code is assigned for the cervical neoplasm.

Treatment Directed at Secondary Site

When a patient is admitted because of a primary neoplasm with metastasis and treatment is directed solely toward the secondary site, the secondary site is designated as the principal diagnosis even though the primary malignancy is still present. A code for the primary malignancy is assigned as an additional diagnosis.

When a patient is admitted because of a primary neoplasm with metastasis and treatment is directed equally toward the primary and secondary sites, the primary malignancy should be designated the principal diagnosis, with an additional code assigned to the secondary neoplasm.

Admission for Complications Associated with a Malignant Neoplasm

Patients with malignant neoplasms often develop complications due to either the malignancy itself or the therapy that they have received. When admission is primarily for treatment of the complication, the complication is coded first, followed by the appropriate code(s) for the neoplasm.

The exception to this guideline is anemia. When the admission/encounter is for management of an anemia associated with the malignancy, and the treatment is only for anemia, the appropriate code for the malignancy is sequenced as the principal or first-listed diagnosis, followed by code **D63.0, Anemia in neoplastic disease.** When the admission/encounter is for management of an anemia associated with an adverse effect of the administration of chemotherapy or immunotherapy, and the only treatment is for the anemia, the anemia code is sequenced first, followed by the appropriate codes for the neoplasm and the adverse effect (T45.1x5-). For example:

- A patient with metastatic, non–small cell lung cancer of the right upper lobe develops anemia following chemotherapy. The patient presents to the oncologist for treatment of anemia of chemotherapy. Assign codes **D64.81, Anemia due to antineoplastic chemotherapy; C34.11, Malignant neoplasm of upper lobe, right bronchus or lung; C79.9, Secondary malignant neoplasm of unspecified site; D63.0, Anemia in neoplastic disease;** and **T45.1x5A, Adverse effect of antineoplastic and immunosuppressive drugs, initial encounter.**

When the admission/encounter is for management of an anemia associated with an adverse effect of radiotherapy, the anemia code should be sequenced first, followed by the appropriate neoplasm code and code **Y84.2, Radiological procedure and radiotherapy as the cause of abnormal reaction of the patient, or of later complication, without mention of misadventure at the time of the procedure.** For example:

- A female patient with cancer of the right breast is seen for treatment of anemia due to radiation therapy. Code **D64.9, Anemia, unspecified,** is assigned first, followed by codes **C50.911, Malignant neoplasm of unspecified site of right female breast,** and **Y84.2, Radiological procedure and radiotherapy as the cause of abnormal reaction of the patient, or of later complication, without mention of misadventure at the time of the procedure.**

When the admission/encounter is for management of an anemia documented as "pancytopenia due to chemotherapy," code D61.810 is assigned for pancytopenia caused by cancer-fighting drugs. In cancer patients, pancytopenia usually occurs due to bone marrow suppression from chemotherapy. Bone marrow suppression (a decreased ability of the bone marrow to manufacture blood cells) is a common side effect of chemotherapy. For example:

- A female patient with cancer of the upper-outer quadrant of the left breast developed pancytopenia following chemotherapy. The patient presents to the oncologist for follow-up of the pancytopenia. The oncologist listed chemotherapy-induced pancytopenia in his diagnostic statement. Assign code **D61.810, Antineoplastic chemotherapy induced pancytopenia,** as the first-listed diagnosis. Assign codes **C50.412, Malignant neoplasm of upper-outer quadrant of left female breast,** and **T45.1x5A, Adverse effect of antineoplastic and immunosuppressive drugs, initial encounter,** as additional diagnoses.

When the admission/encounter is for management of dehydration due to the malignancy or the therapy or a combination of both, and only the dehydration is being treated (intravenous rehydration), the dehydration is sequenced first, followed by the code(s) for the malignancy.

Because the principal diagnosis may be difficult to determine, the focus of treatment can often be used as a guide. For example:

- A patient under treatment for prostate cancer is admitted for chronic constipation that was causing excruciating pain in the stomach and back. An enema was performed, and the patient was given Colace and advised to increase fiber intake. Code **K59.09, Other constipation,** is assigned as the principal diagnosis, and code **C61, Malignant neoplasm of prostate,** is assigned as an additional diagnosis. In this case, the patient was admitted and treated for chronic constipation. Treatment was not directed at the malignancy.

When the admission/encounter is for treatment of a complication resulting from a surgical procedure, designate the complication as the principal or first-listed diagnosis if treatment is directed at resolving the complication. For example:

- A male patient with known adenocarcinoma of the prostate has an outpatient orchiectomy. The physician states that the patient was admitted due to a postoperative complication of postprocedural urethral stricture. Assign code **N99.114, Postprocedural urethral stricture, male, unspecified,** as the principal diagnosis. Assign code **C61, Malignant neoplasm of prostate,** as an additional diagnosis.

Admission or Encounter Involving Administration of Radiation Therapy, Immunotherapy, or Chemotherapy

When an episode of care involves the surgical removal of a neoplasm, primary or secondary site, followed by adjunct chemotherapy or radiation treatment during the same episode of care, the code for the neoplasm should be assigned as the first-listed or principal diagnosis.

When a patient admission/encounter is solely for the administration of chemotherapy, immunotherapy, or external beam radiation therapy, assign code **Z51.0, Encounter for antineoplastic radiation therapy; Z51.11, Encounter for antineoplastic chemotherapy;** or **Z51.12, Encounter for antineoplastic immunotherapy,** as the first-listed or principal diagnosis. When the patient receives more than one of these therapies during the same admission, more than one of these codes may be assigned, in any sequence. Because the patient is still under treatment for the malignancy, even though it may have been removed surgically, an additional code for the malignancy is assigned rather than a code from category Z85.

Note, however, that patients with leukemia are often admitted for a variety of tests or other treatment in addition to chemotherapy. If there is any question about whether the admission is for the sole purpose of chemotherapy, immunotherapy, or external beam radiation therapy, the physician should be consulted.

When the admission or encounter is for the insertion or implantation of radioactive elements (e.g., brachytherapy), assign the appropriate code for the malignancy as the principal or first-listed diagnosis. Code Z51.0 is not assigned in this case.

When a patient is admitted for the purpose of external beam radiation therapy, immunotherapy, or chemotherapy and develops complications such as uncontrolled nausea and vomiting or dehydration, the principal or first-listed diagnosis code is **Z51.0, Encounter for antineoplastic radiation therapy; Z51.11, Encounter for antineoplastic chemotherapy;** or **Z51.12, Encounter for antineoplastic immunotherapy.** Also assign codes for the complications. However, if the purpose of the admission is for insertion or implantation of radioactive elements (e.g., brachytherapy) and the patient develops complications such as uncontrolled nausea and vomiting or dehydration, the principal or first-listed diagnosis is the appropriate code for the malignancy, which is followed by any codes for the complications.

Tumor lysis syndrome (TLS) is a group of serious, potentially life-threatening metabolic disturbances that can occur after antineoplastic therapy or as a result of radiation or corticosteroid therapy. It is often associated with leukemias and lymphomas but is also seen in other hematologic malignancies and solid tumors. Assign code **E88.3, Tumor lysis syndrome,** followed by code T45.1x5- to identify the cause when TLS is drug induced. For example:

• A child is diagnosed with acute myeloblastic leukemia and admitted for chemotherapy. Chemotherapy is administered into a peripheral vein, and the provider diagnoses tumor lysis syndrome secondary to antineoplastic therapy. Code **Z51.11, Encounter for antineoplastic chemotherapy,** is assigned as the principal diagnosis. Also assigned are codes **C92.00, Acute myeloblastic leukemia, not having achieved remission; E88.3, Tumor lysis syndrome; and T45.1x5A, Adverse effect of antineoplastic and immunosuppressive drugs, initial encounter.** Code **3E03305, Introduction of other antineoplastic into peripheral vein, percutaneous approach,** is assigned for the administration of chemotherapy.

When a patient is admitted for the purpose of inserting a port for later administration of chemotherapy but no chemotherapy is given during the same episode of care, the malignancy is designated as the principal diagnosis and code **Z51.11, Encounter for antineoplastic chemotherapy,** is not assigned. When insertion of the port is followed by chemotherapy during the same episode of care, code Z51.11 is assigned as the principal diagnosis, and the malignancy code is assigned as a secondary diagnosis. If an intraperitoneal catheter is inserted for the chemotherapy and chemotherapy is administered during the episode of care, assign code **0WHG33Z, Insertion of infusion device into peritoneal cavity, percutaneous approach,** for the catheter insertion, and code **3E0M305, Introduction of other antineoplastic into peritoneal cavity, percutaneous approach,** for the chemotherapy administration.

An admission for radium implant insertion or for treatment by radioactive iodine (I-131) is not considered an admission solely for a radiotherapy session. The code for the malignant neoplasm is designated the principal diagnosis; code Z51.0 is not assigned.

Encounter to Determine Extent of Malignancy

When the reason for the admission/encounter is to determine the extent of the malignancy or for a procedure such as paracentesis (needle aspiration of the peritoneal cavity) or thoracentesis (needle aspiration of the pleural space between the lungs and chest wall), the primary malignancy or appropriate metastatic site is designated as the principal or first-listed diagnosis, even if chemotherapy or radiotherapy is administered.

Current Malignancy versus Personal History of Malignancy

When a primary malignancy has been excised but further treatment, such as an additional surgery for the malignancy, radiation therapy, or chemotherapy, is directed to that site, the primary malignancy code should be used until treatment is completed.

Codes from category Z85, Personal history of malignant neoplasm, are assigned only when the primary neoplasm has been previously excised or totally eradicated from its site and is no longer under any type of treatment, and there is no evidence of any existing primary malignancy. This guideline applies to both solid and hematopoietic or lymphatic neoplasms, including leukemia.

Malignant Neoplasm Associated with Transplanted Organ

A malignant neoplasm of a transplanted organ should be coded as a transplant complication. A code from category T86, Complications of transplanted organs and tissue, is assigned as the principal diagnosis, followed by code **C80.2, Malignant neoplasm associated with transplanted organ.** An additional code is assigned for the specific malignancy.

Malignant Neoplasm in a Pregnant Patient

Codes from chapter 15 of ICD-10-CM, Pregnancy, Childbirth, and the Puerperium, are always sequenced first on a medical record (see chapter 23 of this handbook). A code from subcategory O9A.1, Malignant neoplasm complicating pregnancy, childbirth, and the puerperium, should be used first, followed by the appropriate code from chapter 2 to indicate the type of neoplasm.

Pathological Fracture Due to a Neoplasm

The sequencing of pathological fractures due to neoplasm is dependent on the focus of treatment, as follows:

- If the focus of treatment is the fracture, a code from subcategory M84.5, Pathological fracture in neoplastic disease, should be sequenced first, followed by the code for the neoplasm.

- If the focus of treatment is the neoplasm with an associated pathological fracture, the neoplasm code should be sequenced first, followed by a code from M84.5 for the pathological fracture. The "code also" note at M84.5 provides this sequencing instruction.

Malignant Ascites

Malignant ascites (R18.0) is the abnormal buildup of fluid in the abdomen caused by malignancy. Diagnostic tests to determine the underlying cause may involve blood tests, ultrasound of the abdomen, and paracentesis. Treatment may include diuretics, therapeutic paracentesis, or other therapies directed at the underlying cause. For example:

- A patient is admitted with pancreatic cancer with massive widespread malignant ascites. The final diagnosis is pancreatic cancer with malignant ascites and metastasis to the retroperitoneum. Therapeutic paracentesis is performed. Assign code **C25.9, Malignant neoplasm of pancreas, unspecified,** as the principal diagnosis. Codes **R18.0, Malignant ascites,** and **C78.6, Secondary malignant neoplasm of retroperitoneum and peritoneum,** should be assigned as secondary diagnoses. Assign code **0W9G3ZZ, Drainage of peritoneal cavity, percutaneous approach,** for the paracentesis.

Malignant Pleural Effusion

Malignant pleural effusions (J91.0) can occur due to impaired pleural lymphatic drainage from a mediastinal tumor (especially in lymphomas) and not because of direct tumor invasion into the pleura. The lymphoma is obstructing the drainage system, which is usually caused by disturbance of the normal Starling forces regulating reabsorption of fluid in the pleural space. The code for the malignancy is assigned first, and the code for the malignant pleural effusion is assigned as an additional diagnosis.

Encounter for Prophylactic Organ Removal

For encounters specifically for prophylactic removal of breasts, ovaries, or another organ due to a genetic susceptibility to cancer or a family history of cancer, the principal or first-listed diagnosis should be a code from category Z40, Encounter for prophylactic surgery. The appropriate codes to identify the associated risk factor (such as genetic susceptibility or family history) should be assigned as additional diagnoses.

If the patient has a malignancy of one site and is having prophylactic removal of another site to prevent either a new primary malignancy or metastatic disease, a code for the malignancy should also be assigned in addition to a code from subcategory Z40.0, Encounter for prophylactic surgery for risk factors related to malignant neoplasms. A Z40.0- code should not be assigned if the patient is having organ removal for treatment of a malignancy, such as the removal of testes for the treatment of prostate cancer.

Coding of Admissions or Encounters for Follow-Up Examinations

Once a malignant neoplasm has been excised or eradicated, periodic follow-up examinations are carried out to determine whether there is recurrence of the primary malignancy or any spread to a secondary site. When there is no evidence of recurrence at either a primary site or a metastatic site, code **Z08, Encounter for follow-up examination after completed treatment for malignant neoplasm,** is assigned as the principal diagnosis. Use an additional code to identify the personal history of malignant neoplasm (Z85.-). Use an additional code to identify any acquired absence of organs (Z90.-). Codes should also be assigned for any diagnostic procedures (such as endoscopy and biopsy) that are carried out.

When there is evidence of recurrence at the primary site, the code for the malignancy is designated as the principal diagnosis. For example, a primary carcinoma of the anterior wall of the urinary bladder that was previously excised but has recurred in the lateral wall is coded to **C67.2, Malignant neoplasm of lateral wall of bladder.**

When there is no recurrence at the primary site but there is evidence of metastasis to a secondary site, a code for secondary neoplasm of that site is assigned along with a code from category Z85. Code Z08 is not assigned.

EXERCISE 28.7

Mark the following statements either true or false.

1. The recurrence of an original primary malignant neoplasm that was previously removed is classified to category Z85, Personal history of malignant neoplasm.   _____

2. If a primary malignant neoplasm was excised previously and the original primary site has not recurred, assign the code for the previous primary malignant neoplasm, using the appropriate code from categories C00 through D49   _____

3. Whenever secondary neoplasms are present, the Z code for identifying personal history of malignant neoplasm can never be sequenced as the principal diagnosis code for Uniform Hospital Discharge Data Set purposes.   _____

TREATMENT OF NEOPLASMS

Treatment of neoplasms consists of surgery, chemotherapy, radiation therapy, and other cancer treatment methods. Surgery generally involves removal of the neoplasm. ICD-10-PCS classifies these surgical procedures to the Medical and Surgical Section, with the most common root operations for these being "Excision," "Resection," "Destruction," and "Extirpation."

Lymph Nodes Excision/Resection

Lymph nodes are often removed as part of the diagnosis or treatment of a malignancy. Removal might involve cutting out one or more individual lymph nodes or an entire lymph-node chain. Each lymph-node level is considered a chain. The resected lymph node(s) is sent to the pathology department to check for metastatic disease.

In ICD-10-PCS, if a part of the lymph-node chain (i.e., individual lymph nodes) is removed, code the removal as an "Excision"; for example, "Excision" is used for the sampling of lymph nodes, such as sentinel nodes. Terms that imply lymph-node excision include "biopsy" and "isolated nodes."

If the intent of the procedure is to remove all of the lymph nodes in an area (i.e., an entire lymph-node chain, rather than isolated nodes), code the removal as a "Resection." The axillary lymph nodes are collectively considered a single body part, and, therefore, multiple procedure codes would not be assigned for the cutting out of various axillary lymph-node levels. Both a radical resection and a modified radical resection imply removal of all of the lymph nodes. Radical procedures involve cutting out everything within a designated anatomical boundary. Note that a radical resection of an organ does not necessarily imply the removal of adjacent nodes; it only implies that the entire organ was resected.

Thermal Ablation

New advancements in radiofrequency thermal ablation have expanded treatment options for some cancer patients. Thermal ablative procedures utilize heat to destroy lung, liver, or renal malignancies. Minimally invasive, image-guided thermal ablation provides effective treatment of localized neoplastic disease and can also be used as an adjunct to traditional surgery, chemotherapy, and/or radiation treatment. Under radiological imaging, a needle-electrode is inserted at the site of the tumor; radiofrequency energy is then applied to destroy the tumor. Thermal ablation can be performed by four different methods: open, laparoscopic, thoracoscopic, and percutaneous. ICD-10-PCS classifies thermal ablative procedures to the Medical and Surgical Section, root operation "Destruction." For example, code **0B5M4ZZ, Destruction of bilateral lungs, percutaneous endoscopic approach,** is assigned for thoracoscopic thermal ablation of both lungs.

Chemotherapy and Immunotherapy

Chemotherapy and immunotherapy are coded to the Administration Section, root operation "Introduction," and to the appropriate body system/region where the chemotherapy or immunotherapy agent is administered (e.g., "central vein," "peripheral vein," "peritoneal cavity"), while character 6, substance, identifies whether an antineoplastic or immunotherapeutic substance was administered. Character 7, qualifier, also provides additional information such as whether high-dose interleukin-2 (IL-2), low-dose IL-2, Clofarabine, or monoclonal antibody was administered. For example, the structure of code **3E03305, Infusion of antineoplastic chemotherapy into peripheral vein,** is as follows:

Character 1 Section	Character 2 Body System	Character 3 Root Operation	Character 4 Body System/ Region	Character 5 Approach	Character 6 Substance	Character 7 Qualifier
3	E	0	3	3	0	5
Administration	Physiological systems and anatomical regions	Introduction	Peripheral vein	Percutaneous	Antineoplastic	Other antineoplastic

Bacillus Calmette-Guerin is a nonspecific immunotherapy agent used in the treatment of melanoma, cancer of the lung, bladder cancer, soft-tissue sarcoma, carcinoma of the colon, and carcinoma of the breast. Interferon is another nonspecific immunotherapy agent used in treating malignancy. Another type of immunotherapy is IL-2, which is used to treat patients with advanced renal cell carcinoma and advanced melanoma. IL-2 therapy can be high dose or low dose. High-dose IL-2 therapy is a hospital inpatient–based regimen usually performed in specialized treatment settings such as the intensive care unit or bone marrow transplant unit. It requires highly specialized oncology professionals to carry out because of the severity of the predictable toxicities, which need extensive monitoring.

Blood brain barrier disruption (BBBD) chemotherapy is a unique option for the delivery of drugs for the treatment of brain tumors and brain metastases. The blood brain barrier (BBB) is an impediment to the delivery of chemotherapy for central nervous system (CNS) malignancies. The BBB is the lining of the small blood vessels in the brain that prevents substances such as toxins or drugs from entering the brain. Patients receiving chemotherapy for brain tumors do not receive adequate doses because antineoplastic drugs cannot cross the BBB through conventional methods of drug delivery. An improved method for drug delivery to the CNS is the infusion of chemotherapy directly into brain arteries through disruption of the BBB. BBBD therapy delivers key drugs and other substances to the brain (i.e., rituximab, trastuzumab, antibodies, or genes), avoiding the long-term cognitive effects of radiotherapy. This technique can deliver 5 to 10 times the concentration of the drug into the brain without the risks of neurotoxicity. Assign code **Z51.11, Encounter for antineoplastic chemotherapy,** as the principal diagnosis when the admission is for chemotherapy with infusion of a substance to disrupt the BBB. This procedure is classified by ICD-10-PCS to the Administration Section, root operation "Introduction," and the BBBD is identified by character 7, qualifier. The structure of the code **3E043GN, Introduction of blood brain barrier disruption substance into central vein, percutaneous approach,** is as follows:

Character 1 Section	Character 2 Body System	Character 3 Root Operation	Character 4 Body System/ Region	Character 5 Approach	Character 6 Substance	Character 7 Qualifier
3	E	0	4	3	G	N
Administration	Physiological systems and anatomical regions	Introduction	Central vein	Percutaneous	Other therapeutic substance	Blood brain barrier disruption

The Viadur (leuprolide acetate) implant is used as palliative treatment for advanced prostate cancer. The device is implanted subcutaneously in the arm and delivers leuprolide acetate continuously over a period of 12 months. Leuprolide acetate lowers testosterone, a hormone that is needed by prostate cancer cells. Assign code **3E013VJ, Introduction of other hormone into subcutaneous tissue, percutaneous approach,** for the insertion of the Viadur implant. The code for the prostate malignancy is designated as the principal diagnosis.

Radiation Therapy

Radiation therapy refers to the radiation procedures performed for cancer treatment. ICD-10-PCS classifies these procedures in a special section strictly for radiology therapy procedures. In this section, the characters have the following meanings:

1. Section.

2. Body system.

3. Modality, which is the basic manner of treatment. Four different modalities are used in this section: "Beam radiation," "Brachytherapy," "Stereotactic radiosurgery," and "Other radiation."

4. Treatment site.

5. Modality qualifier, which further specifies the treatment modality. For example, for "Brachytherapy," additional modality qualifiers specify high dose rate or low dose rate.

6. Isotope, which defines the isotope used, if applicable. For example, isotopes used for "Brachytherapy" include cesium-137, iridium-192, iodine-125, palladium-103, and californium-252.

7. Qualifier.

The structure of the code **DM1198Z, High dose rate (HDR) brachytherapy of right breast using iridium-192 (Ir-192),** is as follows:

Character 1 Section	Character 2 Body System	Character 3 Modality	Character 4 Treatment Site	Character 5 Modality Qualifier	Character 6 Isotope	Character 7 Qualifier
D	M	1	1	9	8	Z
Radiation therapy	Breast	Brachytherapy	Breast, right	High dose rate	Iridium-192	None

Laser Interstitial Thermal Therapy

Thermal therapy can be used to destroy malignancies involving the brain, breast, liver, prostate, and other organs. The energy sources come in many forms, such as laser, microwave, and radiofrequency. The heat source may be extracorporeal (outside the body), extrastitial (outside the tumor), or interstitial (inside the tumor).

Laser interstitial thermal therapy (LITT) is a surgical procedure in which obliteration of soft tissues in the body is performed through elevated temperatures caused by the local absorption of laser energy under magnetic resonance imaging guidance. With this type of therapy, the energy is applied directly to the tumor rather than passing through surrounding normal tissue. The therapy encompasses the whole target but does not extend to surrounding critical structures. LITT may also be performed to remove cancerous lesions from sites such as the head and neck, liver, breast, prostate, and lung. ICD-10-PCS classifies LITT to the Radiation Therapy Section, modality "Other radiation," with the character 5, modality qualifier, of "laser interstitial thermal therapy." The structure of the code **D0Y1KZZ, Laser interstitial thermal therapy of brain stem,** is as follows:

Character 1 Section	Character 2 Body System	Character 3 Modality	Character 4 Treatment Site	Character 5 Modality Qualifier	Character 6 Isotope	Character 7 Qualifier
D	0	Y	1	K	Z	Z
Radiation therapy	Central and peripheral nervous system	Other radiation	Brain stem	Laser interstitial thermal therapy	None	None

Intraoperative Electron Radiation Therapy

Intraoperative electron radiation therapy is a specialized, intensive radiation treatment administered during surgery directly to the cancer tumor or tumor bed. Normal tissue is protected, thereby substantially increasing the effectiveness of the treatment. The code for the malignant neoplasm is designated as the principal diagnosis; code Z51.11 is not assigned. The procedure code for the radiation therapy is assigned from the Radiation Therapy Section, with the modality "Beam radiation," modality qualifier "electrons," and the "intraoperative" value for character 7, qualifier. The structure of the code **DW013Z0, Beam radiation of head and neck using electrons, intraoperative,** is as follows:

Character 1 Section	Character 2 Body System	Character 3 Modality	Character 4 Treatment Site	Character 5 Modality Qualifier	Character 6 Isotope	Character 7 Qualifier
D	W	0	1	3	Z	0
Radiation therapy	Anatomical regions	Beam radiation	Head and neck	Electrons	None	Intraoperative

EXERCISE 28.8

The following exercise reviews the material on neoplasms presented in this handbook. For this exercise, assign procedure codes where applicable.

1. Infiltrating papillary transitional cell
   carcinoma of urinary bladder (neck)
   Percutaneous excision of bladder neck tumor

2. Carcinoma of midesophagus with spread
   to celiac lymph nodes
   Permanent gastrostomy procedure, percutaneous
   approach with synthetic substitute
   Radiotherapy to esophagus using photons 1–10 MeV

3. Malignant carcinoid tumor of small intestine
   Endoscopic excision of tumor of small intestine

4. Carcinoma, scirrhous, female left breast, outer portion
   Open biopsy with frozen section followed
   immediately by left radical mastectomy
   (resection of left breast, left axillary lymph nodes
   and pectoral muscle)

5. Intramural leiomyoma of uterus
   Total vaginal hysterectomy

6. Multiple myeloma

7. Carcinoma of gallbladder with metastasis
   to abdominal lymph nodes and liver
   and peritoneal implants

Exploratory laparotomy with
cholecystectomy, needle
biopsy of peritoneal implant, and intraoperative
electron radiation therapy abdominal lymph nodes

8. Squamous cell carcinoma in situ, floor of mouth
Resection of lesion, floor of mouth (mucosa)

9. Metastatic malignant melanoma from left
lateral chest wall to axillary lymph node

Excision of malignant melanoma
of chest wall (open approach) with radical left
axillary lymphadenectomy (open approach)

10. Metastatic adenocarcinoma of sacrum,
prostatic in origin
Previous prostatectomy

11. A 33-year-old female admitted for prophylactic
removal of both breasts, with documented genetic
susceptibility to breast cancer due to extensive family
history of breast carcinoma
Bilateral mastectomy

12. Seminoma, left testis
Bilateral radical orchiectomy (open approach)

13. Lipoma, right kidney
Percutaneous needle aspiration biopsy of right kidney

14. Chronic lymphocytic leukemia (B-cell), in remission

15. Admitted for chemotherapy (peripheral vein) following
oophorectomy on previous admission for
carcinoma of left ovary

16. Brain metastasis, admitted for chemotherapy
and infusion of substance to disrupt blood brain
barrier (peripheral vein, percutaneous)

17. Ovarian carcinoma with malignant ascites
    and metastasis to the peritoneal cavity
    Percutaneous paracentesis peritoneal cavity

---

18. Patient was diagnosed with glioblastoma multiforme (GBM)
    and admitted for laser interstitial thermal therapy (LITT)
    under MRI guidance. The patient was taken to the OR,
    where the neurosurgeon inserted an MRI-compatible
    laser probe through a guide attached to the cranium
    and then through a small cranial burr hole.
    The probe was then advanced into the tumor
    and positioned under MRI guidance.

---

19. Discharge #1: Patient was diagnosed with a malignant frontal
    lobe glioblastoma of the brain. She subsequently underwent
    open surgical resection of the tumor with insertion of the
    GliaSite® catheter in the cavity created by the tumor excision.
    Discharge #2: Three weeks later, the patient presented
    to the hospital for infusion of high-dose liquid brachytherapy
    (I-125) via the cranial catheter. After therapy, the catheter
    was removed via craniectomy, and the patient was discharged.

---

20. Patient was diagnosed with Philadelphia chromosome positive
    acute lymphocytic leukemia.
    Patient was admitted for antineoplastic chemotherapy.
    A lumbar puncture was performed in the L4–L5 interspace
    using a spinal needle and returning clear fluid.
    Intrathecal methotrexate was instilled, followed by saline.

---

21. Patient was diagnosed with right-lung cancer.
    Patient underwent thoracoscopic removal of lymph nodes for
    biopsy from the right paratracheal stations 2, 4R, 7, 9, and 10R.

Coding OF Injuries, Burns, Poisoning, AND Complications OF Care

CHAPTER 29

Injuries

CHAPTER OVERVIEW

- Injuries, poisoning, and certain other consequences of external causes are found in chapter 19 of ICD-10-CM.

- The primary axis for classifying injuries is the anatomical site.

- The secondary axis is the type of injury.

- The most severe injury is used as the principal diagnosis.

- External cause of morbidity codes indicate how the injury occurred, the intent (accident or intentional), the place where the injury occurred, the status of the patient at the time the injury occurred, and any activity that may have caused or contributed to the injury.

- An External cause code is never a principal diagnosis.

- Multiple External cause codes can be used. The first corresponds to the most serious diagnosis.

- Code child or adult abuse before the associated injuries or conditions resulting from the abuse.

- Fractures make an extensive use of the seventh-character value, which is more detailed than for other injuries.

- Any fracture not specified as open or closed is classified as closed in ICD-10-CM.

- A fracture not indicated as being displaced or not displaced should be coded to displaced.

- Reduction is the most common treatment for fractures.

- If dislocations accompany fractures, they are included in the fracture code.

- Internal injuries, blood vessel and nerve injuries, open wounds, and amputations are also covered in this chapter.

- A traumatic amputation not identified as partial or complete should be coded to complete.

LEARNING OUTCOMES

After studying this chapter, you should be able to:

Use External cause codes to assist in the classification of an injury.

Select the correct seventh-character value for an injury.

Code for procedures related to fractures.

Code for open wounds and other varieties of injuries.

TERMS TO KNOW

External cause codes
indicate external cause of morbidity; used with injury and poisoning codes

Pathological fracture
a fracture caused by bone weakening associated with conditions such as osteoporosis or neoplastic diseases

REMEMBER . . .

This chapter of ICD-10-CM utilizes extensive inclusion and exclusion notes, which make for some long and complicated codes.

INTRODUCTION

Chapter 19 of ICD-10-CM classifies injuries, poisoning, certain early complications of trauma, complications of surgical and medical care, and certain other consequences of external causes. Because this chapter covers such a broad range of conditions, guidelines for the coding of burns, poisoning, adverse effects, and complications of medical and surgical care will be discussed in subsequent chapters of this handbook.

Injuries are classified in the following sections:

S00–S09	Injuries to the head
S10–S19	Injuries to the neck
S20–S29	Injuries to the thorax
S30–S39	Injuries to the abdomen, lower back, lumbar spine, pelvis, and external genitals
S40–S49	Injuries to the shoulder and upper arm
S50–S59	Injuries to the elbow and forearm
S60–S69	Injuries to the wrist, hand, and fingers
S70–S79	Injuries to the hip and thigh
S80–S89	Injuries to the knee and lower leg
S90–S99	Injuries to the ankle and foot
T07	Injuries involving multiple body regions
T14	Injury of unspecified body region
T15–T19	Effects of foreign body entering through natural orifice
T20–T32	Burns and corrosions
T33–T34	Frostbite
T36–T50	Poisoning by, adverse effect of and underdosing of drugs, medicaments and biological substances
T51–T65	Toxic effects of substances chiefly nonmedicinal as to source
T66–T78	Other and unspecified effects of external causes
T79	Certain early complications of trauma
T80–T88	Complications of surgical and medical care, not elsewhere classified

The primary axis for classifying injuries is the anatomical site as indicated in the preceding list; the second axis is determined by type of injury. Chapter 19 of ICD-10-CM uses the S section for coding different types of injuries related to single body regions, and it uses the T section to cover injuries to unspecified body regions as well as poisoning and certain other consequences of external causes. Inclusion and exclusion notes, some of them long and complex, are used extensively in this chapter, and it is important to give careful attention to these if correct code assignments are to be made.

Codes from S00 through T14.9 are for traumatic injuries and should not be used for normal, healing surgical wounds or to identify complications of surgical wounds.

SEVENTH CHARACTERS

Most categories in chapter 19 have seventh-character values that are required for each applicable code. The seventh character must always be the seventh character in the code. For codes that require a seventh character but are not six characters long, the placeholder "x" must be used to fill in the empty characters. Most categories in this chapter have three seventh-character values: "A," initial encounter; "D," subsequent encounter; and "S," sequela. Fractures, which are covered later in this handbook chapter, are the exception. Categories for traumatic fractures have additional seventh-character values.

Although the patient may be seen by a new or different provider over the course of treatment for an injury, assignment of the seventh character is based on whether the patient is undergoing active or subsequent treatment and not whether the provider is seeing the patient for the first time.

For complication codes, active treatment refers to treatment for the condition described by the code even when there may be an earlier precipitating problem. For example, code **T84.50XA, Infection and inflammatory reaction due to unspecified internal joint prosthesis, initial encounter,** is used when active treatment is provided for the infection, even though the condition relates to the prosthetic device, implant, or graft that was placed at a previous encounter.

Seventh Character "A"

The seventh-character value "A," initial encounter, should be used for each encounter in which the patient is receiving active treatment for the condition. Examples of active treatment are surgical treatment to reduce fractures, an emergency department encounter to repair lacerations, wound debridement, and evaluation and management of acute injuries.

Seventh Character "D"

The seventh-character value "D," subsequent encounter, is used for encounters after the patient has completed active treatment of the condition and is receiving routine care for the condition during the healing or recovery phase. For aftercare of an injury, assign the acute injury code with the seventh-character "D" (subsequent encounter). Examples of subsequent care are cast change or removal, an X-ray to check healing status of fracture, removal of external or internal fixation device, medication adjustment, other aftercare, and follow-up visits following treatment of the injury or condition.

Seventh Character "S"

The seventh-character value "S," sequela, is used for complications or conditions that arise as a direct result of a condition, such as scar formation after a burn; the scars are sequelae of the burn. When using the seventh character "S," it is necessary to use both the injury code that precipitated the sequela and the code for the sequela itself. The "S" is added to the injury code, but not the sequela code. The "S" value identifies the injury responsible for the sequela. The specific type of sequela (e.g., scar) is sequenced first, followed by the injury code.

For example:

- A passenger's scalp is lacerated by glass during a car accident. In the emergency department (ED), the patient's laceration is cleaned and sutured. Assign code **S01.02xA, Laceration with foreign body of scalp, initial encounter,** and **V43.61xA, Car passenger injured in collision with sport utility vehicle in traffic accident, initial encounter.**

- The same patient above returns to the ED 10 days later for suture removal. Assign code **S01.02xD, Laceration with foreign body of scalp, subsequent encounter,** and **V43.61xD, Car passenger injured in collision with sport utility vehicle in traffic accident, subsequent encounter.**

- A patient is evaluated by the physician for a keloid scar that developed as a result of a stab wound in right upper arm one year ago. Assign code **L91.0, Hypertrophic scar,** as the first-listed diagnosis, along with code **S41.131S, Puncture wound without foreign body of right upper arm, sequela.**

MULTIPLE CODING OF INJURIES

When coding multiple injuries, each injury should be coded separately unless a combination code is provided, in which case the combination code is assigned. General codes for multiple injuries are provided for use when there is insufficient detail in the medical record to assign a more specific code (as might be the case when a trauma case is transferred promptly to another facility). Codes from category T07, Unspecified multiple injuries, should not be assigned in the inpatient setting unless information for a more specific code is not available.

As discussed in chapter 1 of this handbook, the words "with" and "and" are used in specific ways in ICD-10-CM, and they are used a great deal in chapter 19 of ICD-10-CM. The word "with" means that both sites mentioned in the diagnostic statement are involved in the injury. The word "and," when it appears in a code title, is interpreted as meaning "and/or"—that is, that either or both sites are involved.

In coding injuries, mention of fingers usually takes into account the thumb. However, there are a few separate codes for injuries of the thumb.

When reviewing documentation, keep in mind that terms such as "condyle," "coronoid process," "ramus," and "symphysis" refer to the portion of the bone involved in an injury, not to the bone itself.

SEQUENCING OF INJURY CODES

If admission is due to injury and several injuries are present, the code for the most severe injury, as determined by the provider and the focus of treatment, is designated as the principal diagnosis. If the diagnostic statement is not clear on this point, the physician should be asked to make this determination.

Superficial injuries such as abrasions or contusions are not coded when they are associated with more severe injuries of the same site—only the severe injury should be coded.

When a primary injury results in minor damage to peripheral nerves or blood vessels, the primary injury is sequenced first; then assign additional code(s) for injuries to nerves and spinal cord (such as category S04) and/or injury to blood vessels (such as category S15). When the primary injury is to the blood vessels or nerves, that injury should be sequenced first.

EXTERNAL CAUSE OF MORBIDITY

As mentioned in chapter 11 of this handbook, External cause of morbidity codes (categories V01–Y99) are used with injury codes to provide information about how an injury occurred (cause), the intent (accidental or intentional), the place where the injury occurred, and the status (e.g., military, civilian) of the patient at the time the injury occurred. In the case of a person who seeks care for an injury or other health condition that resulted from an activity, or when an activity contributed to the injury or health condition, activity codes (category Y93) are used to describe the activity.

The codes for poisoning, adverse effect, and underdosing (categories T36–T50) and for toxic effects of substances chiefly nonmedicinal as to source (categories T51–T65) include information on the cause (e.g., the responsible substance) as well as the intent (accidental or intentional). No External cause code from chapter 20 of ICD-10-CM is needed for cause or intent for these codes.

Injuries are a major cause of mortality, morbidity, and disability, and the cost of care related to these conditions contributes significantly to the increased cost of health care. Reporting External cause codes provides data for injury research and evaluation of injury prevention strategies. Although reporting external cause is optional unless mandated by state or insurance carrier regulation, health care providers are strongly encouraged to report External cause codes for all initial treatment of injuries. Guidelines for reporting have been developed, and providers are urged to follow these guidelines so that there is consistency in the data. Use information contained in the official medical record to assign the External cause code(s). These codes are assigned based on physician documentation; however, if the physician does not document External cause information, the coding professional may use documentation available from nonphysicians. If there is a conflict between the physician and nonphysician documentation, the physician's documentation takes precedence.

The External cause code with the appropriate seventh character (initial encounter, subsequent encounter, or sequela) is assigned for each encounter in which the injury or condition is being treated. Most categories in chapter 20 have a seventh-character requirement for each applicable code. While the patient may be seen by a new or different provider over the course of treatment for an injury or condition, assignment of the seventh character for the external cause should match the seventh character of the code assigned for the associated injury or condition for the encounter. For example:

- A three-year-old patient has an initial encounter for injury to the right forearm after the patient was rough housing with a brother. Upon examination, the patient was noted to have suffered a right radial head subluxation. Closed reduction of the dislocation was performed. The provider's final diagnostic statement listed "Nursemaid's elbow." Instructions were given to follow up with the pediatrician in three to five days. The following codes should be assigned: **S53.031A, Nursemaid's elbow, right elbow, initial encounter; W05.2XXA, Accidental twist by another person, initial encounter;** and **Y93.83, Activity, rough housing and horseplay.**

- This same three-year-old patient presents to the pediatrician's office for a follow-up visit. The physician examines the right elbow and determines that the anatomical position is normal. The following codes should be assigned: **S53.031D, Nursemaid's elbow, right elbow, subsequent encounter;** and **W50.2XXD, Accidental twist by another, subsequent encounter.** The activity code is not assigned again because it is used only at the initial encounter for treatment.

Major categories of External cause codes include:

V00–V99	Transport accidents
W00–X58	Other external causes of accidental injury
X71–X83	Intentional self-harm
X92–Y09	Assault
Y21–Y33	Event of undetermined intent
Y35–Y38	Legal intervention, operations of war, military operations, and terrorism
Y62–Y84	Complications of medical and surgical care
Y90–Y99	Supplementary factors related to causes of morbidity classified elsewhere

The selection of appropriate External cause codes for injuries is guided by the Index to External Causes of Injury and by inclusion and exclusion notes in the Tabular List. The codes are found in the Tabular List in alphanumeric order.

External Cause Status

A code from category Y99, External cause status, is assigned to indicate the work status of the person at the time the injury occurred. The status code indicates whether the injury occurred during military activity, whether a nonmilitary person was at work, or whether a student or volunteer was involved in a nonwork activity at the time of the causal event. A code from Y99 should be assigned, when applicable, with other External cause codes, such as transport accidents and falls. Category Y99 codes include status codes for activities done as a hobby, for leisure, and for recreation, as well as volunteer activity and activity of off-duty military personnel.

The external cause status codes are not applicable to poisonings, adverse effects, misadventures, or late effects. Do not assign a code from category Y99 if no other types of External cause codes (cause, activity) are applicable for the encounter. Do not assign code **Y99.9, Unspecified external cause status,** if the status is not stated.

Activity Codes

Assign a code from category Y93, Activity codes, to describe the activity of the patient at the time the injury or other health condition occurred. Codes from category Y93 are used only once, at the initial encounter for treatment. Only one code from Y93 should be recorded on a medical record.

The activity codes are not applicable to poisonings, adverse effects, misadventures, or sequela. Do not assign code **Y93.9, Activity, unspecified,** if the activity is not stated.

Sequencing of External Cause Codes

An External cause code is never used as the principal diagnosis. If the reporting format limits the number of External cause codes that can be used in reporting clinical data, report the code for the cause/intent most related to the principal diagnosis. If the format permits capture of additional External cause codes, the cause/intent, including medical misadventures, of the additional events should be reported rather than the codes for place, activity, or external status.

If two or more events cause separate injuries, an External cause code should be assigned for each. The first-listed External cause code will be selected using the following sequencing hierarchy:

- External cause codes for child and adult abuse take precedence over all other External cause codes.

- External cause codes for terrorism events take priority over all other External cause codes except child and adult abuse.

- External cause codes for cataclysmic events take priority over all External cause codes except those for child and adult abuse and terrorism. Cataclysmic events include storms, floods, hurricanes, tornadoes, blizzards, volcanic eruptions, and earth surface movements and eruptions.

- Transport accidents take priority over all other External cause codes except those for child and adult abuse, terrorism, and cataclysmic events.

- Activity and external cause status are assigned following all causal (intent) External cause codes.

- The first-listed External cause code should correspond to the cause of the most serious diagnosis due to an assault, an accident, or self-harm, following the order of hierarchy listed above.

Transport and Vehicle Accidents

External cause codes for transport accidents (V00–V99) are only assigned if the vehicle involved was moving or running or in use for transport purposes at the time of the accident. A long note at the beginning of this section defines in detail just what is meant by each type of transportation and what vehicles are included. The note also defines the injured person in a motor vehicle accident, such as a passenger, driver, bicyclist, or pedestrian. For example:

S72.309B + V03.10xA + Y93.01 + Y99.8   Open fracture, shaft of femur (pedestrian during recreational walk struck by automobile)

Accidents caused by machines such as agricultural or earth-moving equipment are classified as transport accidents if the pieces of equipment were in operation as transport vehicles when the accidents occurred. Otherwise, they are classified in category W30, Contact with agricultural machinery, or category W31, Contact with other and unspecified machinery, with a fourth character indicating the specific type of equipment.

External Cause of Injury Classified by Intent

Separate External cause codes are provided to classify the external cause of injuries resulting from accident, self-harm, or assault. If the intent is unknown or unspecified, code the intent as accidental intent. All transport accident categories (V00–V99) assume accidental intent. External cause codes for events of undetermined intent should only be used if the record documentation specifies that the intent cannot be determined.

Category Y38, Terrorism, is used to identify injuries and illnesses acquired as a result of terrorism. These codes (Y38.0- through Y38.9-) follow the definition of terrorism established by the U.S. Federal Bureau of Investigation (FBI). Do not classify a death or an injury as terrorist related unless the federal government has designated the incident as terrorism. The definition of terrorism employed by the FBI is found at the inclusion note at the beginning of category Y38: "These codes are for use to identify injuries resulting from the unlawful use of force or violence against persons or property to intimidate or coerce a Government, the civilian population, or any segment thereof, in furtherance of political or social objective." More than one Y38 code may be assigned if the injury is the result of more than one mechanism of terrorism (e.g., destruction of aircraft and firearms). A code from category Y92, Place of occurrence of the external cause, is assigned as an additional code to identify the place of occurrence.

Place of Occurrence

ICD-10-CM provides external cause category Y92, Place of occurrence of the external cause, for use as an additional code to indicate the location of the patient at the time of injury or other condition. Generally, a place of occurrence code is used only once, at the initial encounter for treatment. However, in the rare instance that a new injury occurs during hospitalization, an additional place of occurrence code may be assigned. No seventh-character values are used for category Y92.

Only one code from Y92 should be recorded on a medical record. When the place of occurrence is not specified or is not applicable, code **Y92.9, Unspecified place or not applicable,** is not assigned. Note that codes from category Y92 refer only to the location, not to the activity of the injured person. Separate codes are provided for the activity and status. For example:

W10.0xxA + Y92.520	Fall on escalator in airport building
X03.0xxA + X06.2xxA + Y92.096 + Y93.E9 + Y99.8	Clothing caught fire while burning household trash in backyard of home, causing burn

LATE EFFECTS OF EXTERNAL CAUSES

When the condition code from the main classification is a sequela (late effect) of injury, the associated External cause code must also indicate a late effect or sequela. Sequelae are reported using the External cause code with the seventh-character value "S" for sequela. These codes should be used with any report of a late effect or sequela resulting from a previous injury. A sequela External cause code should never be used with a related current nature of injury code. Late effect External cause codes are used for subsequent visits when a late effect of the initial injury is being treated, and not for subsequent visits for follow-up care (e.g., to assess healing, to receive rehabilitative therapy) when no late effect of the injury has been documented.

For example, a diagnosis of extensive scarring of the face due to an old burn is coded as **L90.5, Scar conditions and fibrosis of skin; T20.00xS, Burn of unspecified degree of head, face, and neck, unspecified site, sequela;** and **X08.8xxS, Exposure to other specified smoke, fire and flames, sequela.** In this example, code T20.00xS indicates that the condition is a late effect of burn of face, head, and neck, and code X08.8xxS indicates that it is a late effect of an accident caused by fire. Note that both codes have the same seventh character "S" for sequela.

EXERCISE 29.1

Assign only the External cause codes in the following exercises. Assume initial encounter unless stated otherwise.

1. Closed fracture, right tibia and fibula, due to fall from bicycle while patient was working as a messenger for a delivery service

2. Injury to deliveryman who got off of a moving pick-up truck not on a public highway because he thought the driver was stopping

3. Multiple facial lacerations to military police officer driving while on duty an automobile that was in a collision with another automobile on expressway

4. Anoxic brain damage due to previous head injury, three years ago, when patient was in traffic accident (struck by car) while walking along highway

5. Injury received by crew member of commercial airplane when he fell at takeoff

6. Injury received by guest passenger in hot-air balloon when balloon made unexpected descent

7. Passenger injured when he accidentally collided with another passenger while getting off a streetcar onto road

8. Railway employee injured when hit by rolling stock while unloading material

9. Passenger injured in accidental

derailment of train

10. Motorcyclist injured in accidental

collision with train

CHILD AND ADULT ABUSE

Expanded codes for child and adult abuse facilitate the gathering of more specific data. Child abuse has become a major concern in the United States. All 50 states, the District of Columbia, and the U.S. territories have mandatory child abuse and neglect reporting laws that require certain professionals and institutions to report suspected maltreatment to a child protective services agency. Each state has its own definitions of child abuse and neglect based on minimum standards set by federal law. Federal legislation provides a foundation for states by identifying a minimum set of acts or behaviors that define child abuse and neglect. Adult abuse is considered to be both underreported and underdiagnosed.

Keep in mind that codes for child and adult abuse are assigned only when the physician documents abuse. Do not interpret narrative descriptions as abuse without the physician's confirmation.

In ICD-10-CM, the first axis of classification of abuse, neglect, or other maltreatment of a child or adult is whether the abuse is confirmed (category T74) or suspected (T76). The selection of the code for confirmed or suspected abuse is based on medical record documentation. The exception to this is code **T74.4, Shaken infant syndrome,** which ICD-10-CM defaults to confirmed abuse.

The fourth character for categories T74 and T76 indicates the type of abuse: neglect or abandonment, physical abuse, sexual abuse, emotional abuse (including bullying and intimidation), forced sexual exploitation, forced labor exploitation, or unspecified maltreatment. The fifth character specifies whether child or adult abuse is involved.

ICD-10-CM does not specify the age limit for the assignment of child abuse codes versus adult abuse codes. The age of majority varies among states. If the patient has reached the age of majority per state guidelines, it would be appropriate to assign the adult abuse codes. In some states, an emancipated minor is considered an adult. For example, if a judge declares a minor emancipated, he or she is usually granted majority status at the same time. Other factors may influence the age of majority as well, such as marriage or participation in the armed forces. In some instances when it is not documented, the provider will need to be queried to determine if the patient is an emancipated minor.

Abuse often results in physical injuries and other medical conditions. When this is the case, sequence first the appropriate code from categories T74 or T76, followed by any accompanying mental health or injury code.

ICD-10-CM classifies confirmed adult and child abuse, neglect, and maltreatment as assault. Any of the assault codes (X92–Y09) may be used to indicate the external cause of any physical injury resulting from the confirmed abuse. In cases of confirmed abuse, use an additional External cause code to identify the perpetrator, if known (Y07.-).

For suspected cases of abuse or neglect, do not report External cause or perpetrator codes. If a suspected case of abuse, neglect, or mistreatment is ruled out during an encounter, code **Z04.71, Encounter for examination and observation following alleged adult physical abuse, ruled out,** or code **Z04.72, Encounter for examination and observation following alleged child physical abuse, ruled out,** should be used. If a suspected case of alleged rape or sexual abuse is ruled out during an encounter, code **Z04.41, Encounter for examination and observation following alleged adult rape, ruled out,** or code **Z04.42, Encounter for examination and observation following alleged child rape, ruled out,** should be used. If a suspected case of forced sexual or labor exploitation is ruled out during an encounter, code **Z04.81, Encounter for examination and observation of victim following forced sexual exploitation,** or code **Z04.82, Encounter for examination and observation of victim following forced labor exploitation,** should be used. No code from category T76 is used for these encounters.

Incidents of documented adult abuse complicating pregnancy, childbirth, and the puerperium, whether suspected or confirmed, are classified to chapter 15 of ICD-10-CM (rather than to T74.- or T76.-), as follows:

O9A.3-   Physical abuse
O9A.4-   Sexual abuse
O9A.5-   Psychological abuse

Codes from O9A.3-, O9A.4-, and O9A.5 should be sequenced first, followed by the appropriate codes (if applicable) to identify any associated current injury due to physical or sexual abuse, as well as a code to identify the perpetrator of the abuse.

Examples of child and adult abuse include the following:

- A patient is seen in the emergency department with a diagnosis of confirmed battered spouse syndrome and with a laceration of the right forehead. She reports that her husband hit her in the face because he was angry when she was late getting ready to go out to dinner. The following codes should be assigned: **T74.11xA, Adult physical abuse, confirmed, initial encounter; S01.81xA, Laceration without foreign body of other part of head, initial encounter; Y04.0xxA, Assault by unarmed fight or brawl, initial encounter; Y07.01, Husband as perpetrator of maltreatment and neglect; and Y99.8, Other external cause status.**

- A four-month-old infant is seen in the emergency department with a diagnosis of shaken infant syndrome. The baby had been unconscious for approximately two hours after being shaken vigorously by the father when he was unable to make the infant stop crying. The diagnostic statement also includes diagnoses of subdural hematoma and bilateral retinal hemorrhage. The following codes should be assigned: **T74.4xxA, Shaken infant syndrome, initial encounter; S06.5x3A, Traumatic subdural hemorrhage with loss of consciousness of 1 hour to 5 hours 59 minutes, initial encounter; H35.63, Retinal hemorrhage, bilateral; Y07.11, Biological father, perpetrator of maltreatment and neglect; and Y99.8, Other external cause status.**

- An elderly woman is brought to the hospital in a state of severe malnutrition. She had been living in an unlicensed care home, where it was suspected she was fed only one meal per day for several months. In the hospital, a gastric feeding tube is placed and high-protein supplements are given for severe caloric deficiency malnutrition. The following codes should be assigned: **T76.01xA, Adult neglect or abandonment, suspected, initial encounter; E41, Nutritional marasmus; Z59.4, Lack of adequate food and safe drinking water; 0DH67UZ, Insertion of feeding device into stomach, via natural or artificial opening; and 3E0G76Z, Introduction of nutritional substance into upper G.I., via natural or artificial opening.**

- A six-month-old infant with heat prostration is brought to the hospital by her parents, who had left her alone in their car while they did their grocery shopping. The parents stated that the child was asleep and they had felt that she would be all right for the short time they would be gone. The physician documents suspected child abandonment. The following codes should be assigned: **T76.02xA, Child neglect or abandonment, suspected, initial encounter, and T67.5xxA, Heat exhaustion, unspecified, initial encounter.**

Subcategory Z62.81, Personal history of abuse in childhood, provides codes to indicate that a patient has a past personal history of abuse in childhood:

Z62.810   History of physical and sexual abuse in childhood
Z62.811   History of psychological abuse in childhood
Z62.812   History of neglect in childhood
Z62.813   History of forced labor or sexual exploitation in childhood
Z62.819   History of unspecified abuse in childhood

Codes from category Z91 are available to indicate that a patient has a past personal history of adult psychological trauma:

Z91.410   History of adult physical and sexual abuse
Z91.411   History of adult psychological abuse
Z91.412   History of adult neglect
Z91.419   History of unspecified adult abuse
Z91.42   History of forced labor or sexual exploitation
Z91.49   History of psychological trauma NEC

There are also counseling codes (category Z69) to provide information regarding encounters for mental health services for the victim or perpetrator of abuse. These codes include counseling for child abuse problems, spousal or partner abuse problems, and other abuse.

FRACTURES

Fractures are classified in different categories or subcategories according to their anatomical locations, as follows:

S02   Fractures of skull and facial bones
S12   Fractures of cervical vertebra and other parts of neck
S22   Fractures of rib(s), sternum, and thoracic spine
S32   Fractures of lumbar spine and pelvis
S42   Fractures of shoulder and upper arm
S49.0–S49.1-   Physeal fractures of shoulder and upper arm
S52   Fracture of forearm
S59.0–S59.2-   Physeal fractures of elbow and forearm
S62   Fracture of wrist and hand level
S72   Fracture of femur
S79.0–S79.1-   Physeal fractures of hip and thigh
S82   Fractures of lower leg, including ankle
S89   Physeal fractures of lower leg
S92.0–S92.8-   Fracture of foot and toe, except ankle
S99.0–S99.2-   Physeal fractures of ankle, foot and toe

Three-character categories indicate more specific sites within these broad groupings, fourth characters usually indicate the bone (e.g., mandible), and fifth characters usually indicate a more specific portion of the bone (e.g., condylar process of mandible). For fractures of the extremities, fourth characters usually indicate a general part of the bone (e.g., upper end of ulna), fifth characters indicate a more specific part of the bone (e.g., olecranon process with intra-articular extension of ulna), and the sixth characters provide information on laterality (e.g., right, left, or unspecified) as well as whether the fracture is displaced or nondisplaced.

In an open fracture, an open wound that communicates with the bone is present. Terms that indicate open fracture include the following: "compound," "infected," "missile," "puncture," and "with foreign body."

Closed fractures do not produce an open wound. They are described by terms such as "comminuted," "depressed," "elevated," "greenstick," "spiral," "simple," and "transverse." Any fracture not specified as open or closed is classified as closed in ICD-10-CM. A comminuted fracture refers to a fracture in which bone is broken, splintered, or crushed into a number of pieces. A "comminuted fracture" is distinguished from a "compound fracture," an open fracture in which the bone is sticking through the skin. (See figure 29.1 for examples of open and closed fractures.)

If ICD-10-CM does not provide codes that identify both site and type of fracture, the fracture site takes precedence over the type of fracture in code assignment. For example, ICD-10-CM provides codes for comminuted fracture of the shaft of bones such as the humerus, tibia, ulna, and fibula, but not for other parts of these bones. If the documentation refers to comminuted fracture of the left distal tibia, assign code **S82.392-, Other fracture of lower end of left tibia.**

A fracture not indicated as either displaced or not displaced should be coded to displaced. Occasionally, a diagnostic statement contains terms that relate to both open and closed fractures. In this case, the code for the open fracture always takes precedence. For example, a diagnosis of com-

FIGURE 29.1   Examples of Open and Closed Fractures

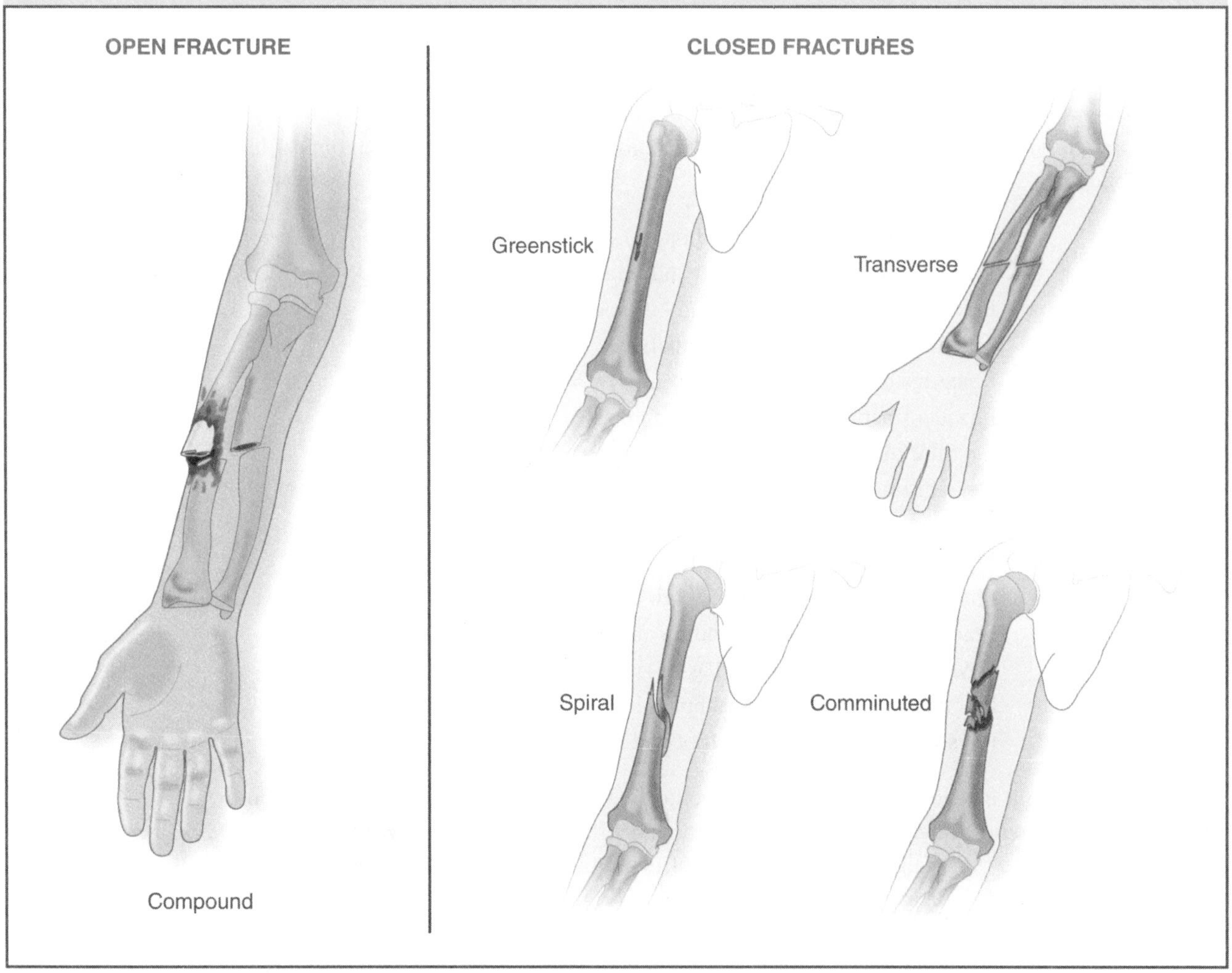

OPEN FRACTURE

Compound

CLOSED FRACTURES

Greenstick

Transverse

Spiral

Comminuted

pound comminuted fracture uses terms that can indicate both open and closed fractures. However, such a fracture would be coded as open because the term "compound" always carries this meaning, even though the term "comminuted" by itself refers to a closed fracture.

The principles of multiple coding of injuries should be followed in coding fractures. Fractures of specified sites are coded individually by site in accordance with both the provisions within categories S02, S12, S22, S32, S42, S49, S52, S59, S62, S72, S79, S82, S89, S92, and S99 and the level of detail furnished by medical record content. Multiple fractures are sequenced in accordance with the severity of the fracture.

Note that a code from category M80, Osteoporosis with current pathological fracture, not a traumatic fracture code, should be used for any patient with known osteoporosis who suffers a fracture—even if the patient had a minor fall or trauma, if that fall or trauma would not usually break a normal, healthy bone.

Seventh-Character Values for Fractures

ICD-10-CM makes extensive use of seventh-character values for fractures. While most categories in chapter 19 have three seventh-character values—"A," initial encounter; "D," subsequent encounter; and "S," sequela—the seventh-character values for fractures are significantly different. More importantly, the actual seventh-character codes vary depending on the bones affected; therefore, it is imperative to review the Tabular List at each category and subcategory level to determine the appropriate code value. For example, codes in category S62, Fracture at wrist and hand level, have six available seventh-character values. In contrast, category S52, Fracture of forearm, has sixteen different seventh-character values (see figure 29.2).

The greater number of seventh-character values does not mean that the concepts of initial encounter, subsequent encounter, and sequela no longer apply. Rather, there are additional axes of classification included in these values. For example, the code values for initial encounter (A, B, C) and subsequent encounter (D–H, J–N, P, Q, R) applicable to category S52, Fracture of forearm (figure 29.2), also distinguish between open (B, C, E, F, H, J, M, N, Q, R) and closed (A, D, G, K, P) fractures. In addition, for subsequent encounters, the code values specify whether the fracture is undergoing routine healing (D–F) or if there is a problem such as delayed healing (G, H, J), nonunion (K–N), or malunion (P–R). For example:

- A patient who suffered a traumatic fracture of the shaft of the left humerus a month earlier is admitted with fever and pain secondary to diverticulitis. The fracture is healing well and is treated minimally.

Principal diagnosis:	K57.92	Diverticulitis of intestine, part unspecified, without perforation or abscess without bleeding
Additional diagnosis:	S42.302D	Unspecified fracture of shaft of humerus, left arm, subsequent encounter for fracture with routine healing

- A young man who fractured the lateral malleolus of the left fibula six weeks previously is admitted for removal of the internal pins under local anesthesia.

Principal diagnosis:	S82.62xD	Displaced fracture of lateral malleolus of left fibula, subsequent encounter for fracture with routine healing

Several different methodologies are used to classify fractures. ICD-10-CM uses the Gustilo classification in the assignment of the seventh-character value for open fractures for categories S52, Fracture of forearm (see figure 29.2); S72, Fracture of femur; and S82, Fracture of lower leg, including ankle. However, do not select the fracture type without provider documentation in the medical record, even though the fracture may be described using the terminology found in the Gustilo classification (figure 29.3). For example, if the documentation reflects an open fracture with a 2-centimeter wound and extensive soft tissue damage, it should not be coded as a Gustilo type III

Figure 29.2   Sample Tabular List Seventh-Character Values

S52 Fracture of forearm

> **Note:** A fracture not indicated as displaced or nondisplaced should be coded to displaced
>
> A fracture not indicated as open or closed should be coded to closed
>
> The open fracture designations are based on the Gustilo open fracture classification

Excludes1: traumatic amputation of forearm (S58.-)

Excludes2: fracture at wrist and hand level (S62.-)

The appropriate 7th character is to be added to each code from category S52

> A - initial encounter for closed fracture
>
> B - initial encounter for open fracture type I or II; initial encounter for open fracture NOS
>
> C - initial encounter for open fracture type IIIA, IIIB, or IIIC
>
> D - subsequent encounter for closed fracture with routine healing
>
> E - subsequent encounter for open fracture type I or II with routine healing
>
> F - subsequent encounter for open fracture type IIIA, IIIB, or IIIC with routine healing
>
> G - subsequent encounter for closed fracture with delayed healing
>
> H - subsequent encounter for open fracture type I or II with delayed healing
>
> J - subsequent encounter for open fracture type IIIA, IIIB, or IIIC with delayed healing
>
> K - subsequent encounter for closed fracture with nonunion
>
> M- subsequent encounter for open fracture type I or II with nonunion
>
> N - subsequent encounter for open fracture type IIIA, IIIB, or IIIC with nonunion
>
> P - subsequent encounter for closed fracture with malunion
>
> Q - subsequent encounter for open fracture type I or II with malunion
>
> R - subsequent encounter for open fracture type IIIA, IIIB, or IIIC with malunion
>
> S - sequela

fracture without physician confirmation. When the documentation reflects an initial encounter for an open fracture, but the Gustilo open fracture type is not specified, ICD-10-CM defaults to the seventh-character value "B" for initial encounter for open fracture type I or II.

Initial Care

The seventh-character value for initial encounter (A, B, C) for traumatic fracture is assigned for each encounter in which the patient is receiving active treatment for the fracture. Examples of active treatment are surgical treatment to reduce fractures, emergency department encounter for acute fracture treatment, and evaluation and management of acute fractures.

Subsequent Care

Codes using a seventh-character value for subsequent care are assigned for encounters after the patient has completed active treatment of the fracture and is receiving routine care for the fracture during the healing or recovery phase. Examples of fracture aftercare are cast change or removal, an X-ray to check healing status of fracture, removal of external or internal fixation device, medication adjustment, rehabilitation, and follow-up visits following fracture treatment.

FIGURE 29.3 Gustilo Classification of Open Fractures

I   Low energy, wound less than 1 cm

II Wound greater than 1 cm with moderate soft tissue damage

III High energy, wound greater than 1 cm with extensive soft tissue damage

    IIIA Adequate soft tissue cover

    IIIB Inadequate soft tissue cover

    IIIC Associated with arterial injury

Subsequent care for complications of fractures, such as malunion and nonunion, should be reported with the appropriate seventh-character values for subsequent care with nonunion (K, M, N) or subsequent care with malunion (P, Q, R). However, if a patient delays seeking treatment for a fracture and presents for initial care for a fracture, malunion or nonunion, the appropriate seventh character for "initial encounter," rather than "subsequent encounter," should be assigned. Care for complications of surgical treatment for fracture repairs during the healing or recovery phase should be coded with the appropriate complication codes rather than the seventh-character values.

Malunion implies that bony healing has occurred but that the fracture fragments are in poor position. Treatment of malunion ordinarily involves surgical cutting of the bone (osteotomy), repositioning the bone, and adding some type of internal fixation device with or without bone graft. Malunion is frequently diagnosed while the fracture is still in a healing state; however, in some cases, surgical intervention is not used in the hope that the patient may not have any functional problems as a result of the malunion.

Nonunion, on the other hand, implies that healing has not occurred and that there is still separation of the bony structures involved in the fracture. Treatment of nonunion usually involves opening the fracture, scraping away intervening soft tissue (usually scar tissue), performing a partial debridement of the bone end, and repositioning the bone. Treating nonunion of a fracture is more complicated and difficult to perform than treating a malunion.

Skull Fractures and Intracranial Injuries

Fractures of skull and facial bones are classified to category S02. Fourth characters indicate the area of the skull (e.g., base) or face (e.g., mandible) fractured. Fifth and sixth characters provide additional specificity, such as the specific bone or the type of fracture. Any associated intracranial injury is coded separately using a code from category S06.

Category S06, Intracranial injury, which includes traumatic injury, is divided into the following subcategories:

S06.0   Concussion

S06.1   Traumatic cerebral edema

S06.2   Diffuse traumatic brain injury

S06.3   Focal traumatic brain injury (with further subdivisions for unspecified; contusion and laceration of right, left, or unspecified cerebrum; traumatic hemorrhage of right, left, or unspecified cerebrum; and contusion, laceration, and hemorrhage of cerebellum or brainstem)

S06.4   Epidural hemorrhage

S06.5   Traumatic subdural hemorrhage

S06.6   Traumatic subarachnoid hemorrhage

S06.8   Other specified intracranial injuries (including injury of right or left internal carotid artery, intracranial portion, and other intracranial injury)

S06.9   Unspecified intracranial injury

If an intracranial injury involves an open wound of the head (S01.-) or a fracture of the skull (S02.-), these are coded separately, as instructed by the notes in the Tabular List. Codes for intracranial injury (S06.-) have additional characters to indicate:

- Whether a loss of consciousness was associated with the injury
- How long the unconscious state lasted
- If the loss of consciousness was greater than 24 hours
  — with return to pre-existing level of consciousness
  — without return to pre-existing level of consciousness with patient surviving
- Whether there was loss of consciousness of any duration with death due to brain injury or due to any other cause, prior to regaining consciousness

Because the type of information above is rarely included in the diagnostic statement, it usually must be obtained through a review of the medical record, particularly the emergency department record and admitting note.

Concussion (S06.0x-) is the most common type of traumatic brain injury. It refers to cerebral bruising that sometimes leads to a transient unconsciousness, often followed by brief amnesia, vertigo, nausea, and weak pulse. The patient may experience severe headache and blurred vision after regaining consciousness. Recovery usually takes place within 24 to 48 hours. Patients with this type of head injury are often dazed, and the physician may have to rely on clinical findings alone to make a diagnosis of concussion. Codes in subcategory S06.0, Concussion, are further specified as "without loss of consciousness," "with loss of consciousness of 30 minutes or less," or "with loss of consciousness of unspecified duration." If the concussion is documented with loss of consciousness of more than 30 minutes, code **S06.0X9, Concussion with loss of consciousness of unspecified duration,** with the appropriate seventh character, is assigned. When there is documentation of concussion with other intracranial injuries classified in category S06, the code for the specified intracranial injury should be assigned instead of a code from subcategory S06.0. In other words, when the head injury is further described as a cerebral laceration or a cerebral contusion, or when it is associated with subdural, subarachnoid, other intracranial hemorrhage, or other specified condition classifiable in category S06, the code for concussion is not assigned.

Postconcussional syndrome (F07.81) includes a variety of symptoms that may occur for a variable period of time following a concussion, sometimes as long as a few weeks. The symptoms most often associated with postconcussional syndrome are headache, dizziness, vertigo, fatigue, difficulty in concentrating, depression, anxiety, tinnitus, heart palpitations, and apathy. Any of these conditions may cause the patient to seek treatment. Code F07.81 is ordinarily not assigned on the initial admission for treatment of the concussion. When the patient is treated for symptoms within 24 to 48 hours of injury and the physician lists a diagnosis as postconcussional syndrome, postcontusional syndrome, or posttraumatic brain syndrome, ask the physician whether the concussion is still in the current state. If it is, it should be coded to S06.0x- rather than F07.81. Posttraumatic headache is often associated with postconcussion syndrome. Use an additional code (G44.3-) to capture any associated acute or chronic posttraumatic headache, if applicable, along with code F07.81.

Vertebral Fractures

Vertebral fractures are classified according to the region of the spine affected: cervical spine (S12.-), thoracic spine (S22.0-), or lumbar spine (S32.0-). Fourth characters at category S12 indicate the vertebra (e.g., first cervical vertebra), while fifth and sixth characters provide additional information on the type of fracture (e.g., stable, unstable, displaced, nondisplaced). Fifth characters at subcategories S22.0 and S32.0 indicate the vertebra (e.g., second thoracic vertebra, third lumbar vertebra, etc.), while sixth characters specify the type of fracture (e.g., wedge compression, stable burst). For example:

S12.030-	Displaced posterior arch fracture of first cervical vertebra
S22.020-	Wedge compression fracture of second thoracic vertebra
S32.031-	Stable burst fracture of third lumbar vertebra

Additional codes are used to report any associated spinal cord injuries, as follows:

S14.0, S14.1-	Cervical spinal cord injury
S24.0, S24.1-	Thoracic spinal cord injury
S34.-	Lumbar spinal cord and spinal nerve injury

If the fracture of the ribs, sternum, and thoracic spine also involve injury of intrathoracic organs, these should be coded separately using codes from subcategory S27.

Fractures of the Pelvis

Fractures of the pelvis are classified to category S32. The pelvis is formed by a group of bones (ischium, ilium, pubis, sacrum, and coccyx) that form a circle that supports the spine and connects the trunk to the lower extremities. Any or all of these bones can be fractured; fractures that involve disruption of the pelvic circle are considered more severe. ICD-10-CM provides codes to identify multiple pelvic fractures with (S32.81-) or without (S32.82-) disruption of the pelvic circle. ICD-10-CM also provides seventh characters to capture whether the fracture is open or closed and to specify the initial or subsequent encounter for care or sequela.

Fractures of the Extremities

Category codes S42, S49, S52, S59, S62, S72, S79, S82, S89, and S92 classify fractures of the extremities. Fourth characters usually indicate a general part of the bone (e.g., upper end of ulna), fifth characters indicate a more specific part of the bone (e.g., olecranon process with intra-articular extension of ulna), and sixth characters provide information on laterality (e.g., right, left, or unspecified) as well as whether the fracture is displaced or nondisplaced. For example:

S42.142B	Displaced fracture of glenoid cavity of scapula, left shoulder, initial encounter for open fracture
S52.044C	Nondisplaced fracture of coronoid process of right ulna, initial encounter for open fracture type IIIA, IIIB, or IIIC

Physeal fractures (subcategories S49.0–S49.1-, S59.0–S59.2-, S79.0–S79.1, S89.0–S89.3-, and S99.0–S99.2-), which include growth plate fractures, refer to a disruption in the cartilaginous physis of long bones that may or may not involve epiphyseal or metaphyseal bone. These fractures account for 15 percent to 20 percent of major long-bone fractures and 34 percent of hand fractures in childhood. Most of these fractures heal well without any further problems. However, some lead to clinically significant shortening and angulation; others lead to disorders due to destruction of epiphyseal circulation, which inhibits development of growth plate or formation of bone bridge. For physeal fractures, assign only the code identifying the type of physeal fracture. Do not assign a separate code to identify the specific bone that is fractured.

There are many different classification systems throughout the world related to physeal fractures, with the Salter-Harris (SH) classification being the preferred system in North America. ICD-10-CM provides fifth characters to capture the SH type of fracture (type I, II, III, or IV), if documented by the physician. For example:

S49.002A   Unspecified physeal fracture of upper end of humerus, left arm, initial encounter for closed fracture

S49.011D   Salter-Harris Type I physeal fracture of upper end of humerus, right arm, subsequent encounter for fracture with routine healing

Multiple fractures of the same bone(s) classified with different fourth-character or fifth-character subdivisions (bone part) within the same three-character category are coded individually by site. For example:

- Initial encounter for nondisplaced comminuted fracture of the shaft of the right humerus, with nondisplaced closed-fracture dislocation of right shoulder involving the greater tuberosity, is coded **S42.354A, Nondisplaced comminuted fracture of shaft of humerus, right arm, initial encounter for closed fracture,** and **S42.254A, Nondisplaced fracture of greater tuberosity of right humerus, initial encounter for closed fracture.**

- Initial encounter closed fractures of the olecranon process and coronoid process of the left ulna are coded **S52.022A, Displaced fracture of olecranon process without intraarticular extension of left ulna, initial encounter for closed fracture,** and **S52.042A, Displaced fracture of coronoid process of left ulna, initial encounter for closed fracture.**

EXERCISE 29.2

Code the following diagnoses. Assume these are for initial encounters unless otherwise noted. Do not assign External cause codes.

1. Comminuted fracture, upper end of left tibia

2. Fracture, left ischium
   Fracture, left second, third, fourth, fifth,
   and sixth ribs

3. Closed fracture of vault of skull with
   subdural hemorrhage; three-hour loss of
   consciousness

4. Open Monteggia's fracture, type II

5. Cerebral concussion
   Brainstem contusion without open wound
   Patient unconscious for almost two hours

6. Trimalleolar fracture, left ankle

7. Closed fracture, lateral condyle,
   left humerus

8. Compound fracture, coronoid process
   of left mandible

9. Compound fracture, type II, shaft of tibia
   and shaft of fibula, left

10. Bilateral compound depressed skull
    fractures
    Bilateral massive cerebral contusion and laceration

Pathological Fractures

Bones weakened by conditions such as osteoporosis or neoplastic disease often develop pathological fractures that occur with either no trauma or only minor trauma that would not result in fracture in a healthy bone. Pathological fractures are classified with musculoskeletal conditions rather than with injuries and are discussed in chapter 22 of this handbook.

Current pathological fractures are reported using categories/subcategories M80, M84.4-, M84.5-, and M84.6-. For example:

- A patient with a chronic vertebral pathological fracture with orders for pain medication is admitted for an unrelated condition. Code **M84.48xA, Pathological fracture, other site, initial encounter for fracture,** is assigned for a chronic vertebral fracture. The seventh-character value "D" is not appropriate because the patient has not completed active treatment.

Compression Fractures

Compression fractures may be due to either disease or trauma. Search the medical record for any recent significant trauma or for any indication of concurrent bone disease that might point to pathological fracture. If the diagnosis cannot be clarified, the physician should be asked to provide further specificity.

Stress Fractures

Stress fractures are different from pathological fractures in that they are due to repetitive force applied before the bone and its supporting tissues have had enough time to absorb such force, whereas pathological fractures are always due to a physiological condition, such as cancer or osteoporosis, that results in damage to the bone. Stress fractures are classified with musculoskeletal conditions rather than with injuries and are discussed in chapter 22 of this handbook.

Periprosthetic Fractures

Periprosthetic fractures are fractures that occur around a prosthesis. Periprosthetic fractures are not complications of the prosthesis, but the result of the same conditions as other fractures—trauma or pathological conditions. These fractures can occur around any prosthesis, but the most common sites are the hip, knee, ankle, shoulder, and elbow. Periprosthetic fractures are classified to category M97, Periprosthetic fracture around internal prosthetic joint.

Fractures Due to Birth Injury

Fractures due to birth injury are not classified in the injury chapter of ICD-10-CM. Instead, they are classified as perinatal conditions (category P13) and are discussed in chapter 26 of this handbook.

PROCEDURES RELATED TO FRACTURES

In the treatment of fractures, the primary goal is to achieve correct bone alignment and maintain alignment until healing is completed and normal function can be restored. Procedures include open and closed reduction, simple manipulation, and application of various types of fixation and traction devices. The type of treatment depends on the general condition of the patient, the presence of any associated injuries, and the type and location of the fracture.

Reduction of Fractures

The most common fracture treatment involves moving bone fragments into as nearly normal an anatomical position as possible, with stabilization to maintain the bone in this position until it is sufficiently healed to prevent displacement. ICD-10-PCS classifies reduction of a displaced fracture to the root operation "Reposition." The application of a cast or splint in conjunction with the "Reposition" procedure is not coded separately. Treatment of a nondisplaced fracture is coded to the procedure performed; for example, casting is classified to the root operation "Immobilization" in the Placement Section.

In an open reduction, the surgeon exposes the bone by extending the open wound over the fracture or making a further incision to work directly with the bone for the purpose of restoring correct alignment. Debridement is often necessary to remove debris or other material that has entered an open fracture site. If irrigation and debridement are done to clean the wound as part of the open reduction, the debridement is not coded separately. In a closed reduction, alignment is achieved without incision to the fracture site. Debridement of the bone is not needed.

Internal Fixation

Internal fixation includes the use of pins, screws, staples, rods, and plates that are inserted into the bone to maintain alignment. When the fractured bone is in good alignment so that no manipulation is necessary, internal fixation may be used to stabilize the bone without any fracture reduction being performed. Internal fixation is also used without reduction when it is necessary to reinsert an internal fixation device because the original is either displaced or broken. An incision is made for the purpose of inserting the internal fixation wires or pins; a code from the root operation "Insertion" is assigned for fixation that is not associated with fracture reduction. Internal fixation can also be used with closed fracture reduction. The small incision necessary to insert the fixation device does not warrant considering the procedure to be an open reduction.

External Fixation

Unlike internal fixation, external fixation is ordinarily noninvasive and includes "Traction" or "Immobilization" by the use of casts or splints. The classification essentially recognizes four types of external fixation devices: monoplanar, ring system, hybrid system, and limb-lengthening device. When "Traction" is performed, a code from the Placement Section, root operation "Traction," is used. External fixation devices may later be removed using the root operation "Removal" in the Medical and Surgical Section. Procedures to take off splints, casts, and braces are classified to the Placement Section, root operation "Removal."

Although "Traction" devices are usually applied by means of Kirschner wires or Steinmann pins, the use of these materials is not considered an internal fixation. "Traction" devices include the following:

- Skin "Traction," such as tape, foam, or felt traction devices applied directly to the skin, with longitudinal force applied to the limb

- Skeletal "Traction" into or through the bone that applies force directly to the long bones (the wires or pins are drilled transversely through the bone and exit through the skin)

- Cervical spinal "Traction," such as Baron's tongs, Crutchfield tongs, and halo skull "Traction"

- Upper-extremity "Traction," such as Dunlap's skin "Traction"

- Lower-extremity "Traction," such as Buck's extension skin "Traction," Charnley's "Traction" unit, Hamilton-Russell's "Traction," balanced suspension "Traction," and fixed skeletal "Traction"

EXERCISE 29.3

Code the following procedures; do not code diagnoses.

1. Traction to right lower extremity with
   traction apparatus

2. Open reduction and debridement
   of Monteggia's fracture, right upper
   extremity, with Rush pin (internal)
   to stabilize ulna

3. Open reduction of fracture, right tibia, with
   Knowles pins (internal) and two-inch screw
   Below-the-knee cast applied

4. Open reduction and Kirschner wire
   fixation (internal) of distal to main
   fragment, fracture of left humerus shaft

5. Open reduction of fracture, left hip,
   with Jewett intramedullary nail fixation (upper femur)

6. Reduction, displaced fracture of right humerus shaft
   (external approach) with cast

7. Open reduction and internal fixation,
   fracture of right mandible

8. Open reduction, fracture of left maxilla and

left zygomatic arch

Closed reduction, nasal bone fracture (external approach)

9. Bifrontal craniotomy with reposition and

debridement of compound skull fractures

Open reduction, right orbital fracture

Tracheostomy (percutaneous)

ADMISSIONS OR ENCOUNTERS FOR ORTHOPEDIC AFTERCARE

Patients who have had fracture reduction usually require aftercare for removal of wires, pins, plates, or external fixation devices. In addition, patients with orthopedic injuries still in the healing stage may be seen primarily for conditions not related to the injury but with some monitoring or clinical evaluation of the injury carried out during the episode of care. Aftercare for traumatic fractures is coded to the acute fracture with the appropriate seventh-character value for subsequent care. The aftercare Z codes should not be used for aftercare of injuries. For aftercare of an injury, the acute injury code is assigned, with the appropriate seventh-character value for subsequent encounter. For example:

• A patient had a right intertrochanteric hip fracture that was repaired through a total hip joint replacement. He is now receiving acute rehabilitation therapy. The patient had a total hip replacement and is now in the healing and recovery phase of treatment for the fracture. Code **S72.141D, Displaced intertrochanteric fracture of right femur, subsequent encounter for closed fracture with routine healing,** should therefore be the principal or first-listed code. Code **Z96.641, Presence of right artificial hip joint,** is assigned as an additional code.

Z codes are provided for admissions or encounters for other (non-fracture-related) orthopedic aftercare, as follows:

Z47.1	Aftercare following joint replacement surgery
Z47.2	Encounter for removal of internal fixation device
Z47.81	Encounter for orthopedic aftercare following surgical amputation
Z47.82	Encounter for orthopedic aftercare following scoliosis surgery
Z47.89	Encounter for other orthopedic aftercare

However, code **Z47.2, Encounter for removal of internal fixation device,** should not be used if the encounter is for removal of the internal fixation device due to infection or inflammatory reaction to an internal fixation device (T84.6-) or a mechanical complication of an internal fixation device (T84.1-). The appropriate code from T84.6- or T84.1- should be used instead.

Z codes are also provided to indicate an orthopedic status when it is significant for the episode of care. Orthopedic status codes include **Z89.23, Acquired absence of shoulder joint; Z89.52, Acquired absence of knee joint; Z89.62, Acquired absence of hip joint; Z96.6-, Presence of orthopedic joint implants; Z96.7, Presence of other bone and tendon implants; Z97.1-, Presence of artificial limb (complete) (partial);** and **Z98.1, Arthrodesis status.** Acquired absence of joint codes are assigned when a patient is awaiting implantation of a joint prosthesis. In a common scenario, the prosthesis is removed due to infection to allow the site time to heal, and the patient is readmitted before completing the joint replacement procedure. The acquired absence codes indicate that the patient has had a prosthesis explanted; however, they can also be used when the current encounter is unrelated to implantation of a new prosthesis.

A code from subcategory Z47.3- is assigned for admissions or encounters involving aftercare following explantation of a joint prosthesis. Aftercare includes admissions for joint replacement surgery where it was necessary to stage the procedure, or for joint prosthesis replacement following a prior explantation of the prosthesis. There may be a medical need to remove an existing joint prosthesis (e.g., due to infection or other problem); however, it may not be possible to replace the prosthesis at the same encounter, thereby requiring a return encounter to insert a new prosthesis.

When the aftercare involves replacement of the hip joint prosthesis following previous explantation, assign code Z47.32. For example:

- A patient developed an infection after a left total hip replacement and was admitted for surgical treatment. At surgery, the prosthesis was removed. An antibiotic impregnated cement spacer was inserted. Because the infection had resolved, the patient was readmitted at six weeks for removal of the antibiotic spacer and revision of the total hip replacement with insertion of a new metal hip prosthesis.

For the initial admission in this example, assign code **T84.52xA, Infection and inflammatory reaction due to internal left hip prosthesis, initial encounter,** as the principal diagnosis. Code **Z96.642, Presence of left artificial hip joint,** should be assigned as an additional diagnosis. Assign code **0SHB08Z, Insertion of spacer into left hip joint, open approach, no qualifier,** and code **0SPB0JZ, Removal of synthetic substitute from left hip joint, open approach, no qualifier.** For the second admission, assign code **Z47.32, Aftercare following explantation of hip joint prosthesis,** as the principal diagnosis. For the procedures performed, assign code **0SRE01Z, Replacement of left hip joint, acetabular surface with metal synthetic substitute, open approach, no qualifier;** code **0SRS01Z, Replacement of left hip joint, femoral surface with metal synthetic substitute, open approach, no qualifier;** and code **0SPB08Z, Removal of spacer from left hip joint, open approach, no qualifier.**

Aftercare codes should be used in conjunction with any other aftercare codes or other diagnosis codes to provide better detail on the specifics of an aftercare encounter visit, unless otherwise directed by the classification. The sequencing of multiple aftercare codes depends on the circumstances of the encounter. For example:

- A patient had a right total hip joint replacement due to degenerative arthritis. He is now receiving physical therapy at home. Codes **Z47.1, Aftercare following joint replacement surgery,** and **Z96.641, Presence of right artificial hip joint,** are assigned for the encounter for therapy. Each code represents a different piece of information regarding the aftercare and is needed to describe the encounter fully.

DISLOCATIONS AND SUBLUXATIONS

Joint dislocation occurs when bones in a joint become displaced or misaligned and the ligaments are damaged. A subluxation is a partial or incomplete dislocation. Dislocation or subluxation associated with fracture is included in the fracture code, and reduction of the dislocation is included in the code for the fracture reduction. Dislocation or subluxation of a joint without associated fracture is classified in the following categories:

S03   Dislocation and sprain of joints and ligaments of head
S13   Dislocation and sprain of joints and ligaments at neck level
S23   Dislocation and sprain of joints and ligaments of thorax
S33   Dislocation and sprain of joints and ligaments of lumbar spine and pelvis

S43   Dislocation and sprain of joints and ligaments of shoulder girdle
S53   Dislocation and sprain of joints and ligaments of elbow
S63   Dislocation and sprain of joints and ligaments at wrist and hand level
S73   Dislocation and sprain of joint and ligaments of hip
S83   Dislocation and sprain of joints and ligaments of knee
S93   Dislocation and sprain of joints and ligaments at ankle, foot, and toe level

The first axis is the general site, such as wrist and hand, with the fifth character indicating a more specific site, such as midcarpal dislocation of the wrist; the sixth-character axis indicates whether the injury is a subluxation or dislocation, and its laterality. Any associated open wound or spinal cord injury is coded separately.

Reduction of dislocation not associated with fracture is coded to the Medical and Surgical Section, root operation "Reposition," with the body part being the appropriate joint (rather than the actual bone, as with procedures to reduce fractures).

INTERNAL INJURIES OF THE CHEST, ABDOMEN, AND PELVIS

Internal injuries of the chest, abdomen, and pelvis are classified to categories S24–S27 and S34–S37. Any associated open wounds are coded separately. For example:

S27.0-	Pneumothorax (traumatic) without mention of open wound
S27.1- + S21.309-	Hemothorax with open wound of front wall of thorax with penetration into thoracic cavity
S36.400-	Injury of duodenum without mention of open wound into cavity
S26.91-	Contusion of heart

Codes from subcategory S37.0, Injury of kidney, are used to describe an internal injury of the kidney caused by trauma. A nontraumatic acute kidney injury is coded **N17.9, Acute kidney failure, unspecified.**

BLOOD VESSEL AND NERVE INJURIES

When a primary injury results in minor damage to peripheral nerves or blood vessels, the primary injury is sequenced first, with additional codes for injuries to nerves and spinal cord (such as category S04) and/or injury to blood vessels (such as category S15). However, when the primary injury is to a blood vessel or nerve, the code for that injury should be sequenced first.

For example, an open wound of the abdominal wall without penetration into the peritoneal cavity, but with rupture of the aorta, would be coded **S35.00-, Injury to abdominal aorta,** with S31.109- as an additional code.

OPEN WOUNDS

Open wounds such as lacerations, puncture wounds, cuts, animal bites, avulsions, and traumatic amputations that are not associated with fracture are coded separately in categories S01, S11, S21, S31, S41, S51, S61, S71, S81, and S91. Fourth characters provide more specificity regarding the body area. Fifth and sixth characters indicate the type of wound, such as laceration, puncture wound, or open bite, and whether there is a foreign body. Any associated injury to internal organs or wound infection is coded separately.

Both cellulitis and osteomyelitis sometimes occur as complications of open wounds. Sequencing of codes for open wounds with these major infections depends on the circumstances of admission. It is important to determine whether the primary condition being addressed is the wound or the resulting infection. For example, a patient who had an open wound of the hand six weeks ago might be seen because osteomyelitis has developed. In this situation, the osteomyelitis would ordinarily be designated as the principal diagnosis, with an additional code for the open wound. A patient who had a slight puncture wound earlier in the week might show evidence of cellulitis at the site. The wound itself did not require any attention. The reason for the encounter is cellulitis, and cellulitis is the principal diagnosis.

AMPUTATIONS

When listed as a diagnosis, traumatic amputation is classified to subcategories S08.1- through S08.8-, S28.1- through S28.2-, S38.1- through S38.2-, S48.0- through S48.9-, S58.0- through S58.9-, S68.0- through S68.7-, S78.0- through S78.9-, S88.0- through S88.9-, and S98.0- through S98.9-, rather than classified as an open wound. ICD-10-CM distinguishes between complete and partial traumatic amputations. An amputation not identified as partial or complete should be coded to complete amputation. For example:

S58.019-	Complete traumatic amputation of arm at elbow
S58.122-	Partial traumatic amputation of left arm below elbow
S88.011-	Complete traumatic amputation of right leg at knee

The term "amputation" is also used for an amputation procedure, which can be performed for a variety of reasons other than the treatment of trauma. Amputation is performed by either disarticulation or cutting through the bone. Amputation procedures are classified in ICD-10-PCS to the Medical and Surgical Section, root operation "Detachment." The body part value is the site of the "Detachment." If applicable, a qualifier is assigned to specify the level where the extremity was detached. "Detachment" procedures are found only in body systems "X" ("anatomical regions, upper extremities") and "Y" ("anatomical regions, lower extremities") because amputations are performed on the extremities, across overlapping body layers (e.g., skin, muscle, bone), and therefore cannot be coded to a specific musculoskeletal body system, such as bones or joints.

The root operation "Detachment" makes use of specific qualifiers that are dependent on the body part value in the "upper extremities" and "lower extremities" body systems. Definitions of the terms used with "Detachment" are shown in table 29.1.

Sample codes include the following:

0X6J0Z0	Disarticulation of right wrist, complete, open
0Y6M0Z0	Complete amputation right foot
0Y6C0Z3	Amputation above right knee, distal shaft of femur
0X680Z2	Midshaft amputation, right humerus

OTHER INJURIES

Superficial injuries such as contusions, blisters, abrasions, superficial foreign bodies, and insect bites are classified to categories S00, S10, S20, S30, S40, S50, S60, S70, S80, and S90. The fourth and fifth characters indicate a more specific site or type of injury. The sixth character indicates laterality. When these injuries are associated with a major injury, such as fracture of the same site, a code for the superficial injury is usually not assigned. Note that the term "superficial" does not refer to the severity of the injury but to the superficial structures affected, that is, those pertaining to or situated near the surface.

TABLE 29.1   Definitions of Terms Used for Qualifiers for "Detachment" Procedures

Body Part	Qualifier Term Definition
Upper arm or upper leg	**High:** Amputation at the proximal portion of the shaft of the humerus or femur
	Mid: Amputation at the middle portion of the shaft of the humerus or femur
	Low: Amputation at the distal portion of the shaft of the humerus or femur
Hand or foot	**Complete:** Amputation through the carpometacarpal joint of the hand or through the tarsometatarsal joint of the foot
	Partial: Amputation anywhere along the shaft or head of the metacarpal bone of the hand or of the metatarsal bone of the foot
Thumb, finger, or toe	**Complete:** Amputation at the metacarpophalangeal/metatarsophalangeal joint
	High: Amputation anywhere along the proximal phalanx
	Mid: Amputation through the proximal interphalangeal joint or anywhere along the middle phalanx
	Low: Amputation through the distal interphalangeal joint or anywhere along the distal phalanx

The presence of a foreign body entering through an orifice is classified in categories T15 through T19. When the foreign body is associated with a penetrating wound, it is coded as an open wound, by site, residual foreign body in soft tissue. A splinter without open wound is classified to superficial injury by body region. A foreign body accidentally left during a procedure in an operative wound is considered to be a complication of a procedure and is coded T81.5-. Codes within T15–T19 that include the external cause do not need an additional External cause code.

EARLY COMPLICATIONS OF TRAUMA

Certain early complications of trauma that are not included in the code for the injury are classified in category T79, Certain early complications of trauma, not elsewhere classified. The fourth-character axis indicates the type of complication, such as air or fat embolism, traumatic secondary and recurrent hemorrhage and seroma, traumatic shock, traumatic anuria, traumatic ischemia of muscle, traumatic subcutaneous emphysema, or traumatic compartment syndrome. Ordinarily, codes from category T79 are assigned as secondary codes, with the code for the injury sequenced first. With today's shorter lengths of stay and increased emphasis on outpatient care, however, the complication itself may occasionally be the reason for an outpatient encounter or admission and is the principal diagnosis in such cases.

Subcategory T79.A, Traumatic compartment syndrome, classifies compartment syndrome secondary to trauma. Nontraumatic compartment syndrome is classified to M79.A-. Acute traumatic compartment syndrome is usually a sequela of a serious injury to the lower or upper extremities, abdomen, or other sites and can lead to significant motor and sensory deficits, pain, stiffness, and deformity when untreated. Acute traumatic compartment syndrome is always associated with fractures, dislocations, and/or crush injuries. Other risk factors for the development of acute traumatic compartment syndrome include vascular injuries and coagulopathy. The diagnosis is established by multiple compartment pressure readings. Traumatic compartment syndrome is coded as follows:

T79.A0   Compartment syndrome, unspecified

T79.A11   Traumatic compartment syndrome of right upper extremity

T79.A12	Traumatic compartment syndrome of left upper extremity
T79.A19	Traumatic compartment syndrome of unspecified upper extremity
T79.A21	Traumatic compartment syndrome of right lower extremity
T79.A22	Traumatic compartment syndrome of left lower extremity
T79.A29	Traumatic compartment syndrome of unspecified lower extremity
T79.A3	Traumatic compartment syndrome of abdomen
T79.A9	Traumatic compartment syndrome of other sites

EXERCISE 29.4

Code the following diagnoses. Assume these are for initial encounters unless otherwise noted. Do not assign External cause codes.

1. Stab wound of abdominal wall, infected

2. Lacerations, left foot, with foreign body

3. Traumatic amputation of left arm and hand above the elbow

4. Traumatic anuria due to injury to kidney

OTHER EFFECTS OF EXTERNAL CAUSES

Categories T66 through T78 classify other and unspecified effects of external causes resulting from exposure to heat or cold, as well as a variety of other conditions due to external causes that are not classifiable elsewhere in ICD-10-CM. Codes from these categories are not assigned when a more specific code for the effect is available. For example, colitis due to radiation is coded **K52.0, Gastroenteritis and colitis due to radiation,** because the effect is identified. Radiation sickness not otherwise specified and with no further information is coded to **T66.-, Radiation sickness, unspecified.** A diagnosis of complication of radiation therapy not otherwise specified and with no further information documented in the medical record is coded to the manifestation (e.g., anemia) and assigned code **Y84.2, Radiological procedure and radiotherapy as the cause of abnormal reaction of the patient, or of later complication, without mention of misadventure at the time of the procedure.**

Code T68.- is assigned for hypothermia, with several exceptions. If hypothermia is due to anesthesia, code T88.51 is assigned. When the hypothermia is not due to low temperature, code **R68.0, Hypothermia not associated with low environmental temperature,** is assigned. An additional code is used to identify the source of exposure, such as exposure to excessive cold of man-made origin (W93) or of natural origin (X31). Three codes are provided for hypothermia of the newborn: **P80.0, Cold injury syndrome; P80.8, Other hypothermia of newborn;** and **P80.9, Hypothermia of newborn, unspecified.**

Category T78, Adverse effects not elsewhere classified, is used to classify a variety of adverse effects, such as anaphylactic reaction/shock, adverse food reactions, angioneurotic edema, unspecified allergy, and Arthus phenomenon.

Anaphylaxis is an immunologic reaction that affects multiple body systems. Reactions can range from mild—with hives, itchiness, swelling of eyes and lips, and some congestion—to life threatening, with airway obstruction and cardiovascular collapse. Shock occurs when there is excessive fluid leakage from the blood vessels into the tissues. Codes from subcategory T78.0 are assigned for both anaphylactic reaction and anaphylactic shock due to adverse food reaction, with a fifth character indicating the type of food involved. For example:

- A patient with a known allergy to tree nuts presents to the emergency department with wheezing and urticaria. The patient is diagnosed with an anaphylactic reaction secondary to eating cookies containing walnuts. Assign code **T78.05xA, Anaphylactic reaction due to tree nuts and seeds, initial encounter.**

Anaphylactic reaction due to correct medicinal substances properly administered is classified to code **T88.6-, Anaphylactic reaction due to adverse effect of correct drug or medicament properly administered,** followed by a code from T36 through T50, with fifth or sixth character 5 to identify the drug. Codes in subcategory T80.5, Anaphylactic reaction due to serum, describe allergic reactions to serum, including blood transfusions, vaccinations, and other serum. Other serum reactions due to the administration of blood and blood products, vaccinations, and other serum are classified to subcategory T80.6. When the anaphylactic reaction is due to an incorrect use of a drug, a medicinal or biological substance, or a toxic material not chiefly medicinal, the reaction is classified as a poisoning, with the poisoning code sequenced first and an additional code of T78.2- assigned to indicate the reaction.

EXERCISE 29.5

Code the following diagnoses and assign External cause codes. Assume these are for initial encounters unless otherwise noted.

1. Heat prostration due to salt
   and water depletion

   _____

2. Frostbite, all toes
   due to cold exposure

   _____

3. Radiation cataract due to excessive exposure
   to microwave radiation

   _____

4. Anaphylactic reaction due to eating peanuts

   _____

LATE EFFECTS OF INJURIES

In coding late effects of injuries, the residual condition or specific type of sequela (such as scar, deformity, or paralysis) is sequenced first, followed by the injury code with the seventh-character value "S," sequela. A seventh-character "S" is also assigned to the External cause of injury code. A current injury code is never used with a late effect code for the same type of injury.

EXERCISE 29.6

Code the following diagnoses and assign External cause codes; sequence the codes according to the principles for coding late effects.

1. Paralysis of right wrist (radial nerve) due to previous accidental self-inflicted laceration of right radial nerve

2. Esophageal stricture due to old lye burn of esophagus

3. Nonunion fracture of neck of left femur suffered in a bar brawl three months ago

4. Posttraumatic scars of cheek due to old accidental lacerations

EXERCISE 29.7

Code the following diagnoses and procedures. Assume these are for initial encounters unless otherwise noted. Assign External cause codes where information is provided.

1. Anterior dislocation of left shoulder, patient thrown from horse she was riding while working as a horse trainer

   Dislocation reduction, external approach

2. Displaced fracture dislocation left humerus, surgical neck; patient caught in avalanche while on vacation skiing at mountain resort

   Open reduction and internal fixation with Rush pin and screws

3. Colles' fracture, right

   Patient fell from chair at home

   Closed reduction with anterior-posterior

   plaster splints (external approach)

---

4. Intracapsular fracture, neck of femur, right

   Patient fell from in-line skates

   Closed reduction with insertion of

   Smith-Petersen nail (percutaneous approach)

---

5. Closed fractures of right upper femur and left ilium

   Fat emboli, posttraumatic

   Patient driving motorcycle on highway

   lost control and overturned

   Open reduction with plate fixation, right upper

   femur, with skeletal traction

   for ilium fracture

---

6. Fracture of base of skull, right side, with right

   subdural hemorrhage without loss of consciousness;

   patient fell from parachute in a voluntary descent

   during military training

---

7. Posttraumatic shortening of left radius

   due to previous comminuted fracture of

   distal end of left forearm, broken in

   accidental crash of snowmobile

---

8. Ruptured spleen, traumatic

   Puncture of left lower quadrant of abdominal wall into peritoneal cavity

   Major contusion to left kidney

   Traumatic shock

   Patient caught in heavy farm machinery

   that he was operating on his farm

Excretory urography with low osmolar contrast

Open splenectomy

9. Cerebral cortex contusion; patient died

from brain injury without regaining consciousness;

patient had fallen through balcony from skyscraper

observation tower while sightseeing

10. Confirmed battered wife syndrome due to severe

beating of chest wall by husband

Multiple contusions over trunk

11. Anoxic brain damage due to previous

intracranial injury with loss of consciousness

three years ago, when patient was accidentally struck by

car while walking along highway

12. Comminuted fracture of the right distal radius

and ulna; child fell from playground equipment;

initial treatment is in the physician's office

Two weeks later, patient had

open reduction and internal fixation

(ORIF) at an acute care hospital

Follow-up visit to the physician's office

for X-rays and postoperative examination

13. A three-year-old child was brought into the hospital

for an evaluation of suspected physical abuse.

The child's older sibling had been beaten severely

by the stepfather, so it was requested that the younger

child be evaluated for abuse. After evaluation, examination,

and interviews, it was determined that the younger

child had not been abused

CHAPTER 30

Burns

CHAPTER OVERVIEW

- Categories T20 through T32 are assigned for all burns and corrosions except radiation-related disorders of the skin and subcutaneous tissue and sunburn.

- ICD-10-CM distinguishes between burns and corrosions. Burn codes are assigned to thermal burns from a heat source. Corrosion codes are for burns due to chemicals.

- Burns are first classified by general anatomical site. A fourth character indicates the type of burn according to depth: first, second, or third degree.

- Codes are sequenced to reflect the degree of the burn. The highest degree takes precedence.

  — Multiple burns on the same site require classification of only the highest degree of burn.

  — Multiple burns at different sites require sequencing the most severe burn first and using additional codes for the burns of other sites.

- The extent of the body surface involved is estimated using the "rule of nines," a guideline that is also used to help code the burn.

- External cause codes are used to classify the place of occurrence as well as:

  — The source of the burns and corrosions, such as fire, electric current, or hot liquid

  — Situations such as accident, assault, and suicide

- Other injuries associated with burns often require additional codes.

- Certain pre-existing conditions might have an impact on the prognosis or care of the patient. These pre-existing conditions should be coded as additional diagnoses.

LEARNING OUTCOMES

After studying this chapter, you should be able to:

Understand the difference between first-, second-, and third-degree burns.

Properly sequence the codes for multiple burns and related conditions.

Understand how the extent of burn is calculated using the "rule of nines."

Identify injuries and illnesses that might be coded in association with the burns.

TERM TO KNOW

Rule of nines
a tool to help physicians estimate the amount of body surface involved in a burn

REMEMBER . . .

Burns heal at different rates. It is possible to have both healed and unhealed burns for the same episode of care.

INTRODUCTION

Codes from categories T20 through T32 are assigned for burns and corrosions except radiation-related disorders of the skin and subcutaneous tissue (categories L55–L59) and sunburn (L55.-). ICD-10-CM distinguishes between burns and corrosions. The burn codes are for thermal burns, except sunburns, that are a result of a heat source (e.g., fire, hot appliance). Burns due to chemicals are classified to corrosion. The guidelines for both burns and corrosions are the same. Nonhealing burns and necrosis of burned skin are coded as acute current burns (categories T20–T28, seventh character "A" for initial encounter or "D" for subsequent encounter). Sequelae (such as scarring or contracture) that remain after a burn has healed are classified as sequela (categories T20–T28, seventh character "S" for sequela). Because burns heal at different rates, a patient may have both healed and unhealed burns during the same episode of care. For this reason, it is possible to use current burn codes as well as late effect burn codes on the same record (when both a current burn and sequelae of an old burn exist).

ANATOMICAL SITE OF BURN

The first axis for classifying burns is the general anatomical site, with a fifth character or sixth character to indicate a more specific site, as follows:

T20–T25　　Burns and corrosions of external body surface, specified by site

T26–T28　　Burns and corrosions confined to eye and internal organs

T30–T32　　Burns and corrosions of multiple and unspecified body regions

When coding burns, assign separate codes for each burn site. Codes for multiple sites and category T30, Burn and corrosion, body region unspecified, should only be used if the location of the burns is not documented. Category T30 is extremely vague and should rarely be used.

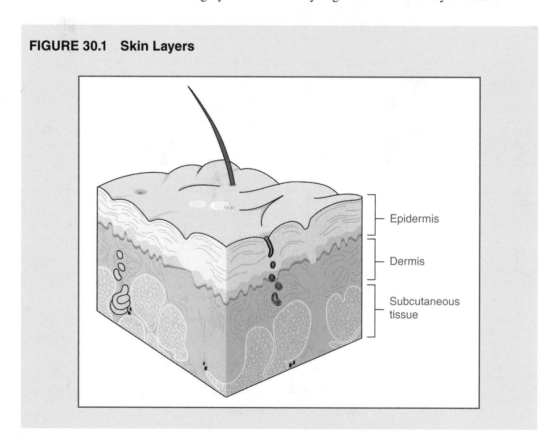

FIGURE 30.1　Skin Layers

Epidermis

Dermis

Subcutaneous tissue

DEPTH OF BURN

For categories T20 through T25, the fourth-character axis indicates the type of burn or corrosion according to depth or degree, as follows:

- First degree (erythema)
- Second degree (blistering)
- Third degree (full-thickness involvement)

First Degree

Damage from first-degree burns is limited to the outer layer of the epidermis, with erythema and increased tenderness. First-degree burns have good capillary refill and do not represent significant injury in terms of fluid replacement needs.

Second Degree

Second-degree burns represent a partial-thickness injury to the dermis, which may be either superficial or deep. Deep second-degree burns heal much more slowly than first-degree burns and are prone to developing infection. The end result of second-degree burns may be hypertrophic scarring.

Third Degree

In third-degree burns, the dermal barrier is lost, and the presence of necrotic tissue creates fluid volume loss with systemic effects on capillaries well away from the burn site. In addition, the burn site establishes an ideal culture medium for infection, which may be life threatening. Blood supply is the critical factor in healing of third-degree burns. Areas rich in blood supply, such as hair follicles and sweat glands, have a better chance for reepithelialization.

Deep third-degree burns are characterized by an underlying necrosis with thrombosed vessels. Codes for burns of this depth are assigned only on the basis of a specific diagnosis made by the physician.

SEQUENCING OF CODES FOR BURNS/CORROSIONS AND RELATED CONDITIONS

When burns and corrosions of the same anatomical site and on the same side are of different degrees (depth), they are classified to the subcategory identifying the highest degree recorded in the diagnosis. A third-degree burn takes precedence over a second-degree burn, and a second-degree burn takes precedence over a first-degree burn. For example, for second- and third-degree burns of right thigh, assign only code T24.311-; no code is assigned for the second-degree burn.

When coding multiple burns, sequence first the code that reflects the burn of the highest degree (most severe), with additional codes for the burns of other sites. For example, a patient is admitted with third-degree burns of the lower leg and first-degree and second-degree burns of the forearm. The following codes should be assigned:

T24.339-   Third-degree burn of lower leg
T22.219-   Second-degree burn of forearm

Burns of the eye and internal organs (T26–T28) are classified by site, but not by degree. The circumstances of the admission will determine the principal diagnosis or first-listed diagnosis if a patient has both internal and external burns.

Codes for burns of "multiple sites" (e.g., **T20.39-, Burn of third degree of multiple sites of head, face, and neck**) should only be assigned when the medical record documentation does not specify the individual sites.

When a patient is admitted for burn injuries and other related conditions such as smoke inhalation and/or respiratory failure, the circumstances of admission govern the selection of the principal or first-listed diagnosis.

When assigning a code for corrosion, the coding professional must first assign a code from categories T51 through T65, Toxic effects of substances chiefly nonmedicinal as to source, to identify the chemical and intent.

SEVENTH-CHARACTER VALUES

Like other injury codes, categories T20 through T28 require the following seventh-character values:

A   Initial encounter
D   Subsequent encounter
S   Sequela

Value "A" (initial encounter) is used for each encounter in which the patient is receiving active treatment for the injury. Examples of active treatment are surgical treatment, emergency department encounter, and evaluation and management of acute injuries. Although the patient may be seen by a new or different provider over the course of treatment for the injury, assignment of the seventh character is based on whether the patient is undergoing active treatment—not on whether the provider is seeing the patient for the first time.

Value "D" (subsequent encounter) is used for encounters after the patient has completed active treatment of the injury and is receiving routine care for the injury during the healing or recovery phase. Examples of subsequent care are medication adjustment, other aftercare, and follow-up visits following injury treatment. The aftercare Z codes should not be used for aftercare for injuries. For aftercare of an injury, assign the acute injury code with the seventh character "D" (subsequent encounter).

Value "S" (sequela) is for use for complications or conditions that arise as a direct result of an injury, such as scar formation after a burn; the scars are sequelae of the burn. When using value "S," it is necessary to use both the code for the sequela itself and the injury code that precipitated the sequela. The specific type of sequela (e.g., scar) is sequenced first, followed by the injury code. The "S" value identifies the injury responsible for the sequela and is added only to the burn or corrosion code, not the sequela code.

Note that using code **Z41.1, Encounter for cosmetic surgery,** is inappropriate for burn patients admitted for repair of scar tissue, skin contracture, or other sequelae. For such patients, a code should be assigned for the condition being treated.

EXTENT OF BURN

Categories T31 and T32 classify burns and corrosions by the extent of body surface involved and the extent of body surface with third-degree burn or corrosion, but not by specific sites. The fourth character indicates the total percentage of body surface involved in all types of burns (T31) or corrosions (T32), including third-degree burns. The fifth character indicates the percentage of the body surface involved in third-degree burns only. Because the fourth character refers to total body surface, the fifth character can never be greater than the total body surface amount. For example, code T31.73 indicates that 70–79 percent of the body surface was involved in some type of burn; the fifth character indicates that third-degree burns were involved in 30–39 percent of the body surface. The fifth character zero (0) is assigned when less than 10 percent of body surface (or no body surface) is involved in a third-degree burn.

The extent of body surface involved in a burn injury is an important factor in burn mortality, and hospitals with burn centers need this information for evaluating patient care management and for preparing statistical data. In addition, third-party payment is often influenced by the extent of the burn. When more than 20 percent of the body surface is involved in third-degree burns, it is advisable to assign an additional code from category T31. Burn centers sometimes use a code from category T31 as a solo code because many of their patients present with such extensive and severe burns involving many sites that coding the sites individually is difficult.

Categories T31 and T32 are based on the classic "rule of nines" for estimating the amount of body surface involved in a burn. Physicians may modify the percentage assignments for head and neck in infants and small children because young children have proportionately larger heads than do adults. The percentage may also be modified for adults with large buttocks, abdomen, or thighs. The rule of nines establishes estimates of body surface involved, as follows:

Head and neck	9 percent
Each arm	9 percent
Each leg	18 percent
Anterior trunk	18 percent
Posterior trunk	18 percent
Genitalia	1 percent

For example, based on this rule a physician can calculate that first-degree burns involve 9 percent of the body surface, second-degree burns involve 18 percent, and third-degree burns involve 36 percent. Adding these together, 63 percent of the body was involved in some type of burn. Code T31.63 (burn of any degree involving 60–69 percent of body surface, with 30–39 percent involved in third-degree burn) could then be assigned. Coding professionals are not expected to calculate the extent of a burn, but understanding the rule of nines may help them recognize when burns are so extensive that the physician should be asked for additional information.

SUNBURN

Sunburn and other ultraviolet radiation burns are classified in chapter 12, Diseases of Skin and Subcutaneous Tissue. Category L55, Sunburn, is assigned for first-degree (L55.0), second-degree (L55.1), and third-degree sunburns (L55.2) or for sunburn of an unspecified degree (L55.9). Sunburn due to other ultraviolet radiation exposure, such as a tanning bed, is classified to category L56, Other acute skin changes due to ultraviolet radiation, or category L57, Skin changes due to chronic exposure to nonionizing radiation.

EXTERNAL CAUSES OF BURNS

External cause codes, including codes from category Y92, Place of occurrence of the external cause, are assigned for burns and corrosions, as discussed in chapter 29 of this handbook, which covers other injuries. The following External cause categories should be used to report source and intent:

X00–X08	Exposure to smoke, fire and flames
X10–X19	Contact with heat and hot substances
X75	Intentional self-harm by explosive material
X76	Intentional self-harm by smoke, fire and flames
X77	Intentional self-harm by steam, hot vapors and hot objects
X96	Assault by explosive material
X97	Assault by smoke, fire and flames
X98	Assault by steam, hot vapors and hot objects

ASSOCIATED INJURIES AND ILLNESSES

When a burn is described as infected, two codes are required. The code for the burn is sequenced first, with an additional code for the infection. For example, Initial encounter, *Staphylococcus* infection, second-degree burn of abdominal wall, is coded to T21.22xA + L08.89 + B95.8.

Other injuries frequently occur with burns, and other conditions are sometimes caused by burns. Examples of such injuries include the following:

- Smoke inhalation often occurs in cases of burns due to combustible products (category T59). It is caused by inhalation or exposure to hot gaseous products of combustion and can cause serious respiratory complications. Code J68.9 is assigned for smoke inhalation due to chemical fumes and vapors. Code J70.5 is assigned to describe a smoke inhalation injury not otherwise specified. Use an additional code to identify any associated respiratory conditions, such as acute respiratory failure. When a patient presents with a burn injury and another related condition, such as smoke inhalation or respiratory failure, the circumstances of admission determine the selection of the principal or first-listed diagnosis.

  For example, a child who was rescued from a burning house has no obvious burns, but soot is present about his nose and mouth. The patient is intubated and ventilated for less than 48 hours because of the risk of airway edema from the smoke. The provider diagnoses smoke inhalation. Code **T59.811A, Toxic effect of smoke, accidental (unintentional), initial encounter,** is assigned as the principal diagnosis. Assign code **J70.5, Respiratory conditions due to smoke inhalation,** as a secondary diagnosis, and code **X00.1xxA, Exposure to smoke in uncontrolled fire in building or structure, initial encounter,** for the external cause of the injury. Also assign codes **5A1945Z, Respiratory ventilation, 24–96 consecutive hours,** and **0BH17EZ, Insertion of endotracheal airway into trachea, via natural or artificial opening,** for the airway management secondary to the toxic effects of smoke.

- Electrical burns, such as those caused by high-tension wires, may cause ventricular arrhythmias (I49.-) that require immediate attention.

- Certain substances from plastic products may produce hydrogen cyanide. Toxic effect of hydrogen cyanide is coded to T57.3-.

- Traumatic shock (T79.4-) is often present at the time of admission or may occur later.

Pre-existing conditions may also have an impact on the burn patient's prognosis and care management and therefore should be coded as additional diagnoses when they otherwise meet criteria for reportable diagnoses. Examples of potentially harmful pre-existing conditions that should be reported include the following:

- Cardiovascular disorders (such as angina, congestive heart failure, or valvular disease) may increase ischemia and precipitate myocardial infarction in a patient with extensive second-degree or third-degree burns. Pulmonary wedge monitoring may be necessary in these cases.

- Asthma, chronic bronchitis, and other chronic obstructive pulmonary diseases may require ventilation therapy.

- Peptic ulcers, either gastric or duodenal, and ulcerative colitis are pre-existing conditions that may lead to gastrointestinal bleeding and require treatment along with the burn.

- Pre-existing kidney disease increases the risk of tubular necrosis and renal failure in patients with third-degree burns or extensive second-degree burns.

- Alcoholism may pose a threat of alcohol withdrawal syndrome, requiring prophylactic treatment for delirium tremens.

- Diabetes mellitus slows the healing process, and diabetes mellitus with stated manifestations can further complicate the management of burn cases.

EXERCISE 30.1

Code the following diagnoses, including External cause codes. Assume that the incidents are for the initial encounter unless otherwise stated.

1. First-degree burn of lower left leg and second-degree burns of left foot when adding wood to bonfire at beach resort while on vacation

2. First-degree burns of face and both eyes, involving corneas, eyelids, nose, cheeks, and lips, due to accidental lye spill at home

3. Burns over 38 percent of body, with 10 percent of body involved in third-degree burns and 28 percent involved in second-degree burns; paid firefighter burned in forest fire

4. Acid burns to left cornea from nitric acid

5. Subsequent encounter with nonhealing first- and second-degree burns of back that occurred five weeks ago when patient's clothing caught fire in kitchen accident in his home

6. Food service employee sustained first-degree and second-degree burns, thumb and two fingers, right, from kitchen fire in nursing home while cooking, initial encounter

7. Farm employee admitted with severe shock
   due to third-degree burns of back
   due to uncontrolled barn fire, initial encounter

   _____

8. First-, second-, and third-degree burns
   of body; 10 percent first degree, 15 percent second
   degree, and 32 percent (over the trunk) third degree;
   patient is crew member of ferry boat steamship
   on which boiler exploded

   _____

9. Severe sunburn of face, neck, and
   shoulders; patient spent most of the
   day at the beach

   _____

10. Infected friction burn of left thigh due to
    rope burn while water skiing barefoot at
    Lake Berryessa

   _____

11. First-degree burns of back of left hand
    due to hot tap water in home where
    patient was visiting

   _____

12. Superficial burns (dermatitis) of face and chest
    from a tanning bed

   _____

13. Bilateral corneal flash burn due to welding torch
    (Welder's eye/photokeratitis)

   _____

14. Release of skin contracture due to
    third-degree burns of the right hand
    that occurred in a house fire five years ago

   _____

CHAPTER 31

Poisoning, Toxic Effects, Adverse Effects, and Underdosing of Drugs

CHAPTER OVERVIEW

- A condition caused by drugs or other ingested substances can be considered as an adverse effect, a toxic effect, or a poisoning.

- Underdosing refers to taking less of a medication than is prescribed by a provider or a manufacturer's instruction.
  - Underdosing codes should never be assigned as the principal or first-listed codes.
  - If the reduction in the prescribed dose of the medication results in a relapse or an exacerbation of the medical condition for which the drug is prescribed, then the medical condition itself should be coded first.

- An adverse effect is one caused by a correctly prescribed and used drug.
  - A code indicating the nature of the adverse effect is assigned first.
  - The combination code (T36–T50) that includes the adverse effect and the responsible substance follows.

- Poisoning is a condition caused by the incorrect use of a drug or another substance.
  - A code from categories T36 through T65 is sequenced first.
  - This is followed by the code for the manifestation of the poisoning.
  - When no intent of poisoning is indicated, the code for accidental poisoning should be assigned.

- Interactions of properly used therapeutic drugs and alcohol or nonprescription drugs are considered instances of poisoning.

- Codes for poisoning, adverse effects, and underdosing are found in the ICD-10-CM Table of Drugs and Chemicals.

- No additional External cause code is required for poisoning, toxic effect, adverse effect, and underdosing codes.

- Acute conditions caused by alcohol or drug abuse are considered poisonings, but chronic conditions are not.

- The late effects of poisoning, adverse effects, and underdosing are coded with the seventh character "S" for sequela.

LEARNING OUTCOMES

After studying this chapter, you should be able to:

- Differentiate between adverse effects and poisoning.
- Locate codes associated with poisoning and adverse effects.
- Code for poisoning due to substance abuse.
- Code for late effects for adverse reactions and poisoning.

TERMS TO KNOW

Adverse effect
classification of a condition caused by a drug or another substance when used correctly

Poisoning
classification of a condition caused by a drug or another substance when used incorrectly

Toxic effect
classification of a condition caused by ingestion or contact with a harmful substance

Underdosing
classification of a condition caused by taking less of a medication than is prescribed by a provider or a manufacturer's instruction

REMEMBER . . .

A condition caused by the use of a drug may be classified as either an adverse effect or a poisoning. The determination is based only on whether or not the substance was correctly prescribed and properly administered.

INTRODUCTION

CHAPTER 31

*Poisoning,
Toxic Effects,
Adverse
Effects, and
Underdosing
of Drugs*

Conditions due to drugs and medicinal and biological substances are classified to categories T36 through T50. Codes in these categories are combination codes that specify both the responsible substance and whether it is a poisoning (including the intent, e.g., accidental), an adverse effect, or an underdosing, with the fifth or sixth character used to specify the following:

1 Poisoning, accidental (unintentional)

2 Poisoning, intentional self-harm

3 Poisoning, assault

4 Poisoning, undetermined

5 Adverse effect

6 Underdosing

Toxic effects of substances chiefly nonmedicinal as to source are classified to categories T51 through T65. Similar to categories T36 through T50, codes in categories T51 through T65 are combination codes that specify the responsible substance as well as the intent (e.g., accidental). However, adverse effect and underdosing are not applicable to toxic effects. As with other categories in chapter 19 of ICD-10-CM, categories T33 through T65 require seventh-character values, as follows: "A" for initial encounter, "D" for subsequent encounter, and "S" for sequela. These values are described in more detail in chapter 29 of this handbook.

The condition is classified as an adverse effect when the correct substance was administered as prescribed. When the substance was used incorrectly, it is classified as a poisoning with the appropriate fifth or sixth character 1–4, depending on the intent of the poisoning (e.g., accidental). A condition classified as an adverse effect may be clinically the same as a condition classified as a poisoning, and the responsible drug may be the same for both; the determination of whether the condition is a poisoning or an adverse effect is based on the manner in which the substance was used. The coding distinction between adverse effects of drugs administered correctly and poisoning facilitates the collection of data on adverse effects that result from the correct use of drugs, and on the extent to which incorrect use results in patient care problems.

Note that using the prescribed medication less frequently or in smaller amounts than prescribed or instructed by the manufacturer is not coded as poisoning, but rather as underdosing.

When the drug was correctly prescribed and properly administered, a code for the nature of the adverse effect is sequenced first, followed by an additional code(s) for the adverse effect of the drug (T36–T50, with a fifth or sixth character 5—e.g., T36.0x5-). The adverse effects of therapeutic substances correctly prescribed and properly administered (toxicity, synergistic reaction, side effect, and idiosyncratic reaction) may be due to (1) differences among patients, such as age, sex, disease, and genetic factors, and (2) drug-related factors, such as type of drug, route of administration, duration of therapy, dosage, and bioavailability. Drug adverse effect manifestations can range from minor or temporary effects to more serious and sometimes permanent damage. Examples of adverse effect manifestations include rash, tachycardia, delirium, gastrointestinal hemorrhage, vomiting, hepatitis, renal failure, and respiratory failure.

When the condition results from the interaction of two or more therapeutic drugs, each used correctly, it is classified as an adverse effect, and each drug is coded individually, unless the combination code is listed in the Table of Drugs and Chemicals.

When the condition is a poisoning, the poisoning code (e.g., T36.0x1-) is sequenced first, followed by additional codes for all manifestations. Poisoning codes have an associated intent, and code selection is based on the circumstance of the poisoning. When no intent of poisoning is indicated, the code for accidental poisoning should be assigned. The codes for undetermined poisoning (fifth or sixth character 4) are reserved for use when there is specific documentation in the record that the intent of the poisoning cannot be determined. The following are examples of how a diagnosis of coma due to codeine is coded based on documentation of the intent of the poisoning:

CHAPTER 31

Poisoning,
Toxic Effects,
Adverse
Effects, and
Underdosing of
Drugs

<u>T40.2x1A</u> + R40.20	Coma due to accidental poisoning due to codeine
<u>T40.2x2A</u> + R40.20	Coma due to codeine taken in a suicide attempt
<u>T40.2x4A</u> + R40.20	Coma due to overdose of codeine, cause unknown
<u>T40.2x1A</u> + R40.20	Coma due to poisoning due to codeine

If there is also a diagnosis of abuse of or dependence on the substance, the abuse or dependence is also coded.

Because codes in categories T36 through T65 include the responsible substances as well as the external cause, no additional External cause code is required for these codes. However, if the intent of the underdosing is known, External cause codes may be used to report failure in dosage during medical and surgical care (Y63.6–Y63.9) or patient's underdosing of medication regimen (Z91.12- or Z91.13-).

The consequences of harmful substances ingested or coming into contact with a person are classified as toxic effects. Most are assigned to categories T51 through T65, Toxic effects of substances chiefly nonmedicinal as to source; the exception is contact with and (suspected) exposure to toxic substances (Z77.-). Code examples include the following:

T57.2x1-	Chronic manganese toxicity
T57.0x1-	Toxicity due to exposure to arsenical pesticide
Z77.090	Toxicity due to asbestos exposure

Toxic effect codes should be sequenced first, followed by the appropriate code(s) to identify all the associated manifestations of the toxic effect, such as respiratory conditions due to external agents (J60–J70). Similar to the codes for poisoning, toxic effect codes are combination codes that include the substance and indicate the associated intent by the use of the following fifth or sixth characters:

1 accidental

2 intentional self-harm

3 assault

4 undetermined

Also similar to the codes for poisoning, when no intent is indicated, the code for accidental intent (fifth or sixth character 1) should be assigned. The codes for undetermined intent (fifth or sixth character 4) are reserved for use when the record specifically documents that the intent of the toxic effect cannot be determined.

A diagnostic statement of toxic effect, toxicity, or intoxication due to a prescription drug, such as digitalis or lithium, without any further qualification usually refers to an adverse effect of a correctly administered prescription drug. The adverse effect should be coded as such unless medical record documentation indicates otherwise. The following terms in the medical record usually indicate correct usage and identify the condition as an adverse effect:

- "Allergic reaction"
- "Cumulative effect of drug" (toxicity)
- "Hypersensitivity to drug"
- "Idiosyncratic reaction"
- "Paradoxical reaction"
- "Synergistic reaction"

When the medical record documents an error in dosage or administration, the condition should be coded as a poisoning. Terms that usually identify the condition as a poisoning include the following:

530

CHAPTER 31

*Poisoning,
Toxic Effects,
Adverse
Effects, and
Underdosing
of Drugs*

- "Wrong medication given" or "wrong medication taken"
- "Error made in drug prescription"
- "Wrong dosage given" or "wrong dosage taken" (unless specified as underdosing, or lower dosage than prescribed)
- "Intentional drug overdose"
- "Nonprescribed drug taken with correctly prescribed and properly administered drug"

The poisoning code is sequenced first, followed by the code for the manifestation. This sequencing is based on the chapter-specific guideline providing such direction. Therefore, it applies even if the poisoning may have already been addressed.

For example, a patient is seen in the emergency department in a coma and suffering from acute respiratory failure due to a drug overdose. The patient undergoes a gastric lavage for the drug overdose. The patient is also intubated, connected to an invasive mechanical ventilator, and transferred to another hospital for continued toxicology management and treatment of the acute respiratory failure. The poisoning is still sequenced as the principal diagnosis at the receiving hospital.

When a condition is the result of the interaction of a therapeutic drug used correctly with a nonprescription drug or with alcohol, it is classified as a poisoning. Poisoning codes are also assigned for each drug. For example, a diagnosis of coma identified as an adverse reaction to Valium taken correctly but associated with the intake of two martinis is coded as follows:

T51.0x1A	Poisoning due to alcohol, accidental
T42.4x1A	Poisoning due to Valium, accidental
R40.20	Coma

Taking a larger or more frequent dosage than prescribed is classified as a poisoning. Note that taking a lower amount or discontinuing the use of a prescribed medication is not classified as either a poisoning or an adverse reaction, but rather as underdosing. Discontinuing the use of a prescribed medication on the patient's own initiative (not directed by the patient's provider) is also classified as an underdosing. Underdosing codes should never be assigned as the principal or first-listed code. If the reduction in the prescribed dose of the medication results in a relapse or an exacerbation of the medical condition for which the drug is prescribed, then the medical condition itself should be coded first.

For example, a patient was prescribed Amiodarone to control his atrial fibrillation. The patient quit taking his prescribed medication on his own one week ago, because he said the medication made him nauseous. He is now admitted for control of atrial fibrillation and medication adjustment. The atrial fibrillation is coded as the principal diagnosis and the underdosing code as an additional diagnosis, as follows:

I48.91	Atrial fibrillation
T46.2x6A	Underdosing of Amiodarone
Z91.14	Patient's noncompliance with medication

Figure 31.1 illustrates a process for coding adverse effects of drugs or poisoning.

LOCATION OF CODES ASSOCIATED WITH POISONING, ADVERSE EFFECTS, AND UNDERDOSING

Codes for poisonings, adverse effects, and underdosing are located most easily by referring to the ICD-10-CM Table of Drugs and Chemicals (see figure 31.2). Drugs and other chemicals are listed in alphabetical order in the left column of the Table, with the first column to the right listing the accidental poisoning code for that substance. The remaining columns provide codes for poisoning for the other external circumstances (intentional self-harm, assault, and undetermined), for adverse effect, and for underdosing.

529

CHAPTER 31

*Poisoning,
Toxic Effects,
Adverse
Effects, and
Underdosing of
Drugs*

If a specific drug cannot be located in the Table, it can usually be found by either the generic name or the drug class or type (e.g., antibiotic). The hospital pharmacist can also be a valuable source of information.

Codes should not be assigned directly from the Table of Drugs and Chemicals without verification in the Tabular List. The Table is extensive and very detailed, but it does not take into account

FIGURE 31.1 Decision Tree for Coding Adverse Effects of Drugs or Poisoning Due to Drugs or Medicinal or Biological Substances

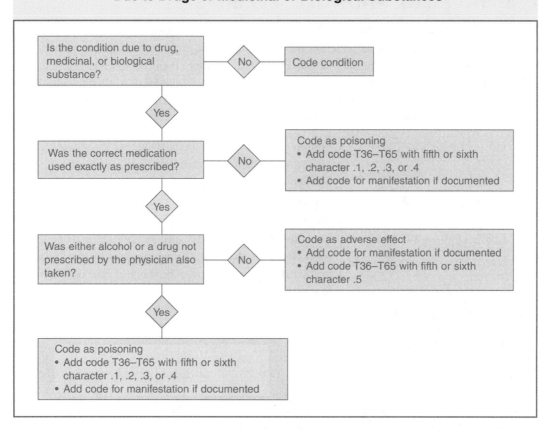

FIGURE 31.2 Excerpt from ICD-10-CM Table of Drugs and Chemicals

Substance	Poisoning, Accidental (Unintentional)	Poisoning, Intentional Self-Harm	Poisoning, Assault	Poisoning, Undetermined	Adverse Effect	Underdosing
Acetylphenylhydrazine	T39.8x1	T39.8x2	T39.8x3	T39.8x4	T39.8x5	T39.8x6
Acetylsalicylic acid (salts)	T39.011	T39.012	T39.013	T39.014	T39.015	T39.016
-enteric coated	T39.011	T39.012	T39.013	T39.014	T39.015	T39.016
Acetylsulfamethoxypyridazine	T37.0x1	T37.0x2	T37.0x3	T37.0x4	T37.0x5	T37.0x6
Achromycin	T36.4x1	T36.4x2	T36.4x3	T36.4x4	T36.4x5	T36.4x6
-ophthalmic preparation	T49.5x1	T49.5x2	T49.5x3	T49.5x4	T49.5x5	T49.5x6
-topical NEC	T49.0x1	T49.0x2	T49.0x3	T49.0x4	T49.0x5	T49.0x6
Aciclovir	T37.5x1	T37.5x2	T37.5x3	T37.5x4	T37.5x5	T37.5x6

532

CHAPTER 31

Poisoning,
Toxic Effects,
Adverse
Effects, and
Underdosing
of Drugs

the instructional notes in the Tabular List. For example, the Table lists codes from category T36, Poisoning by, adverse effect of and underdosing of systemic antibiotics, but the exclusion note indicating that codes from subcategory T45.1 should be used for antineoplastic antibiotics is found only by looking up category T36 in the Tabular List.

GUIDELINES FOR ASSIGNMENT OF CODES FOR POISONING, ADVERSE EFFECTS, UNDERDOSING, AND TOXIC EFFECTS

When two or more drugs or medicinal or biological substances are reported as being responsible for a poisoning, an adverse effect, an underdosing, or a toxic effect, code each substance individually, unless the same code would describe the causative agent for more than one adverse reaction, poisoning, underdosing, or toxic effect. In other words, assign as many codes as needed to completely describe all responsible substances; however, when a code identifies more than one responsible substance, assign that code only once. For example:

I49.1 + T46.0x5A + T42.4x5A	Supraventricular premature beats secondary to use of digitalis and Valium, both used as prescribed, initial encounter
R50.83 + T50.A15A	An infant with a high fever due to correct administration of DTap vaccine
R68.2 + L29.9 + T42.3x5A	Patient suffering from dry mouth and itching as a result of taking phenobarbital as prescribed by his physician (either R68.2 or L29.9 may be the principal or first-listed code)

ENVIRONMENTAL TOXINS

Subcategory T65.82, Toxic effect of harmful algae and algae toxins, describes toxic effects of exposure to harmful algae bloom, such as toxic effect of blue-green algae bloom, brown tide, cyanobacteria bloom, Florida red tide, *Pfiesteria piscicida*, and red tide. *Karenia brevis* (*K. brevis*) is a microscopic, fast-growing marine alga species that creates blooms called red tides and produces a powerful toxin known as brevetoxin. When shellfish feed on *K. brevis*, brevetoxin becomes concentrated in the shellfish. Individuals who eat shellfish contaminated with brevetoxin develop neurotoxic shellfish poisoning. This type of food poisoning leads to severe gastrointestinal and neurological symptoms. Assign code Z77.121 to describe possible contact with and exposure to harmful algae and algae toxins. This code may be assigned when the patient may have been in the vicinity of algae bloom but has not developed symptoms, or when the patient has symptoms suspicious of exposure to algae bloom but a definitive cause of the symptoms has not been confirmed.

Environmental exposure to brevetoxin can also affect people who swim in an ocean polluted by brevetoxins or who inhale brevetoxins in the air. Symptoms can include irritation of the eyes, nose, and throat; tingling of the lips and tongue; coughing; wheezing; and shortness of breath. For example, a patient develops severe abdominal pain, vomiting, and a tingling sensation in the fingers after eating shellfish. The patient is diagnosed with neurotoxic shellfish poisoning due to red tides. Assign code **T65.821A, Toxic effect of harmful algae and algae toxins, accidental (unintentional), initial encounter.**

CHAPTER 31

*Poisoning,
Toxic Effects,
Adverse
Effects, and
Underdosing of
Drugs*

EXERCISE 31.1

Code the following diagnoses, assuming that the drug involved was taken correctly unless otherwise specified. Assume these are initial encounters.

1. Coma due to acute barbiturate intoxication, attempted suicide

2. Two-year-old patient ingested an unknown quantity of mother's Enovid

3. Syncope due to hypersensitivity to antidepressant medication

4. Hypokalemia resulting from reaction to Diuril given by mistake in physician's office

5. Diplopia due to allergic reaction to antihistamine, taken as prescribed

6. Lethargy due to unintentional overdose of sleeping pills

7. Electrolyte imbalance due to interaction between lithium carbonate and Diuril, both taken as prescribed

8. Parkinsonism, secondary to correct use of haloperidol

9. Cerebral anoxia resulting from barbiturate overdose, suicide attempt

10. Toxic encephalopathy due to excessive use of aspirin

11. Ataxia due to Valium (taken as prescribed) consumed with three martinis

534

CHAPTER 31

Poisoning,
Toxic Effects,
Adverse
Effects, and
Underdosing
of Drugs

12. Allergic dermatitis due to slow-acting insulin

_____

13. Coumadin intoxication due to accumulative

   effect resulting in gross hematuria

_____

14. Severe bradycardia due to accidental

   double dose of digoxin

_____

15. Generalized convulsions due to accidental

   Darvon overdose

_____

16. Light-headedness resulting from interaction

   between Aldomet and peripheral

   vasodilating agent (both taken as prescribed)

_____

17. Uncontrolled hypertension due to patient having

   reduced his antihypertensive medication

   (patient could not afford it)

_____

UNSPECIFIED ADVERSE EFFECT OF DRUGS

ICD-10-CM provides code **T88.7-, Unspecified adverse effect of drug or medicament,** to identify adverse reactions when the nature of the reaction is not specified. Use an additional code from categories T36 through T50, with fifth or sixth character 5 if applicable, to identify the responsible drug. Code T88.7- may be used in the outpatient setting, but only when no sign or symptom of the adverse effect is documented. The use of code T88.7- for inpatient reporting is inappropriate. If the patient is exhibiting symptoms or signs, the code for that condition should be assigned. If the adverse condition cannot be identified, one of the following codes should be assigned:

R82.5   Elevated urine levels of drugs, medicaments and biological substances
R82.6   Abnormal urine levels of substances chiefly nonmedicinal as to source
R89.2   Abnormal level of other drugs, medicaments and biological substances in
        specimens from other organs, systems and tissues
R89.3   Abnormal level of substances chiefly nonmedicinal as to source in specimens
        from other organs, systems and tissues

ICD-10-CM provides subcategories T50.90-, Poisoning by, adverse effect of and underdosing of unspecified drugs, medicaments and biological substances, and T50.91-, Poisoning by, adverse effect of and underdosing of multiple unspecified drugs, medicaments and biological substances, for instances when the medical documentation does not specify the drug(s) or substance(s) responsible for the poisoning, adverse effect, or underdosing.

POISONING DUE TO SUBSTANCE ABUSE OR DEPENDENCE

CHAPTER 31

*Poisoning,
Toxic Effects,
Adverse
Effects, and
Underdosing of
Drugs*

An acute condition due to a reaction resulting from the interaction of alcohol and one or more drugs or due to a drug involved in abuse or dependence is classified as a poisoning. Additional codes are assigned for both the acute manifestation of the poisoning and the dependence or abuse. For example:

T40.1x1A + J81.0 + F11.20   Acute pulmonary edema due to accidental heroin overdose in a patient who is heroin dependent

Chronic conditions related to alcohol or drug abuse or dependence are not classified as poisoning. The code for the chronic condition is sequenced first, followed by a code for the abuse or dependence. For example:

K70.30 + F10.20   Alcoholic cirrhosis of the liver; chronic alcohol dependence
K70.10 + F10.20   Alcoholic hepatitis; chronic alcohol dependence, episodic
F14.14   Drug-induced depressive state due to cocaine abuse

EXERCISE 31.2

Code the following diagnoses and procedures. Assign External cause codes where appropriate. Assume these are initial encounters.

1. Muscle cramps of leg due to occupational use of arsenic pesticide

2. Systemic hypocalcemia and hypokalemia due to use of lye in household chores

3. Bradycardia due to ingestion of oleander leaves

4. Patient, a known cocaine abuser, was admitted with acute respiratory failure due to crack/cocaine overdose. Patient was placed on mechanical ventilation for 20 hours.

5. Patient admitted with dialysis dementia secondary to aluminum toxicity (aluminum acetate solution) due to renal dialysis therapy

CHAPTER 31 :

Poisoning,

Toxic Effects,

Adverse

Effects, and

Underdosing

of Drugs

LATE EFFECTS OF POISONING, ADVERSE EFFECTS, AND UNDERDOSING

When coding late effects of a poisoning, the code for the responsible drug or substance is sequenced first (the code from categories T36 through T65), with the seventh character "S" for sequela, followed by the specific type of sequela (e.g., brain damage).

When coding late effects of an adverse effect, assign a code for the nature of the adverse effect (sequela) first, followed by the code for the responsible drug or substance (T36–T50, with fifth or sixth character 5), with the seventh character "S" for sequela.

Long-term chronic effects of a prescription drug taken over a period of time—and still being taken at the time the chronic effects arise—are coded as current adverse effects. For example, steroid-induced diabetes may be classified as an adverse effect of correctly administered medication, a poisoning, or a late effect of poisoning. If a patient who develops steroid-induced diabetes and is currently taking steroids as prescribed, the condition is coded as an adverse effect (E09.- + T38.0x5A). However, if the patient experiences delayed effects that arose or remain long after the steroid was discontinued, code E09.- is assigned first, followed by code T38.0x5S.

Other examples of coding adverse and late effects of a prescription drug may include:

G93.9 + T36.0x5A   Brain damage due to allergic reaction to penicillin (current medication)

G93.9 + T36.0x5S   Brain damage due to allergic reaction to penicillin (use of medication discontinued six months ago)

EXERCISE 31.3

Code the following diagnoses, sequencing the codes correctly. Assign External cause codes where appropriate.

1. Extrapyramidal disease resulting from previous overdose of Thorazine in an attempted suicide six months ago

2. Bilateral neural deafness resulting from accidental overdose of streptomycin administered in physician's office two years ago

3. Anoxic brain damage secondary to previous accidental overdose of Nembutal nine months ago

4. Secondary parkinsonism due to poisoning by lithium carbonate four years ago

5. Patient with a diagnosis of acute systolic congestive heart failure was recently discharged with a prescription for digoxin 200 mcg once daily as well as instructions to follow a low-fat and low-sodium diet and avoid alcohol and caffeine. Two weeks later, patient was seen in the emergency department with shortness of breath on minimal exertion and severe edema. On questioning, patient admitted to having reduced digoxin to every other day because it is too expensive. Diagnosis: Relapse of acute systolic congestive heart failure due to low dose of digoxin.

CHAPTER 32

Complications of Surgery and Medical Care

CHAPTER OVERVIEW

- Categories T80 through T88 in ICD-10-CM cover complications of medical and surgical care that are not already classified elsewhere.

- Complications that occur in a specified body site are classified in the chapter of ICD-10-CM for that site.

- Intraoperative and postprocedural complication codes are found within the body system chapters, with codes specific to the organs and structures of that body system.

- Postcare conditions must meet certain criteria to be classified as complications.

  — There must be an unexpected or abnormal occurrence.

  — There must be a documented relationship between the condition and the care.

  — There must be an indication that it is a complication.

- There are several instructional notes (in particular, exclusion notes) related to complications.

- When coding, look for a subterm indicating postoperative or iatrogenic condition.

- Look to the main term **Complications** if no subterms are found in the particular entry for the condition.

- Complications involving an internal device, an implant, or a graft are classified first.

- It is important to distinguish between admission for complications and admission for routine and scheduled aftercare.

INTRODUCTION

Categories T80 through T88 are provided in ICD-10-CM for complications of medical and surgical care that are not classified elsewhere. Categories T80 through T85 and T88 require a seventh-character value to specify initial encounter ("A"), subsequent encounter ("D"), or sequela ("S"), similar to other codes in chapter 19 of ICD-10-CM. Refer to chapter 29 in this handbook for a more detailed explanation on the use of seventh characters. As a reminder, assignment of the seventh character is based on whether the patient is undergoing active or subsequent treatment and not whether the provider is seeing the patient for the first time. For complication codes, active treatment refers to treatment for the condition described by the code, even though it may be related to an earlier precipitating problem. For example, **T82.7xxA, Infection and inflammatory reaction due to other cardiac and vascular devices, implants and grafts, initial encounter,** is used when active treatment is provided for the infection, even though the condition relates to a vascular device, implant, or graft that was placed at a previous encounter.

Note that not all conditions that occur following surgery or other patient care are classified as complications. Complications are determined by multiple criteria. First, the condition or occurrence must exceed routine expectations for the surgical or medical care. For example, a major amount of bleeding is expected with joint replacement surgery; hemorrhage should not be considered a complication of this procedure unless the bleeding is particularly excessive. In addition, a cause-and-effect relationship between the care provided and the condition must be documented, including some indication that the condition is a complication—as opposed to a postoperative condition in which no complication is present, such as an artificial opening status or an absence of an extremity. In some cases, the cause-and-effect relationship is implicit, as in a complication due to the presence of an internal device, an implant, or a graft or due to a transplant.

Code assignment for postprocedural complications is based on the provider's documentation of the relationship between the complication and the procedure. The coding professional cannot make this determination and should always query the provider for clarification when a postprocedural complication is not documented clearly. The guideline regarding a code assignment's being based on the provider's documentation of the relationship between the condition and the care or procedure extends to any complications of care, regardless of the chapter in which the code is located. Note that the term "complication" as used in ICD-10-CM does not imply that improper or inadequate care is responsible for the problem.

No time limit is defined for the development of a complication. It may occur during the hospital episode in which the care was provided, shortly thereafter, or even years later. When a complication occurs during the episode in which the operation or other care was given, it is assigned as an additional code. When a complication develops later and is the reason for the hospital admission or encounter, it is designated as the principal or first-listed diagnosis. Complications of surgical and medical care are classified in ICD-10-CM as follows:

- Complications that occur in a specified body site are classified in the chapter of ICD-10-CM for that site.

- Complications that affect multiple sites or body systems are generally classified in categories T80 through T88. Additional codes are assigned as appropriate to identify the specific condition resulting from the complication.

- Intraoperative and postprocedural complication codes are found within the body system chapters of ICD-10-CM, with codes specific to the organs and structures of that body system. These codes should be sequenced first, followed by a code(s) for the specific complication, if applicable.

- Complications of abortion, pregnancy, labor, or delivery are classified in chapter 15 of ICD-10-CM.

It is imperative to use the Alphabetic Index carefully and follow all instructional notes. Exclusion notes are fairly extensive in this section and often direct the coding professional elsewhere. There are several basic exclusions from categories T80 through T88 that must be observed:

- Complications of medicinal agents, such as adverse effects, poisoning, and toxic effects of drugs and chemicals

- Any encounters with medical care for postoperative conditions in which no complications are present, such as artificial opening status, closure of external stoma, or fitting and adjustment of external prosthetic device

- Burns and corrosions from local applications and irradiation

- Mechanical complication of respirator or ventilator

- Postprocedural fever

- Complications of the condition for which surgery was performed

- Complications of surgical procedures during pregnancy, childbirth, and the puerperium

- Specified conditions classified elsewhere, such as ostomy complications, postlaminectomy syndrome, postgastric surgery syndromes, or postmastectomy lymphedema syndrome

- Any condition classified elsewhere in the Alphabetic Index when described as being due to a procedure or medical care (Note that the adjective "iatrogenic" is often used to indicate that the condition is a result of treatment.)

- Injury codes from chapter 19 should not be assigned for injuries that occur during, or as a result of, a medical intervention. Assign the appropriate complication code(s).

When assigning codes in categories T80–T88, Complications of surgical and medical care NEC, use an additional code to identify the specific complication if the additional code provides greater specificity as to the nature of the condition. If, however, the complication code describes the condition fully, no additional code is necessary.

LOCATING COMPLICATION CODES IN THE ALPHABETIC INDEX

First refer to the main term for the condition and look for a subterm indicating a postoperative or another iatrogenic condition. For example:

Adhesion(s) . . .
-postoperative (gastrointestinal tract) K66.0
--with obstruction K91.30 . . .
--pelvic peritoneal N99.4 . . .
-vagina N99.2 . . .
Colostomy . . .
-malfunctioning K94.03

When no relevant entry can be found under the main term for the condition, refer to the main term **Complications** and look for an appropriate subterm, such as one of the following:

- The nature of the complication, such as "foreign body," "accidental puncture," or "hemorrhage"

- The type of procedure, such as "colostomy," "dialysis," or "shunt"

- The anatomical site or body system affected, such as "respiratory system"
- General terms, such as "mechanical," "infection," or "graft"

Examples include the following entries from the Alphabetic Index:

Complication(s) (from) (of) . . .

-cardiac . . .

--device, implant or graft T82.9 . . .

---infection or inflammation T82.7 . . .

---mechanical

----breakdown T82.519 . . .

----displacement T82.529 . . .

-postmastoidectomy NEC H95.19-

POSTOPERATIVE CONDITIONS NOT CLASSIFIED AS COMPLICATIONS

Certain conditions resulting from medical or surgical care are residual conditions of a procedure, but no complicating factor is involved. For example, postlaminectomy syndrome often occurs following laminectomy, but it is a sequela of the procedure, not a complication. The extensive exclusion list at the beginning of the T80–T88 series is helpful in making some of these distinctions. Other examples include:

K56.52	Postoperative intestinal or peritoneal adhesions with complete obstruction
K94.12 + B95.4	Infection of enterostomy due to group C *Streptococcus*
N73.6	Postoperative pelvic adhesions (female)

Some conditions that occur postoperatively are not classified as complications, nor do they have special codes to indicate that they are postoperative in nature. For example, postoperative pain not associated with a specific postoperative complication is assigned to the appropriate postoperative pain code in category G89. A code for postoperative pain is assigned only if the pain is not routine or if the postoperative pain was not expected immediately after surgery. In addition, the postoperative pain must meet the guidelines for a reportable diagnosis.

Patients are frequently admitted from outpatient surgery with pain and/or nausea and vomiting, but these are common symptoms during postoperative recovery and are not coded to categories T80 through T88 unless the physician identifies them specifically as complications of the surgery. The principal diagnosis is the symptom or other condition that occasions the postoperative admission.

Sometimes, the patient is admitted because of a general concern rather than because of specific symptoms. Although physicians may state that the admission is for observation, this type of situation is ordinarily not coded to category Z03, Encounter for medical observation for suspected diseases and conditions ruled out. If no specific condition is identified, the principal diagnosis is admission for postprocedural aftercare (Z48.-).

Postoperative anemia is rarely considered to be a complication of surgery. When the physician documents postoperative anemia due to blood loss, code **D62, Acute posthemorrhagic anemia,** is assigned, but no complication code is assigned unless the physician documents excessive bleeding as a complication. The fact that blood is administered during a surgical procedure does not indicate a postoperative anemia. Transfusions are sometimes given as a prophylactic replacement to avoid postoperative anemia. Anemia is not assigned solely because the patient received a transfusion; the physician must document the condition.

A diagnosis of postoperative hypertension often means only that the patient has a pre-existing essential hypertension or an elevated blood pressure. If the physician clearly identifies hypertension as a postoperative complication, code **I97.3, Postprocedural hypertension,** is assigned.

EXERCISE 32.1

Code the following diagnoses. Do not assign External cause codes.

1. Postoperative fever

2. Postoperative esophagitis

3. Colostomy malfunction

4. Postleukotomy syndrome

5. Postoperative peritoneal adhesions

6. Postoperative blind loop syndrome

COMPLICATIONS AFFECTING SPECIFIC BODY SYSTEMS

ICD-10-CM classifies many intraoperative and postprocedural complication codes within the body system chapters with codes specific to the organs and structures of that body system. These codes should be sequenced first, followed by a code(s) for the specific complication, if applicable. Intraoperative and postprocedural complications and disorders are classified within body system chapters to the categories listed below:

D78	Spleen
E36 and E89	Endocrine system
G97	Nervous system
H59	Eye and adnexa
H95	Ear and mastoid process
I97	Circulatory system
J95	Respiratory system
K91 and K94	Digestive system
L76	Skin and subcutaneous tissue
M96 and M97	Musculoskeletal system
N99	Genitourinary system

The above categories (except for E89 and K94) provide additional characters to specify complications such as intraoperative or postprocedural hemorrhage (subcategory D78.2), postprocedural hematoma (code D78.31 or D78.32), postprocedural seroma (code D78.33 or D78.34), or accidental puncture and laceration (e.g., inadvertent rents, tears, or lacerations) during a procedure. In addition, codes distinguish whether the conditions resulted from a procedure on the specified organ or from complications of other procedures. For example:

- Hemorrhage after repair of spleen laceration is coded to **D78.21, Postprocedural hemorrhage of spleen following a procedure on the spleen.**

- Hematoma after repair of spleen laceration is coded to **D78.31, Postprocedural hematoma of spleen following a procedure on the spleen.**

- Accidental laceration of the spleen secondary to colectomy is coded to **D78.12, Accidental puncture and laceration of spleen during other procedure.**

Several of the categories listed above provide additional specificity for certain other procedures or other complications besides intraoperative or postprocedural hemorrhage, seroma, and hematoma, and accidental puncture and laceration. Category E89, Postprocedural endocrine and metabolic complications and disorders, not elsewhere classified, is further subdivided to provide specific codes for the following types of complications:

E89.0	Postprocedural hypothyroidism
E89.1	Postprocedural hypoinsulinemia
E89.2	Postprocedural hypoparathyroidism
E89.3	Postprocedural hypopituitarism
E89.40	Asymptomatic postprocedural ovarian failure
E89.41	Symptomatic postprocedural ovarian failure
E89.5	Postprocedural testicular hypofunction
E89.6	Postprocedural adrenocortical (-medullary) hypofunction
E89.810	Postprocedural hemorrhage of an endocrine system organ or structure following an endocrine system procedure
E89.811	Postprocedural hemorrhage of an endocrine system organ or structure following other procedure
E89.820	Postprocedural hematoma of an endocrine system organ or structure following an endocrine system procedure
E89.821	Postprocedural hematoma of an endocrine system organ or structure following other procedure
E89.89	Other postprocedural endocrine and metabolic complications and disorders

Category G97, Intraoperative and postprocedural complications and disorders of nervous system, not elsewhere classified, includes additional codes for problems related to spinal or lumbar puncture and ventricular shunting, such as cerebrospinal fluid leak from spinal puncture (G97.0), other reaction to spinal and lumbar puncture (G97.1), and intracranial hypotension following ventricular shunting (G97.2).

Category H95, Intraoperative and postprocedural complications and disorders of ear and mastoid process, not elsewhere classified, provides additional codes for problems related to postmastoidectomy, such as chronic inflammation (H95.11-), granulation (H95.12-), mucosal cyst (H95.13-), and other disorders (H95.19-), as well as postprocedural stenosis of the external ear canal (H95.81-).

Category I97, Intraoperative and postprocedural complications and disorders of circulatory system, not elsewhere classified, also includes codes for conditions such as postcardiotomy syndrome (I97.0), other postprocedural cardiac functional disturbances (I97.11–I97.191), postmastectomy lymphedema syndrome (I97.2), postprocedural hypertension (I97.3), intraoperative cardiac functional disturbances (I97.71–I97.791), and other complications such as intraoperative or postprocedural cerebrovascular infarction (I97.81–I97.821).

Category J95, Intraoperative and postprocedural complications and disorders of respiratory system, not elsewhere classified, includes specific codes for several other complications, such as the following:

J95.00–J95.09	Tracheostomy complications
J95.1, J95.2	Acute pulmonary insufficiency following thoracic surgery (J95.1) and following nonthoracic surgery (J95.2)
J95.3	Chronic pulmonary insufficiency following surgery
J95.4	Chemical pneumonitis due to anesthesia
J95.5	Postprocedural subglottic stenosis
J95.81-	Postprocedural pneumothorax
J95.82-	Postprocedural respiratory failure
J95.83-	Postprocedural hemorrhage of a respiratory system organ or structure following a procedure
J95.84	Transfusion-related acute lung injury (TRALI)
J95.85-	Complication of respirator, which includes ventilator-associated pneumonia (see chapter 18 of this handbook for a more detailed discussion)
J95.86-	Postprocedural hematoma and seroma of a respiratory system organ or structure following a procedure

Code J95.4 is assigned for chemical pneumonitis due to anesthesia and includes postprocedural aspiration pneumonia and Mendelson's syndrome when they result from a procedure. An additional code for adverse effect, if applicable, is assigned to identify the anesthesia (T41.-, with fifth or sixth character 5). Do not assign a code from category J69, Pneumonitis due to solids and liquids, with code J95.4 because J95.4 fully describes the nature of the complication.

Code K91.86 is used to report the retention of gallstones following cholecystectomy. This condition is not uncommon following a laparoscopic cholecystectomy because gallstones may fall into the bile duct, abdominal cavity, or abdominal wall, causing a later obstruction or infection. Code **K91.86, Retained cholelithiasis following cholecystectomy,** is assigned in this situation.

Category M96, Intraoperative and postprocedural complications and disorders of musculoskeletal system, not elsewhere classified, includes specific codes for the following conditions:

M96.0	Pseudarthrosis after fusion or arthrodesis
M96.1	Postlaminectomy syndrome, not elsewhere classified
M96.2, M96.3	Kyphosis postradiation (M96.2) and postlaminectomy (M96.3)
M96.4	Postsurgical lordosis
M96.5	Postradiation scoliosis
M96.6-	Fracture of bone following insertion of orthopedic implant, joint prosthesis, or bone plate

ICD-10-CM differentiates between cardiac functional disturbances that occur intraoperatively during cardiac or other type of surgery (I97.7-) and postprocedural cardiac functional effects following cardiac or other surgery (I97.1-). For example:

K81.0 + I97.191 + I49.9	Acute cholecystitis; postoperative cardiac arrhythmia (same admission)
I97.130 + I50.9	Heart failure following cardiac surgery performed during previous admission; patient discharged one month ago
I97.131 + I50.21	Acute systolic heart failure on second postoperative day following cholecystectomy
I97.710	Cardiac arrest during cardiac bypass surgery

EXERCISE 32.2

Code the following diagnoses. Do not assign External cause codes.

1. Cataract fragments in left eye following cataract surgery

   _____

2. Headache due to lumbar puncture

3. Post-iridectomy plateau iris syndrome

4. Seroma of saphenous vein following cardiac bypass surgery

5. Postprocedural hypertension

6. 35-year-old female patient presents to physician's office with complaints of flushing, sleeplessness, headache, and lack of concentration after having had uterine artery embolization for uterine leiomyoma a few months ago. Physician diagnoses patient with premature postsurgical menopause.

COMPLICATIONS FOLLOWING INFUSION, TRANSFUSION, AND THERAPEUTIC INJECTION

Category T80 includes the following complications following infusion, transfusion, and therapeutic injection:

T80.0	Air embolism
T80.1	Vascular complications
T80.2-	Infections
T80.3-	ABO incompatibility reaction due to transfusion
T80.4-	Rh incompatibility reaction
T80.A-	Non-ABO incompatibility reaction
T80.5-	Anaphylactic shock due to serum
T80.6-	Other serum reactions (e.g., intoxication, protein sickness, serum rash, serum sickness, serum urticaria)
T80.81-	Extravasation of vesicant agents
T80.89-	Other complications
T80.9-	Unspecified complication

Codes T80.211- and T80.212- distinguish between systemic and local infections due to central venous and pulmonary artery catheters. Examples of central venous catheters include the Hickman catheter, peripherally inserted central catheter (PICC), port-a-cath, umbilical venous catheter, and triple lumen catheter. A pulmonary artery catheter is also known as a Swan-Ganz catheter or a right heart catheter. Central line–associated bloodstream infections are systemic infections and are coded to T80.211-. A local infection due to a central venous or pulmonary artery catheter is assigned code T80.212-. Local infections include exit- or insertion-site infections, port or reservoir infections, or tunnel infections, which are laboratory-confirmed bloodstream infections not due to an infection at another site. When there is a documented infection due to a central venous or pulmonary artery catheter, but the infection is not specified as to whether it is systemic or local, assign code T80.219-.

Code T80.22- describes an acute infection following a transfusion, infusion, or injection of blood and blood products. Transfusion-transmitted infections include any infectious organism (bacteria, virus, parasite, or other) transmitted through transfusion, infusion, or injection of blood or blood products (whole blood, red blood cells [RBCs], plasma, platelets, or other). Code T80.22- should be used for acute infections, not for chronic cases. In addition, if the transfusion-transmitted infection has specifically been identified as human immunodeficiency virus (HIV), assign a code for the HIV disease first.

ICD-10-CM provides codes to report transfusion reactions due to blood or blood product incompatibility, as follows:

T80.30–T80.39	ABO incompatibility reaction due to transfusion of blood or blood products
T80.40–T80.49	Rh incompatibility reaction due to transfusion of blood or blood products
T80.A0–T80.A9	Non-ABO incompatibility reaction due to transfusion of blood or blood products

These codes also provide information on the different types of hemolytic transfusion reactions, including both acute hemolytic transfusion reaction and delayed hemolytic transfusion reaction. A hemolytic transfusion reaction is a systemic response by the body to the administration of blood that is incompatible with the recipient's blood, resulting in destruction of RBCs. This condition can lead to acute renal failure and/or disseminated intravascular coagulation.

Anaphylactic reactions following transfusion of blood and blood products (T80.51-) are attributed to soluble substances in donor plasma. The most common transfusion reactions are fever, chills, pruitus, or urticaria, which can resolve without specific treatment or complications. For example:

- A patient presented with complaints of dizziness, weakness, and fatigue. The provider documented weakness and fatigue due to acute anemia due to blood loss, and the patient subsequently received two units of packed RBCs into the peripheral vein. During the administration of the second unit, she developed fever, hoarseness, and facial edema and was treated with IV Benadryl. Assign code **D62, Acute posthemorrhagic anemia,** as the principal diagnosis. Codes **T80.51xA, Anaphylactic reaction due to administration of blood and blood products, initial encounter,** and **T45.8x5A, Adverse effect of other primarily systemic and hematological agents, initial encounter,** should be assigned as additional diagnoses. Assign procedure code **30233N1, Transfusion of nonautologous red blood cells into peripheral vein, percutaneous approach.**

Please note that other transfusion-related problems are coded to other chapters, such as hemochromatosis due to repeated blood cell transfusions (E83.111), transfusion-associated circulatory overload (E87.71), post-transfusion purpura (D69.51), and post-transfusion fever (R50.84).

Code T80.52- is used to report anaphylactic reactions due to vaccination, and code T80.59- is reserved for anaphylactic reactions due to other serum. Although an anaphylactic reaction to vaccine is rare, it can develop when a person with preformed IgE antibodies to a vaccine constituent is given a vaccine containing that substance. The IgE-mediated reactions are usually caused by vaccine components other than the immunizing agent. Serum sickness is a reaction similar to an allergy. It involves an immune system reaction to certain medications, injected proteins used to treat immune conditions, or antiserum (the liquid part of blood that contains antibodies that help protect against infectious or poisonous substances). Codes T80.61-, T80.62-, and T80.69- describe other serum reactions due to the administration of blood and blood products, other serum reaction due to vaccination, and other serum reaction, respectively.

Extravasation is the accidental infiltration of intravenously infused drugs into the surrounding tissue. Vesicants are chemically active substances, such as certain antineoplastic drugs, that can produce blistering on direct contact with the skin or mucous membrane. In milder cases, extravasation can cause pain, reddening, or irritation at the site of the infusion needle. In severe cases, tissue damage may involve tissue necrosis and lead to loss of the limb. The following codes are assigned to describe complications following extravasation of vesicant agent:

T80.810-   Extravasation of vesicant antineoplastic chemotherapy

T80.818-   Extravasation of other vesicant agent

COMPLICATIONS DUE TO PRESENCE OF INTERNAL DEVICE, IMPLANT, OR GRAFT

Categories T82 through T85 classify conditions that occur only because an internal device, implant, or graft is present. These complications are classified according to the body system, as follows:

T82   Complications of cardiac and vascular prosthetic devices, implants and grafts

T83   Complications of genitourinary prosthetic devices, implants and grafts

T84   Complications of internal orthopedic prosthetic devices, implants and grafts

T85   Complications of other internal prosthetic devices, implants and grafts

Complications of this type are classified first according to whether they are mechanical or nonmechanical in nature. A mechanical complication is one that results from a failure of the device, implant, or graft, such as breakdown, displacement, leakage, or other malfunction. These are classified by the type of mechanical complication and the type of device involved. For example:

T82.111-   Defective cardiac pulse generator

T82.49-   Obstruction of arteriovenous dialysis catheter

T82.511-   Breakdown of surgically created arteriovenous shunt

T83.39-   Perforation of uterus by intrauterine contraceptive device

T84.195-   Protrusion of intramedullary nail in left femur

T85.621-   Displacement of peritoneal dialysis catheter

Subcategory T84.0, Mechanical complications of internal joint prosthesis, classifies a range of complications involving prosthetic joint implants, with additional characters to identify the specific joint (e.g., right knee, left hip). The specific mechanical complications are indicated as follows:

T84.01-   Broken internal joint prosthesis

T84.02-   Dislocation of internal joint prosthesis

T84.03-   Mechanical loosening of internal prosthetic joint

T84.05-   Periprosthetic osteolysis of internal prosthetic joint

T84.06-   Wear of articular bearing surface of internal prosthetic joint

T84.09-   Other mechanical complication of internal joint prosthesis

Infection and inflammatory reactions due to the presence of a device, an implant, or a graft that is functioning properly are classified to the following codes and subcategories:

T82.6-	Infection and inflammatory reaction due to cardiac valve prosthesis
T82.7-	Infection and inflammatory reaction due to other cardiac and vascular devices, implants and grafts
T83.5-	Infection and inflammatory reaction due to prosthetic device, implant and graft in urinary system
T83.6-	Infection and inflammatory reaction due to prosthetic device, implant and graft in genital tract
T84.5-	Infection and inflammatory reaction due to internal joint prosthesis
T84.6-	Infection and inflammatory reaction due to internal fixation device
T84.7	Infection and inflammatory reaction due to other internal orthopedic prosthetic devices, implants and grafts
T85.7-	Infection and inflammatory reaction due to other internal prosthetic devices, implants and grafts

Additional codes should be assigned to identify the infection.

Code **T82.7-, Infection and inflammatory reaction due to other cardiac and vascular devices, implants and grafts,** is used for infections due to arterial, dialysis, or peripheral venous catheters or an infusion catheter not otherwise specified. Bloodstream infections due to central venous and pulmonary artery catheters should be assigned code T80.211- rather than code T82.7-.

Codes in subcategory T83.51, Infection and inflammatory reaction due to urinary catheter, should have additional codes for the specific infection, such as cystitis or sepsis, and for the responsible organism if that information is available. Examples of codes assigned from categories T82 through T85 include the following:

T82.7xxA	Infected pacemaker pocket, initial encounter
T85.71xA + B96.20	*Escherichia coli* infection due to peritoneal dialysis catheter, initial encounter
T83.511A + N30.11	Chronic interstitial cystitis with hematuria due to indwelling urethral catheter, initial encounter

Subcategories T82.8, T83.8, T84.8, and T85.8 classify other complications due to the presence of an internal prosthetic device, implant, or graft. Also included in these subcategories are nonmechanical complications, with additional characters indicating embolism, fibrosis, hemorrhage, pain, stenosis, or thrombosis. When the complication is documented as postoperative pain due to the presence of a device, an implant, or a graft left in a surgical site, an additional code from category G89 is used to identify acute (G89.18) or chronic (G89.28) pain due to presence of the device, implant, or graft.

Code T82.857- is assigned for occlusion of a coronary bypass graft unless occlusion is identified by the physician as being due to arteriosclerosis. Arteriosclerotic occlusions of a coronary artery bypass graft or transplanted heart are classified to subcategories I25.7 and I25.8, with additional characters to indicate the type of graft (autologous vein, autologous artery, nonautologous biological graft, transplanted heart, bypass graft of transplanted heart, and other coronary bypass graft). Occlusion of the coronary artery when there is no history of bypass graft is classified as arteriosclerosis of native coronary arteries (I25.10–I25.119).

TRANSPLANT COMPLICATIONS

Category T86, Complications of transplanted organs and tissue, is reserved for transplant complications such as failure, infection, rejection, or malignancy associated with organ transplant, with the fourth, fifth, or sixth character indicating the organ involved. When infection is present, a code from categories B95 through B97 should be assigned as an additional code. A transplant complication code is assigned only if the complication affects the function of the transplanted organ. Additional codes are assigned to identify other transplant complications, such as acute graft-versus-host disease (D89.810), malignancy associated with organ transplant (C80.2), or post-transplant lymphoproliferative disorders (D47.Z1). Two codes are required to fully describe a transplant complication: the appropriate code from category T86 and a secondary code that identifies the complication. For example:

T86.09 + D89.810	Acute graft-versus-host disease resulting from complications of bone marrow transplant
T86.19 + C80.2 + C64.9	Malignant neoplasm of transplanted kidney
T86.858 + D47.Z1	Lymphoproliferative disorder post intestinal transplant

Code T86.5 describes complications of stem cell transplants. Stem cell transplants can be performed using the patient's own stem cells (autologous stem cell transplant) or donor stem cells (allogeneic stem cell transplant). Most stem cell transplantation procedures are performed using stem cells collected from the peripheral blood. Complications can develop from a stem cell transplant, including graft-versus-host disease, stem cell (graft) failure, organ damage, cataracts, secondary cancers, and death.

Pre-existing conditions or conditions that develop after the transplant are not coded as complications unless they affect the function of the transplanted organs. Post-transplant surgical complications that do not relate to the function of the transplanted organ are classified to the specific complication. For example, a postsurgical infection is coded as a postoperative wound infection, not as a transplant complication. However, infections affecting the function of transplanted organs are classified to category T86, such as **T86.812, Lung transplant infection.** Post-transplant patients who are seen for treatment unrelated to the transplanted organ are assigned a code from category Z94, Transplanted organ and tissue status, to capture the transplant status of the patient. A code from category Z94 should never be used with a code from category T86 for the same organ.

For conditions that affect the function of the transplanted kidney—other than chronic kidney disease (CKD)—a code from subcategory T86.1 should be assigned, along with a secondary code that identifies the condition. Patients with CKD following a transplant should not be assumed to have transplant failure or rejection unless it is documented by the provider. Patients who have undergone kidney transplant may still have some form of CKD because the transplant may not fully restore kidney function. Therefore, the presence of CKD alone does not constitute a transplant complication. If documentation supports the presence of failure, infection, rejection, or another transplant complication, then it is appropriate to assign a code from subcategory T86.1, Complications of kidney transplant, followed by the appropriate CKD code (N18.-). For patients with CKD following a kidney transplant who do not have a transplant complication such as failure or rejection, code **Z94.0, Kidney transplant status,** should be assigned instead of a code from subcategory T86.1. For example:

- A patient with end-stage kidney disease due to a congenital anomaly of the urinary tract status post deceased-donor right renal transplantation was admitted with delayed graft function and persistent severe hyperkalemia, which required intermittent hemodialysis of less than six hours per day. For the principal diagnosis, assign code **T86.19, Other complication of kidney transplant,** for the delayed graft function. Assign codes **N18.6, End stage renal disease; Q64.9, Congenital malformation of urinary system, unspecified; Z99.2, Dependence on renal dialysis;** and **E87.5, Hyperkalemia,** as additional diagnoses. Assign code **5A1D70Z, Performance of urinary filtration, intermittent, less than 6 hours per day,** for the hemodialysis.

COMPLICATIONS OF REATTACHMENT AND AMPUTATION

Complications of reattached extremities and amputated stump are classified to category T87. Complications of reattached extremities are classified by whether they relate to the upper extremity (T87.0x-) or the lower extremity (T87.1x-). The sixth character indicates laterality. Complications of other reattached body parts are classified to code T87.2.

Complications of amputated stump include neuroma (T87.30-T87.34), infection (T87.40-T87.44), necrosis (T87.50-T87.54), dehiscence of amputation stump (T87.81) and other complication of amputation stump (T87.89). Code T87.89 includes amputation stump contracture, contracture of next proximal joint, flexion, edema, and hematoma. The fifth characters for subcategories T87.3- through T87.5- specify whether the condition is of the upper or lower extremity, as well as laterality. Phantom limb syndrome is a relatively common condition after amputation whereby the patient has the perception of sensations, usually including pain, in an arm or a leg after the limb has been amputated. Phantom limb syndrome is not coded to category T87, but to code G54.6 or G54.7, depending on whether or not there is associated pain.

EXERCISE 32.3

Code the following diagnoses and procedures. Do not assign External cause codes. Assume the encounter is an initial one.

1. Leakage of breast prosthesis

2. Intrauterine contraceptive device imbedded in uterine wall

3. Erosion of skin by protruding pacemaker electrodes

4. Bone marrow transplant with rejection syndrome
   Acute graft-versus-host disease

5. Displaced lens implant, right eye

6. Complication of transplanted intestine
   Malignant neoplasm of colon related to intestinal transplant

7. Broken right hip joint prosthesis after fall

8. A 60-year-old woman with type 2 diabetes had a right above-the-knee amputation two months ago due to severe diabetic circulatory problems in the limb. The stump had developed an abscess with *Staphylococcus aureus* cultured.

9. Kidney transplant failure with chronic kidney disease,
   stage IV

---

10. A patient with severe single-vessel coronary artery disease
    had cardiac catheterization and angioplasty with attempts
    to pass a stent into the right coronary artery.
    During manipulation of the wire, the wire broke off and
    became stuck in the right coronary artery and in the aorta.
    A snare was used to catch the wire and pull it out.

COMPLICATIONS OF PROCEDURES NOT CLASSIFIED ELSEWHERE

Category T81, Complications of procedures, not elsewhere classified, is used to classify a miscellaneous group of postoperative complications. Additional codes are not usually required because the complication code itself provides sufficient specificity. Category T81 requires a seventh character to be added to each code to specify initial encounter ("A"), subsequent encounter ("D"), or sequela ("S"). Examples of codes in category T81 include:

T81.11-   Postoperative cardiogenic shock
T81.31-   Disruption of external operation (surgical) wound
T81.83-   Persistent postprocedural fistula

Cardiogenic shock is attributable to a weakened heart that is not able to pump enough blood to organs of the body. Causes of cardiogenic shock include myocardial infarction, pericardial tamponade, and heart failure. Assign code **T81.11x, Postprocedural cardiogenic shock,** for cardiogenic shock due to surgery. Postoperative infections originating in the wound, lungs, or blood/vascular catheter may lead to septic shock. Code **T81.12x, Postprocedural septic shock,** is assigned for postoperative septic shock. Refer to chapter 14 of this handbook for additional information on coding postprocedural septic shock and sepsis due to a postprocedural infection. Assign code **T81.19x, Other postprocedural shock,** for postsurgical hypovolemic shock (the most common type of postoperative shock), which occurs when large amounts of fluids are lost because of hemorrhage or severe dehydration. For example:

- A patient developed refractory cardiogenic shock, which required temporary peripheral veno-venous extracorporeal membrane oxygenation (ECMO) support, after undergoing aortic valve (mechanical) replacement due to severe aortic stenosis. Assign code **I35.0, Nonrheumatic aortic (valve) stenosis,** as the principal diagnosis. Assign code **T81.11xA, Postprocedural cardiogenic shock, initial encounter,** as an additional diagnosis. Assign codes **02RF0JZ, Replacement of aortic valve with synthetic substitute, open approach,** and **5A1522H, Extracorporeal oxygenation, membrane, peripheral veno-venous,** for the procedures.

Wound dehiscence involves partial or total disruption of any or all layers of an operative wound site. Common causes of wound dehiscence include excess tension on the sutured edges, necrosis of the wound edges, seroma or hematoma causing pressure on the wound, and wound infection. ICD-10-CM provides codes to distinguish between disruption of internal (T81.32-) and external (T81.31-) surgical wounds as well as a disruption of a traumatic injury wound repair (T81.33-). For example:

- An eight-year-old patient had a lower leg traumatic laceration that was sutured several weeks ago. The patient was seen in the emergency department two weeks after the sutures were removed because of disruption of the wound repair. Code T81.33xA is assigned for this encounter.

COMPLICATIONS OF FOREIGN BODY ACCIDENTALLY LEFT DURING SURGERY

Subcategory T81.5, Complications of foreign body accidentally left in body following procedure, is assigned for situations in which there is an unintended retention of a foreign object (e.g., sponge) in a patient after surgery or another procedure. The occurrence of unintended retention of objects at any point after the surgery ends should be captured regardless of setting. However, do not assign a code from subcategory T81.5 when the provider intentionally leaves a foreign body during surgery to avoid subjecting the patient to the additional risk of removal.

The National Quality Forum's "Serious Reportable Events in Healthcare—2011 Update" provides an implementation guideline for unintended retention of a foreign object in a patient after surgery or other invasive procedure. According to this guideline, reportable events include:

- Occurrences of unintended retention of objects at any point after the surgery/procedure ends, regardless of setting (postanesthesia recovery unit, surgical suite, emergency department, patient bedside) and regardless of whether the object is to be removed after discovery
- Unintentionally retained objects (including such things as wound packing material, sponges, catheter tips, trocars, guide wires) in all applicable settings

The National Quality Forum report also provides the following definition: "Surgery ends after all incisions or procedural access routes have been closed in their entirety, device(s) such as probes or instruments have been removed, and, if relevant, final surgical counts confirming accuracy of counts and resolving any discrepancies have concluded and the patient has been taken from the operating/procedure room."

Subcategory T81.5 is further subdivided to specify the complication due to the foreign body, such as adhesions (T81.51-), obstruction (T81.52-), perforation (T81.53-), other complication (T81.59-), or unspecified complication (T81.50-). Sixth characters specify whether the foreign body was accidentally left following surgical operation ("0"); following infusion or transfusion ("1"); following kidney dialysis ("2"); following injection or immunization ("3"); following endoscopic examination ("4"); following heart catheterization ("5"); following aspiration, puncture, or other catheterization ("6"); following removal of catheter or packing ("7"); following other procedure ("8"); or following unspecified procedure ("9"). For example:

- At surgery, a suture broke away from the needle and the needle was lost. Multiple attempts to find it were unsuccessful. An X-ray did not reveal the needle and the chest was closed. Another X-ray showed that the needle was positioned to the right of the aortic valve. The chest is reopened but the needle still cannot be located. The surgeon decides that further search for the needle would cause the patient harm, so the chest is closed, and the patient is transferred to the ICU in stable condition. In this instance, do not assign code **T81.500A, Unspecified complication of foreign body accidentally left in body**

following surgical operation, initial encounter, because the surgeon made the decision to leave the needle to avoid harm to the patient.

- A patient was admitted for right hip hemiarthroplasty due to femoral neck fracture. While in postanesthesia care, postoperative radiographs revealed a loose cement fragment in the joint. The patient is returned to surgery for exploration with removal of the cement fragment. In this example, code **T81.590A, Other complication of foreign body accidentally left in body following surgical operation, initial encounter,** should be assigned because surgery had ended, and the patient had to be returned to surgery to remove the cement fragment.

Acute reaction to foreign substance (rather than foreign body) accidentally left during a procedure is coded to subcategory T81.6, rather than subcategory T81.5. Category T81 also provides codes for complications of artery following a procedure, such as mesenteric artery (T81.710-), renal artery (T81.711-), other artery (T81.718-), or unspecified artery (T81.719-).

OTHER COMPLICATIONS OF SURGICAL AND MEDICAL CARE NOT CLASSIFIED ELSEWHERE

Category T88, Other complications of surgical and medical care, not elsewhere classified, is used to classify a number of specific conditions that may occur following almost any type of procedure. For example:

T88.0- Sepsis following immunization
T88.1- Generalized vaccinia
T88.2- Shock due to anesthesia
T88.4- Failed or difficult intubation

COMPLICATIONS VERSUS AFTERCARE

As discussed earlier, it is important to differentiate between an admission for a complication of surgery or medical care and one for aftercare. An admission for aftercare is usually planned in advance to take care of an expected residual or to carry out follow-up activity, such as removal of pins or plates placed during earlier orthopedic surgery. Aftercare is classified to categories Z42 through Z51. The aftercare Z codes should not be used for aftercare of injuries. For aftercare of an injury, the acute injury code is assigned with the appropriate seventh-character value for subsequent encounter (see chapter 29 of this handbook).

Subcategory Z48.0, Encounter for attention to dressings, sutures and drains, distinguishes between encounters for change or removal of nonsurgical wound dressing (Z48.00), for change or removal of surgical wound dressing (Z48.01), for removal of sutures (Z48.02), and for removal of drains (Z48.03).

Be careful not to assign complication codes for routine aftercare encounters. For example:

Z47.2   Admitted for removal of pins from femur
Z47.33 Admitted for replacement of knee prosthesis following explantation of infected joint prosthesis
Z46.89 Patient visit for removal of cast

EXERCISE 32.4

Code the following diagnoses, some of which identify complications and some of which identify aftercare. Assume the encounter is an initial one. Do not assign External cause codes or procedure codes.

1. Admitted for removal of internal fixation
   nail in right forearm that has extruded into surrounding
   tissue, causing severe pain

2. Admitted for closure of colostomy

3. Admitted for adjustment of breast prosthesis

4. Admitted for removal of displaced breast prosthesis

STATUS POST

The term "status post" used in diagnostic statements is sometimes interpreted by coding professionals to mean that there is a postoperative complication; however, the term is rarely intended to carry this meaning. Status post usually indicates that the patient underwent the procedure at some time in the past. A status post condition is usually classified in the Z80–Z87 series. However, this status is coded only if the status post condition is significant for the current episode of care. If it is currently insignificant, the condition is not assigned such a code.

SURGICAL OR MEDICAL CARE AS EXTERNAL CAUSE

As with certain other ICD-10-CM chapter 19 codes, some of the complication of care codes include the external cause (the type of procedure that caused the complication) as well as the nature of the complication. Therefore, no External cause code indicating the type of procedure is necessary for these codes. For example, code **M96.621, Fracture of humerus following insertion of orthopedic implant, joint prosthesis, or bone plate, right arm,** includes the nature of the complication (fracture) as well as the type of procedure that caused the complication (insertion of orthopedic implant, joint prosthesis, or bone plate).

In addition, ICD-10-CM provides three sets of External cause codes to indicate medical or surgical care as the cause of a complication:

Y62–Y69   Misadventures to patients during surgical and medical care

Y70–Y82   Medical devices associated with adverse incidents in diagnostic and therapeutic use

Y83–Y84   Surgical and other medical procedures as the cause of abnormal reaction of the patient, or of later complication, without mention of misadventure at the time of the procedure

Codes from categories Y62 through Y69 are used only when the condition is stated to be due to a misadventure of medical or surgical care. These categories include failure of sterile precautions during surgical and medical care (Y62.0–Y62.9), failure in dosage (Y63.0–Y63.9), contaminated medical or biological substances (Y64.0–Y64.9), other misadventures (Y65.0–Y65.53), other specified misadventure (Y65.8), nonadministration of surgical and medical care (Y66), and unspecified misadventure (Y69).

Code Y65.51 is assigned when the wrong operation (procedure) is performed on the correct patient and includes a wrong device implanted into a correct surgical site. Code Y65.52 is assigned for performance of an operation (procedure) on a patient not scheduled for surgery. This includes performance of a procedure intended for another patient and performance of a procedure on the wrong patient. Code Y65.53 is assigned for performance of the correct operation (procedure) on the wrong side/body part. Examples using External cause codes to indicate misadventures to patients during surgical and medical care as the cause of a complication include the following:

J70.0+Y63.2   Radiation pneumonitis due to adverse reaction to overdose of radiotherapy

T81.89x-+Y65.51   Left femoral component inserted into right leg instead of right femoral component during total knee replacement

Categories Y70–Y82 are used to report breakdown or malfunction of medical devices during use, after implantation, or with ongoing use. The codes are used to report adverse incidents with the following types of devices:

Y70   Anesthesiology devices
Y71   Cardiovascular devices
Y72   Otorhinolaryngological devices
Y73   Gastroenterology and urology devices
Y74   General hospital and personal-use devices
Y75   Neurological devices
Y76   Obstetric and gynecological devices
Y77   Ophthalmic devices
Y78   Radiological devices
Y79   Orthopedic devices
Y80   Physical medicine devices
Y81   General- and plastic-surgery devices
Y82   Other and unspecified medical devices

Codes from categories Y83 and Y84 are used when the condition is described as due to medical or surgical care but without mention of misadventure. Because of the potential legal problems that may develop from reporting some external cause codes, the facility should give careful thought to formulating policies and guidelines for their use. Never make an assumption that there has been a misadventure; such codes should be assigned only when there is a clear-cut diagnostic statement to this effect by the physician.

EXERCISE 32.5

Code the following diagnoses. Do not assign External cause or Z codes. Assume the encounter is an initial one.

---

1. Infected injection site, left buttock

---

2. Sloughing of skin graft due to rejection of
pedicle graft to right arm

3. Headache due to lumbar puncture

4. Postoperative cardiac arrest occurring in operating room
during closure of abdomen, with successful resuscitation

5. Persistent vomiting following gastrointestinal surgery

6. Air embolism resulting from intravenous infusion

7. Thrombophlebitis of antecubital vein of the
upper arm resulting from intravenous infusion

8. Hypovolemic shock due to surgery
this morning

9. Persistent postoperative fistula

10. Cardiac insufficiency resulting from
mitral valve prosthesis, in place for three years

11. Perforation of coronary artery by
catheter during cardiac catheterization

12. Displacement of cardiac pacemaker
electrode

13. Phantom limb with pain following surgical amputation

14. Neuroma of stump following surgical
amputation of left leg

15. Methicillin-susceptible *Staphylococcus aureus*
infection of transplanted kidney

16. A patient with leukemia is admitted to the hospital after
noting feelings of palpitations and shortness of breath.
The patient has an infusion catheter in place for the administration
of chemotherapy. A chest X-ray shows that the tip of the infusion
catheter had broken off and traveled to the pulmonary artery.

17. A 13-year-old male status post open reduction internal fixation
of a right radial shaft fracture is admitted with bowing and angulation
(malunion) of the fracture site secondary to a bent plate
(internal fixation device). The physician states that vigorous activity
on the child's part caused the plate to break and plans to reinsert
a six-hole plate for fixation of the fracture.

Final Review Exercise

Final Review Exercise

The final review exercise draws on concepts presented throughout this handbook. Read each brief summary below and assign codes for all diagnoses and procedures, including codes for external causes and locations of occurrence as needed. For the purposes of this assignment, accept narrative statements (for example, conditions, procedures, or other therapy) as though listed in a diagnostic statement.

In day-to-day practice, many hospitals have opted through their internal coding policies not to collect data on minor services, such as casting or traction, and noninvasive diagnostic services performed in the inpatient setting, such as X-rays, electrocardiograms (EKGs), computerized tomography (CT) scans, and ultrasounds. For this reason, codes for these minor services have been omitted from the answers. ICD-10-PCS codes for outpatient procedures have also been omitted because the Health Insurance Portability and Accountability Act (HIPAA) code set standard for procedures performed in the outpatient setting is CPT/HCPCS. If you are using the *without Answers* version of this handbook, ask your instructor for the answers.

1. A patient was admitted with complaint of a dull ache and occasional acute pain in the right calf. Examination revealed swelling and redness of the calf as well as a slight fever. The patient gave a history of having been on Premarin therapy for the past 20 years and stated that she has always followed the doctor's instructions for its use. Venous plethysmography revealed the presence of a thrombus. The estrogen therapy dosage was modified, and the patient was discharged with a diagnosis of deep vein thrombosis and thrombophlebitis of the right femoral vein due to supplemental estrogen therapy. She will be seen in the physician's office in one week and will be followed regularly over the next several months.

   Code(s):

2. A patient was admitted to the hospital because he was suffering acute abdominal pain. He was also found to be intoxicated, and his medical history indicated that he has been alcohol dependent for several years with episodic binging every three to four months. The current binge apparently started three days ago. The abdominal pain proved to be due to alcohol-induced acute pancreatitis, and he was treated with nasogastric suction, administration of IV fluids, and pain control. The patient was observed for possible withdrawal reaction with standby orders; multiple vitamins were given.

   Code(s):

3. A patient with a four-year history of anorexia nervosa was seen in the physician's office because of significant weight loss over the past three months, going from 82 pounds down to 53 pounds. She was admitted to increase body weight and to be given nutrition counseling because of her severe malnutrition.

Code(s):

4. A patient was admitted through the emergency department following a fall from a ladder while painting the outside of his single-family house. He had contusions of the scalp and face and an open type I intertrochanteric fracture of the right femur. The fracture site was debrided, and an open reduction with internal fixation was carried out.

Code(s):

5. A patient who underwent a modified radical mastectomy of the left breast six months earlier because of carcinoma now has metastasis to the bone. She was admitted for a transfusion of nonautologous packed red blood cells (via peripheral vein) to treat aplastic anemia, probably due to her treatment by chemotherapy. She was discharged with a hemoglobin count of 11.5 and will be followed as an outpatient.

Code(s):

6. A patient was admitted for cholecystectomy because of chronic cholecystitis. Before she went to the operating room the next morning, nursing personnel noted that she had apparently developed a urinary tract infection, and laboratory tests confirmed a diagnosis of urinary tract infection due to *E. coli*. Because of the infection, the surgery was canceled, antibiotic therapy was instituted, and the patient was discharged on the third hospital day to continue antibiotic therapy at home. She will be seen in the physician's office in three weeks, and surgery will be rescheduled.

Code(s):

7. A patient who recently underwent an oophorectomy because of adenocarcinoma of the ovary was admitted to the hospital for chemotherapy. Shortly after administration of the therapy, the patient developed a fever and chills and on the second day she had a productive cough. Chest X-rays indicated an acute pneumonia, and sputum culture was positive for *Klebsiella*. Antibiotics were administered, and the patient was discharged on the fifth hospital day after the chemotherapy was administered via peripheral vein.

Code(s):

8. A patient who had noticed significant abdominal enlargement over a period of several weeks without a change in her dietary habits was admitted for exploratory laparotomy. Surgery revealed a large malignant ovarian tumor, and the left ovary was resected. The pelvic cavity was explored thoroughly for any evidence of metastatic spread, but none was noted. Chemotherapy treatments were started (via peripheral vein) on the day prior to discharge, and the patient was scheduled to continue therapy on an outpatient basis.

Code(s):

9. A female patient who had undergone surgery for carcinoma of the right breast two months earlier has since been on a program of chemotherapy. On a routine office visit yesterday, the physician noted that she had become severely dehydrated as a result of this program, and she was admitted for IV therapy for rehydration. Her regular chemotherapy session (via peripheral vein) was carried out on the third day.

Code(s):

10. A patient was admitted with abdominal pain and complaints of melena noted for the past two days. Examination revealed an acute diverticulitis of the colon. Laboratory studies reported a significant hypokalemia. The provider documented hypokalemia, and the patient was placed on oral potassium. Bleeding from the diverticulitis subsided within a few days on conservative treatment, and the patient was discharged to be followed on an outpatient basis.

Code(s):

11. A patient was admitted with complaints of severe joint pain affecting both hands and hips. The physician's diagnosis indicated rheumatoid arthritis with sympathetic inflammatory myopathy.

Code(s):

12. A patient who was two months pregnant contracted rubella. On her next prenatal visit to the doctor's office (at 9 weeks' gestation), it was decided to admit the patient for therapeutic abortion because of the probability of abnormality of the fetus. Complete abortion was carried out by D & C.

Code(s):

13. Increasing fetal stress was noted during labor. The patient was transferred to the surgical suite, where a classic cesarean delivery was performed. A full-term normal male was delivered at 38 weeks.

Code(s):

14. A patient was admitted with systolic heart failure, acute on chronic congestive heart failure, and unstable angina. The unstable angina was treated with nitrates, and IV Lasix was administered to manage the heart failure. Both conditions improved, and the patient was discharged to be followed on an outpatient basis.

Code(s):

15. A patient was admitted for observation and evaluation for possible intracranial injury following a collision with another car while he was driving to work. The patient had minor bruises on both the right and left upper back and abrasions of the skin of the left upper arm. The bruises did not appear to need any treatment; the abrasions were swabbed with disinfectant, and Neosporin was applied. Intracranial injury was ruled out.

Code(s):

16. A patient was brought to the emergency department following a burn injury experienced in a fire at the garage where he works. He was admitted and treated for first-degree and second-degree burns of the forearm and third-degree burn of the back.

Code(s):

564

17. A patient was admitted because of suspected
carcinoma of the colon. Exploratory laparotomy
was carried out, and a significant mass was
discovered in the sigmoid colon. The sigmoid
colon was resected and end-to-end anastomosis
accomplished. Small nodules were noted on
the liver, and a needle biopsy of the liver was
performed during the procedure. The pathology
report confirmed adenocarcinoma of the sigmoid
colon with metastasis to the liver.

Code(s):

18. A patient was discharged following prostate
surgery with an indwelling urethral catheter in
place. He was readmitted with urinary sepsis due
to methicillin-resistant *Staphylococcus aureus*
(MRSA) due to the presence of the catheter.
The physician confirmed the diagnosis of sepsis
due to MRSA. The catheter was removed and
the patient started on antibiotic therapy. The
patient's condition improved over several days,
and he was discharged without an indwelling
catheter.

Code(s):

19. A patient 25 weeks pregnant was diagnosed
as having an iron-deficiency anemia and was
admitted for transfusion of nonautologous
packed red blood cells (via peripheral vein).

Code(s):

20. A patient was admitted with occlusion (due to plaque) of the right common carotid artery, and open carotid endarterectomy was carried out with extracorporeal circulation (continuous cardiac output) used throughout the procedure.

Code(s):

21. A patient was admitted in a coma due to acute cerebrovascular thrombosis with cerebral infarction; the coma cleared by the fourth hospital day. Aphasia and hemiparesis were also present. The aphasia had cleared by discharge, but the hemiparesis was still present.

Code(s):

22. A patient was admitted with severe abdominal pain that began two days prior to admission and progressed in severity. Esophagogastroduodenoscopy (EGD) revealed an acute gastric ulcer, but no signs of hemorrhage or malignancy were noted. The provider documented acute gastric ulcer, and the patient was put on a medical regimen, including a bland diet, and was advised not to take aspirin.

Code(s):

23. A patient with type 1 diabetes mellitus with hyperglycemia was admitted for regulation of insulin dosage. The patient had been in the hospital three weeks earlier for an acute ST elevation myocardial infarction of the inferolateral wall, and an EKG was performed to check its current status.

Code(s):

566

24. A patient who was treated seven weeks ago at Community Hospital for an acute anterolateral myocardial infarction is now admitted to University Hospital for surgical repair of an atrial septal defect resulting from the recent infarction. Following thoracotomy, the defect was repaired with a nonautologous tissue graft; cardiopulmonary bypass (extracorporeal circulation, continuous cardiac output) was used during the procedure. The patient was discharged in good condition, to be followed as an outpatient.

Code(s):

25. A patient with bilateral mixed conductive and sensorineural hearing loss was admitted for cochlear implantation. Bilateral multiple channel implants were inserted through an open approach, and the patient was discharged, to be followed as an outpatient.

Code(s):

26. A patient who underwent a right kidney transplant three months ago is admitted for biopsy because of an increased creatinine level discovered on an outpatient visit. Percutaneous biopsy revealed chronic rejection syndrome. The patient was discharged on a modified medication regimen, to be followed closely as an outpatient.

Code(s):

27. A patient was admitted with a displaced fracture of the shaft of the right femur. Closed reduction was carried out and a cast was applied.

Code(s):

28. A patient who has had recurrent attacks of angina was seen in his physician's office because he felt that the anginal attacks seemed to be occurring more frequently and to be more severe and more difficult to control. He had not had a thorough evaluation previously, and bypass surgery had not been recommended in the past. He was admitted to the hospital for diagnostic studies to determine the underlying cause of this unstable angina. He underwent combined right- and left-heart catheterization, which revealed significant atherosclerotic heart disease. He was advised that coronary artery bypass surgery was indicated, but he did not want to make a decision without further discussion with his family. He was discharged on antianginal medication and will be seen in the doctor's office in one week.

Code(s):

29. The patient discussed in the preceding case returned to the hospital for bypass surgery. His angina is under control with the antianginal medications he was prescribed. Reverse right greater saphenous vein grafts were brought from the aorta to the obtuse marginal and the right coronary artery; the left internal mammary artery was loosened and brought down to the left anterior descending artery to bypass this obstruction. The gastroepiploic artery was used as a pedicled graft to bypass the circumflex. Extracorporeal circulation (continuous cardiac output) and intraoperative pacemaker were used during the procedure and discontinued afterward.

Code(s):

30. A patient was brought to the hospital by ambulance after a fall from the scaffolding while working on the construction of a new bank building. He had struck his head and experienced a brief period of unconsciousness (approximately 45 minutes). On examination, he was found to have an open skull fracture with cerebral laceration and contusion. The skull fracture was reduced after debridement, and the patient was transferred to the intensive care unit, where he stayed for four days. He was discharged on the 10th day in good condition and advised to avoid any strenuous activity and to see his physician in one week.

Code(s):

31. A patient was admitted for corrective surgery for a keloid of the left hand due to a burn experienced in a brush fire one year ago. Radical excision of the scar was carried out, and the defect was covered with a full-thickness graft taken from the left upper arm. The patient was discharged in good condition, to be seen in the physician's office in two weeks.

Code(s):

32. A patient was brought to the emergency department by ambulance at 1:00 a.m. by her husband, who stated that they had been to a dinner party at a friend's home earlier in the evening. His wife had two martinis before the meal and several glasses of wine with the meal. At bedtime she took Valium that her physician had ordered prn for nervousness and inability to sleep. Shortly thereafter, the husband noticed that she appeared to be somewhat stuporous, became worried about her condition, and brought her to the emergency department. The provider documented accidental overdose secondary to Valium taken with alcohol.

Code(s):

33. A patient was admitted to the hospital with an admitting diagnosis of acute hip pain. There was no history of trauma; she stated that she had simply stood up from her chair, immediately experienced acute pain in the left leg, and fallen back into the chair. She has had osteoporosis for several years and is also known to have diabetes. An X-ray revealed a fracture of the lower third of the shaft of the femur. A routine preoperative chest X-ray showed a few strands of atelectasis and a small cloudy area that may have represented mild pleural effusion. A cast was applied to the leg to immobilize the fracture. Her blood sugars were monitored and remained normal throughout the stay. The physician documented spontaneous fracture secondary to osteoporosis.

Code(s):

34. A patient with a five-year history of emphysema was brought to the hospital's emergency department in acute respiratory failure. Endotracheal intubation was carried out in the emergency department, and the patient was placed on mechanical ventilation. She was then admitted to the ICU, where she remained on the ventilator for three days and then was taken off the ventilator without a weaning period. She was discharged on the fifth hospital day.

Code(s):

35. A patient in acute respiratory failure was brought to the hospital by ambulance with a ventilator in place. In the ambulance, an endotracheal tube was inserted into the patient. He had a long history of congestive heart failure, and studies confirmed that he was in congestive failure, with pleural effusion and acute pulmonary edema. The patient was treated with diuretics, and his cardiac condition was brought back into an acceptable range. He continued on ventilation for four days and was weaned on the fifth day. The physician was questioned regarding the reason for the admission, and she indicated that the patient was admitted for the acute respiratory failure.

Code(s):

570

36. A five-year-old child was brought to the emergency department after the mother found the child playing with an open bottle of her prescription sedatives. She could not tell if the child had taken any pills, but she wanted the child evaluated for possible problems. The child was evaluated, and no evidence of poisoning or any other signs or symptoms were found. The mother was reassured, and the child was taken home.

Code(s):

37. A patient with hypertensive and diabetic end-stage renal disease who is on chronic dialysis is admitted because of disequilibrium syndrome (electrolyte imbalance) caused by the dialysis.

Code(s):

38. A patient who has had arteriosclerotic disease of the right lower extremity with intermittent claudication for three years recently progressed to ulceration and is now admitted with ulceration and gangrene of the toes of the right foot resulting from the arteriosclerosis. A tarsometatarsal amputation of the right foot was performed, and the patient left the operating room in good condition.

Code(s):

39. A two-year-old child with a severe cough was admitted to the hospital with a history of having experienced malaise, loss of appetite, and cough for several days. In addition to the cough, he was experiencing some shortness of breath, and a chest X-ray showed an acute pneumonia. Sputum cultures showed *B. pertussis*. He was started on IV antibiotics and became afebrile on the fifth hospital day. A repeat chest X-ray was negative on the sixth hospital day, and the cough had partially cleared. He was discharged on the eighth day to be cared for at home and followed as an outpatient.

Code(s):

40. A 10-year-old boy was admitted because of severe cellulitis of the left leg. He had gone on a hiking trip in the nearby forest with his Boy Scout troop a week earlier. He stated that there was a good deal of thorny brush and that he had several minor thorn punctures of the left leg but had experienced no problem with them. The day before admission, he had developed a painful, reddened, and swollen area that had become worse during the night. A diagnosis of cellulitis due to *Streptococcus* A was made, and antibiotics were administered. The wound itself was evaluated but did not appear to need specific treatment. The area on the leg progressively healed. The patient was discharged to continue the antibiotic series at home and will be seen in the physician's office in one week.

Code(s):

41. An unconscious diving instructor was admitted with concussion, skull fracture, and subdural hematoma after jumping from a high diving board and hitting the side of the pool at the gymnasium where he worked. Drainage of the subdural space was carried out by incision, and the fracture was reduced. The patient left the operating room in fair condition but died from his brain injury the following day without having ever regained consciousness.

Code(s):

42. A patient was admitted because of increasing confusion and memory loss, which his family was unable to deal with. The patient was disoriented and unable to furnish any information. He was diagnosed as having senile dementia with Alzheimer's disease and was transferred to a nursing home.

Code(s):

43. Newborn twin girls, both living, were delivered in the hospital at 35 completed weeks, with extremely low birth weight of 850 grams for twin #1 and 900 grams for twin #2. Both were transferred to the neonatal intensive care nursery with a diagnosis of extreme immaturity.

Code(s):

44. A patient with a long history of angina pectoris came to the emergency department complaining of increasing anginal pain that he could not relieve with nitroglycerin and rest. The pain occurred again about an hour prior to arrival at the ED and subsequently increased in severity. Cardiac catheterization done recently showed some occlusion of the right coronary artery. It was decided to go ahead with a percutaneous transluminal coronary angioplasty (PTCA), administering a thrombolytic agent to a coronary artery, in the hope of averting what appeared to be an impending myocardial infarction. The procedure was carried out without incident and the infarction was averted, but the patient did have an occlusion of the coronary artery.

Code(s):

45. A patient was admitted to the hospital with unstable angina that had been increasing in severity since the previous day. He was placed on bed rest and telemetry, and IV nitroglycerin was administered. An EKG showed some paroxysmal tachycardia as well, and so IV heparin was added to his medication program. His angina returned to its normal status, and the tachycardia was not shown on repeat studies at the end of one week. The patient was discharged to be seen by a visiting nurse over the next two weeks to supervise his medication regimen, and an appointment with his physician was made for two weeks later.

Code(s):

46. A patient who had been HIV-positive for several years was seen in his physician's office with skin lesions over his back suggestive of HIV-related Kaposi's sarcoma. He was admitted for incisional biopsy, which confirmed the diagnosis.

Code(s):

47. A patient was admitted through the emergency department with acute right flank pain and was taken to surgery for removal of a ruptured appendix. At the time of the appendectomy, generalized peritonitis was observed along with some suspicious nodules on the head of the pancreas. A needle biopsy was performed while the abdomen was open; a diagnosis of carcinoma of the pancreas head was made on the basis of the pathological examination.

Code(s):

574

48. A patient with a long history of type 2 diabetes mellitus was admitted in hyperosmolar coma with blood sugars out of control. Modification of the insulin regimen was instituted, and the patient was monitored carefully throughout her stay. The coma cleared on the first hospital day, and the patient's blood sugar levels were brought into control over the next four days. In addition to this acute metabolic condition, she was also diagnosed with diabetic chronic kidney disease with stage 2 chronic kidney disease while in the hospital. The patient was discharged on a modified insulin regimen and will be followed by a visiting nurse until the diabetes stabilizes.

Code(s):

49. A patient was admitted with a severe stage 3 pressure ulcer on the left buttock, with extensive necrotic tissue and gangrene. She was taken to the operating room, where the surgeon carefully excised the necrotic tissue (skin). The ulcer site was then treated with antibiotic ointment and gauze bandage, and the patient was returned to the nursing unit, where the wound was monitored carefully and additional antibiotic treatment was administered. By the fourth day, healing was beginning to close the area, but treatment was continued until discharge on the seventh day. The family was advised to use an egg crate mattress and to turn the patient regularly. The patient was scheduled for an outpatient visit in one week.

Code(s):

50. A patient with a diagnosis of morbid obesity, type 1 diabetes, and stage 3 chronic kidney disease underwent a laparoscopic lap band procedure eight weeks ago. She now presents to the gastrointestinal clinic for gastric band adjustment. The gastric band was adjusted by introducing a saline solution into a small access port placed just under the skin.

Code(s):

Appendix A

APPENDIX A   Coding and Reimbursement

Clinical coding systems assign distinct alphanumeric values to medical diagnoses, procedures and surgery, signs and symptoms of disease and ill-defined conditions, poisoning and adverse effects of drugs, and complications of surgery and medical care. Such systems serve an important function for physician reimbursement, hospital payments, quality review, benchmarking measurement, and the collection of general medical statistical data. In addition, coding accuracy is critical for ensuring accurate risk adjustment and, correspondingly, reliable comparative quality ratings.

Reimbursement is based on claims and documentation filed by providers using medical diagnosis and procedure codes. Depending on the type of provider and payer, different combinations of coding systems are used in payment models to reimburse providers for the care rendered to patients. The coding systems in use currently in the United States are the following:

- ICD-10-CM diagnosis codes
- ICD-10-PCS procedure codes
- Current Procedural Terminology (CPT)
- Health Care Procedure Coding System (HCPCS) level II codes

Essentially all providers and all payers use the ICD-10-CM system for diagnosis reporting. For reporting procedures, however, the Health Insurance Portability and Accountability Act (HIPAA) designates different standards. ICD-10-PCS is the standard for hospitals when reporting surgery and procedures for inpatients. CPT and HCPCS are the standards for hospital reporting of outpatient procedures, and for reporting all physician and other nonhospital provider services.

MEDICARE AND MEDICAID REIMBURSEMENT

Medicare and Medicaid are federal programs managed by the Centers for Medicare & Medicaid Services (CMS). They have different payment models based on the provider. The discussion below focuses primarily on Medicare, as the variation in state Medicaid programs is too great to discuss in detail here. Medicare reimburses most providers on a prospective payment system (PPS) basis, in which payment is made based on a predetermined, fixed amount. CMS uses separate PPSs for reimbursement to acute care inpatient hospitals, hospital outpatient services, inpatient psychiatric facilities, inpatient rehabilitation facilities, long-term care hospitals, home health agencies, hospice agencies, and skilled nursing facilities.

Physicians and Nonhospital Providers

Medicare and Medicaid reimburse physicians and other nonhospital providers/suppliers for services rendered to beneficiaries on a fee-for-service (FFS) basis. CMS develops fee schedules for physicians, ambulance services, and clinical laboratory services and for durable medical equipment, prosthetics, orthotics, and supplies. These fee schedules are driven by the CPT or HCPCS codes. However, diagnosis codes may also be used to determine coverage or medical necessity for medical items and services that are "reasonable and necessary" for a variety of purposes.

Hospitals

Medicare reimburses hospitals on a PPS basis, in which payment is made based on a predetermined, fixed amount. The payment amount for a particular service is derived based on the

577

classification system of that service (for example, diagnosis-related groups [DRGs] for acute care inpatient hospital services).

Acute Care Inpatient Hospitals

Under the inpatient PPS, each inpatient admission to an acute care inpatient hospital is categorized into a DRG. Each DRG has a payment weight assigned to it, based on the average resources used to treat Medicare patients in that DRG. The DRGs use principal diagnosis, secondary diagnoses, and procedures using ICD-10-CM and ICD-10-PCS codes to group clinically similar patients using similar resources. Each inpatient admission can be grouped to only one of over 700 DRGs. As of October 1, 2007, CMS revised the DRG groupings by resequencing the groups and refining the list of secondary diagnoses that were considered to affect the severity of a case. This system is called Medicare Severity Diagnosis-Related Groups (MS-DRGs). All secondary diagnoses are classified based on the degree of severity: complication/comorbidity (CC), major complication/comorbidity (MCC), or non-CC/MCC. The principal diagnosis, along with the presence or absence of CCs or MCCs, and the procedure may affect the DRG classification. Therefore, it is crucial that the codes are sequenced correctly to ensure accurate reimbursement.

Hospital Outpatient Services

Under the outpatient PPS (OPPS), hospital outpatient services, certain Medicare Part B services furnished to hospital inpatients who have no Part A coverage, and partial hospitalization services furnished by community mental health centers are classified into groups called ambulatory payment classifications (APCs). Services in each APC are similar clinically and in terms of the resources they require. A payment rate is established for each APC. Depending on the services provided, hospitals may be paid for more than one APC for an encounter. There are more than 700 individual APCs.

In most cases, the unit of payment under the OPPS is the individual service or procedure (using CPT or HCPCS codes). Services are assigned to APCs based on similar clinical characteristics and similar costs. The payment rate and copayment calculated for an APC apply to each service within the APC. Sometimes, new services are assigned to New Technology APCs, which are based solely on similarity of resource use until clinical and cost data are available to permit assignment to a clinical APC.

Most services are paid separately, including, but not limited to, the following:

- Most surgical, diagnostic, and nonsurgical therapeutic procedures
- Blood and blood products
- Most clinic and emergency department visits
- Some drugs, biologicals, and radiopharmaceuticals
- Brachytherapy sources
- Corneal tissue acquisition costs

Partial hospitalization for psychiatric services is paid on a per diem basis, with the payment rates dependent on the number of individual services provided to the patient on one day. The payment represents the expected cost of a day of intensive mental health care in a hospital outpatient department (OPD) or community mental health center (CMHC). There are two APCs for partial hospitalization furnished by hospital OPDs and two APCs for partial hospitalization furnished by CMHCs, all based on intensity of day.

Within each APC, payment for ancillary and supportive items and services is packaged into payment for the primary independent service. Separate payments are not made for a packaged service that is considered an integral part of another service paid under the OPPS.

Inpatient Psychiatric Facilities

Inpatient services furnished in psychiatric hospitals—as well as general hospitals' psychiatric units exempt from prospective payment—are paid by Medicare on a per diem PPS base rate adjusted by factors for facility and patient characteristics that account for variation in patient resource use. Patients are classified to MS-DRGs based on the principal ICD-10-CM psychiatric diagnosis, and a comorbidity adjustment is calculated based on certain diagnosis codes. Each inpatient admission can be grouped to only one of 17 psychiatric DRGs. Note that the list of comorbidities is different from the CC/MCC list for acute care inpatient hospital MS-DRGs.

Inpatient Rehabilitation Facilities

The inpatient rehabilitation facility (IRF) PPS uses information from a patient assessment instrument (IRF PAI) to classify patients into distinct groups based on clinical characteristics and expected resource needs. A case-mix adjusted payment for varying numbers of days of IRF care is made using case-mix groups (CMGs). Separate payments are calculated for each group, including the application of case- and facility-level adjustments. Payment is calculated on a per discharge basis. The IRF PAI requires diagnosis codes to report the etiologic diagnosis as well as secondary diagnoses. The etiologic diagnosis refers to the original problem leading up to the condition requiring rehabilitation. Secondary diagnoses considered comorbidities are arrayed into three tiers based on whether the costs associated with the specific comorbidity are high, medium, or low.

Long-Term Care Hospitals

The Medicare PPS for long-term care hospitals (LTCHs) applies to hospitals that have an average inpatient length of stay greater than 25 days. These hospitals are paid on a per discharge system with a DRG-based patient classification system that reflects the differences in patient resources and costs in LTCHs. These DRGs are referred to as MS-LTC-DRGs. Similar to MS-DRGs, they are driven by the principal diagnosis, secondary diagnoses, and procedures identified by ICD-10-CM and ICD-10-PCS codes.

Critical Access Hospitals

Critical access hospitals (CAHs) are recognized by Medicare as a separate provider type with its own regulations and a separate payment method from other types of hospitals. To qualify as a CAH, a hospital must meet several criteria, the most important of which are the following:

- Location in a rural area more than a 35-mile drive from the nearest hospital or CAH or more than a 15-mile drive in areas with mountainous terrain or only secondary roads

- No more than 25 inpatient beds

- Average annual length of stay of 96 hours or less per patient for acute care

CAHs are not subject to the inpatient or outpatient PPS. Instead, CAHs may choose to be paid by Medicare under the "Standard Payment Method" or the "Optional Payment Method." Under the standard method, payments for outpatient CAH facility services are made at 101 percent of reasonable costs, and professional services are billed under the Medicare Physician Fee Schedule (PFS). Under the optional method, the Medicare Administrative Contractor is billed for both facility and professional services furnished to outpatients by a physician or practitioner who has reassigned his or her billing rights to the CAH.

Home Health Agencies

Under prospective payment, Medicare pays home health agencies a predetermined base payment. The payment is adjusted for the health condition and care needs of the beneficiary. The adjustment for the health condition, or clinical characteristics, and service needs of the beneficiary is referred to as the case-mix adjustment. A case-mix adjusted payment for up to 60 days of care is made using one of 153 home health resource groups.

Effective January 1, 2020, CMS implemented a new payment model for the home health PPS, the Patient-Driven Groupings Model (PDGM). PDGM relies more heavily on clinical characteristics and other patient information to place home health periods of care into meaningful payment groups. The PDMG relies on five main case-mix variables: admission source, timing, clinical grouping, functional impairment level, and comorbidity adjustment. This results in over 400 possible case-mix adjusted payment groups into which a 30-day period can be placed. Clinical groups are intended to reflect the primary reason for home health services, which are defined by the principal diagnosis identified by the ICD-10-CM code reported on the claim. Under PDGM, functional impairment levels are determined based on assessments made using the Outcome and Assessment Information Set (OASIS). A comorbidity adjustment category is based on the presence of secondary diagnoses. A home health–specific comorbidity list was developed with broad clinical categories used to group comorbidities within the PDGM.

Hospice Agencies

Medicare pays hospice agencies a daily rate for each day a beneficiary is enrolled in the hospice benefit. The daily payments are made regardless of the amount of services furnished on a given day and are intended to cover costs that the hospice incurs in furnishing services identified in the beneficiary's plan of care. Payments are made based on the following levels of care required to meet beneficiary and family needs:

- Routine home care
- Continuous home care
- Inpatient respite care
- General inpatient care

Skilled Nursing Facilities

Skilled nursing facilities (SNFs) are paid by Medicare on a per diem PPS covering all costs (routine, ancillary, and capital) related to the services. Effective October 1, 2019, per diem payments for each admission are calculated using a new case-mix classification model called the Patient Driven Payment Model (PDPM). Under PDPM, payment is determined through the combination of six payment components: physical therapy, occupational therapy, speech-language pathology, non-therapy ancillary services, and nursing. SNF providers complete the Minimum Data Set, Version 3 (MDS 3.0) Resident Assessment Instrument. MDS assessments are used to classify patients into payment categories under the Patient Driven Payment Model (PDPM). The patient's primary diagnosis ICD-10-CM code on the MDS 3.0 is used to classify the patient into one of ten PDPM clinical categories.

MEDICARE ADVANTAGE PLANS

In addition to the Medicare payment models based on the type of provider listed previously, Medicare Advantage (MA) plans are available. MA plans are run by private companies under contract to Medicare. These plans cover hospital inpatient as well as physician services. In some instances, they may also cover other services not covered by traditional Medicare. Medicare uses a risk adjustment model to adjust compensation for the costs of taking care of MA members using Hierarchical Condition Categories (HCCs). The HCC model uses ICD-10-CM diagnosis codes to predict medical and drug spending. There are more than 80 HCCs, which are correlated to ICD-10-CM diagnosis codes. CMS's model is accumulative, meaning that more than one HCC can be assigned to a patient. It's important to note that there are two types of HCCs: one for CMS and another one for the commercial payer population.

COMMERCIAL PAYER REIMBURSEMENT

Commercial payers determine their own rules for payment and reimbursement based on fee schedules or negotiated contracts. Some commercial payers have negotiated contracts that are based on diagnosis codes, procedure codes, a combination of both, or other payment models such as DRGs.

Appendix B

Reporting of the Present on Admission Indicator

The present on admission (POA) indicator is a data element required for Medicare claims reporting. The POA indicator provides information on whether a diagnosis was present at the time of a patient's admission. The Medicare POA requirement applies to all diagnosis codes involving inpatient admissions to general acute care hospitals (except for critical care access hospitals, Maryland waiver hospitals, long-term care hospitals, cancer hospitals, and children's inpatient facilities). Some states (e.g., Maryland) have additional regulatory requirements for POA reporting. State guidelines for public health and quality reporting may differ from the national Medicare reporting requirements. In addition, several commercial health plans require POA reporting by contractual agreement with the hospital.

It is important that the POA indicator be reported correctly because it is significant in quality-of-care reporting and analysis and potentially significant for medicolegal and reimbursement issues. A select number of hospital-acquired conditions (HACs) are not recognized by the Medicare severity diagnosis-related group (MS-DRG) system if the condition is the only complication/comorbidity (CC) or major complication/comorbidity (MCC). In other words, if the only CC/MCC reported is one of the HACs, the case will not be assigned to the higher-weighted MS-DRG.

The POA indicator should be reported for principal and secondary diagnosis codes and External cause of injury codes based on a review of the provider's documentation. Distinguishing between pre-existing conditions and complications enhances the use of administrative data for outcomes reporting. Secondary diagnoses may be chronic illnesses that have been in existence for some time, or they may have developed after admission. Unless the POA indicator is reported, it is not easy to determine the difference between pre-existing conditions and complications when analyzing only the ICD-10-CM codes.

DEFINITION

The term "present on admission" means "present at the time the order for inpatient admission occurs." Conditions or adverse events that occur prior to an inpatient admission are considered to be present on admission. Present on admission conditions or adverse events include any that occur in the emergency department, observation, clinic, or outpatient surgery prior to inpatient admission.

DOCUMENTATION

The usefulness of POA data for quality-of-care, medicolegal, and reimbursement issues is dependent on the provider's accurate and complete medical record documentation. "Provider" in this context refers to the physician or any qualified health care practitioner who is legally accountable for establishing the patient's diagnosis, similar to the definition used for code assignment. Do not include documentation from nurses or other allied health professionals who are not legally accountable for establishing the patient's diagnosis (except for the reporting of pressure ulcer staging and body mass index).

The provider must resolve any inconsistent, missing, conflicting, or unclear documentation before the appropriate POA indicator may be selected. Resolving inconsistencies may necessitate querying the provider for clarification.

There is no required time frame as to when a provider must identify or document a condition to be present on admission. In some clinical situations, it may not be possible for a provider to make a definitive diagnosis (or a condition may not be recognized or reported by the patient) for a period of time after admission. In some cases, it may be several days before the provider arrives at a definitive diagnosis. This does not mean that the condition was not present on admission. Determination of whether the condition was present on admission is based on the applicable POA guideline or the provider's best clinical judgment.

GUIDELINES

Guidelines for the selection of POA indicators are included in the *ICD-10-CM Official Guidelines for Coding and Reporting* as appendix I. The POA guidelines are not intended to replace any guidelines in the main body of the official guidelines, nor are they intended to provide guidance on when a condition should be coded. Rather, the POA guidelines are intended to show how to apply the POA indicator to the final set of diagnosis codes already selected.

The guidelines are not intended to be a substitute for a provider's clinical judgment as to whether a condition was or was not present on admission. Issues related to the linking of signs and symptoms, timing of test results, or findings should be referred to the provider for clarification.

REPORTING OPTIONS

There are five options for reporting all diagnoses:

Code	Definition
Y	Yes (Present at the time of inpatient admission.)
N	No (Not present at the time of inpatient admission.)
U	Unknown (Documentation is insufficient to determine if condition is present on admission.)
W	Clinically undetermined (Provider is unable to clinically determine whether condition was present on admission or not.)
Unreported/not used	Exempt from POA reporting (This option is the only circumstance in which the POA field is left blank. The condition must be on the list of ICD-10-CM codes for which this field is not applicable.)

Conditions Present on Admission

Assign "Y" as the POA reporting option for the following circumstances:

- Condition explicitly documented as being present on admission.

- Condition diagnosed prior to inpatient admission (e.g., hypertension, diabetes mellitus, asthma).

- Condition diagnosed during the admission but clearly present (but not diagnosed) before admission (e.g., a patient with a lump in her breast is admitted and has a biopsy, and the pathology report reveals carcinoma of the breast).

- Condition diagnosed as possible, probable, suspected, or rule out at the time of discharge and, based on signs, symptoms, or clinical findings, condition is suspected during admission (e.g., a patient is admitted with chest pain, transferred to another facility, and discharged as possible myocardial infarction).

- Condition that developed during an outpatient encounter prior to a written order for inpatient admission (e.g., a patient falls while in the emergency department, sustains a fracture, and is subsequently admitted as an inpatient).

- Condition diagnosed as impending or threatened, based on symptoms or clinical findings that were present on admission (e.g., a patient with a known history of coronary atherosclerosis is now admitted for treatment of impending myocardial infarction; the final diagnosis is documented as "impending" myocardial infarction).

- Condition reported with a code that includes multiple clinical concepts, and all the clinical concepts included in the code are present on admission (e.g., a duodenal ulcer that perforates prior to admission).

- Condition reported with the same ICD-10-CM code representing two or more conditions during the same encounter, and all conditions were present on admission (e.g., bilateral unspecified age-related cataracts).

- Single code that only identifies the chronic condition and not the acute exacerbation (e.g., acute exacerbation of chronic leukemia).

- Chronic condition, even if it is not diagnosed until after admission (e.g., lung cancer is diagnosed during hospitalization).

- Condition in which the final diagnosis includes comparative or contrasting diagnoses, and both are present or suspected at the time of admission (e.g., a patient is admitted with severe abdominal pain, nausea, and vomiting, with the admitting diagnosis of acute pyelonephritis versus diverticulum of the colon; the patient is discharged and sent home).

- Infection codes that include the causal organism, if the infection (or signs of the infection) is present on admission, even though the culture results may not be known until after admission (e.g., a patient is admitted with severe cough, fever, and congestion and his culture of sputum reveals staphylococcal infection; the patient is diagnosed with staphylococcal pneumonia).

- Congenital conditions and anomalies (except for categories Q00–Q99, Congenital anomalies, which are on the exempt list). Congenital conditions are always considered to be present on admission.

- Condition present at birth or that develops in utero, including conditions that occur during delivery (e.g., injury during delivery).

- External cause code representing an external cause of morbidity that occurred prior to inpatient admission (e.g., the patient fell out of bed at home).

Conditions Not Present on Admission

Assign "N" as the POA reporting option for the following circumstances:

- Condition the provider explicitly documents as not present at the time of admission (e.g., a patient develops a vascular catheter infection a few days after the insertion of the catheter).

- Condition reported as an inconclusive final diagnosis based on signs, symptoms, or clinical findings that were not present on admission (e.g., a patient develops a fever after surgery, and the final diagnosis includes "possible postoperative infection").

- Condition diagnosed as impending or threatened and based on symptoms or clinical findings that were not present on admission (e.g., a patient is admitted to the hospital for prostate surgery and postoperatively develops chest pain; the final diagnosis includes "impending myocardial infarction").

- Condition reported with a code that includes multiple clinical concepts, and at least one of the clinical concepts included in the code is not present on admission (e.g., chronic obstructive pulmonary disease with acute exacerbation, and the exacerbation is not present on admission; gastric ulcer that does not start bleeding until after admission; asthma patient develops status asthmaticus after admission).

- Conditions reported with the same ICD-10-CM code representing two or more conditions during the same encounter, and any one of the conditions was not present on admission (e.g., traumatic secondary and recurrent hemorrhage and seroma are assigned to a single code, T79.2, but only one of the conditions was present on admission).
- External cause code representing an external cause of morbidity that occurs during inpatient hospitalization (e.g., a patient falls out of the hospital bed during his stay, or he experiences an adverse reaction to a medication administered after inpatient admission).

Unclear Documentation

Assign "U" as the POA indicator when the medical record documentation is unclear as to whether the condition was present on admission. Coding professionals are encouraged to query the providers when the documentation is unclear. It is important to note that "U" should not be routinely assigned but should be used only under very limited circumstances, such as when the provider is not available to provide clarification.

Conditions Clinically Undetermined

Assign "W" as the POA indicator when the medical record documentation indicates that it cannot be clinically determined whether the condition was present on admission. For example, a patient is admitted in active labor, and during the stay a breast abscess is noted when she attempts to breastfeed. The provider is unable to determine if the abscess was present on admission.

It is important to distinguish between the reporting options "U" and "W." For example, if the provider is queried and is not able to determine whether the condition was present on admission, report using "W." In contrast, if the documentation is not available and the provider is not queried, or the provider is not available to provide a response, report using "U." Make every attempt to limit the number of "U" options reported, as this may potentially be construed as an error or treated as "N" for Medicare payment purposes.

Conditions Exempt from POA Reporting

A list of categories and codes exempt from the POA requirement may be found on the Centers for Medicare & Medicaid Services (CMS) website at www.cms.gov/Medicare/Medicare-Fee-for-Service-Payment/HospitalAcqCond/Coding. The codes and categories on this exempt list are intended for circumstances regarding the health care encounter or factors that influence the health status but do not represent a current disease or injury. These codes and categories describe conditions that are always present on admission.

Examples include injury, poisoning, and certain other consequences of external causes with the seventh character "S," personal and family history codes, and encounter for immunization Z codes.

The codes and categories on the exempt list are the only codes that are exempt from POA reporting. The list of exempt codes is updated every year based on the new codes implemented for the year.

Special Considerations

For obstetric patients, whether or not delivery occurs during the current hospitalization does not affect assignment of the POA indicator. The determining factor for POA assignment is whether the pregnancy complication or obstetric condition described by the code is present at the time of admission. If the obstetric code includes information that is not a diagnosis, do not consider that information in the POA determination. If the obstetric code includes more than one diagnosis (e.g., category O11, Pre-existing hypertension with pre-eclampsia) and any one of the diagnoses identified by the code was not present on admission, assign "N."

Newborns are not considered to be admitted until after birth; therefore, any condition that is present at birth or that develops in utero is considered to be present at admission.

EXERCISE B.1

Assign the appropriate POA indicator for the following scenarios:

1. A patient is treated in observation, falls out of bed, and breaks a hip. The patient is subsequently admitted as an inpatient to treat the hip fracture. What is the POA indicator for the fracture?   _____

2. A patient is admitted to the hospital for coronary artery bypass surgery. Postoperatively, he develops a pulmonary embolism. What is the POA indicator for the pulmonary embolism?   _____

3. A patient is admitted in active labor. She is known to have a gastric ulcer under medical management. After delivering the baby, she complains of melena and is noted to have bleeding from the gastric ulcer. What is the POA indicator for bleeding from the gastric ulcer?   _____

4. A single liveborn infant is delivered in the hospital. The physician documents neonatal tachycardia. What is the POA indicator for the neonatal tachycardia?   _____

5. A patient is admitted with fever, weakness, severe malaise, and coughing. She is diagnosed with pneumonia. She deteriorates rapidly and is transferred to the intensive care unit with severe sepsis. On physician query, the physician documents that he cannot determine whether the patient had sepsis on admission because she deteriorated so quickly. What is the POA indicator for the severe sepsis?   _____

EXERCISE B.2

Locate the POA exempt list on the CMS website. Write an "X" next to each code below that is exempt from POA reporting.

1. O80   Encounter for full-term uncomplicated delivery   _____

2. O60.10   Preterm labor with preterm delivery, unspecified trimester   _____

3. Z99.2   Dependence on renal dialysis   _____

4. V00.311- Fall from snowboard   _____

5. Y30.-   Falling, jumping or pushed from a high place, undetermined intent   _____

Appendix C

APPENDIX C

Case Summary Exercises

Therese M. Jorwic, MPH, RHIA, CCS, CCS-P, FAHIMA, and Janatha R. Ashton, MS, RHIA

CONTENTS

About This Appendix 594

1 Symptoms, Signs, and Ill-Defined Conditions 596

2 Infectious and Parasitic Diseases. 602

3 Endocrine, Nutritional, and Metabolic Diseases. 604

4 Mental Disorders. 607

5 Diseases of the Blood and Blood-Forming Organs and Certain Disorders Involving the Immune Mechanism. 611

6 Diseases of the Nervous System and Sense Organs 614

7 Diseases of the Respiratory System. 617

8 Diseases of the Digestive System 623

9 Diseases of the Genitourinary System 633

10 Diseases of the Skin and Subcutaneous Tissue 640

11 Diseases of the Musculoskeletal System and Connective Tissue 643

12 Complications of Pregnancy, Childbirth, and the Puerperium 649

13 Abortion and Ectopic Pregnancy 659

14 Congenital Anomalies. 661

15 Perinatal Conditions 665

16 Diseases of the Circulatory System 670

17 Neoplasms 680

18 Injuries. 691

19 Burns. 704

20 Poisoning, Toxic Effects, Adverse Effects, and Underdosing of Drugs 707

21 Complications of Surgery and Medical Care 715

ABOUT THIS APPENDIX

The case summary exercises in this appendix are based on the actual medical records of both inpatients and outpatients. The patients described often have multiple conditions that may or may not be related to the current episode of care. Some exercises include several episodes of care for the same patient in various settings.

How to Use This Appendix

The case summary style of the exercises requires you to consider the patient's condition as well as all relevant information provided: medical history, reason for admission or encounter, laboratory results, procedures performed, and diagnoses listed. In all exercises, you need to apply pertinent coding principles and official coding guidelines in making code assignments and designating the principal diagnosis and procedure for each episode of care.

Each exercise includes a brief summary and a diagnosis statement that should be read carefully. You may assume that all diagnoses and procedures that are mentioned and that should be coded have been approved by the patient's physician. Be sure to sequence the principal diagnosis and principal procedure first.

After referring to the appropriate ICD-10-CM and ICD-10-PCS coding manuals, fill in the codes that you think should be assigned (including any appropriate codes for external causes and locations of occurrence as needed) in the space provided next to each case summary. For inpatient care and the outpatient and ambulatory care settings, assign and sequence codes according to the *ICD-10-CM Official Guidelines for Coding and Reporting*. Use the *ICD-10-PCS Official Coding Guidelines* for inpatient procedures.

The sequence of this appendix corresponds to chapters 13 through 33 of the handbook and progresses from simpler to more difficult areas. It is recommended that you will have read all of the chapters (1–33) of the handbook before you begin the case summary exercises in this appendix. You may, however, complete the exercises in any order after you have learned the basic coding principles and understand how to apply official coding guidelines.

About the Answers

Answers are provided in the right-hand column of the *with Answers* version of the handbook. (Ask your instructor for the answers if you are using the *without Answers* version.) The right-hand column lists the appropriate codes for each exercise, with the codes for the principal diagnosis and principal procedure sequenced first. Explanatory comments discuss why certain codes are appropriate while others are not, and why some conditions listed in the case summaries are not coded at all. The comments also indicate how principal diagnosis and procedure codes were designated and which symptoms are inherent to certain conditions and so are not coded separately.

ICD-10-PCS is the Health Insurance Portability and Accountability Act (HIPAA) standard for the reporting of inpatient procedures by hospitals. For outpatient encounters, ICD-10-PCS codes are typically not reported when a claim is submitted. However, a hospital may choose to collect ICD-10-PCS codes for outpatient procedures for internal or non-claim-related purposes. In addition, hospitals may report ICD-10-PCS procedure codes for outpatient services for specific payers under contractual agreements or as required by their state data reporting regulations.

In day-to-day practice, many hospitals have opted through their internal coding policies not to collect data on noninvasive (without contrast) diagnostic services performed in the inpatient setting, such as X-rays, electrocardiograms (EKGs), computerized tomography (CT) scans, and ultrasounds. In addition, minor noninvasive services such as application of splints and traction are typically not reported. For this reason, codes for these minor services have been omitted from the answers.

The codes and comments in the answers reflect the latest *ICD-10-CM Official Guidelines for Coding and Reporting* (2021 edition) and *ICD-10-PCS Official Coding Guidelines* (2021 edition). Specific guidelines are referenced in parentheses by section and guideline number.

1. SYMPTOMS, SIGNS, AND ILL-DEFINED CONDITIONS

1. **Inpatient admission:** The patient, an elderly man, was admitted through the emergency department for severe urinary retention. In the emergency department, it was also determined that his hypertension was accelerated. He had been hospitalized three months earlier for identical problems, and he said he had not taken any of his medications since the last hospitalization, as he could not afford the cost. The urinary retention was relieved by placement of a Foley catheter. Medications were started, and the hypertension improved rapidly. The patient was evaluated for the extent of benign prostatic hypertrophy. Transurethral resection of the prostate was recommended, but it was refused by the patient.

   Discharge diagnoses: (1) Hypertensive urgency, (2) acute urinary retention secondary to benign hypertrophy of the prostate, (3) noncompliance with treatment program.

Code(s):

2. **Inpatient admission:** The patient was admitted for recurrent epistaxis that did not respond to nasal packing in the emergency department. He was status post myocardial infarct seven weeks earlier, with no current symptoms. An EKG was performed to evaluate the status of the MI. The patient also suffered from a deviated nasal septum. Multiple attempts were made to stop the bleeding with more packing, but none was successful for more than a few hours. Therefore, the following procedures were performed: (1) anterior and posterior nasal packing, (2) endoscopic ethmoidal artery ligation, (3) endoscopic septoplasty. He was transfused via peripheral vein with two units of packed red cells during the operation.

Discharge diagnoses: (1) Severe and recurrent epistaxis, (2) post myocardial infarct, (3) deviated nasal septum.

Code(s):

3. **Inpatient admission:** The reason for the patient's admission was substernal chest pain with some arm involvement. A combined right and left selective low osmolar contrast coronary angiography with fluoroscopy and a bilateral low osmolar contrast pulmonary angiography were performed. No coronary artery disease or pulmonary embolus was found.

Discharge diagnosis: Chest pain without occlusive coronary artery disease.

Code(s):

4. **Inpatient admission:** The patient, a 19-year-old man, was transferred from another hospital with intractable headache. The accompanying CT scan was normal, but clinical symptomatology was suggestive of subarachnoid hemorrhage. Lumbar puncture, non-contrast bilateral internal carotid cerebral arteriogram, and contrast cerebral MRI were all normal. When the findings were discussed with the patient, he became increasingly belligerent. Although his headaches were only somewhat improved, he refused further treatment and was discharged for follow-up with his own physician.

Discharge diagnosis: Headache.

Code(s):

5. **Inpatient admission:** The patient has a known diagnosis of prostatic cancer. He started having fevers approximately one week earlier. The fevers did not respond to outpatient antibiotics. Blood and urine cultures showed no growth. He was admitted for workup of the fevers with possible prostatic abscess formation. There were no obvious signs of infection or abscess on a transrectal ultrasound of the prostate. An iodine-123 radioisotope bone scan of the body revealed no skeletal metastases. The antibiotic therapy was changed, and he was given an IV push. He improved and was discharged.

Discharge diagnoses: (1) Fever of unknown origin, (2) cancer of the prostate.

Code(s):

6. **Inpatient admission:** The two-year-old patient had an acute onset of fever and some shaking chills at home. He was thought to have experienced a febrile seizure and was admitted for workup and treatment. There was some infiltrate in the right lung per chest X-ray. All laboratory work was within normal limits. He was observed during his stay. No problems were noticed, and he remained afebrile after the first day. He was discharged for office follow-up.

Discharge diagnosis: Rule out febrile seizure.

Code(s):

7. **Inpatient admission:** The patient was admitted through the emergency department with possible acute cholecystitis. She had severe abdominal pain and a markedly elevated white count. A gallbladder ultrasound, cholecystogram, and contrast intravenous pyelogram were all normal. The next day her pain was almost gone, and the white blood count dropped to nearly normal. It was not felt worthwhile to continue the workup.

    Discharge diagnoses: (1) Abdominal pain, (2) leukocytosis.

    Code(s):

8. **Inpatient admission:** The patient, an obese male, was admitted with generalized abdominal pain suggestive of early appendicitis, although he had a normal white count and normal differential. An intravenous pyelogram and X-ray of the lower gastrointestinal tract with barium enema were negative. All laboratory studies were normal. He improved while in the hospital without a definite cause for his pain ever being identified. He was placed on a low-fat, 1,500-calorie diet prior to discharge.

    Discharge diagnoses: (1) Abdominal pain of undetermined origin, generalized; (2) obesity.

    Code(s):

9. **Outpatient clinic visit:** This patient with type 2 diabetes was seen by his primary care physician for evaluation of an inconclusive liver function scan and abdominal pain. The physician ordered a CT scan of the liver and advised the patient to return in one week.

    Discharge diagnosis: Abnormal liver function, upper right quadrant abdominal pain, and diabetes mellitus.

    Code(s):

10. Inpatient admission: The patient, a woman with type 1 diabetes, was admitted because of increased swelling of the right foot that was determined to be an abscess. *Staphylococcus aureus* grew from the abscess. She underwent a percutaneous incision and drainage of the foot abscess. Her course in the hospital otherwise was essentially unremarkable. The foot gradually improved with antibiotic therapy, hyperbaric oxygen therapy, and daily whirlpool therapy.

Discharge diagnoses: (1) Abscess right foot, (2) type 1 diabetes mellitus.

Code(s):

11. Inpatient admission: The child was admitted with a fever and lethargy. The admitting diagnosis was "rule out sepsis." When admitted, he was responsive but lethargic. The physical examination was within normal limits except for the left eardrum, which was reddened. He was placed on intravenous antibiotics after the full septic workup was complete. Improvement was evident by the next day, when he was alert, active, and started on feedings. He became afebrile and was discharged on oral antibiotics for otitis media, with sepsis ruled out.

Discharge diagnoses: (1) Fever, (2) otitis media.

Code(s):

12. Inpatient admission: The patient, a 10-month-old male, presented with acute stridor and respiratory distress. His mother felt that he had possibly choked on a peach. Nothing was seen on chest X-ray. A rigid bronchoscopy ruled out foreign body, but the findings were consistent with croup. He was discharged on medication to follow up with his pediatrician in one week.

Discharge diagnosis: Croup.

Code(s):

13. **Emergency department visit:** A 26-year-old male, involved in a car crash, was taken to the local emergency department (ED) in a coma, where he was diagnosed with a traumatic brain injury with loss of consciousness of one hour. Glasgow coma scale (GCS) was 6 on arrival in the ED. Patient was transferred to a trauma center for further care.

Discharge diagnosis: Traumatic brain injury.

Code(s):

2. INFECTIOUS AND PARASITIC DISEASES

1. **Inpatient admission:** This HIV-positive patient was admitted with skin lesions on the chest and back. Excisional biopsies were taken, and the pathological diagnosis was Kaposi's sarcoma. Leukoplakia of the lips and splenomegaly were also noted on physical examination.

   Discharge diagnoses: (1) HIV infection; (2) Kaposi's sarcoma, back and chest; (3) leukoplakia; (4) splenomegaly.

   Code(s):

2. **Inpatient admission:** The patient underwent an outpatient laparoscopic-assisted cholecystectomy for cholecystitis and was admitted the next day because of a flare-up of chronic hepatitis C. The chronic hepatitis C was secondary to intravenous drug use. With medication, the chronic hepatitis C was controlled, and the woman was discharged.

   Discharge diagnoses: (1) Chronic hepatitis C, (2) IV drug dependence.

   Code(s):

3. **Inpatient admission:** An elderly male patient with a history of benign hypertension became extremely febrile the day before admission. On admission, he was extremely lethargic with a possible septic urinary tract infection. He was pan cultured and started on IV antibiotics and fluids. *Pseudomonas* showed in the urine culture. The next day, his mind was quite clear and the fever defervesced from an initial 104.6 to 99.0 degrees. However, he had gross hematuria. As the IV fluids were decreased, he resumed his usual hypertensive state. By the third hospital day, the urine had cleared and he was discharged on oral antibiotics, with septicemia ruled out.

   Discharge diagnoses: (1) Urinary tract infection due to *Pseudomonas,* (2) gross hematuria, (3) benign essential hypertension.

   Code(s):

4. **Inpatient admission:** The patient, with arterio-sclerotic coronary heart disease and type 2 diabetes mellitus, came to the hospital with symptoms that were believed to represent sepsis. She was placed on antibiotics, and the symptoms improved. ST- and T-wave changes were evident on an EKG. The patient's glucose showed marked elevation, thought to be secondary to the sepsis. The blood sugars were brought under control with an adjustment of her insulin therapy and an appropriate diet.

   Discharge diagnoses: (1) Arteriosclerotic coronary heart disease, (2) uncontrolled type 2 diabetes mellitus, (3) questionable sepsis.

   Code(s):

5. **Outpatient clinic visit:** The HIV-infected patient was suffering from an acute lymphadenitis due to his HIV infection. The glands in the neck area were most affected. Antibiotics were prescribed, but the patient refused antiretroviral treatment at this time. He was of the opinion that his religion would eventually make antiretroviral medication unnecessary. Another consideration was his narcotic dependency. He was encouraged to continue participation in support groups for people with narcotic addiction and HIV.

   Diagnoses: (1) Acute lymphadenitis secondary to HIV infection, (2) narcotic dependence, (3) refusal of medication due to religious reasons.

   Code(s):

6. **Inpatient admission:** The patient is an 85-year-old female who presented to the emergency department (ED) with increasing shortness of breath, hypoxia, productive cough, and progressive weakness. She acutely deteriorated in the ED and was emergently sent to the intensive care unit (ICU). In the ICU, the patient was intubated, mechanically ventilated for four days, and started on broad-spectrum antibiotics.

   Diagnoses: (1) Septic shock, (2) acute respiratory failure, (3) *Hemophilus influenzae* pneumonia.

   Code(s):

3. ENDOCRINE, NUTRITIONAL, AND METABOLIC DISEASES

1. **Inpatient admission:** The patient was admitted for an evaluation of her adrenal malfunction. She had a four-year history of hypertension and hypokalemia with evidence of primary aldosteronism. A non-contrast CT scan of the abdomen also suggested a left adrenal mass. She was discharged and was to return for a left adrenalectomy the following week.

   Discharge diagnoses: (1) Probable adrenal mass, left; (2) hypertension and hypokalemia probably due to primary aldosteronism.

   Code(s):

2. **Inpatient admission:** The patient was admitted for severe malnutrition and hematuria secondary to amyotrophic lateral sclerosis. Because of her malnutrition, a nasogastric feeding tube was placed under fluoroscopy and nutritional substance was administered later. During her stay, the hematuria cleared spontaneously, and she was discharged to home care.

   Discharge diagnoses: (1) Malnutrition, (2) hematuria secondary to amyotrophic lateral sclerosis.

   Code(s):

3. **Inpatient admission:** The patient fell at his single-family home and was unable to get up. Neighbors found him several hours later, and he does not remember any circumstances surrounding the event. Blood sugars were monitored, and a diagnosis of diabetes mellitus was given. It became rapidly evident to the attending physician that, even with dietary restriction, the patient would need insulin therapy to lower his blood sugar level. Insulin therapy was started. The only other positive finding was beta-*Streptococcus* group B, which grew from the urine culture and was treated with oral antibiotics.

   Discharge diagnoses: (1) New onset type 2 diabetes mellitus, out of control; (2) urinary tract infection with beta-*Streptococcus*.

   Code(s):

4. **Outpatient clinic visit:** The patient with type 2 diabetes was status post cadaveric kidney and pancreatic transplants. He was being seen for follow-up of a recent amputation of the foot due to a nonhealing, gangrenous ulcer on his left foot secondary to diabetic peripheral vascular disease. The operative site was healing very nicely, and there was no evidence of infection.

   Diagnoses: (1) Status post left foot amputation, (2) status post kidney and pancreas transplants, (3) diabetes mellitus.

   Code(s):

5. **Inpatient admission:** The patient, an elderly woman with type 2 diabetes mellitus, developed hypoglycemia at the nursing home and was symptomatic. In the emergency department, her decreased blood sugar was treated with intravenous D5W. A urinary tract infection was also present and was treated with antibiotics. The urine culture grew *Klebsiella*, sensitive to Cipro. She then developed mild congestive heart failure, probably secondary to the hypoglycemic reaction, which responded to oxygen and rest. Her Diabeta regimen was restarted at a lower dosage.

   Discharge diagnoses: (1) Congestive heart failure secondary to hypoglycemia, (2) type 2 diabetes mellitus, (3) urinary tract infection.

   Code(s):

6. **Inpatient admission:** The patient, a young male with type 1 diabetes, was brought in a comatose state to the emergency department by friends. He was admitted with ketoacidosis and was resuscitated with saline hydration via insulin drip. After regaining consciousness, he reported that the morning of admission he was experiencing nausea and vomiting and decided not to take his insulin because he had not eaten. He was treated with intravenous hydration and insulin drip. By the following morning, his laboratory work was within normal range and he was experiencing no symptoms.

   Discharge diagnoses: (1) Diabetic ketoacidosis, (2) juvenile-onset diabetes.

   Code(s):

606

7. **Inpatient admission:** The patient with type 1 diabetes mellitus seriously out of control was admitted for regulation of insulin dosage. He had a recently abscessed right molar, which was determined, in part, to be responsible for the elevation of his blood sugar. The patient had been in the hospital three weeks earlier for an acute transmural myocardial infarction of the infero-posterior wall, and an EKG was performed to check its current status.

Discharge diagnoses: (1) Myocardial infarction, (2) abscessed tooth, (3) uncontrolled type 1 diabetes mellitus.

Code(s):

8. **Outpatient clinic visit:** A 57-year-old Hispanic male presented to the Medical Eye Service clinic for a retinal evaluation of diabetic retinopathy. He reported vision that fluctuated only in the morning and poorer vision in the right eye. He was diagnosed with type 2 diabetes mellitus 15 years ago and is currently taking Glucophage. He was diagnosed with diabetic retinopathy and advised to schedule grid laser treatment at his earliest convenience.

Diagnosis: Severe nonproliferative diabetic retinopathy, OD greater than OS.

Code(s):

4. MENTAL DISORDERS

1. **Outpatient clinic visit:** The patient was seen to evaluate his progress in dealing with his long-standing alcoholism. In addition, he had a passive-aggressive personality disorder and was dependent on Librium. He was actively participating in Alcoholics Anonymous and stated he would continue to participate. He apparently now had some alcoholic liver damage and was referred to an internist for further investigation of that condition.

   Diagnoses: (1) Alcohol dependence; (2) passive-aggressive personality disorder; (3) drug dependence, Librium; (4) alcoholic liver damage.

Code(s):

2. **Outpatient clinic visit:** The patient, a young female, was brought in by her sister. She has had periods of severe depression for many years. Her medications consisted of Lithium, Synthroid, and Maxalt for depression, hypothyroidism, and migraine headaches, respectively. During the past week, however, she became manic, running all her credit cards to the limit, getting inappropriately involved in a woman's suicide attempt, quitting her job, and trying to take over the pulpit at church. On the day of the clinic visit, she threatened to strike a neighbor with a lead pipe. She was to be admitted for Lithium adjustment.

   Diagnoses: (1) Bipolar disorder, manic type; (2) hypothyroidism; (3) migraine headaches.

Code(s):

3. **Inpatient admission:** The woman was brought in by police for observation of a suspected mental condition. They found her roaming the streets, and she seemed disoriented and confused. She was treated for scabies, body lice, and cellulitis of the right foot. Her mental status cleared rapidly. The only psychiatric disorder found was moderate intellectual disability.

Discharge diagnoses: (1) Moderate intellectual disability; (2) scabies; (3) body lice; (4) cellulitis, right foot.

Code(s):

4. **Outpatient clinic visit:** This 59-year-old male patient with a history of paranoid schizophrenia has had constant conflict with his family and coworkers for years. His wife reported that he was in danger of losing his job because he threatened his supervisor's life. He recently spent the night in jail after an altercation with a neighbor. Medication was prescribed, and he was to return for follow-up in one week.

Diagnosis: Schizophrenia, paranoid type, chronic with acute exacerbation.

Code(s):

5. **Outpatient clinic visit:** An 18-year-old patient was described by his mother as recently having periods of depression, throwing temper tantrums, and stealing from neighbors. He had a history of type 1 diabetes and sometimes refused to take his insulin or follow his diet. His speech, best described as "baby talk," had also become worse during the previous two months. A prescription was written for his depression.

Diagnoses: (1) Depression, (2) borderline personality disorder, (3) delayed speech development, (4) type 1 diabetes mellitus.

Code(s):

6. **Inpatient admission:** The patient was brought to the emergency department by the police and admitted to psychiatric service. Police requested an evaluation after the man was disorderly and aggressive at the scene of an automobile accident in which he was involved. He was admitted with a diagnosis of probable dementia.

Discharge diagnoses: (1) Organic brain syndrome with presenile dementia, (2) probably Alzheimer's disease with dementia.

Code(s):

7. **Inpatient admission:** The patient, with a four-year history of anorexia nervosa, was seen in the physician's office because of significant weight loss over the past three months, going from 82 pounds down to 53 pounds. She was admitted to increase body weight and to be given nutritional counseling because of her severe malnutrition.

Discharge diagnosis: Anorexia nervosa, severe malnutrition.

Code(s):

610

8. **Inpatient admission:** The patient was admitted with possible pyelonephritis. Her complaints were bilateral flank pain and chills. A contrast intravenous pyelogram was normal. Within two days of admission, the character of her pain changed somewhat in that it became primarily in the right upper quadrant. The physician documented in the progress notes that significant features of conversion hysteria were present and accounted for the patient's symptoms. On the third hospital day, the patient's IV was discontinued, liver function tests were rechecked, and antibiotics were discontinued. Later that day, she left abruptly, saying she would not return.

Discharge diagnoses: (1) Right upper quadrant abdominal pain, (2) conversion disorder.

Code(s):

9. **Psychiatry clinic visit:** The HIV-infected patient, who had a long history of cocaine addiction, started using cocaine again. Several months ago, he was admitted for treatment of *Pneumocystis carinii* pneumonia. Presently, severe depression brought him to the clinic. He and the physician had an extensive discussion about returning to Narcotics Anonymous and also joining an AIDS support group. A prescription for Prozac was given for his depression.

Diagnoses: (1) Severe depression, (2) cocaine addiction, (3) HIV infection.

Code(s):

10. **Outpatient clinic visit:** Patient is a 34-year-old male who came back from a tour of duty in Iraq. Since his return, his family has noticed he is often anxious, has a short temper, and has been drinking excessively. His family persuaded him to seek professional counseling, during which he was diagnosed with post-traumatic stress disorder, given a prescription for Paxil, and scheduled for once-a-week therapy sessions at the mental health clinic.

Diagnoses: (1) Acute post-traumatic stress disorder, (2) anxiety disorder due to alcohol abuse.

Code(s):

5. DISEASES OF THE BLOOD AND BLOOD-FORMING ORGANS AND CERTAIN DISORDERS INVOLVING THE IMMUNE MECHANISM

1. **Inpatient admission:** The patient had a congenital aplastic anemia that had been responding well to treatment. She was admitted for observation following a full-mouth extraction for multiple dental caries with pulp exposure and pyorrhea in outpatient surgery. She had only minimal bleeding following surgery. However, it was believed to be necessary to admit her for monitoring. She was discharged the next day with her blood counts remaining at acceptable levels.

   Discharge diagnosis: Aplastic anemia.

   Code(s): _____

2. **Inpatient admission:** The patient, who had sickle-cell anemia, presented to the emergency department with a two- to three-day history of severe right leg and arm pain. After she was admitted, parenteral narcotics were administered and the pain improved. The blood counts returned to a stable level within 24 hours.

   Discharge diagnosis: Sickle-cell pain crisis.

   Code(s): _____

3. **Inpatient admission:** The patient was an elderly woman visiting her physician with complaints of heart palpitations. A routine office evaluation revealed significant anemia. She had not been eating well because she had recently moved from her home of 30 years. After admission to the hospital, a cardiology consultation suggested that the palpitations were probably due to the anemia. During the gastrointestinal workup, mild gastritis was revealed. After a transfusion of two units of packed red blood cells into the peripheral vein (percutaneous approach), her hemoglobin returned to normal range. The patient was discharged to the nursing home with a prescription for Zantac to control her gastritis.

   Discharge diagnoses: (1) Nutritional anemia, (2) gastritis.

   Code(s): _____

4. Inpatient admission: The patient had locally advanced bladder cancer. He had excellent response to chemotherapy treatments administered prior to admission, with only a small amount of residual disease noted in the bladder. He was admitted with increasing nausea, anorexia, fevers, and constipation. His calcium levels were found to be elevated. A slight decrease was achieved with IV hydration, and the calcium levels continued to fall with IV pamidronate. Because he was asymptomatic, further workup was not indicated, and he was discharged.

Discharge diagnoses: (1) Hypercalcemia, (2) bladder cancer.

Code(s):

5. Inpatient admission: The patient was diagnosed with Coombs-negative hemolytic anemia four years earlier. Since diagnosis, her disease course waxed and waned. During some bouts, she had 15 to 20 blood transfusions of two to three units of packed red blood cells each. This admission was for splenectomy. The plan also called for removing a kidney stone on the left side, which was identified on her preadmission workup. Both surgeries, total splenectomy and laparoscopic pyelolithotomy, were performed without incident. Her postoperative recovery also went smoothly.

Discharge diagnoses: (1) Hypersplenism secondary to acquired hemolytic anemia; (2) stone, left kidney.

Code(s):

6. Inpatient admission: A 50-year-old man receiving Coumadin therapy was admitted with hematemesis secondary to acute gastritis. A prolonged prothrombin time was reported, secondary to the anticoagulant effect of the Coumadin therapy. The patient was admitted because of the acute gastritis with bleeding.

Discharge diagnosis: Acute gastritis due to Coumadin therapy.

Code(s):

7. **Outpatient clinic visit:** A 59-year-old female patient presents to the oncologist with oat cell lung cancer of the right upper lobe and anemia. Patient had recently undergone a chemotherapy treatment.

   Diagnoses: (1) Anemia due to carcinoma, (2) oat cell lung carcinoma.

   Code(s):

8. **Inpatient admission:** The patient, a woman with a diagnosis of cell-mediated immune deficiency with thrombocytopenia and eczema, was admitted for incision and drainage of a foot abscess. Her course in the hospital was essentially unremarkable. The foot gradually improved with intermittent hyperbaric oxygen therapy and daily whirlpool therapy. *Staphylococcus aureus* grew from the abscess.

   Discharge diagnoses: (1) Abscess right foot, (2) cell-immune deficiency with thrombo-cytopenia and eczema.

   Code(s):

6. DISEASES OF THE NERVOUS SYSTEM AND SENSE ORGANS

1. **Ophthalmology clinic visit:** The HIV-infected patient complained of difficulty focusing while reading. His examination revealed no evidence of retinopathy. He did have early presbyopia, for which "drugstore readers" were recommended.

   Diagnoses: (1) Presbyopia, (2) HIV infection.

   Code(s):

2. **Inpatient admission:** The patient was under medical management for long-standing, bilateral mild stage primary open-angle glaucoma, as well as age-related bilateral macular degeneration. Three days previously, an abnormally high intraocular pressure developed. The patient was treated successfully as an outpatient. The next day, another pressure spike occurred, and the patient was admitted for further management. He was treated medically for two days, and both the pressure and visual acuity improved sufficiently for discharge.

   Discharge diagnoses: (1) Acute primary open-angle glaucoma, (2) macular degeneration, (3) intraocular pressure.

   Code(s):

3. **Inpatient admission:** The patient previously suffered anterior dislocation of the left hip, which was reduced; however, this was followed by numbness and weakness in the left femoral nerve distribution. Evaluation indicated that she would benefit from surgery. A left femoral nerve external (percutaneous) neurolysis was carried out successfully.

   Discharge diagnosis: Mononeuritis, femoral nerve.

   Code(s):

4. **Inpatient admission:** The patient, a teenager, was admitted for evaluation and control of his intractable seizures. On days one, three, and four, seizures were recorded per video EEG. His video EEGs were consistent with epileptiform discharges of right temporal lobe origin. Dilantin and phenobarbital dosages were adjusted, and the patient was discharged in satisfactory condition.

   Discharge diagnosis: Partial complex epilepsy localized to the right temporal lobe.

   Code(s):

5. **Ambulatory surgery:** The patient was brought in for surgical intervention of a mature, symptomatic cataract in the left eye and high intraocular pressures despite medical therapy. An external trabeculectomy and phacoemulsification were performed.

   Diagnoses: (1) Primary open-angle glaucoma, severe stage left eye, moderate stage right eye; (2) cataract, left eye.

   Code(s):

6. **Inpatient admission:** The patient, an 18-month-old boy, was admitted with right orbital cellulitis. He was started on antibiotics and seemed to be improving. However, the day after admission, a slight exophthalmos was noticed. A non-contrast CT scan of the head showed increasing edema of the eye orbit with filling of ethmoid sinuses. The medications were changed. A right endoscopic complete ethmoidectomy was performed because the ethmoid sinuses were filled on the right side. The infant improved and was discharged in satisfactory condition.

   Discharge diagnoses: (1) Right orbital abscess; (2) exophthalmos, right orbital edema; (3) acute ethmoidal sinusitis.

   Code(s):

7. **Inpatient admission:** The elderly male patient, with type 1 diabetes, developed weakness of the right arm and leg. The weakness worsened; eventually, he fell and was unable to move. When brought to the emergency department, he was able to speak but unable to use his right arm or leg. A consultation after admission suggested either an acute left-sided cortical stroke or a TIA. Diagnostic radiographic procedures were scheduled; however, he completely recovered before the procedures could be completed and was able to ambulate with no neurological deficits within 24 hours of admission. He was discharged and will have a workup performed for cerebrovascular insufficiency as an outpatient.

   Discharge diagnoses: (1) Probable transient ischemic attack, (2) diabetes mellitus.

   Code(s):

8. **Inpatient admission:** The patient, an elderly female nursing home resident, was under medical management for chronic senile dementia and postherpetic neuralgia. She also had a history of renal cyst. She was admitted with nausea and emesis, which cleared after several days. She also complained of increasing nasal sinus congestion and headache. She was treated with antibiotics and decongestants for sinusitis. Recovery was uneventful, and she was returned to the nursing home for further care.

Discharge diagnoses: (1) Postherpetic neuralgia, (2) sinusitis, (3) chronic senile dementia.

Code(s):

9. **Neurology clinic visit:** The patient, a 23-month-old right-handed girl, has congenital mitral stenosis. After a cardiac catheterization six months earlier, she had a large middle cerebral artery infarct. She is being followed for left arm paralysis, residuals of the cerebrovascular accident. She appeared to be making progress with weekly physical therapy. The muscle strength, tone, and stretch reflexes were improved, but she had some decrease in light touch sensation.

Diagnoses: (1) Paralysis, left arm; (2) congenital mitral stenosis.

Code(s):

10. **Inpatient admission:** A 50-year-old female with terminal metastatic breast cancer is admitted to the hospital because of severe neck pain. The pain has worsened over the past week in spite of increasing amounts of oral pain medications. She is admitted for pain management and is initially given p.o. morphine 10–15 mg q. 4–6 hours p.r.n. for severe pain. During the next morning, she continues to complain of severe pain and is given IV (via peripheral vein) morphine 2 mg, which relieves her pain. Eventually, her pain subsides and the morphine is gradually tapered off. She is discharged and referred to the pain clinic for further outpatient care.

Diagnosis: Severe neck pain due to bone metastasis from malignant neoplasm of right breast.

Code(s):

7. DISEASES OF THE RESPIRATORY SYSTEM

1. **Inpatient admission:** The patient, a 51-year-old woman with acute respiratory failure secondary to an acute exacerbation of chronic obstructive bronchitis, was brought to the emergency department (ED) by emergency medical services. In the ED, she was intubated and placed on mechanical ventilation. On admission, it soon became apparent that she had suffered severe, irreversible hypoxic encephalopathy. On day 5, she was weaned from the ventilator and extubated; however, significant neurological function was never regained. In accordance with her advance directive, tube feedings were discontinued. She became febrile and dyspneic. Antibiotics were started to provide comfort and relief of her pneumonia. She expired on day 13.

   Discharge diagnoses: (1) Acute respiratory failure with hypoxia secondary to chronic obstructive bronchitis, (2) pneumonia, (3) encephalopathy.

   Code(s):

2. **Inpatient admission:** The elderly patient came to the emergency department complaining of shortness of breath and nausea. It was apparent that she was suffering from congestive heart failure and respiratory failure, and she was admitted for immediate treatment of the acute respiratory failure. Before any diagnostic work could be accomplished, she died.

   Discharge diagnoses: (1) Acute respiratory failure, (2) congestive heart failure.

   Code(s):

3. **Inpatient admission:** The patient was admitted after visiting the emergency department for shortness of breath, chest pain, hypoxia, and a white blood cell count of 32,600. The patient had a history of chronic obstructive pulmonary disease (COPD). Interstitial infiltrate at the right middle and lower lobes of the lung was seen on chest X-ray. Sputum culture grew *Streptococcus pneumoniae.* He tolerated the antibiotics, and the symptoms improved significantly.

Discharge diagnoses: (1) Right lower lobe pneumonia due to *Streptococcus pneumoniae,* (2) acute exacerbation of chronic obstructive lung disease.

Code(s):

4. **Inpatient admission:** The patient, a young man, came to the emergency department after being ill for at least three weeks. He initially had a head cold and sore throat, followed by fever, difficulty swallowing, chills, and brown sputum. Because of severe lymphadenopathy in the neck, as well as other stated symptomatology, he was admitted. A huge left tonsil confluent with the surrounding tissues and covered with exudate was also noted on the physical examination. This appeared to represent a peritonsillar abscess and severe tonsillitis. A throat culture showed a heavy growth of beta-*Streptococcus* group C. Intravenous antibiotics were given with success, and he was discharged.

Discharge diagnoses: (1) Severe tonsillitis with beta-*Streptococcus* group C, (2) probable left peritonsillar abscess.

Code(s):

5. **Inpatient admission:** A patient with type 1 diabetes was admitted with a right heel ulcer that had failed a number of outpatient therapies. Also, because the patient was hypoxic on admission with a history of COPD, he was given supplemental oxygen. He coughed up sputum, and a chest X-ray showed a mild increase in interstitial markings. Consequently, he was treated for acute bronchitis with erythromycin, which provided good results. Gradually, the foot ulcer healed. But the hypoxia persisted, and an increase in his oxygen therapy was helpful. He was to be followed by home health services.

Discharge diagnoses: (1) Diabetic foot ulcer, right heel; (2) acute bronchitis; (3) diabetes mellitus; (4) history of COPD.

Code(s):

6. **Inpatient admission:** The patient, a man in extremely poor health due to chronic obstructive pulmonary disease and chronic alcoholism, was admitted for severe shortness of breath, a PO_2 of 42, abdominal pain, and what appeared to be impending delirium tremens. He was placed on Ventolin and Solu-Medrol. Librium was also given to prevent delirium tremens. A colonoscopy was performed because of a past history of polyps, with no recurrence found. It was felt that the patient had mild colitis. On discharge, he was no longer dyspneic at rest. He was to start taking Zantac for colitis and to continue Solu-Medrol.

Discharge diagnoses: (1) Chronic lung disease with acute bronchospasm, (2) impending delirium tremens, (3) alcohol dependence, (4) colitis, (5) history of adenomatous colon polyps.

Code(s):

7. **Inpatient admission:** The patient, a 13-month-old girl, had two apnea alarms within the past few hours. After the last discharge from this hospital for apnea, an apnea alarm was ordered. Because of continued alarms, the mother returned the child to the hospital. The patient was placed on a cardiac apnea monitor with event record mode. There were no alarms noted during hospitalization. She was discharged home with an apnea monitor with event record mode in place.

   Discharge diagnosis: Rule out apnea.

   Code(s):

8. **Inpatient admission:** The patient, a three-year-old boy, was admitted for evaluation of fever, cough, and persistent pulmonary interstitial infiltrate. A chest tube was placed on the right side for drainage. The child's condition was consistent with pneumonia and aspiration of mucus. On the day after chest tube insertion, the chest X-ray was clear, and the chest tube was pulled. He was placed on aspiration precautions and antibiotics. He was to be followed up as an outpatient.

   Discharge diagnosis: Pneumonia secondary to aspiration of mucus.

   Code(s):

9. **Inpatient admission:** The patient, a five-year-old male, was seen as an outpatient for chronic asthmatic bronchitis with exacerbation without improvement. He was admitted for further treatment and on physical examination was also found to have bilateral suppurative otitis media. After being placed in a croup tent and treated with antibiotics, his temperature gradually returned to normal, and he improved.

   Discharge diagnoses: (1) Asthmatic bronchitis, (2) acute suppurative otitis media.

   Code(s):

10. **Inpatient admission:** The patient was admitted after she developed progressive dyspnea and wheezing, intractable to ambulatory care management. The provisional admitting diagnosis was status asthmaticus. Her history showed that she was status post mastectomy for breast cancer and still had some residual lymphedema in the left upper extremity. In the hospital, she received low-flow oxygen, antibiotics, bronchodilators, and IV steroids, as well as her usual medications for hypertension and hypothyroidism.

Discharge diagnoses: (1) Status asthmaticus, (2) hypertension, (3) hypothyroidism, (4) status post breast cancer with lymphedema.

Code(s):

11. **Inpatient admission:** The patient, an elderly woman, was known to have congestive heart failure, arteriosclerotic heart disease, and chronic obstructive pulmonary disease. She had no history of coronary artery bypass grafting. She developed increased shortness of breath, dyspnea on exertion, temperature elevation, and productive cough. These problems were felt to represent congestive heart failure and pneumonia. She was admitted for cultures, IV antibiotics, pulmonary toilet, and increased diuresis. Her initial non-contrast chest film showed congestive heart failure and bilateral lung infiltrates. In discussing this case with the pulmonary consultant, the physician felt it was wise to transfer the patient to another hospital so that both pulmonary and cardiology staff could work together with this patient.

Discharge diagnoses: (1) Arteriosclerotic heart disease, (2) congestive heart failure, (3) pneumonia, (4) chronic obstructive lung disease.

Code(s):

12. **Inpatient admission:** The patient, a 94-year-old man with known arteriosclerotic coronary artery disease, no history of bypass, and exacerbation of end-stage chronic obstructive bronchitis, was admitted with a provisional diagnosis of acute respiratory failure. He was treated with IV antibiotics and pulmonary toilet. Although his long-term prognosis was poor, he was improved upon discharge.

Discharge diagnoses: (1) Arteriosclerotic coronary artery disease, (2) end-stage chronic obstructive bronchitis, (3) angina, (4) acute respiratory failure.

Code(s):

13. **Inpatient admission:** The patient, a five-week-old infant, had been discharged from the hospital following her birth without any complaints. She was now admitted through the emergency department, where she was found to be febrile and lethargic and to have a weak cry. Dry mucous membranes were also noted. The admission diagnosis was "rule out sepsis." She was given STAT respiratory treatment and IV fluids, followed by intravenous antibiotics. Urine cultures grew *Enterococcus.* Blood cultures were negative. Sputum cultures grew *Mycoplasma pneumoniae.* She gradually improved and was weaned from the oxygen tent. She improved rapidly and was discharged three days following admission.

    Discharge diagnoses: (1) Right lower lobe pneumonitis due to *Mycoplasma pneumoniae,* (2) fever, (3) dehydration, (4) urinary tract infection.

    Code(s):

14. **Inpatient admission:** The patient, an 18-month-old male, was admitted with reactive airway disease versus viral pneumonia. His symptoms of wheezing and congestion had become increasingly worse over the past few days. He had been healthy since birth except for congenital pulmonary stenosis, which was evaluated during this admission. He was placed on medications and oxygen. Blood culture and viral panel were negative. He was to be followed by the pulmonary clinic.

    Discharge diagnoses: (1) Acute exacerbation of reactive airway disease, (2) mild pulmonary stenosis.

    Code(s):

15. **Inpatient admission:** A 76-year-old female with known Hodgkin intrathoracic lymphoma was admitted for malignant pleural effusion. She had previously undergone thoracentesis with symptomatic relief. Because of the recurrence of the effusion, video-assisted thoracoscopic (VAT) surgery was carried out, along with left pleurodesis and the injection of talc.

    Discharge diagnoses: (1) Malignant pleural effusion, (2) Hodgkin intrathoracic lymphoma.

    Code(s):

8. DISEASES OF THE DIGESTIVE SYSTEM

1. **Inpatient admission:** Three weeks after undergoing a gastric bypass, this patient was admitted because of continuous vomiting and severe dehydration. Radiological and laboratory studies provided no indication of problems with the previous surgery or other abnormalities. Rehydration was accomplished. On close observation, it appeared that she was eating too fast and too much.

   Discharge diagnoses: (1) Exogenous morbid obesity with recent gastric bypass, (2) dehydration due to continuous vomiting.

   Code(s):

2. **Inpatient admission:** The elderly nursing home patient was admitted with aspiration pneumonitis. She was unable to swallow or eat as a result of a stroke, which occurred two months earlier. She was experiencing progressive aspiration and weight loss. It was hoped that anchoring a feeding tube would alleviate the situation. Therefore, a percutaneous gastrostomy with placement of a feeding tube with endoscopic guidance was performed.

   Discharge diagnoses: (1) Difficulty swallowing secondary to cerebrovascular infarction, (2) impending malnutrition, (3) aspiration pneumonia.

   Code(s):

3. **Inpatient admission:** The patient was transferred from facility A, where he experienced 12 hours of hematemesis requiring transfusions with 14 units of red blood cells and 6 units of fresh-frozen plasma. Upon admission to facility B, a gastroscopic examination revealed a 4- by 2-centimeter gastric ulcer with visible vessels. He was taken to the operating room, where a hemigastrectomy with Billroth I anastomosis of the duodenum was performed.

   Discharge diagnosis: Bleeding gastric ulcer.

   Code(s):

4. Inpatient admission: The patient's admitting diagnosis was acute pancreatitis. Findings on a CT scan performed prior to admission were consistent with acute and chronic pancreatitis and pancreatic duct calculi. Multiple stones were noted on endoscopic retrograde cholangiopancreatography (ERCP); one of them was big enough to occlude the pancreatic duct. There was generalized stenosis of the pancreatic duct. (During ERCP, a stent was put in place to bypass the area of obstruction. The patient improved immediately.) Extracorporeal shock wave lithotripsy (ESWL) then achieved partial fragmentation of the stone. Because of abdominal pain, a second ESWL was required and, again, achieved only partial fragmentation of the stone. The patient underwent another ERCP, which identified multiple stones and pancreatic duct stenosis with occlusion of the previously placed stent. During the procedure, the obstructed area was passed through, but there was still a 2-millimeter area of pancreatic duct stenosis. A balloon was inserted to dilate this area endoscopically. There were multiple stones, and the occluded stent was removed and replaced with a new one beyond the area of obstruction. No puncture of the skin or mucous membrane was necessary to remove or replace the occluded stent.

Discharge diagnoses: (1) Acute and chronic pancreatitis, (2) pancreatic calculi.

Procedures: (1) ERCP with pancreatic duct stent insertion, (2) ESWL (pancreatic stone) on two separate occasions, (3) ERCP with prolonged dilation of pancreatic duct and removal of occluded stent and replacement with a new, single-pigtail stent.

Code(s):

5. Outpatient visit: The patient came in complaining of severe abdominal pain. Abdominal scout film showed scoliosis and some degenerative changes in the lumbar spine. However, a high osmolar contrast abdominal CT scan showed extensive diverticulosis involving the descending and sigmoid portions of the colon, with obvious evidence of diverticulitis.

Diagnosis: Diverticulitis.

Code(s):

6. **Inpatient admission:** The 86-year-old woman was admitted with rectal bleeding. She was also massively dehydrated, with a BUN of 124. On admission, some IV fluids and transfusions of whole blood via a peripheral vein were administered because her initial hemoglobin was 9.5 and later dropped to 7.4. On colonoscopy, multiple ulcers of the rectum, consistent with ulcerative proctitis, were found and brush biopsies were taken. The tissue was negative for neoplastic disease, and the patient was started on steroid enemas, with resolution.

Discharge diagnoses: (1) Rectal bleeding, (2) dehydration, (3) acute blood loss anemia, (4) ulcerative proctitis.

Code(s):

7. **Inpatient admission:** The patient, a 20-year-old female, presented to the emergency department complaining of bilateral arm and shoulder pain, "yellow eyes," and dark urine. The emergency department evaluation revealed profound jaundice with markedly elevated liver function tests. The patient was admitted for further evaluation. A non-contrast gallbladder ultrasound was negative for gallstones. Hematological studies indicated sickle-cell disease, which could be contributing to the jaundice. Because the liver function gradually improved, it was felt that she could be further evaluated as an outpatient for probable acute hepatitis B.

Discharge diagnosis: Jaundice secondary to sickle-cell disease versus acute hepatitis B.

Code(s):

8. **Inpatient admission:** The patient was admitted for evaluation of guaiac-positive stools. All sites that could be visualized on esophagogastroduodenoscopy (EGD) were within normal limits except a small area in the gastric fundus, which was excised for biopsy. A colonoscope was then inserted to 35 centimeters, and diverticula were noted. Because of narrowing resulting from edema due to diverticulitis, it was not possible to pass the scope farther. The tissue report showed benign acute and chronic gastritis but no ulcer.

Discharge diagnoses: (1) Occult blood in stool of undetermined origin, (2) diverticulosis with diverticulitis of colon, (3) acute and chronic gastritis.

Code(s):

9. **Inpatient admission (episode 1):** Because the patient had a 20-year history of severe complicated ulcerative colitis, he was admitted for surgical intervention. A total abdominal colectomy with ileostomy was performed. The postoperative recovery was without incident.

Discharge diagnosis: Ulcerative colitis.

Code(s):

Inpatient admission (episode 2): Three months after surgery, the patient was again admitted for a percutaneous endoscopic endorectal pull-through with excision of the submucosal portion of the rectum with endoscopic formation of a loop ileostomy via the existing ileostomy. This procedure was further treatment for the long-standing and intractable ulcerative colitis.

Discharge diagnosis: Ulcerative colitis.

Code(s):

Inpatient admission (episode 3): Four months after the second surgery, the patient was admitted for ileostomy closure. An incision was made around the stoma, the intestine was pulled out of the abdominal wall, and the ends were excised. Anastomosis was secured by staples. He had no symptoms of ulcerative colitis. The postoperative course was uneventful.

Discharge diagnosis: Status post ileostomy closure.

Code(s):

10. **Inpatient admission:** The patient experienced rectal pain for several months due to a 2.5-centimeter mass on the anterior rectal wall. An open excision of the mass was performed, and a frozen section revealed an inflammatory lesion without evidence of malignancy. The final pathology report showed the tissue to represent a granuloma of the rectum.

    Discharge diagnosis: Rectal granuloma.

Code(s):

11. **Inpatient admission:** The patient, a woman with chronic right upper-quadrant abdominal pain, was admitted for possible pancreatitis after two episodes of vomiting clear fluid. Pain medications were started, and a nasogastric (NG) tube was placed for drainage, with intermittent suction. The NG tube was pulled three days after admission, and the patient was discharged to follow up with her physician one week later.

    Discharge diagnosis: Pancreatitis.

    Principal procedure: Insertion, nasogastric tube.

Code(s):

12. **Inpatient admission:** The patient, a man with a long history of alcohol dependence with resultant alcoholic cirrhosis, was admitted with red, coffee-ground hematemesis. An emergent esophagogastroduodenoscopy revealed bleeding esophageal varices, which were excised. The varices are secondary to the alcoholic cirrhosis. No problems were identified in the stomach or duodenum. He was transfused via peripheral vein in his left arm with multiple units of packed red cells and frozen plasma, and yet the bleeding continued. He was returned to surgery, and an esophagoscopy was performed to sclerose the bleeding esophageal varices a second time.

Discharge diagnoses: (1) Upper gastrointestinal bleed, (2) esophageal varices, (3) Laennec's cirrhosis, (4) alcohol dependence.

Principal procedure: Control of esophageal bleeding by excision of varices.

Code(s):

13. **Inpatient admission:** The patient, a 35-year-old male, was admitted for possible gastritis. He had undergone a cadaveric renal transplant for end-stage renal disease secondary to focal membranous glomerulonephritis two years earlier. On endoscopic examination of the lower esophagus and stomach, patchy erythemas were seen in the stomach and brush biopsies of the stomach were taken. A linear erosion was noted at the gastroesophageal junction with recent bleeding. The impression was mild reflux esophagitis and mild antral duodenitis. As his dietary intake improved, his physical condition improved as well.

Discharge diagnoses: (1) Reflux esophagitis with bleeding, (2) duodenitis.

Code(s):

14. **Inpatient admission:** The patient recently underwent an ultrasound that showed a filling defect in the gallbladder, thought to represent a cholelithiasis. The physician concluded that the woman's symptoms were suggestive of cholecystitis and that cholecystectomy was in order. On admission, a laparoscopic cholecystectomy with lysis of adhesions around the gallbladder was carried out, followed by a contrast intraoperative cholangiogram. A proctologist was consulted due to the presence of persistent rectal pain. A mild anal fissure was identified on flexible sigmoidoscopy. An excisional needle biopsy of the liver was performed due to an abnormal liver function study times 3. The pathology report indicated that the liver tissue was normal.

Discharge diagnoses: (1) Chronic cholecystitis and cholelithiasis, (2) anal fissure, (3) abnormal liver function studies.

Code(s):

15. **Inpatient admission:** The male patient came in complaining of headache, nausea, vomiting, and chest pain. The impression on admission was possible coronary artery disease and probable viral gastroenteritis. Only a small, sliding hiatal hernia was found on air contrast upper GI. No ischemia was found on cardiac evaluation. The patient gradually improved and was discharged two days later to follow up with his family physician in one week for gastroenteritis and further evaluation of the hiatal hernia.

Discharge diagnoses: (1) Probable viral gastroenteritis, (2) hiatal hernia.

Code(s):

16. **Inpatient admission:** The patient, a woman with a long history of Crohn's disease, was admitted with abdominal cramping, vomiting, and diarrhea of sudden onset. Admitting orders included all current medications for Crohn's disease. Her amylase was 241 on admission, and she had a slightly elevated white blood count. Both returned to normal with treatment for pancreatitis, and the abdominal problems also slowed down. She was to be followed as an outpatient.

Discharge diagnoses: (1) Pancreatitis, (2) Crohn's disease.

Code(s):

17. **Physician office visit (episode 1):** The patient, an elderly woman, came in for severe epigastric abdominal pain. She had some nausea but no vomiting. She was referred for further studies to rule out cholecystitis and localized ulcer perforation.

Diagnosis: Possible cholecystitis and/or perforated gastric ulcer.

Code(s):

Inpatient admission (episode 2): An ultrasound was negative and an upper GI endoscopy failed to yield a diagnosis. Therefore, the patient was admitted for further evaluation because of the continued severity of her abdominal pain. An exploratory laparotomy was performed and immediately revealed a perforated appendix lying in a subhepatic space with abscess. An appendectomy was performed. The abscess cleared postoperatively with administration of high doses of intravenous antibiotics.

Discharge diagnosis: Appendicitis with perforation and subhepatic abscess.

Code(s):

18. **Inpatient admission:** The patient was admitted with vague abdominal pain, and a workup was carried out. All laboratory findings were within normal limits, except for a slightly elevated white blood cell count. The patient requested transfer to another hospital close to his home for further evaluation. The patient was transferred with a working diagnosis of diverticulitis versus colon tumor.

Discharge diagnosis: Diverticulitis versus tumor of colon.

Code(s):

19. **Inpatient admission:** The patient, an eight-year-old boy, was brought to the hospital from school because of persistent cyclical vomiting with accompanying abdominal pain. He was admitted for observation and monitoring of vital signs. Laboratory work was within normal limits, vital signs remained stable, the abdomen remained flat and soft, and there was no muscle guarding or tenderness. He was discharged the following day in an improved condition.

Discharge diagnoses: (1) Cyclical vomiting syndrome, (2) abdominal pain.

Code(s):

20. **Inpatient admission:** The patient had a history of recurrent infections in the perianal area. He was seen two days earlier in the physician's office for a perianal abscess and anal fistula. The prescribed medication and enemas did not alleviate the situation, so he was admitted for surgical intervention. In surgery, an anal fistulotomy was performed on the skin of the perineum with drainage of the perianal abscess. The patient responded to further treatments of antibiotics and diet and was to be followed in the office.

Discharge diagnoses: (1) Perianal abscess, (2) anal fistula.

Code(s):

21. **Inpatient admission:** The patient is status post heart transplantation six months earlier. Since then, he had been admitted numerous times for fever and diarrhea, presumably due to cytomegalovirus. On this occasion, he was admitted for further evaluation of fever and diarrhea. Stool and blood cultures were negative. A single, shallow erosion in the colon was viewed and excised for biopsy on colonoscopy. Internal, bleeding hemorrhoids were also visualized. The pathology report showed moderate, nonspecific, chronic colitis with no diagnostic evidence of cytomegalovirus. Chronic colitis was determined to be the cause of the patient's symptomatology. The patient was also followed by endocrinology for his diabetes, and no changes were recommended in his medication. His diarrhea improved, medication and diet were prescribed for bleeding hemorrhoids and chronic colitis, and he was released.

Discharge diagnoses: (1) Chronic colitis; (2) bleeding internal hemorrhoids; (3) diabetes mellitus, type 1; (4) status post heart transplant.

Code(s):

22. **Inpatient admission:** The patient had undergone cardiac transplantation about three years earlier. On this occasion, he came to the emergency department with a three-day history of right lower quadrant pain. The white blood cell count was elevated, and a small-bowel X-ray examination showed some dilated small bowel loops but no free air. He was admitted, and an abdominal gastrointestinal ultrasound showed a mass measuring about 5 by 5 by 4 centimeters, which was presumed to be an appendiceal cyst. He underwent an ultrasound-directed percutaneous right lower quadrant aspiration; only a few drops of material were collected for diagnostic examination. Blood cultures were sterile, leukocytosis improved, and he remained afebrile with gradually decreasing pain. He was discharged on antibiotics and was to return in a few weeks for an interval appendectomy.

Discharge diagnoses: (1) Probable appendiceal cyst, (2) status post cardiac transplantation.

Procedure performed: Ultrasound-directed aspiration of appendiceal mass.

Code(s):

9. DISEASES OF THE GENITOURINARY SYSTEM

1. **Inpatient admission:** The patient, an 83-year-old woman, was admitted after coming to the emergency department complaining of fever, confusion, and lethargy. Urine and blood cultures were positive for *E. coli.* Sepsis and urinary tract infection were diagnosed. The patient slowly responded to IV antibiotic therapy, but she began to experience vomiting episodes with abdominal pain. These episodes were probably related to her hiatal hernia with reflux esophagitis. The vomiting seemed to improve with medications and diet. The patient was discharged one week following admission on oral Keflex and Zantac to follow up as an outpatient.

   Discharge diagnoses: (1) Urinary tract infection, (2) gram-negative sepsis secondary to diagnosis 1, (3) hiatal hernia with reflux esophagitis.

   Code(s):

2. **Inpatient admission:** The patient was admitted for abnormal uterine bleeding. An ultrasound performed prior to admission suggested a possible bicornuate uterus. Because of her morbid obesity, a hysteroscopy with dilation and curettage was performed. Findings indicated a single cavity without any septum, polyps, or submucous fibroids. The patient was seen by the dietitian and discharged on a 1,500-calorie diet to reduce her weight.

   Discharge diagnoses: (1) Morbid obesity, (2) abnormal uterine bleeding unrelated to menstruation.

   Code(s):

3. **Inpatient admission:** The patient, a young man with hypertensive heart disease and end-stage renal disease, was admitted for placement of an arteriovenous fistula in his left arm to prepare for hemodialysis. The AV fistula was accomplished between the left radial artery and cephalic antebrachial vein in the lower arm. A single 4-hour intermittent hemodialysis session was provided to treat the end-stage chronic kidney disease.

   Discharge diagnoses: (1) Hypertensive heart disease and nephrosclerosis, (2) end-stage chronic kidney disease.

Code(s):

4. **Inpatient admission:** The patient had a history of frequent episodes of severe chronic interstitial cystitis. Despite previous treatment, she has had no resolution of her symptoms. She was admitted for and received an open partial cystectomy and bilateral ileoureterostomy.

   Discharge diagnosis: Severe, chronic interstitial cystitis.

Code(s):

5. **Inpatient admission:** The patient had chronic kidney disease secondary to malignant hypertension and was status post insertion of a left arteriovenous fistula six months earlier. He presented with exacerbation of his renal condition and was admitted for evaluation and hemodialysis. His medications were adjusted, and he received several 5-hour intermittent hemodialysis sessions during this admission. His condition stabilized, and he was discharged in an improved state.

   Discharge diagnoses: (1) End-stage renal disease associated with malignant hypertension, (2) exacerbation of kidney disease.

Code(s):

6. **Inpatient admission:** The patient had end-stage renal disease and chronic kidney disease secondary to hypertension. He was admitted for a cadaveric renal transplant. He underwent a single 4-hour renal hemodialysis session prior to transplant. The left donor kidney was placed in the right iliac fossa. Postoperative recovery was uneventful.

Discharge diagnosis: End-stage renal disease resulting from hypertension.

Code(s):

7. **Inpatient admission:** The patient became ill the day before admission with nausea, vomiting, dysuria, and hematuria. Initial laboratory work included a urinalysis report of red blood cells too numerous to count, and a repeat urinalysis the following day reported the same results. On contrast retrograde pyelogram of both kidneys, the ureters, and the bladder, hydronephrosis of the right kidney and possibly some secondary hydronephrosis with obstruction of the ureteropelvic junction were seen. Spontaneously, the hematuria and other symptoms cleared. The patient was to be referred to a urologist for follow-up.

Discharge diagnosis: Hematuria and hydronephrosis possibly due to idiopathic ureteropelvic obstruction.

Code(s):

8. **Physician office visit (episode 1):** The patient, an elderly man, has had carcinoma of the bladder with numerous recurrences since 2007. On his annual bladder checkup, an obstructive prostate with urinary retention was present, but no evidence of a recurrence of the carcinoma was found. He was to be admitted for further evaluation of the prostatic obstruction.

Diagnoses: (1) Prostatic obstruction with urinary retention, (2) no evidence of recurrence of bladder carcinoma.

Code(s):

Inpatient admission (episode 2): On cystoscopy, a mild urethral stricture and an obstructive prostate with urinary retention were found. The urethra was dilated, and the patient underwent transurethral prostatectomy (TURP) without complication. The pathology report showed benign prostatic hypertrophy.

Discharge diagnoses: (1) Urethral stricture secondary to benign prostatic hypertrophy (BPH), (2) urinary retention, (3) history of carcinoma of the bladder.

Code(s):

9. **Inpatient admission:** The nursing home patient had frequent urinary tract infections and numerous courses of antibiotics. The most recent urine culture grew *Pseudomonas aeruginosa*, resistant to all oral antibiotics. The patient was admitted for IV antibiotic therapy. Significant in her history was the placement about three years earlier of a cardiac pacemaker for conduction defects. It was working satisfactorily during her hospitalization. Because the cultures continued to show *Pseudomonas* after IV antibiotics were given, a cystoscopy was performed. The patient still had a bladder infection with erythema of the bladder wall. Urine cultures were obtained at that time, and the report showed a high colony count of *Pseudomonas* that was then susceptible to oral antibiotics. She was discharged on oral Cipro.

Discharge diagnoses: (1) Bladder infection, resistant to oral antibiotics; (2) pacemaker in situ.

Code(s):

10. **Inpatient admission:** The patient was experiencing heavy, abnormal uterine bleeding and abdominal pain. On vaginal examination, there was bright red blood in the vagina and the left adnexa was enlarged. The woman was admitted and taken to surgery, where an exploratory laparotomy revealed a left follicular ovarian cyst. While the surgeon was examining the left ovary, the cyst spontaneously ruptured. An ovarian cystectomy was performed without complication. The postoperative course was uneventful, and the patient was discharged.

   Discharge diagnosis: Ruptured left follicular ovarian cyst.

   Code(s):

11. **Inpatient admission:** The male patient was admitted with severe colic secondary to a left ureteral calculus. A cystoscopy was performed, and a stone extracted. On retrograde pyelography, no stone was seen in the ureter or kidney. However, the pathology report indicated that only a small fragment of the stone was retrieved. Postoperatively, the patient did well at first but then began having severe colic again. He was returned to surgery for another cystoscopy. The remainder of the stone was located in the distal left ureter and extracted. The postoperative course was uncomplicated.

   Discharge diagnosis: Left ureteral calculus.

   Code(s):

12. **Inpatient admission:** The patient, a woman with insignificant past medical and surgical history, was to be a living related kidney donor for her brother, a patient with end-stage renal disease secondary to hypertension. She was prepared for surgery the day of admission, but the surgery was canceled due to her brother's active hepatitis C infection.

   Discharge diagnoses: (1) Kidney donor, (2) procedure canceled.

   Code(s):

13. **Inpatient admission:** The patient was previously evaluated and found to be a suitable kidney donor for his eight-year-old son. A total unilateral left donor nephrectomy was performed without complication, and the patient was discharged.

    Discharge diagnosis: Donor nephrectomy.

    Code(s):

14. **Inpatient admission:** The patient, a young woman, was admitted with a two-day history of dysuria, frequency, and urgency, with onset of severe flank pain on the evening prior to admission. A laboratory workup confirmed pyelonephritis, and she was immediately started on intravenous medications and fluid. Urine cultures grew *Enterobacter aerogenes,* which was sensitive to several antibiotics.

    Discharge diagnoses: (1) Acute pyelonephritis, (2) abdominal and flank pain.

    Code(s):

15. **Inpatient admission:** The patient was admitted for a hysterectomy. Prior to admission, a diagnostic workup showed extensive endometriosis involving the uterus, ovaries, and fallopian tubes. Because the patient had asthma, she was seen by the pulmonary consult service and cleared for surgery. A total abdominal hysterectomy and a bilateral salpingo-oophorectomy were performed without complication. Postoperatively, the patient did well and was discharged.

    Discharge diagnoses: (1) Endometriosis of uterus, ovaries, and fallopian tubes; (2) asthma.

    Code(s):

16. **Inpatient admission:** The patient, a young woman, was admitted for treatment of a persistent, symptomatic right adnexal mass. The cystic mass was about 5 centimeters and presumed to be ovarian in origin. An exploratory laparotomy was performed, with right ovarian cystectomy. Pathological findings confirmed a follicular cyst. The patient's postoperative course was unremarkable, and she was discharged.

Discharge diagnosis: Follicular cyst, right ovary.

Code(s):

17. **Inpatient admission:** A patient with irregular but heavy menstruation and hirsute of face and abdomen was seen for an X-ray that was suggestive of ovarian mass. An exploratory laparotomy was performed with wedge biopsy of both ovaries; results were consistent with primary polycystic ovary syndrome. The patient was started on oral contraceptives to decrease testosterone levels.

Discharge diagnosis: Polycystic ovary syndrome.

Code(s):

18. **Inpatient admission:** The patient had a four-month history of gross hematuria. A kidney ultrasound showed lesion of bladder. A cystoscopy confirmed lesion of trigone bladder. The patient was then admitted for open radical cystoprostatectomy with urinary diversion due to infiltrative mucinous adenocarcinoma. Once the bladder, prostate, and seminal vesicles were removed, an ureteroenteric anastomosis was performed to connect the ureters to a newly created ileostomy.

Discharge diagnosis: Adenocarcinoma trigone bladder.

Code(s):

10. DISEASES OF THE SKIN AND SUBCUTANEOUS TISSUE

1. **Inpatient admission:** The female patient was admitted for treatment of an open wound of the scalp with cellulitis of the scalp and left ear. The wound was the result of a cut two days before admission. Excisional debridement of both the scalp and the left ear was carried out in the operating room. The patient was treated with antibiotics during her two-day stay. She was discharged on oral antibiotics in an improved condition.

   Discharge diagnosis: Cellulitis of scalp and ear secondary to scalp laceration.

   Code(s):

2. **Inpatient admission:** The patient, a young man with spina bifida of the lumbar region, was admitted for excision of a sacral pressure ulcer. He had a ventriculoperitoneal shunt in place on the right side for hydrocephalus. The lesion was successfully fulgurated without complication.

   Discharge diagnoses: (1) Stage 3 pressure ulcer, sacrum; (2) lumbar spina bifida; (3) status post placement of a ventriculoperitoneal shunt for hydrocephalus.

   Code(s):

3. **Inpatient admission:** The female patient was admitted from the nursing home with a large stage 3 sacral pressure ulcer, which was treated with excisional debridement and a skin pedicle flap-graft closure of the back. She had chronic lymphocytic B-cell leukemia, which required peripheral vein transfusions with three units of whole blood. She was stabilized and returned to the nursing home.

   Discharge diagnoses: (1) Pressure ulcer, sacrum; (2) chronic lymphocytic leukemia.

   Code(s):

4. **Inpatient admission:** The patient, an elderly man, had an acute onset of swelling, erythema, and tenderness in the left anterior neck. He was admitted for evaluation and IV antibiotic therapy, with provisional diagnoses of thyroiditis and cellulitis. Radiological findings showed a large, mixed-density, soft-tissue mass in the left lower neck consistent with cellulitis. The mass appeared to involve the soft tissue of the neck but not the thyroid gland. Abscess formation could not be excluded, although none was directly visualized. His symptomatology responded well to antibiotic therapy.

   Discharge diagnoses: (1) Cellulitis, (2) possible abscess.

Code(s):

5. **Inpatient admission:** The patient's admitting diagnoses were abdominal pain and ventral wall hernia. The woman presented for hernia repair. At the time of surgery, she was noted to have numerous mid-abdominal adhesions of the peritoneum, mostly in the area of a previous midline scar. Sharp lysis of the extensive adhesions was undertaken, and then the hernia was repaired. Postoperatively, the patient did very well.

   Discharge diagnoses: (1) Ventral wall hernia, (2) abdominal adhesions.

Code(s):

6. **Inpatient admission:** The patient was admitted for intravenous antibiotic treatment of cellulitis of the left leg secondary to a minor scratch. By the third hospital day, the erythema was much improved. During the entire hospitalization, the patient, a known opioid drug abuser, exhibited considerable drug-seeking behavior and requested narcotics, especially IV morphine. All narcotics were discontinued on the third hospital day, and he exhibited no withdrawal symptoms. He was discharged for follow-up in the physician's office.

   Discharge diagnoses: (1) Cellulitis, left leg; (2) drug abuse; (3) scratch, left leg.

Code(s):

7. **Inpatient admission:** A patient was diagnosed with radiation recall dermatitis of the right chest after starting amoxicillin for urinary tract infection due to *E. coli*. Medical history indicated administration of extra-beam radiation to the area one year ago in treatment of poorly differentiated squamous cell carcinoma of right lung. The provider documented that the dermatitis at the previously irradiated chest was the result of the prescribed antibiotic use. The amoxicillin was discontinued and the patient was started on a different antibiotic.

Discharge diagnoses: (1) Dermatitis of right chest, (2) urinary tract infection, (3) current primary carcinoma of right lung, (4) history of radiation.

Code(s):

8. **Inpatient admission:** A patient was admitted for incision and drainage of chin abscess. A blade was used to open the draining area. A small amount of purulent material was expressed. The area was bluntly dissected widely around the abscess pocket, and the wound was drained of fluid.

Discharge diagnosis: Incision and drainage of MRSA abscess of the skin.

Code(s):

9. **Outpatient visit:** A patient was seen for six-month swelling and tenderness of the left cheek. Excised skin and subcutaneous tissue of the area resulted in a diagnosis of hyaline necrosis, a hallmark for lupus profundus.

Discharge diagnosis: Lupus erythematosus profundus

Code(s):

11. DISEASES OF THE MUSCULOSKELETAL SYSTEM AND CONNECTIVE TISSUE

1. **Inpatient admission:** The patient had experienced increasingly severe pain in his left arm, left shoulder, and neck for two months. Magnetic resonance imaging performed prior to admission showed evidence of a C7–T1 disc herniation. His only other health problem was benign hypertension, which was controlled with medications. He was admitted for a cervical laminotomy and complete cervical discectomy of the cervical thoracic disc, which were performed by oblique, muscle-splitting incision. His postoperative course was unremarkable, and he was discharged after two days.

   Discharge diagnoses: (1) Cervical disc herniation, C7–T1; (2) benign essential hypertension.

   Code(s):

2. **Outpatient encounter (episode 1):** The patient's complaints were neck pain that radiated into both arms, hand pain with numbness and clumsiness, and electric shock–type pains down her body when she bent down. A magnetic resonance imaging scan showed marked spinal stenosis at C3–C4 and C5–C6. She was to be admitted for repair of the spinal stenosis.

   Diagnosis: Spinal stenosis.

   Code(s):

   Inpatient admission (episode 2): The patient was admitted for repair of spinal stenosis. An excision of discs at C3–C4 and C5–C6 with fusion was carried out using an anterior approach. A graft of bone was excised from the right iliac crest.

   Discharge diagnosis: Severe cervical spine stenosis.

   Code(s):

3. **Inpatient admission:** The patient, a 33-year-old woman, had a history of low back pain. She recently developed intractable left sciatic pain and paresthesia. Lumbar magnetic resonance imaging procedures, performed prior to admission, showed progressive lumbosacral disc herniation on the left. She was also receiving medications for gastric ulcers and asthma, and these were continued during the hospital stay. A lumbosacral microdiscectomy was performed for a protruded lumbosacral disc herniation, which also had a subligamentous extrusion. The patient recovered with resolution of symptoms and was discharged to follow up with her physician in one week.

Discharge diagnoses: (1) Lumbosacral disc extrusion, (2) gastric ulcers, (3) asthma.

Code(s):

4. **Inpatient admission:** The teenage patient had complained of left hip pain for the past three weeks. The pain started after a fall that occurred while he was playing basketball in a gym. X-rays revealed a grade I, slipped capital femoral epiphysis of the left hip. The hip was pinned percutaneously, and the postoperative course was uneventful.

Discharge diagnosis: Slipped capital femoral epiphysis, left hip.

Code(s):

5. **Inpatient admission:** An emergency open repair of a right rotator cuff tear was performed on this patient after she was crushed between a sliding patio door and its frame at her apartment. Exploration revealed a torn right rotator cuff and ruptured deltoid muscle, right shoulder. Open repair of the rotator cuff tendon and repair of the ruptured deltoid muscle were accomplished. The patient recovered and was discharged to follow-up in one week.

Discharge diagnoses: (1) Tear, right rotator cuff; (2) rupture, deltoid muscle.

Code(s):

6. **Inpatient admission:** The patient, status post cadaveric renal and pancreas transplants with type 2 diabetes and diabetic peripheral angiopathy, had a nonhealing ulcer on his left heel with muscle necrosis that had been debrided three weeks earlier. He came to the emergency department complaining of a three-day history of left foot pain, fever, and foul-smelling discharge from the ulcer. He was admitted, and a left below-the-knee amputation of the lower leg at the distal portion of the tibia and fibula was performed.

Discharge diagnosis: Diabetic gangrene of the left foot.

Code(s):

7. **Inpatient admission:** The patient, an elderly man with chest pain, was admitted to rule out acute myocardial infarction. Two weeks prior to admission, he had a respiratory infection that caused excessive coughing. On evaluation, there was no evidence of cardiac problems, and his chest pain was believed to be due to costochondritis secondary to excessive coughing.

   Discharge diagnosis: Costochondritis.

   Code(s):

8. **Inpatient admission:** The patient, an elderly woman, had severe pain in her left hip. The pain started after a hip fracture five years ago, when she was injured in an automobile accident. Her admission diagnoses were traumatic arthritis and ankylosis of the left hip. She also had a pacemaker and had type 2 diabetes. A total hip replacement was performed without complication.

   Discharge diagnoses: (1) Arthritis and ankylosis secondary to old hip fracture, left side; (2) diabetes mellitus.

   Code(s):

9. **Inpatient admission:** The patient's right knee had bothered him for several months. He had a very painful chronic, indolent, septic prepatellar bursa. It was treated with many antibiotics, cleared up, and then recurred. He was currently admitted for surgical intervention. The site was incised and drained, and then the prepatellar bursa was partially excised. He was referred for physical therapy on discharge.

   Discharge diagnosis: Septic joint, bacterial, right knee.

   Code(s):

10. **Inpatient admission:** For two weeks, the patient had been complaining of left sciatica and had failed outpatient management with bed rest and pain medications. A magnetic resonance imaging procedure confirmed L5–S1 disc herniation on the left. She was hospitalized at complete bed rest with conservative management and pain medications as needed. She received good pain relief with IV pain medication and an epidural spinal space steroid injection. She was discharged for physical therapy follow-up.

Discharge diagnosis: Intractable pain secondary to herniation of the L5–S1 disc, with S1 radiculopathy.

Code(s):

11. **Inpatient admission:** The patient was admitted with traumatic arthritis of the left hip due to an old fracture of the femoral neck suffered in a car accident. She underwent a partial hip resurfacing of the femoral head with placement of resurfacing device. The surgery and postoperative course were without complication.

Discharge diagnosis: Posttraumatic left hip arthritis.

Code(s):

648

12. **Inpatient admission:** The patient, a 12-year-old female, had a history of scoliosis secondary to neurofibromatosis, type 1, and had been treated with a brace for four years. She was now admitted for surgical repair of the progressive scoliosis. A posterior approach anterior column lumbar fusion of T2–L3 using Isola instrumentation interbody fusion device and right iliac crest bone grafting was performed. Her postoperative course was uneventful.

    Discharge diagnosis: Thoracolumbar scoliosis secondary to neurofibromatosis, type 1.

    Code(s):

13. **Inpatient admission:** A 59-year-old man was admitted for reverse total shoulder arthroplasty to treat severe degenerative joint disease of the right glenohumeral joint and supraspinatus tear of the right shoulder. The glenoid and humeral components were placed after ensuring adequate bone support.

    Discharge diagnoses: (1) Supraspinatus tear, (2) degenerative joint disease of shoulder.

    Code(s):

14. **Inpatient admission:** A patient was seen for spontaneous rupture of the flexor digitorum profundus tendon of the left little finger. The area was opened for exploration; the proximal end of the tendon was repaired with sutures.

    Discharge diagnosis: Rupture of the tendon of left little finger.

    Code(s):

12. COMPLICATIONS OF PREGNANCY, CHILDBIRTH, AND THE PUERPERIUM

1. **Inpatient admission (episode 1):** The patient was admitted with pregnancy at 38 weeks' gestation. A repeat low transverse cervical cesarean section and elective open bilateral tubal ligation were performed. A 3,300-gram male infant was delivered; Apgar scores were 9 and 10. The postoperative course was unremarkable. On day 3, the mother's staples were removed, and both the mother and the baby were discharged.

   Discharge diagnoses: (1) Term pregnancy delivered, (2) elective tubal ligation.

   Code(s):

   Inpatient admission (episode 2): The patient underwent a cesarean section seven days earlier. She had an intramuscular abscess/infection of the operative wound at the time she was admitted through the emergency department with a temperature of 101 degrees and minimal drainage of the incision. IV Kefzol was started, but she continued to spike up to a temperature of 101.8 degrees. The antibiotic therapy was changed, and the patient defervesced.

   Discharge diagnosis: Postoperative wound infection.

   Code(s):

2. **Inpatient admission:** This type 1 diabetic patient on insulin was status post a low transverse cesarean delivery 12 days earlier. The day before admission, she noticed a large amount of bloody discharge from her cesarean wound. She was taken to the operating room, where the wound was opened and a very large hematoma was evacuated from the abdominal subcutaneous tissue. The wound was drained and packed. Three days later, a secondary wound closure was accomplished.

Discharge diagnoses: (1) Postpartum hematoma, (2) diabetes mellitus.

Code(s):

3. **Inpatient admission:** The patient, a 39-year-old female, gravida II, para 1, was admitted in active labor at 39 weeks' gestation. She was dilated to 5 centimeters approximately six hours following admission. Pitocin augmentation was started, and she progressed to complete dilation. Low forceps were used due to arrested active phase of labor. There was no episiotomy, but there was a second-degree perineal laceration (perineum and vaginal wall) that was repaired with 3-0 Dexon. A male infant was delivered weighing 2,835 grams, with Apgar scores of 9 and 9. The patient had indicated before delivery that she desired a sterilization procedure. Following delivery, a laparoscopic bilateral tubal ligation was accomplished.

Discharge diagnoses: (1) Delivery at term, (2) perineal laceration, (3) elective sterilization.

Code(s):

4. **Inpatient admission:** The admitting diagnoses were intrauterine pregnancy at 29 weeks' gestation, premature rupture of membranes with a slow leak of amniotic fluid 12 days prior to admission, and chorioamnionitis. The patient was placed under bed rest, observation, and corticosteroids. However, the patient went into premature labor and was admitted. Radiological findings revealed a vertex right occiput transverse presentation with a compound presentation of a fetal hand. Because the patient had a temperature of 101.4 degrees, chorioamnionitis was presumed and antibiotics were started. On a subsequent examination, the fetus was found to be presenting vertex left occiput anterior with right hand compound presentation. The right hand was reducible and was pushed up toward the left side of the fetal body. Following a prolonged second stage, a female infant with Apgar scores of 5 and 7 was delivered spontaneously over an intact perineum. A prior cesarean vertical section scar was found to be intact.

Discharge diagnoses: (1) Delayed delivery following premature rupture of membrane, compound presentation, (2) chorioamnionitis.

Code(s):

5. **Inpatient admission:** The patient, gravida II, para 1, was admitted in labor with a 27-week pregnancy. The fetus was in a complete breech position. Labor ceased within a few hours after admission, but the patient was observed closely because she had a history of recurrent pregnancy loss. By the second day, contractions recurred and she rapidly progressed to complete dilation. Because the breech presentation resulted in obstructed labor, an emergent low cervical cesarean section was performed, and a female infant was delivered with Apgar scores of 9 and 9. The postpartum course was uneventful, and the patient was discharged in good condition on the third postoperative day.

Discharge diagnosis: Preterm delivery, complicated by breech presentation.

Code(s):

6. **Inpatient admission:** The patient, gravida 2, para 1, was admitted at 37 weeks' gestation with spontaneous rupture of membranes and contractions every two to three minutes. She had a history of congenital heart block with pacemaker, which the physician documented was under control by the pacemaker and was not affecting the pregnancy. Because there was no descent, even though the patient was pushing adequately, three attempts at forceps delivery were made with no success due to cephalopelvic disproportion. Because of failure of forceps due to bony pelvic obstruction, a primary low transverse cesarean section was performed. A live single male was delivered. The postoperative course was uneventful.

Discharge diagnosis: Cesarean delivery of term, live infant, complicated by bony pelvis and cephalopelvic disproportion and failed forceps.

Code(s):

7. **Inpatient admission:** The patient was admitted with an intrauterine pregnancy at 34 weeks' gestation in preterm labor. The provider determined that the patient had false labor that ceased spontaneously, and she was discharged the next day.

Discharge diagnosis: Preterm labor.

Code(s):

8. **Inpatient admission:** The patient, at 10 weeks' gestation, was admitted for severe dehydration due to hyperemesis gravidarum. The patient had glaucoma, and treatment with eye drops was continued during the patient's stay. She responded well to IV fluid hydration and antiemetics. The provider documented that the glaucoma did not affect the pregnancy.

Discharge diagnoses: (1) Hyperemesis gravidarum with dehydration, (2) glaucoma.

Code(s):

9. **Inpatient admission:** The patient was admitted with a nonviable fetus at 27½ weeks' gestation. An ultrasound prior to admission showed severe renal malformations in the dysmorphic fetus. A pediatric urology consult concluded fetal nonviability secondary to severe oligohydramnios, enlarged kidneys, and a nonoperable candidate. A Prostin capsule was placed intravaginally, and the patient went on to have spontaneous expulsion of a stillborn female. The patient was discharged the following day.

Discharge diagnoses: (1) Spontaneous vaginal delivery of stillborn fetus with multiple congenital anomalies (pregnancy), (2) oligohydramnios.

Code(s):

10. **Inpatient admission:** When admitted, this woman, with trichorionic/triamniotic triplet gestation at 28 weeks, was thought to have had premature rupture of membranes. She was placed on magnesium sulfate after rupture of membranes was ruled out. Tocolysis was continued until she underwent spontaneous rupture of membranes one week later. During labor, internal fetal heart rate monitoring using electronic transducer through the cervix was carried out. She had a rapid vaginal delivery with liveborn triplets. The fetal monitoring electrode was removed.

Discharge diagnosis: Spontaneous vaginal delivery of liveborn triplets.

Code(s):

11. **Inpatient admission:** The patient, a 44-year-old female, gravida I, para 0, was admitted for management of an intrauterine fetal death at 23 weeks. On a routine office visit 10 days earlier, no fetal heartbeat was heard. An ultrasound confirmed the suspicions. She elected to have medical induction of labor via intravenous infusion via the arm rather than waiting for a spontaneous delivery and was admitted. A Pitocin drip was started and some contractions were obtained, but the cervix remained unchanged. Dilation and curettage were performed, and she was discharged that afternoon.

   Discharge diagnoses: (1) Intrauterine fetal death at 23 weeks, (2) macerated fetus, (3) elderly primigravida.

   Code(s):

12. **Inpatient admission:** The 14-year-old patient (gravida I, para 0) was pregnant at 25 weeks' gestation when she was admitted with abdominal pain and questionable labor. On examination she was 50 percent effaced and tight fingertip dilated with cephalic presentation. She was placed on Terbutaline. By the next day, she was without discomfort or contractions and was discharged.

   Discharge diagnosis: Premature labor.

   Code(s):

13. **Inpatient admission:** The young patient, gravida I, para 0, ab 0, at 43 weeks' gestation, presented in labor and labored poorly but succeeded in reaching 4 to 5 centimeters dilation. Augmentation with Pitocin resulted in no change after several hours, and a primary lower uterine segmental cesarean section was performed due to prolonged labor, with birth of a 7-pound, 5-ounce female. The patient did well after delivery and was discharged on the fourth postoperative day.

   Discharge diagnoses: (1) Post-term, intrauterine pregnancy; (2) failure to progress in labor due to secondary uterine inertia, with prolonged first stage.

   Code(s):

14. **Inpatient admission:** The patient, gravida 2, para 1, was admitted at approximately 25½ weeks' gestation with a history of contractions for 24 hours. She was contracting every four to six minutes. Radiological findings showed an intrauterine fetal death of fetus 1 of the triplet pregnancy (monochorionic) but also showed that the other two fetuses were progressing normally. The contractions stopped and then started again. The patient was given magnesium sulfate for tocolysis but contracted through the magnesium and was placed on Ritodrine. Because she then developed a fever with suspected chorioamnionitis and was in active labor, a primary low cervical cesarean section delivered three male monochorionic fetuses, two liveborn and one stillborn. Postoperatively, the patient did well on antibiotics.

Discharge diagnoses: (1) Cesarean delivery of triplets (two liveborn and one stillborn) at 25½ weeks, (2) chorioamnionitis.

Code(s):

15. **Inpatient admission:** The young patient in the 37th week of gestation was admitted with contractions occurring every few minutes. The cervix was 25 percent effaced with a 6-centimeter dilation. Although she had undergone a previous cesarean section, she wished a trial at vaginal delivery. The membranes were artificially ruptured. Six hours later, she was tried on intravenous Pitocin augmentation and within the hour progressed to complete dilation and began pushing. She pushed for two hours and was unable to progress satisfactorily due to arrested active phase of labor. She was taken to surgery, where a repeat low transverse cervical cesarean section was performed for obstructed labor due to cephalopelvic disproportion. A healthy, single, liveborn female was delivered. The postpartum course was uneventful.

Discharge diagnoses: (1) Intrauterine pregnancy at term, (2) previous cesarean section, (3) cephalopelvic disproportion (CPD).

Code(s):

16. **Inpatient admission:** The patient, in her 25th week of gestation, was transferred from another hospital with complete effacement, complete dilation, and occasional contractions. She underwent a primary low cervical cesarean section with preoperative diagnoses of preterm labor, advanced cervical dilation, and failed magnesium tocolysis. Findings included a live male infant weighing 880 grams. The patient's postoperative course was uneventful except for the occurrence of hemorrhoids, which were successfully treated with suppositories.

    Discharge diagnoses: (1) Intrauterine pregnancy at 25 weeks, (2) preterm labor.

    Code(s):

17. **Inpatient admission:** The patient was admitted in active labor at term (38 weeks' gestation). She had multiple sclerosis, which had been exacerbated by the pregnancy. In the delivery room, she spontaneously delivered a liveborn female infant over a midline episiotomy without complication.

    Discharge diagnoses: (1) Spontaneous vaginal delivery of term, live female; (2) multiple sclerosis.

    Code(s):

18. **Physician office visit:** The patient came in for her routine prenatal checkup. She was a primigravida in her first trimester. There were no complications.

    Diagnosis: Normal pregnancy at 10 weeks.

    Code(s):

19. Physician office visit: The patient came in for her routine prenatal checkup. She was a primigravida in her first trimester. She complained of hyperemesis. She had been unable to eat and had lost 2 pounds since her last visit. Medication was prescribed. She was instructed to call the office immediately if there were no improvement within 12 hours. She was to be rescheduled for a return visit the following week.

Diagnosis: First trimester pregnancy complicated by mild hyperemesis gravidarum.

Code(s):

20. Inpatient admission: The patient was admitted in labor with an estimated 39-week gestation. When she was approximately 7 to 8 centimeters dilated, an amniotomy was performed that revealed meconium-stained liquor. She rapidly progressed to complete cervical dilation. Fetal distress due to meconium necessitated delivery. The infant's head was visible and in the occiput anterior position. Low forceps were applied, a midline episiotomy was performed, and the infant was successfully delivered. The midline episiotomy was repaired.

Discharge diagnoses: (1) Term delivery of liveborn infant, (2) meconium-stained liquor, (3) fetal stress.

Code(s):

21. Inpatient admission: The patient, a young woman with estimated gestation of 29 weeks, was admitted for gestational diabetes. It was decided that close monitoring of her blood sugars was in order and the possibility of starting insulin should receive consideration. Throughout her stay, she had no problems or complications. She was maintained on an 1,800-calorie diet. Her blood sugars were borderline abnormal, and a trial at diet control was to be instituted before further consideration was given to the use of insulin.

Discharge diagnoses: (1) Gestational diabetes; (2) intrauterine pregnancy, 29 weeks.

Code(s):

22. **Inpatient admission:** The patient, with an estimated 37-week gestation, was admitted in labor. Her prenatal course was uncomplicated, except for mild pre-existing hypertension. The labor was also uneventful, and the membranes spontaneously ruptured. A 7-pound, 3-ounce viable male was delivered. The delivery was spontaneous and vaginal, with a midline episiotomy, which extended into a third-degree, IIIa laceration. The third-degree laceration of the perineum and the anal sphincter were sutured. Following delivery, the mother was stable, with no apparent complications.

    Discharge diagnoses: (1) Spontaneous vaginal delivery of term male infant, (2) third-degree perineal laceration.

    Code(s):

23. **Inpatient admission:** The patient, with an estimated gestation of 39.5 weeks, presented with spontaneous rupture of the membranes and irregular contractions. Her previous pregnancy was delivered by cesarean vertical section. At first, labor failed to progress despite irregular contractions, and she was started on Pitocin via peripheral IV. She then moved ahead with labor and pushed for approximately 45 minutes. The baby was delivered spontaneously, with the help of a midline episiotomy.

    Discharge diagnoses: (1) Term pregnancy delivered of liveborn male infant, (2) previous cesarean section.

    Code(s):

13. ABORTION AND ECTOPIC PREGNANCY

1. **Inpatient admission:** The 22-year-old patient was at 10 weeks' gestation with an intrauterine pregnancy. She stated that this pregnancy was the result of a rape and did not wish to carry it to term. Inpatient admission was needed for additional counseling for the sexual assault. A complete abortion was accomplished with a dilation and curettage. There were no complications.

   Discharge diagnoses: (1) Elective abortion, (2) history of rape.

   Code(s):

2. **Inpatient admission:** The patient, at 12 weeks' gestation, wished to have the pregnancy terminated following studies showing the fetus to be anencephalic. An intrauterine saline injection produced an incomplete abortion. This procedure was followed by a dilation and curettage.

   Discharge diagnosis: Therapeutic abortion secondary to fetal abnormality.

   Code(s):

3. **Inpatient admission:** The patient was admitted following a spontaneous abortion, which she experienced earlier in the day. On examination, it appeared that the abortion was incomplete, and she was bleeding heavily. A dilation and curettage was performed.

   Discharge diagnosis: Incomplete spontaneous abortion.

   Code(s):

4. **Obstetrics clinic visit:** The patient had an elective abortion performed at another facility two days earlier. She visited the clinic because of pelvic pain, fever, and non-bloody discharge. She was given antibiotics.

   Diagnosis: Acute endometritis following abortion.

   Code(s):

660

5. Obstetrics clinic visit: The 35-year-old patient wished to electively terminate a pregnancy because of her hyperthyroidism, which has been difficult to control. She was at 10 weeks' gestation. A complete abortion resulted from the vacuum aspiration curettage.

Diagnoses: (1) Therapeutic abortion, complete; (2) hyperthyroidism.

Code(s):

6. Inpatient admission: The young patient was transferred in from another hospital, where she had been treated for a lacunar infarction. She was making a good recovery at the other hospital until the day before she was transferred, when she became agitated and aggressive and complained of abdominal pain without significant findings on examination. Her husband suggested the possibility of pregnancy, and an HCG assay confirmed the condition, with pregnancy estimated at 6 weeks. After a series of discussions with the patient and family, it was decided to proceed with an abortion. She was admitted here for the abortion. A complete abortion was accomplished with vacuum aspiration curettage. Her mental status improved, and she was discharged.

Discharge diagnosis: Elective abortion, complete, secondary to lacunar cerebral infarction.

Code(s):

7. Inpatient admission: The patient, known to be in early pregnancy, was admitted with acute abdominal pain. Ultrasound revealed a right tubal pregnancy. The tubal pregnancy was removed laparoscopically via a small incision in the abdomen. The patient was discharged the next day in good condition. She was to be seen in the doctor's office in two weeks.

Discharge diagnosis: Ectopic pregnancy.

Code(s):

14. CONGENITAL ANOMALIES

1. **Inpatient admission:** The 27-year-old patient was admitted for a cardiac pacemaker implant for her atrioventricular heart block, presumably congenital. A skin incision into the chest wall was made, and a dual chamber synchronous pacemaker was inserted into a subcutaneous pocket. The right atrioventricular transvenous leads were inserted percutaneously. She was kept on bed rest until she was stable and then discharged.

   Discharge diagnosis: Atrioventricular heart block, probably congenital in origin.

2. **Inpatient admission:** The patient, an infant, was admitted for open repair of bilateral undescended intraabdominal testes. In the operating room, he underwent bilateral orchiopexies. On the second postoperative day, a diffuse paralytic ileus was visualized on a KUB study. The infant began vomiting secondary to the obstruction caused by the ileus. A nasogastric (NG) tube was placed, and he was maintained on nasogastric suction and IV hydration for the following two days. On postoperative day 4, the tube was manually removed, and the patient was discharged. The postoperative ileus extended this admission by two days.

   Discharge diagnoses: (1) Undescended testes; (2) postoperative ileus, secondary to bilateral orchiopexies.

Code(s):

Code(s):

3. **Inpatient admission:** The patient, a six-week-old infant, was admitted for evaluation of a fever. She was placed on IV antibiotics, and blood cultures grew coagulase-negative *Staphylococcus*. The provider documented "Staph sepsis." Because a murmur was noticed on physical examination, an echocardiogram was done. This revealed physiological peripheral branch pulmonary artery stenosis and a small left-to-right atrial shunt, most likely a patent foramen ovale. Based on these findings, the provider diagnosed patent foramen ovale and pulmonary artery stenosis.

Discharge diagnoses: (1) Coagulase-negative, community-acquired staphylococcal sepsis; (2) peripheral pulmonary artery stenosis; (3) patent foramen ovale.

Code(s):

4. **Inpatient admission:** The patient, a two-month-old male infant, was referred for evaluation of a faulty airway. The mother reported that he had had noisy breathing since birth and that it had worsened recently. Severe to moderate laryngomalacia was identified on a flexible bronchoscopy. A supraglottostomy with repair of the larynx was performed without complication during the procedure or afterward. The patient received antibiotics postoperatively and was discharged in good condition.

Discharge diagnosis: Laryngomalacia.

Code(s):

5. **Inpatient admission:** The patient, a 14-year-old male, had congenital honeycomb lung and type 1 diabetes. On admission, right heart failure due to left heart failure was present. His breathing was labored, and lower extremity edema was evident. Recently, his oxygen requirements increased dramatically, he ran intermittent fevers, and he consumed large amounts of liquids. With diuretics, significant reduction of the pitting edema was achieved. Antidepressants were added to his medication regimen to help address his depression, agitation, and anxiety. Humidified oxygen mask, alternating percussion, and postural drainage helped his breathing. The insulin dosage and type were adjusted. He was discharged on a diabetic diet in stable condition.

Discharge diagnoses: (1) Right heart failure due to left heart failure, (2) honeycomb lung, (3) type 1 diabetes mellitus, (4) depression.

Code(s):

6. **Inpatient admission:** This four-year-old patient has a diverticulum of the left ventricle. She had a pulmonary artery band inserted four years ago for another congenital defect. Shortly after the prior surgery, she had a stroke and now has a residual paralysis of the right arm. Currently, she was admitted with labored breathing and shortness of breath. Her lungs showed infiltrates on chest X-ray, and sputum culture showed presence of *Klebsiella*. She was placed on antibiotics and continuous oxygen therapy for pneumonia, and she slowly improved. She required feeding by nursing staff because her right side is dominant. During this admission, her congenital problem was reevaluated by diagnostic testing. She was discharged in satisfactory condition.

Discharge diagnoses: (1) *Klebsiella* pneumonia; (2) monoplegia; (3) diverticulum, left ventricle.

Code(s):

7. **Inpatient admission:** The patient, a two-year-old male, had congenital bilateral clubfoot and atretic spinal cord at level T11–L4. He needed a walker to ambulate, using mostly the upper extremities to get around. He was admitted for repair of a left tibial torsion. A tibial rotational osteotomy was performed, with insertion of pins. He was placed in a splint postoperatively and was changed to a long leg cast the next day. The patient was discharged subsequently to follow up with the orthopedic surgeon in one week.

Discharge diagnosis: Atretic spinal cord at T11–L4 with left tibial torsion.

Code(s):

8. **Inpatient admission:** The patient, a 20-month-old girl, was admitted for correction of a left talipes equinovarus clubfoot. Shortly after admission, she started running a fever and it became apparent that she had acute otitis media. She was placed on antibiotics and discharged. Surgery was to be rescheduled at a later date.

Discharge diagnoses: (1) Talipes equinovarus, left; (2) bilateral otitis media.

Code(s):

9. **Inpatient admission:** The patient, a teenage male, was referred by his orthodontist for surgical correction of multiple congenital deformities. Examination revealed maxillary hypoplasia and maxillary asymmetry. He was found to have an excessive crossbite, with the maxillary midline several millimeters to the right. Surgical correction was indicated, and the plan was to perform both maxillary and mandibular osteotomies to achieve the amount of movement needed. During surgery, it was possible to move the left maxilla into its desired position without a mandibular osteotomy being performed. Postoperatively, he did very well, and the occlusion was good.

Discharge diagnoses: (1) Maxillary hypoplasia, (2) maxillary asymmetry, (3) excessive crossbite.

Procedure performed: Segmental maxillary osteotomy.

Code(s):

10. **Inpatient admission:** The patient, a 10-month-old infant, had congenital extrahepatic biliary atresia. She was admitted for a liver transplant workup and at admission was in chronic liver failure. The workup included a chest X-ray, KUB study, Doppler ultrasound of liver, and EKG, as well as an upper GI endoscopy of the esophagus, stomach, and duodenum.

Discharge diagnoses: (1) Extrahepatic biliary atresia; (2) placed on liver transplant list, stage II.

Code(s):

15. PERINATAL CONDITIONS

1. **Inpatient admission:** The patient, a preterm, newborn male triplet (1,720 grams), was delivered by cesarean section, as were the other two liveborn males. He initially required supplemental oxygen and a nasal prong CPAP for transient tachypnea. He was weaned five hours after birth. The one-minute Apgar score was 6, and the five-minute score was 8. He was also treated for diaper dermatitis. A circumcision was performed prior to discharge.

   Discharge diagnoses: (1) Premature male triplet, (2) transient tachypnea, (3) diaper dermatitis.

   Code(s):

2. **Inpatient admission:** The patient, a one-day-old, 2,200-gram infant, was born prematurely at 34 weeks' gestation. She was transferred from another hospital for evaluation of a right congenital diaphragmatic hernia. At Hospital A, just before transfer, intubation was required due to respiratory distress. The ventilatory support was continued at Hospital B for three days. When the infant was stabilized, the right diaphragmatic hernia was repaired via an open approach. She progressed rapidly and was discharged on the second postoperative day.

   Discharge diagnoses: (1) Prematurity, (2) diaphragmatic hernia, (3) respiratory distress syndrome.

   Code(s):

3. **Inpatient admission:** The patient, a newborn female infant, was delivered spontaneously at term. She was noticed to be jaundiced on the initial screening labs. Lab tests showed the total bilirubin was increased, and she was started on a single session of phototherapy under bilirubin lights. She progressed rapidly and was discharged to home with the mother.

   Discharge diagnoses: (1) Term female newborn, (2) neonatal jaundice.

Code(s):

4. **Inpatient admission:** The patient, a preterm male infant, was delivered vaginally at approximately 29 weeks' gestation. He weighed 1,855 grams at birth. Initially he did well; however, on the evening of birth, he was noted to have dusky spells when feeding. During that night, he developed tachypnea. Due to abnormal heart sounds, tachypnea, and dusky spells, an echocardiogram was performed. It showed a patent foramen ovale. The patient did well and was released the next day, to follow up with a pediatric cardiologist on an outpatient basis.

   Discharge diagnoses: (1) Premature, single, male newborn; (2) patent foramen ovale.

Code(s):

5. **Inpatient admission:** The patient, a newborn preterm male infant delivered by cesarean section, weighed 2,300 grams at birth and had Apgar scores of 8 and 9. Shortly after birth, an increased respiratory rate, effort, and grunting required that he be placed on oxygen. A classical hyaline membrane disease then developed, consistent with his 32- to 33-week gestational age and size. A catheter was percutaneously placed in the umbilical vein and advanced into the inferior vena cava immediately to allow ease in administration of IV fluids and medication. A right pneumothorax, identified on chest X-ray, was immediately needle aspirated, and a chest tube was placed. Subsequently, he was transferred to the neonatal intensive care unit at another hospital.

   Discharge diagnoses: (1) Prematurity, (2) hyaline membrane disease, (3) spontaneous right pneumothorax.

   Procedures performed: (1) Umbilical vein catheter placement, (2) right chest tube placement, (3) aspiration of pleural space (thoracentesis).

Code(s):

6. **Inpatient admission:** The patient was delivered prematurely by cesarean section and weighed 1,750 grams. She had multiple problems, including microcephaly due to congenital Zika virus and congenital heart disease. The infant's mother had been infected with Zika virus while pregnant. This newborn was transferred to another hospital for further evaluation and intensive pediatric care.

Discharge diagnoses: (1) Prematurity, (2) microcephaly due to Zika virus, (3) congenital heart disease.

Code(s):

7. **Inpatient admission:** The patient, a six-day-old female, was admitted with respiratory distress, wheezes, and a heart murmur. She was intubated on admission and improved on the ventilator. She was extubated 48 hours later. Community-acquired respiratory syncytial viral (RSV) bronchiolitis was diagnosed. Other treatment included antibiotics and aerosols. An echocardiogram indicated a ventricular septal defect. She was to return at a later date for further evaluation.

Discharge diagnoses: (1) Respiratory syncytial viral bronchiolitis, (2) ventricular septal defect, (3) respiratory distress.

Code(s):

8. **Inpatient admission:** The patient, an 11-month-old male infant, had congenital cytomegalovirus infection. Because of distorted, loud, and rattling breathing, he was admitted for evaluation of his hypertrophied tonsils and adenoids. Treatment for congenital cytomegaloviral infection was continued throughout the admission. In surgery, a microrigid laryngoscopy, a microrigid bronchoscopy, and an external adenotonsillectomy were performed. No abnormalities were noted on laryngoscopy or bronchoscopy. The patient's postoperative course was uncomplicated.

Discharge diagnoses: (1) Hypertrophied adenoids and tonsils, (2) congenital cytomegalovirus infection.

Code(s):

9. **Inpatient admission:** The patient, an 11-month-old male, was found to have a dysplastic kidney on the right side. Because the kidney was not functioning, he was admitted for surgical removal. An open right, simple nephrectomy was performed. The procedure was uncomplicated, as was the postoperative course. The pathology report showed the kidney to be both dysplastic and multicystic.

Discharge diagnosis: Right multicystic dysplastic kidney.

Code(s):

10. **Inpatient admission:** The patient, a 7-pound, 6-ounce male infant, was delivered vaginally to a 31-year-old woman (gravida 2, para 0–1) at 43 weeks' gestation. The mother's pregnancy was uncomplicated, labor lasted 24 hours, and the delivery was spontaneous. Apgar scores were 5 and 7. Due to transient tachypnea and a continued oxygen requirement, the infant was taken to the special care nursery. His overall condition improved rapidly with oxygen and adjustments in body fluids.

Discharge diagnoses: (1) Post-term newborn male, (2) transient tachypnea of the newborn.

Code(s):

11. **Inpatient admission:** The patient, a three-week-old male, was admitted through the emergency department with a three-day history of upper respiratory tract infection (URI). Following admission, he was observed not breathing for short periods during sleep. Antibiotics were started for the URI, and he was observed closely. He had been followed in the outpatient clinic for failure to thrive. All evaluative workups were negative, and no active disease other than the respiratory infection was found. The URI cleared, but the apneic episodes continued. The URI was determined to be community acquired. He was to be transferred to the children's hospital for more detailed studies of his episodic sleep apnea and failure to thrive.

Discharge diagnoses: (1) Failure to thrive, (2) acute upper respiratory tract infection, (3) apnea.

Code(s):

12. **Inpatient admission:** The infant was born in the hospital to a 36-year-old primigravida woman at an estimated 34 weeks' gestation. The mother's pregnancy was complicated by maternal hypertension and gestational diabetes. The infant was delivered by a primary cesarean section due to fetal distress and metabolic acidemia resulting from the mother's failure to progress at labor. The infant was placed on oxygen by nasal prong following birth in response to fetal distress. The oxygen was removed when heart rate, breathing, and blood gases returned to normal. The infant's blood sugars were low following birth, and an infusion of intravenous glucose was initiated until the blood sugars stabilized.

    Discharge diagnoses: (1) Premature newborn male with birth weight of 1,880 grams, (2) transient hypoglycemia.

    Code(s):

13. **Inpatient admission:** The patient, a preterm male infant, was born the day before admission in another hospital. He weighed 2,608 grams and had Apgar scores of 7 and 9. He was noted to have elevated temperature. WBCs were also elevated. He was transferred for investigative studies. A urinary tract infection was confirmed with a urine culture that was positive for *E. coli*, and the infection was treated with intravenous antibiotics. Left hydronephrosis was confirmed by bilateral renal ultrasound. Suspected septicemia was ruled out when all blood cultures were negative prior to institution of antibiotic therapy.

    Discharge diagnoses: (1) Urinary tract infection, (2) congenital hydronephrosis, (3) prematurity.

    Code(s):

16. DISEASES OF THE CIRCULATORY SYSTEM

1. **Inpatient admission (episode 1):** The reason for this woman's admission was repair of a 4.7-centimeter infrarenal abdominal aortic aneurysm. She also had arterial hypertension. Because of her strong family history of aneurysms, she wished to have her aneurysm removed on an elective basis rather than waiting for it to follow its natural course. At surgery, via an open approach, the aneurysm sac was cut open, the aneurysm was excised, and a 16-millimeter Dacron graft was placed. The procedure was successful, and the patient was discharged on the fifth postoperative day.

   Discharge diagnoses: (1) Infrarenal abdominal aortic aneurysm, (2) arterial hypertension.

   Code(s):

   Physician office visit (episode 2): The patient presented for routine follow-up examination of an abdominal aortic aneurysm repair with graft replacement. She was doing well, with only mild discomfort. The midline incision was well healed. Femoral and distal pulses were palpable bilaterally. She was to return in three months.

   Diagnosis: Status post aortic aneurysm.

   Code(s):

2. **Inpatient admission:** The patient was admitted for workup of right carotid artery stenosis. A carotid duplex performed as an outpatient procedure at another facility showed 80 percent stenosis on the right side and 40 percent on the left. A nonselective low osmolar carotid arteriography of the internal and external carotid arteries bilaterally, conducted the day after admission, showed only a 50 percent stenosis of the right common carotid artery. The external carotids were found to be small, but there was no significant internal carotid disease on either side. Therefore, because the patient was asymptomatic, it was felt that surgery would present a higher risk of stroke than treating her medically.

   Discharge diagnoses: (1) Carotid artery disease, stenosis.

   Code(s):

3. **Inpatient admission:** This patient was admitted for repair of a left common carotid stenosis. Two months earlier, an endarterectomy of a right carotid stenosis had been performed. Six months earlier, she had suffered a cerebral hemorrhage that resulted in apraxia and oropharyngeal phase dysphagia, both of which required additional nursing assistance during this encounter. The open left endarterectomy was successfully accomplished, and the patient was discharged on the fourth hospital day.

   Discharge diagnoses: (1) Left carotid stenosis, (2) residuals of old cerebrovascular accident.

   Code(s):

4. **Inpatient admission:** The patient was admitted with recurrent unstable angina that could not be controlled with sublingual nitroglycerin. There was no history of bypass or angioplasty in the past. On left cardiac catheterization with coronary arteriography with low osmolar contrast, a narrowing in the left anterior descending coronary artery and a stenotic area in an intermediate branch were identified. A successful percutaneous transluminal coronary angioplasty (PTCA) of both vessels was carried out.

   Discharge diagnoses: (1) Unstable angina secondary to coronary arteriosclerosis, (2) chronic total occlusion of coronary artery.

   Code(s):

5. **Inpatient admission:** The patient received his first pacing system 15 years earlier because of congenital complete heart block and severe bradycardia. At the time of admission, he was experiencing these conditions again, plus fatigue secondary to pacemaker pulse generator malfunction. He was admitted for insertion of a new generator. After he was prepped for surgery, the old pacemaker was removed via an incision into the subcutaneous pocket, and a new dual chamber pacing device was inserted and connected to the existing leads. The postoperative period was uncomplicated.

Discharge diagnosis: Malfunctioning pacemaker.

Code(s):

6. **Inpatient admission:** The patient came to the emergency department because she was unable to speak well. She was admitted because she appeared to be somewhat aphasic. Following admission, she was found to be in longstanding persistent atrial fibrillation. A CT scan of the head showed only some probable old defects, and the aphasia was thought to probably be due to a recent cerebral embolus. By the fifth day, she was stable and able to go home. The aphasia had cleared, and the fibrillation was controlled with medication.

Discharge diagnoses: (1) Cerebral embolism, (2) atrial fibrillation.

Code(s):

7. **Inpatient admission:** The patient was admitted for severe aortic valve stenosis and left ventricular hypertrophy. The aortic valve was replaced with a prosthesis via open approach. The patient was successfully weaned from the cardiopulmonary bypass (extracorporeal cardiac) machine. An intraoperative echocardiogram revealed appropriate functioning of the prosthesis.

Discharge diagnoses: (1) Aortic stenosis and calcification, (2) left ventricular hypertrophy.

Code(s):

8. **Inpatient admission:** The admission diagnoses were aortic and mitral insufficiency. The patient also had HIV infection. A bacterial endocarditis, involving the aortic and mitral valves, had developed five months before admission and was treated and resolved with antibiotics. Procedures performed were mitral and aortic valve replacement with prosthesis via open approach and cardiopulmonary bypass (extracorporeal cardiac) during the procedure. The patient improved considerably during the next two days with medications and was transferred to the rehabilitation hospital.

   Discharge diagnoses: (1) Aortic and mitral insufficiency, (2) HIV infection.

   Code(s):

9. **Inpatient admission:** The patient was admitted with atypical chest pain and aching of the left upper extremity. Following admission, she had episodic visual blurring and dizziness. A myocardial infarction was ruled out. Neurological checks were unremarkable, except for a questionable small infarct in the left occipital lobe. Her long-term aspirin therapy was increased, and within two days she was fully ambulatory and asymptomatic.

   Discharge diagnoses: (1) Atypical chest pain of unclear etiology, (2) transient ischemic attacks.

   Code(s):

10. **Inpatient admission:** The patient, a young woman, was admitted with pain and edema in the left leg, which had started two days earlier when she drove home from Florida without stopping. Findings on a venous Doppler ultrasound of the pelvic and leg region were consistent with thrombosis. She was discharged on Coumadin.

    Discharge diagnosis: Iliac vein thrombosis on the left, acute.

    Code(s):

11. **Inpatient admission:** The patient was brought to the hospital emergency department with burning, low sternal, epigastric pain. While in the ED, she developed respiratory distress and subsequent acute type 1 myocardial infarction with cardiopulmonary arrest. She was resuscitated, and maneuvers involved in this activity included intubation, mechanical ventilation, and defibrillation. Chest X-rays confirmed pulmonary edema and high output congestive heart failure. EKGs confirmed acute subendocardial myocardial infarction in progress. The patient was then admitted and remained on the ventilator for approximately 24 hours, with gradual improvement. She was transferred to another hospital for further workup and treatment.

    Discharge diagnoses: (1) Acute myocardial infarction, (2) pulmonary edema, (3) congestive heart failure, (4) cardiopulmonary arrest.

    Code(s):

12. **Inpatient admission:** The patient was admitted for evaluation of a three-month history of fever, fatigue, and headaches. She received consultation from the rheumatology service, which recommended biopsy of the temporal arteries. The left temporal artery was negative for inflammation. The right temporal artery, however, showed inflammation of the intima. The histologic picture was compatible with arteritis. Prednisone was given, and the headaches subsided.

    Discharge diagnoses: (1) Right temporal arteritis; (2) open biopsy, right and left temporal arteries.

    Code(s):

13. **Inpatient admission:** The patient, who had a history of type 2 diabetes managed with oral antidiabetic medication, was admitted for treatment of a stroke. The major manifestations were ptosis on the right; moderate expressive aphasia; right-to-left disorientation; and a slow, shuffling gait. On a CT scan of the head, a low-density area was seen at the posterior limb of the left internal capsule and the left posterior parietal subcortical white matter. No hemorrhage was viewed. Gradually, the manifestations improved and then resolved. The patient also had a right midfoot ulcer that required bedside debridement (using a Versajet) by the physician. She was discharged to be followed up by a home health nurse.

    Discharge diagnoses: (1) Cerebrovascular infarction of a thromboembolic source, left posterior artery; (2) type 2 diabetes; (3) diabetic foot ulcer.

    Code(s):

14. **Inpatient admission:** The patient had a three-month history of progressive cyanosis of the fingers and toes. Due to sudden and dramatic progression of symptoms, she was admitted. A right upper-extremity arteriogram with low osmolar contrast revealed complete absence of arterial flow to all proximal phalanges. The findings were thought to be consistent with vasculitis. A percutaneous vascular biopsy of the artery of the right hand was performed to confirm this diagnosis. The report indicated changes consistent with chronic inflammation and necrotizing vasculitis. On vascular surgery consultation, it was felt that her gangrene would demarcate without surgical intervention. There was gradual improvement in pain, and she was switched to oral medications.

    Discharge diagnoses: (1) Necrotizing vasculitis, (2) digital gangrene.

    Code(s):

15. Inpatient admission: The patient was transferred from another hospital for evaluation of a possible recurrent pulmonary embolism and right lower-extremity pain and swelling determined to be deep vein thrombosis (prior to transfer). A left pulmonary arteriogram with high osmolar contrast confirmed an acute left pulmonary embolus, and heparin was started. Ultrasound of the right lower extremity demonstrated an acute thrombosis of the right femoral vein. Bilateral mammograms were taken to evaluate a right breast lump with discharge that was found on physical examination. The finding was a suspicious density in the upper outer quadrant of the right breast. The patient was to be referred to the gynecology clinic for follow-up of this problem after discharge. All medications were adjusted, and she showed much improvement.

Discharge diagnoses: (1) Deep venous thrombosis, right leg; (2) recurrent pulmonary embolism; (3) lump, right breast.

Code(s):

16. Inpatient admission: A patient, who had peripheral vascular disease and rest pain, came in for a second opinion about possible reconstruction of right femorotibial artery occlusive disease. An angiogram of the right lower extremity with low osmolar contrast demonstrated a peroneal vessel that would allow reconstruction. Following an evaluation, he was scheduled to undergo the procedure. However, because he had no other significant diseases or active cardiac ischemia, he was felt to be at low risk for a distal reconstruction. The patient was discharged prior to the procedure due to the development of an upper respiratory infection. The procedure was to be rescheduled in two weeks.

Discharge diagnoses: (1) Right femorotibial artery occlusion, (2) URI.

Code(s):

17. Inpatient admission: The patient was admitted with probable acute type 1 myocardial infarction and chronic atrial fibrillation. He was admitted to the critical care unit and was administered several medications. A cardiology consultation confirmed an acute inferolateral myocardial infarction on echocardiogram, and the patient was transferred to another hospital for cardiac catheterization.

Discharge diagnoses: (1) Acute myocardial infarction, (2) atrial fibrillation.

Code(s):

18. **Inpatient admission:** The patient, an elderly man, was transferred from a nursing home. He had had nondominant left-sided hemiplegia since suffering a cerebral thrombosis about three months earlier. He was doing well until the day of admission. A CT scan of the head showed an acute cerebral hemorrhage. He was treated and improved somewhat but then had increased problems secondary to extension of the bleeding. Another CT scan showed a large hematoma in the right basal ganglia. With consultation, it was decided that only supportive care was needed, and the patient was returned to the nursing home.

Discharge diagnoses: (1) Acute cerebral hemorrhage, (2) right basal ganglia hematoma, (3) previous cerebral thrombosis with residual left-sided hemiplegia.

Code(s):

19. **Inpatient admission:** The patient, a female resident of a nursing home, was transferred because of nausea and vomiting. She also had type 1 diabetes mellitus and arteriosclerotic cardiovascular disease. An upper GI X-ray showed esophageal obstruction. She was then admitted with provisional diagnoses of esophageal obstruction versus hiatal hernia versus esophagitis. A gastroscopy was performed to evaluate the stomach, and a partial obstruction due to stricture to the level of the distal esophagus was viewed and dilated. The patient improved without further symptoms. Her blood sugar levels rose to 500 on the third day of admission, and the diabetes was diagnosed as out of control. Her insulin was increased twice in an attempt to lower her blood sugar to baseline. The long-term outlook was not good because the patient was not a candidate for definitive surgery. The esophageal stricture was thought to have resulted from a previous cerebrovascular accident.

Discharge diagnoses: (1) Esophageal stricture; (2) arteriosclerotic cardiovascular disease; (3) uncontrolled diabetes mellitus, type 1.

Code(s):

20. Inpatient admission: The patient was admitted through the emergency department with substernal chest pain, thought to represent unstable angina. He got pain relief with nitroglycerin. The next morning, he asked to be discharged because he had no insurance and could not afford to be in the hospital. Because his physician did not agree with his decision, the patient signed himself out against medical advice. He promised to see the cardiologist immediately and take his medications.

Discharge diagnosis: Angina, probably unstable.

Code(s):

21. Inpatient admission: The patient, who had no history of bypass or angioplasty, was admitted with recurrent angina, which could not be controlled with medications and ultimately resulted in an acute type 1 ST elevation myocardial infarction of the anterior wall. On combined right and left cardiac catheterization with coronary cineangiography with low osmolar contrast, a narrowing in the left anterior descending coronary artery and stenoses in the left circumflex and distal right coronary artery were found. A successful three-vessel coronary artery bypass graft was carried out. The left internal mammary was used to bypass the left anterior descending, and a reverse segment of the left saphenous vein graft was used to bypass the left circumflex and distal right coronary arteries. The left greater saphenous vein was harvested via a percutaneous endoscopic procedure.

Discharge diagnoses: (1) Anterior acute myocardial infarction, (2) coronary arteriosclerosis.

Procedure: Three-vessel coronary artery bypass graft.

Code(s):

22. Inpatient admission: The patient was admitted for a planned exploratory laparotomy and a possible excision of a cystic mass in the pelvis. Shortly after admission, however, she developed bigeminal pulse. The anesthesiologist believed that she should not have surgery. The surgery was canceled, and she was referred to her internist.

Discharge diagnoses: (1) Bigeminal pulse, (2) pelvic mass.

Code(s):

23. **Inpatient admission:** The patient, an elderly woman, had a rather sudden onset of severe pleuritic chest discomfort that brought her to the emergency department. She had been undergoing a series of radiation therapy treatments for history of endometrial carcinoma. She was admitted for further evaluation. A right pulmonary angiogram with high osmolar contrast confirmed the diagnosis of single subsegmental pulmonary embolism in the right lower lobe. She was treated with heparin and later Coumadin. Coumadin was to be continued on discharge. The patient was to return for her regular radiation therapy treatment as scheduled.

Discharge diagnoses: (1) Pulmonary embolism, (2) history of endometrial carcinoma of the uterus.

Code(s):

24. **Inpatient admission:** The patient was transferred from another hospital for treatment of an acute type 1 ST elevation inferior wall myocardial infarction. She also had hypercholesterolemia and benign hypertension; treatment of these conditions was continued during the hospital stay. A left cardiac catheterization with coronary angiogram and arteriography using low osmolar contrast was performed and revealed coronary arteriosclerosis. It was determined that she would benefit from a percutaneous transluminal coronary angioplasty. The angioplasty was performed on the left coronary artery. She tolerated the procedure well and was to continue her medical treatment after discharge.

Discharge diagnoses: (1) Acute inferior myocardial infarction, (2) coronary arteriosclerosis, (3) hypercholesterolemia, (4) benign essential hypertension.

Code(s):

17. NEOPLASMS

1. **Inpatient admission:** The elderly woman's admitting diagnosis was carcinoma of the stomach with metastasis to the ovaries. An exploratory laparotomy was performed for the purpose of excising the gastric tumor, but it was so densely attached to other structures that it could not be resected. However, a total abdominal hysterectomy and bilateral salpingo-oophorectomy were accomplished, and the patient returned to her room in fair condition. Palliative systemic chemotherapy infusions were given. On the third postoperative day, a large right pleural effusion developed, and a chest tube was percutaneously placed in the right pleural cavity for drainage. Cytology for malignant cells in the pleural effusion was negative. The patient remained stable and wanted to return to her home. The chest tube was removed before discharge.

   Discharge diagnoses: (1) Carcinoma of the stomach metastatic to the ovaries, (2) pleural effusion.

   Code(s):

2. **Inpatient admission:** The patient underwent a hemicolectomy and splenectomy a year earlier for excision of a primary adenocarcinoma of the colon. Recently, he developed abdominal pain. He was admitted with a questionable liver lesion. An ultrasound of the liver, a CT scan of the abdomen, and an exploratory laparotomy with needle biopsy of the liver were performed. The findings indicated inoperable adenocarcinoma of the liver.

   Discharge diagnosis: Adenocarcinoma of the colon metastatic to the liver, unresectable.

   Code(s):

3. **Inpatient admission:** The patient was admitted through the emergency department with severe shortness of breath. She had a history of left upper lobe, non–small cell carcinoma, which had been treated with radiation. Recently, a recurrence in the left supraclavicular area of the lung was found, and she received palliative radiation therapy. She also had a history of severe chronic obstructive bronchitis and had used home oxygen for several years. Her medications were increased for the chronic obstructive pulmonary disease, and she improved sufficiently for discharge.

Discharge diagnoses: (1) Chronic obstructive pulmonary disease with acute exacerbation, (2) recurrent non–small cell lung cancer.

Code(s):

4. **Inpatient admission:** On a previous admission, the patient was diagnosed with poorly differentiated papillary serous cystadenocarcinoma of the right ovary. She was admitted for, and received, her fifth chemotherapy treatment (into central vein) with Taxol and Cisplatin.

Discharge diagnosis: Papillary serous cystadenocarcinoma, stage III.

Code(s):

5. **Inpatient admission:** The patient was seen in the outpatient clinic, where an X-ray revealed compression fractures of T6 and T8. He gave no history of trauma. He was admitted for further evaluation to determine the etiology of the pathological fractures. Bone marrow aspirate from the vertebrae and biopsies revealed multiple myeloma. During the stay, he went into fluid overload and developed some chest heaviness with runs of ventricular tachycardia. The tachycardia necessitated his transfer to cardiac level II to rule out myocardial infarction. Myocardial infarct was ruled out, and he was discharged after stabilization. He was to be followed up by the oncology clinic.

Discharge diagnoses: (1) Multiple myeloma; (2) compression fractures, T6 and T8; (3) fluid overload; (4) tachycardia.

Code(s):

6. **Physician office visit:** The 63-year-old patient made her annual visit to her gynecologist. She had no complaints. Examination revealed a 6- to 7-centimeter mass at the vaginal apex. She was to be scheduled for an exploratory laparotomy.

   Diagnosis: Vaginal mass.

   Code(s):

7. **Inpatient admission:** The patient was admitted for workup of an abdominal mass. An esophago-gastroduodenoscopy with ultrasound of the abdomen demonstrated a complex cystic solid mass in the pancreas, which had invaded the portal vein. The mass was most consistent with carcinoma of the pancreas. The patient refused colonoscopy, biopsy, and surgery. Therefore, she was discharged with medication and was to follow up with her local physician for palliative treatment of carcinoma.

   Discharge diagnosis: Probable carcinoma of the pancreas with extension to the portal vein.

   Code(s):

8. **Inpatient admission (episode 1):** The patient had a rapidly progressing, drug-resistant, primitive melanotic neuroectodermal tumor (PNET) metastatic to the left femur. He was admitted for fixation of a pathological fracture of the left femur. An open reduction with internal fixation of the left proximal femur with intramedullary nail insertion was performed.

   Discharge diagnoses: (1) PNET metastatic to the femur; (2) pathological fracture, neck of the left femur.

   Code(s):

Inpatient admission (episode 2): The patient was readmitted for management of a right-sided pleural effusion. A right-sided thoracentesis was accomplished, and he had some relief of his breathing. Cytology confirmed the pleural effusion was malignant. A closed biopsy of the right lung confirmed metastasis to the lung. The patient improved and was discharged to follow up in his physician's office.

Discharge diagnoses: (1) Malignant pleural effusion, (2) PNET metastatic to the left femur and right lung.

Code(s):

Inpatient admission (episode 3): The patient was again admitted with the admission diagnosis of severe hypoxemia. He had massive bilateral pulmonary metastases. It was hoped that he could be relieved by chest tube drainage; however, it was obvious from his chest X-ray that removing a small amount of lung fluid would not affect the overall clinical situation. In consultation with the family, it was decided that only terminal care should be provided. He had significant hemoptysis the second day of hospitalization and was in a comatose state until his death that evening.

Discharge diagnoses: (1) Hypoxemia and hemoptysis secondary to malignant pleural effusion, (2) coma, (3) primitive melanotic neuroectodermal tumor metastatic to the left femur and lungs. Primary unknown.

Code(s):

9. **Inpatient admission:** The patient was admitted for chemotherapy. She had ovarian papillary serous cystadenocarcinoma, stage III. Three months earlier, diaphragmatic and omental masses were positive as well. She received Taxol and Cisplatin percutaneously via central vein IV without difficulty. She was to return in three weeks for her next treatment.

Discharge diagnosis: Stage III papillary serous cystadenocarcinoma with metastases to the diaphragm and omentum.

Code(s):

10. **Inpatient admission:** The patient was admitted for removal of an abdominal aortic aneurysm. When the abdomen was opened, carcinoma of the esophagus was found. Because the patient was elderly and the aneurysm was small, the surgeon decided not to repair it or to excise the neoplasm. Prior to discharge, a percutaneous endoscopic gastrostomy tube was inserted to ensure adequate caloric intake. The patient recovered without difficulty and was discharged to home with family.

   Discharge diagnoses: (1) Aortic aneurysm, (2) carcinoma of esophagus.

   Code(s):

11. **Outpatient visit:** The patient complained of dyspnea on exertion, moderate night sweats, and intermittent fevers. On routine chest X-ray, a mass was visualized in the mediastinum. He was to be scheduled for a CT scan.

   Diagnosis: Probable neoplastic disease.

   Code(s):

12. **Inpatient admission (episode 1):** The patient was admitted for evaluation of a mediastinal mass. On CT scan of the thorax, a large mass was identified in the anterior superior portion. Multiple pulmonary nodules were also seen. Excisional needle biopsies of nodules in the lungs, obtained during an exploratory thoracotomy, were positive for yolk sac tumor. The first of a series of five chemotherapy treatments was administered percutaneously via central vein IV prior to discharge.

   Discharge diagnosis: Yolk sac tumor of mediastinum with metastases to both lungs.

   Code(s):

Inpatient admission (episode 2): This admission was for a second cycle of chemotherapy (into central vein) for the yolk sac tumor of the mediastinum. The patient had minimal nausea and vomiting and was discharged following his treatment.

Discharge diagnosis: Yolk sac tumor of mediastinum with metastases to both lungs.

Code(s):

13. **Inpatient admission:** The female patient had melanoma for a number of years. She had undergone a primary resection 10 years ago without recurrence, but one year ago, melanoma was discovered in her axilla and she underwent axillary dissection. A few months later, she presented with sacral pain, and a bone scan revealed left femoral neck and right midfemur sites of metastasis. She had hepatic and adrenal metastases as well. She was admitted for the fifth course of chemotherapy, which was given percutaneously into central vein IV.

Discharge diagnosis: Metastatic melanoma left and right femur, liver, and adrenal gland.

Code(s):

14. **Outpatient clinic visit:** The patient, an elderly woman, returned to the clinic for follow-up of her right malignant extramedullary ileal plasmacytoma. On a recent MRI, it was evident that the neoplasm, which was previously irradiated, had grown. Although she had failed current radiotherapy, there was no evidence that the neoplasm had spread outside its original location. She was started on medication and was to be scheduled for pelvic MRI.

Diagnosis: Malignant ileal plasmacytoma.

Code(s):

686

15. **Inpatient admission:** The female patient had had abdominal pain for several months and infertility for three years. On hysterosalpingo-gram taken before admission, a right tubal occlusion and questionable uterine myoma were visualized. She was admitted for a myomectomy. During the procedure, multiple adhesions were noted from the tubes to a previous myomectomy site, and lysis was carried out. It was felt that the constriction of the tubes by the adhesions might be the cause of the infertility. On the third postoperative day, the staples were removed and the patient went home.

    Discharge diagnoses: (1) Symptomatic leiomyoma, (2) infertility, (3) adhesions.

    Code(s):

16. **Inpatient admission:** The patient was admitted for treatment of a moderately differentiated adenocarcinoma of the endometrium and myometrium. The diagnosis was made after a diagnostic D & C performed a month earlier. She was taken to surgery, where a laparotomy was performed through a midline incision. Exploration revealed no palpable nodes. A total abdominal hysterectomy and bilateral salpingo-oophorectomy were performed without incident or complication. Frozen section of the myometrium showed only minimal invasion at less than one-third of the depth. The postoperative course was benign, and the patient was discharged.

    Discharge diagnosis: Adenocarcinoma of the endometrium, moderately well differentiated, with minimal myometrial involvement.

    Code(s):

17. Outpatient surgery (episode 1): The patient had a persistent left lung infiltrate on X-ray and subsequently had left pleural effusion. Thoracentesis and bronchoscopy with brush biopsy of the left lung were performed. Tissue studies yielded no diagnosis. The patient was to be admitted for further evaluation.

Diagnosis: Left pleural infiltrate on X-ray, pleural effusion.

Code(s):

Inpatient admission (episode 2): The patient was taken to surgery, where a thoracoscopy with decortication and left pleural excisional biopsy were performed. The final specimen report showed moderately differentiated epidermoid carcinoma of the left lung. The patient's first course of electron beam radiation therapy was given prior to discharge.

Discharge diagnosis: Primary carcinoma of lung.

Code(s):

18. Inpatient admission: The patient developed right-sided tinnitus two years earlier, followed by a precipitous loss of hearing on the right side. A preadmission MRI scan identified a large acoustic neuroma. Because hearing on the right was totally lost, it was decided to excise the neuroma using an open radiosurgical destruction technique. The tumor was dissected completely. There were no postoperative complications, and the patient was discharged in satisfactory condition.

Discharge diagnosis: Acoustic neuroma on the right.

Code(s):

19. **Inpatient admission:** The patient, an elderly right-handed woman, was transferred from a nursing home with left hemiparesis and a diagnosis of suspected brain tumor. She underwent a CT-guided stereotactic biopsy without complications. The frozen-section diagnosis was glioblastoma. She was to come back for radiation therapy the following week, and in the meantime she was to be transferred back to the nursing home for further management. She had continued left hemiparesis, which prevents her from being managed at home.

Discharge diagnoses: (1) Primary glioblastoma, right temporal lobe; (2) left hemiparesis.

Code(s):

20. **Inpatient admission:** The patient, an elderly woman, entered the hospital with a history of weight loss, anorexia, dysphagia, and rectal bleeding. She had also fallen many times at home. A fecal impaction was diagnosed from an abdominal CT scan following admission. Preparation for colonoscopy took about three days, and when the colonoscopy was finally accomplished, the impaction had cleared and no abnormalities were seen. A hiatal hernia was found on esophagogastroduodenoscopy, and two meningiomas were identified on magnetic resonance imaging of the head. She was started on Zantac for the hiatal hernia. It seemed that most of her generalized symptoms were secondary to the fecal impaction. The falling episodes are most likely related to the meningiomas, although they showed no mass effect. Neurological consultation was to be obtained as an outpatient. The patient was discharged on stool softeners for prevention of fecal impaction and Zantac for hiatal hernia.

Discharge diagnoses: (1) Meningiomas, (2) fecal impaction, (3) hiatal hernia.

Code(s):

21. **Inpatient admission:** The patient was admitted with severe back pain. He had prostate cancer excised in 2006. An MRI performed prior to admission showed metastasis to the S1, S2, and S3 areas of the spine. A fine-needle aspiration biopsy of the sacrum was performed, and the report confirmed that metastatic adenocarcinoma, consistent with a prostatic primary, was strongly positive. A bilateral open scrotal orchiectomy was performed without complication. Megavoltage beam radiation treatments (photons 9 MeV) to the operative site were started, and the pain came under control with intravenous morphine. The patient was discharged with pain well controlled on oral medications.

    Discharge diagnosis: Metastatic prostate cancer.

    Code(s):

22. **Inpatient admission:** This 14-year-old patient was admitted to the hospital with a diagnosis of glioblastoma multiforme. The patient is now admitted to undergo a blood brain barrier disruption and percutaneous intra-arterial chemotherapy via the right internal carotid artery and, two days later, via the right basilar artery.

    Discharge diagnosis: Glioblastoma multiforme, admit for chemotherapy.

    Code(s):

23. **Outpatient encounter:** A patient presented to the outpatient imaging department for a "high risk" screening mammogram. The physician documented that she is postmenopausal and nulliparous. In addition, the patient has a sister who is currently being treated for breast cancer.

    Diagnoses: (1) Screening mammogram, bilateral; (2) postmenopausal; (3) nulliparous.

    Code(s):

24. Outpatient encounter: The patient has small-cell lung cancer that is in complete remission. The patient is now being seen for prophylactic cranial irradiation therapy, using photons 1–10 MeV.

Diagnoses: (1) Small-cell lung cancer, in remission; (2) radiation therapy.

Code(s):

25. Inpatient admission: The patient presents with a mass in the submandibular gland, which proves to be an adenoid cystic carcinoma. During the course of treatment, the patient has a bilateral radical resection of the level I lymph nodes.

Diagnoses: (1) Adenoid cystic carcinoma of right submandibular gland, (2) removal of lymph nodes.

Code(s):

18. INJURIES

1. **Inpatient admission:** The patient was struck in the face with a softball during a recreational ball game with no loss of consciousness. The result was severe compound fractures of the left ethmoid sinus and frontal sinus bones. The fractures were debrided, and open reduction was carried out. Initially, the postoperative course was uneventful, and the nasal packs, sutures, and nasal splint were removed. However, on the eighth day, the patient became confused and combative. A lumbar puncture was grossly positive for submeningitis. Improvement was rapid with antibiotics and intravenous steroids.

   Discharge diagnoses: (1) Compound nasal, ethmoid, and frontal sinus fractures; (2) post-operative meningitis.

   Procedures: Open reduction of compound fractures of the ethmoid and frontal sinus bones.

Code(s):

2. **Inpatient admission:** The patient, an elderly woman, was cleaning the bathroom and fell backward into the bathtub at her home. She was admitted with possible compression fractures of the lumbar spine. She had several similar falls in the past due to frequent transient ischemic attacks. She lives alone in a single-family residence. X-rays of the spine showed some degenerative disk disease of L4 and L5, but there were no fractures. She was treated for pain and released after two days.

Discharge diagnoses: (1) Lumbar sprain injury to back, (2) probable transient ischemic attack.

Code(s):

3. **Inpatient admission:** The patient was carrying a bicycle up an outside stairway at his house when he fell from the stairway into the alley. An X-ray of the lumbosacral spine taken in the emergency department showed an L4 fracture, and X-ray of the upper arm revealed a nondisplaced comminuted fracture of the shaft of the right humerus. An L4–L5 bilateral posterior foraminotomy with fusion and a bone graft (obtained from the iliac crest) to the posterior column L4–L5 facet joints were performed. The fracture of the humerus was treated with application of a sling and immobilization for five days.

Discharge diagnoses: (1) Fracture, L4; (2) nondisplaced fracture, humerus.

Code(s):

4. Inpatient admission: The patient was admitted following a fall from a ladder at home while watering flower boxes in the garden, in which she sustained numerous injuries. X-rays showed a nondisplaced fracture of the right humeral neck. A splint was applied, but no other treatment was required. There were contusions on her forehead, thighs, and knees, as well as small abrasions of her forehead and right thigh. The patient received pain medications because of the contusions. The abrasions were superficial and healed without treatment and without evidence of infection.

Discharge diagnoses: (1) Nondisplaced fracture, anatomical neck, right humerus; (2) contusions of forehead, thighs, and knees; (3) abrasions on forehead and right thigh.

Code(s):

5. Inpatient admission: The patient was admitted with diagnoses of probable rib fractures and pneumonia. She slipped and fell in the bathtub of her single-family home while taking a shower about four days before admission and had experienced increasingly severe upper back and neck pain. Just prior to admission, she began running a fever, felt short of breath, and developed inspiratory chest wall pain. No rib fractures were identified on chest X-ray, but right upper lobe pneumonia was evident. Sputum culture grew *Klebsiella*. The patient was started on antibiotics and the pneumonia improved. Back pain was relieved by pain medication and bed rest.

Discharge diagnoses: (1) Right upper lobe pneumonia, (2) cervical and thoracic back strain.

Code(s):

6. **Emergency department visit:** The patient and her husband had been drinking heavily, became intoxicated, and had an argument when they got home to their second-floor apartment. During the argument, he shoved her and she fell in the bedroom against the corner of the waterbed, striking her left upper back and chest. She came to the emergency department complaining of severe pain and difficulty breathing. She was found to have subcutaneous emphysema due to the fractures of the ninth and tenth ribs. The ribs were strapped, and she was given a prescription for pain medication. She was released to be followed up as an outpatient.

   Diagnoses: (1) Fractured left ribs, ninth and tenth posteriorly; (2) subcutaneous emphysema; (3) alcohol abuse with intoxication.

   Code(s):

7. **Inpatient admission:** The patient, an elderly woman, was admitted following a fall off her porch at her single-family home while sweeping leaves off the porch. A femoral intertrochanteric fracture was diagnosed in the emergency department, and she was admitted. An open reduction with internal fixation was carried out. As anticipated, postoperative transfusions of three units of packed red blood cells via peripheral vein for blood loss were required during surgery. The blood loss resulted in a drop in hemoglobin and hematocrit, which were monitored daily. Her postoperative recovery went smoothly, and she was transferred to the skilled nursing unit for rehabilitation.

   Discharge diagnoses: (1) Closed fracture, right femur; (2) acute blood loss anemia.

   Code(s):

8. **Inpatient admission:** Three weeks before admission, the patient, a construction worker, sustained a perilunate dislocation along with closed fractures of the third metacarpal and proximal middle phalanx bones of the left hand in an accident. The accident occurred when he went to sleep at the wheel and the dump truck he was driving overturned in the median of the interstate; no other vehicles were involved. Immediately after the accident, the patient was seen in a local emergency department, where the metacarpal fracture was reduced and casted and the proximal phalanx was reduced and splinted. The perilunate dislocation was not reduced at that time. He was now admitted to this hospital, where a closed reduction of the perilunate dislocation was carried out after X-rays confirmed there was no fracture and the phalangeal and metacarpal fractures remained in good alignment. A short arm cast was applied, and he was discharged.

Discharge diagnoses: (1) Closed right perilunate dislocation, (2) healing fractures of the metacarpal shaft and proximal phalanx on the right.

Code(s):

9. **Inpatient admission:** The patient fell from a tree that he was pruning on his farm. He was able to drive himself to the hospital, but it was apparent on admission that his left arm was fractured. He underwent an open reduction and internal fixation of a fracture of the proximal humerus and an open reduction and internal fixation of the comminuted fractures of the radial and ulnar shafts. He recovered without incident and was discharged to follow up in one week.

Discharge diagnoses: (1) Comminuted left radius and ulnar shaft fractures, (2) displaced left proximal humerus fracture.

Code(s):

10. **Inpatient admission:** The patient fell in her apartment after tripping over her cat while carrying a laundry basket to the washer. She was brought in by ambulance and admitted with a fracture of the shaft of right femur. An open reduction with internal fixation was performed. A postoperative fever developed, and a chest X-ray showed severe atelectasis as the cause of the fever. Respiratory therapy gave instructions on incentive spirometry, antibiotics were initiated, and the patient was discharged to a nursing home.

    Discharge diagnoses: (1) Closed fracture, femur; (2) postoperative fever and atelectasis.

    Code(s):

11. **Inpatient admission:** The patient was admitted after a box fell on his head at the service garage where he works. A CT scan of the head was negative for any abnormalities, but hourly neurological checks were made to rule out an intracranial injury. No injury was found. A small abrasion on his upper right arm, where the box scraped the skin, was cleansed and Neosporin applied.

    Discharge diagnosis: Observation for possible intracranial injury.

    Code(s):

12. **Inpatient admission:** The patient, a seven-year-old male, sustained a high-velocity gunshot wound in a drive-by shooting. He was riding his bike in his neighborhood street. He was brought to the emergency department with a massive hemorrhage from the left groin due to the gunshot wound. He also sustained major lacerations of the femoral artery and femoral vein at the hip level, in addition to a bullet lodged in the femur. The patient was immediately taken to surgery. The following procedures were performed via incision: (1) left internal iliac to femoral artery bypass graft with reverse saphenous vein graft; (2) left popliteal to femoral vein bypass graft with greater saphenous vein graft; (3) removal of bullet from the femur; (4) insertion of pins in fracture, left femur.

Discharge diagnoses: (1) Lacerations of left common femoral artery and femoral vein, with massive hemorrhage; (2) gunshot wound to left groin with high-velocity rifle; (3) bullet lodged in femur; (4) open, nondisplaced, type IIIC nondisplaced subtrochanteric fracture of left femur.

Code(s):

13. **Inpatient admission:** The patient, a 10-year-old boy, was admitted through the emergency department after being struck by an automobile while riding his bicycle in the street in front of his home. His injuries were fractures of the left tibia and fibula, a 4-centimeter laceration and superficial abrasions on the left side of the head, and a 1-centimeter-deep laceration on the right earlobe. The fractures were reduced via incision, and an intramedullary Rush rod was placed in the left tibia. The earlobe and head lacerations were sutured.

Discharge diagnoses: (1) Simple fractures, left tibia and fibula; (2) right ear laceration; (3) left parietooccipital laceration.

Code(s):

14. **Emergency department visit (episode 1):** The patient had been drinking heavily in recent weeks. While visiting the area, he reduced his alcohol intake during the past 24 hours and suffered a seizure. In the emergency department, he seemed to be normal. No neurological or physical abnormalities were noted, and he was released after receiving Dilantin.

Diagnosis: Seizure, probably due to decrease in alcohol consumption.

Code(s):

Inpatient admission (episode 2): The patient returned to his room at a local motel, had another seizure, and then fell in the bathroom. He was again brought to the emergency department and found to have a dislocated shoulder. Several attempts were made to replace the shoulder to its proper position. Because this reduction was not successful, he was admitted. With medications to control alcohol withdrawal and seizures along with IV fluids, he became mentally clear. A closed reduction of the dislocated shoulder was performed. The injury became a difficult management problem because the patient would not leave the orthopedic appliance on, and the next day a heavy plaster cast was placed on the shoulder to ensure correct positioning and activity reduction.

Discharge diagnoses: (1) Alcohol withdrawal seizure, (2) left shoulder dislocation.

Code(s):

15. **Emergency department visit (episode 1):** The 14-year-old patient was brought to the emergency department with severe pain and swelling of his left ankle. He sustained the injury when he fell off his skateboard on the grade school playground. An X-ray showed a simple trimalleolar fracture of his left ankle. The fracture was reduced, and he was placed in a long leg cast.

Diagnosis: Severe pain and swelling, left ankle, associated with trimalleolar fracture.

Code(s):

Orthopedic clinic visit (episode 2): The patient was status post trimalleolar fracture of the left ankle. He had been in the cast since sustaining the injury three weeks earlier. He had no complaints regarding the fracture, but he had worn down the cast. The cast breakdown extended the length of the sole of the foot. The long leg cast was removed, and the skin was intact. X-rays showed a healing fracture with no change in the reduction. Therefore, he was placed back into a short leg walking cast.

Diagnosis: Aftercare, healing left trimalleolar fracture.

Code(s):

Orthopedic clinic visit (episode 3): The patient is status post trimalleolar fracture of the left ankle. The fracture now appears to be well healed. The cast was removed. There is no swelling or redness. No additional follow-up is anticipated.

Diagnosis: Aftercare, status post left trimalleolar fracture.

Code(s):

16. **Inpatient admission:** The patient fractured her left knee several years earlier when she was thrown off a horse. Since then, she had undergone realignment and debridement procedures of the undersurface of the patella. At the time of admission, she was severely disabled with multiple effusions, pain, crepitation, and inability to bear weight on the leg. She was taken to surgery and underwent an uneventful total patellectomy. The knee was immobilized with a cast, and she was discharged.

    Discharge diagnosis: Left patellofemoral arthritis.

Code(s):

17. **Inpatient admission:** The woman suffered a displaced fracture dislocation of her right ankle. The injury happened when she jumped off her single-family home front porch in an attempt to catch her fleeing dog, who was being given a bath. She underwent an open reduction and internal fixation of the fracture and was treated with elevation, bed rest, analgesics, and antibiotics. She was released in stable condition.

    Discharge diagnosis: Trimalleolar fracture dislocation, right ankle.

Code(s):

18. **Inpatient admission:** The patient was shopping at a retail food warehouse when a gallon can of tomatoes fell on his head from a shelf about 15 feet overhead. He was briefly unconscious and disoriented. X-rays of his skull showed a depressed parasagittal skull fracture with considerable parasagittal depression. He was admitted and taken to surgery, where a craniectomy was performed, with elevation of the depressed skull fracture.

    Discharge diagnosis: Depressed skull fracture.

    Code(s):

19. **Inpatient admission:** The patient fractured her left patella when she suffered a fall into a hole while golfing on the public golf course. She was taken to surgery, where an open reduction and internal fixation were performed without complication. By the second postoperative day, she was ambulatory on crutches and ready for discharge.

    Discharge diagnosis: Closed fracture, left patella.

    Code(s):

20. **Physician office visit:** The patient went to see his physician after falling off a moving motorcycle. He complained of leg pain, and the physician noted swelling in the right lower extremity. The physician felt that a fracture of the tibia was probable and referred the patient for X-ray to confirm or rule out. For reasons unknown, the patient did not report to the hospital radiology department and did not return to see the physician as instructed.

    Diagnosis: Suspected fracture, right tibia.

    Code(s):

21. **Inpatient admission:** A six-month-old infant was admitted with listlessness, nausea and vomiting, and extremely pale skin. The physician diagnosed the patient with heat prostration and suspected child abandonment. The baby was admitted and rehydrated with intravenous fluids.

    Discharge diagnoses: (1) Heat prostration, (2) suspected child abandonment.

    Code(s):

19. BURNS

1. **Inpatient admission:** The patient sustained flash burns when his clothing caught fire. Someone had thrown gasoline onto the park cooking grill by which he was cooking. He suffered second-degree burns to the face, neck, and upper chest, with some first- and second-degree burns on the left forearm. All in all, 12 percent of the total body surface area was burned. The wounds were treated with antibiotics and pain medications. Physical therapists debrided the burned areas and provided hydrotherapy. The wounds continued to heal, and the patient was discharged.

Discharge diagnoses: (1) Second-degree burns, face, neck, and upper chest; (2) first- and second-degree burns, left forearm; (3) 12 percent of body surface affected by burns.

Code(s):

2. **Inpatient admission:** The patient was brought to the emergency department after being burned. He had been clearing and burning brush in a field at his farm when a gust of wind moved the fire to his tractor. There was an explosion because of the gasoline fumes, and he caught fire. He was treated with IV fluids, antibiotics, and pain medications. All in all, 14 percent of the total body surface was affected by the burns, of which 4 percent was third degree. He was transferred to a burn treatment center for surgical debridement and skin grafting.

Discharge diagnoses: (1) First- and second-degree burns of the face, right ear, right forearm, and right thumb; (2) third-degree burn of the left hand.

Code(s):

3. Inpatient admission (episode 1): The patient was admitted with burns of her right hand and fingers up to the wrist. She had reached into hot water, not realizing the temperature, while canning on her farm. She was taken to surgery, where an excisional debridement of the burns was carried out to prepare the wound for the graft. A split thickness skin graft was applied over the dorsum and volar aspects of the hand. The postoperative recovery was without infection or other complication.

Discharge diagnosis: Second- and third-degree burns, right hand and fingers (3 percent of total body surface burned, 2 percent affected by third degree burn).

Code(s):

Physician office visit (episode 2): Both the burns and the surgical site on this woman's hand seem to be healing nicely. There was no evidence of infection. The area was rebandaged. Antibiotics were continued, and she was to return the following week.

Diagnosis: Second- and third-degree burns, right hand and fingers.

Code(s):

20. POISONING, TOXIC EFFECTS, ADVERSE EFFECTS, AND UNDERDOSING OF DRUGS

1. **Inpatient admission:** The patient, a 33-year-old male, was admitted through the emergency department after an overdose of Dilantin. His gait was ataxic and he had nausea, vomiting, and blurry vision. His Dilantin level was 48. He had AIDS-related complex (ARC), well documented from previous hospitalizations. He also had posttraumatic epilepsy, which resulted from an intracranial injury received in a previous motor vehicle accident. On questioning, he admitted to taking an additional 400 milligrams of Dilantin accidentally on the day of admission. Over the next four days, the Dilantin level gradually decreased to 16.1, and the regular dosage was restarted. It was clear that the current dosage was adequate in preventing seizures without significant side effects.

   Discharge diagnoses: (1) Dilantin toxicity, (2) HIV positive, (3) posttraumatic epilepsy.

   Code(s):

2. **Outpatient clinic visit:** The patient came in because of a new rash on his body. The thrush, previously diagnosed and being treated with Dapsone, is improving.

   Diagnoses: (1) Skin rash due to an allergic reaction to Dapsone taken internally as prescribed, (2) thrush.

   Code(s):

3. **Inpatient admission:** The patient underwent an autologous bone marrow transplantation for choriocarcinoma 13 days earlier. He was readmitted four hours after discharge with a rash, which changed character to an urticarial type of eruption. A skin biopsy of the right lower arm revealed superficial perivascular infiltrate consistent with urticaria. The patient had been started on vancomycin the morning prior to admission. Vancomycin was discontinued, and the urticaria cleared spontaneously.

Discharge diagnoses: (1) Vancomycin allergy with an urticarial reaction, (2) choriocarcinoma.

Code(s):

4. **Inpatient admission:** The patient, a 73-year-old male, was admitted for upper and lower gastrointestinal endoscopy for gastrointestinal bleeding. The patient was given atropine and, shortly thereafter, the preoperative evaluation showed a heart rate on three occasions of 35, 36, and 37. The patient normally had a heart rate in the upper 40s and had never had one in the 30s. The procedure was canceled due to his bradycardia, and a cardiac evaluation was to be obtained prior to rescheduling. The slow heart rate may have been a reaction to atropine because it occurred shortly after administration of the drug.

Discharge diagnoses: (1) Gastrointestinal bleed, (2) slow heart rate due to atropine correctly administered.

Code(s):

5. **Inpatient admission:** The patient, a 46-year-old with AIDS, was recently discharged after workups for fever and weight loss, which were negative. He was readmitted because of histoplasmosis. Amphotericin B was started, and he tolerated the treatment well. Because the patient needed to continue treatment with this medication at home over a fairly long period of time, a Hickman catheter was inserted into the superior vena cava to facilitate administration. He also had severe granulocytopenia, thought to be due to AZT, which was discontinued.

   Discharge diagnoses: (1) Acquired immuno-deficiency syndrome; (2) disseminated histoplasmosis; (3) granulocytopenia, possibly due to AZT.

   Code(s):

6. **Inpatient admission:** The patient was admitted in an altered mental state, showing some confusion as well as ataxia, jaundice, and dizziness. Her husband reported that he felt that the problem related to a massive overusage of an herbal tea given to her by a "healer." She was told to use about a tablespoon per day in a cup of tea but instead had been drinking about a gallon a day. She had a fibroid mass diagnosed about one year earlier but refused conventional treatment. Instead, she was trying to cure it with the tea. After checking with the Poison Control Center, it was determined that the phenylbutazone in this particular brand of tea was probably what was causing her problems. Her mental status returned to its baseline state within 48 hours, and the other problems related to herbal tea consumption disappeared in the same time frame. The presence of a huge uterine mass was confirmed on CT scan, and surgery was offered but refused.

   Discharge diagnoses: (1) Central nervous and digestive system problems secondary to herbal tea intoxication, (2) uterine mass.

   Code(s):

7. **Inpatient admission:** The patient, a young man, collapsed on the street after leaving a bar. An ambulance brought him to the emergency department in severe respiratory distress, which escalated to respiratory failure. He was endoscopically intubated, ventilatory support was initiated, and he was admitted. Respiratory arrest ensued. He died within three hours of admission. Autopsy findings indicated lethal levels of Valium, cocaine, marijuana, and ephedrine.

   Discharge diagnosis: Respiratory failure secondary to overdoses of multiple substances.

   Code(s):

8. **Inpatient admission:** The patient was admitted for a transurethral resection of the prostate (TURP) for benign prostatic hypertrophy. He was taken to the operating room, but immediately following the induction with general anesthesia, atrial fibrillation developed. The procedure was canceled and the atrial fibrillation treated. It was determined that the arrhythmia was due to the anesthetic.

   Discharge diagnoses: (1) Benign prostatic hypertrophy, (2) atrial fibrillation secondary to anesthesia.

   Code(s):

9. **Inpatient admission:** The patient was admitted with nausea and vomiting for the past 24 hours. He was found to have an elevated digoxin level, and, after adjustment of dosage, the level came down and the nausea and vomiting ceased. On questioning, he seemed to be taking the digoxin correctly. A new prescription was written, and the patient's digoxin level was to be monitored.

   Discharge diagnosis: Digoxin toxicity.

   Code(s):

10. **Inpatient admission:** The patient was admitted with moderate persistent asthma, which had become intractable to management on an ambulatory care basis. The medications consisted of antibiotics, bronchodilators, and IV steroids. Unfortunately, her stay was prolonged because of an allergic reaction to two of the medications. Celestone and prednisone caused jitteriness and anxiety to the extent that Lorazepam was necessary.

    Discharge diagnoses: (1) Severe asthma, (2) medication allergy.

    Code(s):

11. **Inpatient admission:** The patient came to the outpatient area with swelling and discoloration of the right arm. She was admitted with a provisional diagnosis of axillary vein thrombosis. A venogram of the right arm showed nearly complete obstruction of the axillary vein with an intraluminal clot. She gave a history of having started on birth control pills recently, and it was felt that the drug (Orval) was the cause of the thrombosis. She was taken off the birth control pills and started on IV anticoagulation. When discharged, her prothrombin time was in the therapeutic range, and the arm pain and edema were better.

    Discharge diagnosis: Right axillary vein thrombosis.

    Code(s):

12. Inpatient admission: The patient, an elderly woman, was admitted with shortness of breath, dyspnea on exertion, fever, and productive cough. These problems were felt to represent lobar pneumonia. She was admitted for cultures and intravenous antibiotics. A chest film showed bilateral lung infiltrates. Erythromycin and Bactrim (also known as sulfamethoxazole and trimethoprim) were given intravenously. However, diarrhea resulted. These drugs were discontinued; when she was switched to Ceftin, her condition showed rapid improvement.

Discharge diagnoses: (1) Lobar pneumonia, (2) diarrhea.

Code(s):

13. Inpatient admission: The patient, a young woman, was brought to the emergency department via ambulance. She was suffering from acute alcohol intoxication. She admitted, however, that she had also ingested a handful of Compazine and Advil (ibuprofen), thinking they were vitamins and aspirin. In the emergency department, she was treated with charcoal and Narcan and admitted for observation. A psychiatric consultation was obtained, and the psychiatrist deemed the patient stable and not dangerous to herself or others. The patient agreed to obtain drug and alcohol treatment and was discharged.

Discharge diagnoses: (1) Acute alcohol intoxication; (2) multiple substance overdose, Compazine, Advil, and alcohol.

Code(s):

14. Inpatient admission: The patient was admitted with subdural hematoma that appeared to be related to the anticoagulant she had been on for some time. She underwent an initial CT scan of the brain, which confirmed the subdural hematoma. She had been on chronic Coumadin therapy and had also been taking aspirin as prescribed by her physician for a left lower-extremity deep venous thrombosis. Her Coumadin and aspirin were held, and the prothrombin time was measured on a daily basis. The Coumadin was adjusted, and the aspirin was discontinued. The physician was queried and confirmed that the subdural hematoma was a result of the bleeding disorder caused by the Coumadin. Her condition at discharge was good.

Discharge diagnoses: (1) Subdural hematoma secondary to medications; (2) chronic deep venous thrombosis, left leg.

Code(s):

15. Inpatient admission: The patient fractured her left patella when she fell down the basement steps in her single-family home. An open reduction was performed with internal fixation yesterday. During recovery, she had problems with nausea, vomiting, and urinary retention secondary to morphine administration. The pain medication was changed to Demerol, and the symptoms subsided by the second day. The patient was discharged in satisfactory condition the same day.

Discharge diagnoses: (1) Closed fracture, left patella; (2) allergic reaction to morphine.

Procedure: Open reduction of patellar fracture with internal fixation.

Code(s):

16. **Inpatient admission:** A patient was scheduled for outpatient knee arthroscopy. The patient had been sedated, then intubated, and anesthesia was started. The surgeon injected the patient's knee with Bupivacaine. However, prior to the insertion of the arthroscopic trocars, the patient began having trouble breathing. The patient subsequently went into cardiopulmonary arrest and a code blue was called. The patient was resuscitated and admitted to the ICU, where she continued to receive ventilator support through the previously placed intubation. Twelve hours later, the patient was transferred to Hospital B for further intensive evaluation and consultation.

Discharge diagnoses: (1) Adverse reaction to Bupivacaine, (2) cardiopulmonary arrest secondary to #1, (3) anoxic encephalopathy, (4) diabetes with neuropathy, (5) hypertension, (6) osteoarthritis, knees.

Code(s):

21. COMPLICATIONS OF SURGERY AND MEDICAL CARE

1. **Inpatient admission:** The patient was suffering an acute rejection episode involving her left cadaveric renal transplant. She had undergone the transplant three months earlier for end-stage renal disease (ESRD) due to focal glomerulonephritis. An endoscopic-guided percutaneous biopsy of the transplanted kidney was performed, and it was deemed suitable for her to go home after a pulse of steroids.

   Discharge diagnosis: Kidney transplant rejection.

   Code(s):

2. **Inpatient admission:** The admitting diagnosis was revision of hip arthroplasty. The patient had undergone a total left hip arthroplasty five weeks earlier for osteoarthritis. The prosthesis worked well until the previous week, when she heard a pop. X-rays taken on admission showed a superior displacement of the left acetabular cup, which continued to migrate proximally despite bed rest. The left acetabular component of the prosthesis was moved back to the correct location and recemented in place. Three days after surgery, the patient had a hemoglobin of 10.9 and was transfused with two units of packed red blood cells. Hemoglobin count improved, and the patient was discharged on the fifth postoperative day.

   Discharge diagnoses: (1) Superior displacement, left acetabular cup prosthesis; (2) acute blood loss anemia.

   Code(s):

3. Inpatient admission: The patient was admitted for removal of a left knee prosthesis, which had caused persistent pain since it was placed three years earlier. A recurrent thrombophlebitis was also present in the right lower extremity and was currently being treated with Coumadin. The left knee prosthesis was examined via incision, and there was necrotic tissue of the bone ends (tibia and fibula), which was debrided. Components of the prosthesis were noted to be loosened, and the prosthesis was removed and replaced. Physical therapy was started, and the patient was discharged on antibiotics.

Discharge diagnoses: (1) Necrosis, bone; (2) malfunctioning left knee prosthesis; (3) thrombophlebitis, right leg.

Code(s):

4. Inpatient admission: Two months before admission, the patient completed 37 X-ray therapy treatments following resection of his tongue for removal of primary squamous cell carcinoma. He was admitted for evaluation and therapy of spontaneous extraoral drainage from an exposed bone plate of the left mandible. After debridement of the affected site via incision, he was discharged for follow-up care at the referring hospital.

Discharge diagnosis: Osteoradionecrosis of left mandible.

Code(s):

5. **Inpatient admission:** The patient underwent a laryngoscopy with biopsy in the ambulatory surgery area, and a primary neoplasm of the false vocal cords was confirmed. In the recovery room, she developed acute respiratory insufficiency and was placed on oxygen. Because of the severity of the respiratory insufficiency, she was admitted. By the third hospital day, her blood gases returned to normal, and she was discharged.

   Discharge diagnoses: (1) Carcinoma of vocal cords, (2) postoperative respiratory insufficiency.

   Code(s):

6. **Inpatient admission:** The patient was admitted because of a displaced T tube, which was partially out of the common bile duct. The T tube was blocked by a malignant tumor of the pancreas, which caused the tube to buckle and leak. The patient was transferred to another hospital for care.

   Discharge diagnoses: (1) Bile in peritoneum due to T tube partially out of common duct; (2) tumor, head of pancreas.

   Code(s):

7. **Inpatient admission:** The admission diagnoses were possible uterine septum and adnexal mass. A left ovarian cystic mass, which was thought to be an endometrioma and a uterine septum, was confirmed on hysteroscopy and laparoscopy. In the course of evaluation, a perforation of the left uterine horn occurred. Laparotomy was performed, and the cystic mass was excised from the ovary. The abdominal cavity was copiously irrigated and the uterine perforation repaired. Pathological findings identified the cystic mass as a dermoid cyst of the ovary.

   Discharge diagnoses: (1) Dermoid cyst, left ovary; (2) uterine septum; (3) inadvertent puncture, left uterine horn.

   Code(s):

ICD-10-CM and ICD-10-PCS Coding Handbook, without Answers, 2021 Revised Edition

718

8. Inpatient admission: The patient underwent a cystoscopy, with endoscopic passage of a stone basket up the left ureter and a contrast retrograde pyelogram of the kidneys, ureters, and bladder the day before admission. After release, she experienced terrible pain in the ureteral area and had to be admitted for pain control. A repeat intravenous pyelogram was normal, and laboratory studies were all within normal limits. By the end of the second day, her pain was controlled with oral medications, and she was discharged.

Discharge diagnosis: Postoperative pain of undetermined cause.

Code(s):

9. Inpatient admission: The patient underwent a cold conization of the cervix and fractional dilatation and curettage for postmenopausal bleeding in the outpatient surgery center. The surgery was uncomplicated, and the operative site was dry at the conclusion of the procedure. An examination of tissue rendered a pathological diagnosis of severe cervical dysplasia, CIN-III. Within two hours postoperatively, there was excessive bleeding and a vaginal pack was placed. She bled through the pack and was then admitted for suture repair of site of the previous cervical biopsy. Postoperatively, she remained dry with no further problems and was discharged in good condition.

Discharge diagnoses: (1) Severe cervical dysplasia, CIN-III; (2) postoperative bleeding.

Code(s):

10. Inpatient admission: The patient had a subtrochanteric stress fracture of the left femur, which had been repaired with pin insertion three weeks earlier. She returned with an infection of the operative wound site and delayed healing of the fracture. A wide excisional debridement of the infection site of the soft tissue was carried out via incision. No definite infection could be demonstrated within the bone. Cultures of the operative wound grew *Staphylococcus aureus,* sensitive to everything, and the patient was maintained on IV antibiotics until discharge.

Discharge diagnosis: Deep soft tissue infection, left thigh.

Code(s):

11. Inpatient admission: The patient underwent a cervical discectomy and fusion last year. The pain improved for a few months but has recurred. He was readmitted for further surgery. A left C3–C4, C5–C6, and C6–C7 posterior cervical decompressive laminectomy with foraminotomy was performed. There was considerable postoperative pain, well out of proportion to what would be expected for this surgery. He remained in the hospital the week following surgery, primarily to receive intramuscular pain medications.

Discharge diagnoses: (1) Cervical spondylosis, (2) severe postoperative back pain.

Code(s):

12. **Inpatient admission:** A month earlier, the patient had undergone open reduction and internal fixation of a traumatic fracture of the left femur. She came to the emergency department with a severe and deep infection of the left thigh. She was admitted and taken to surgery immediately, where a wide excisional debridement of the subcutaneous tissue of the infection was carried out and hardware was removed from the upper portion of the femur. Cultures of fixation pins grew *Staphylococcus aureus,* and she was maintained on IV oxacillin. She was to continue antibiotics at home after discharge.

    Discharge diagnosis: Staphylococcal infection due to orthopedic fixation device.

    Code(s):

13. **Inpatient admission:** This acutely ill patient was admitted with fever, weakness, and chills. He had undergone a bilateral herniorrhaphy four days before admission. He is now experiencing some urgency on urination and dysuria. On admission to the hospital, the operative incisions were slightly red and tender and the abdomen somewhat distended. Blood cultures and wound cultures revealed a heavy growth of *Staphylococcus aureus,* which also grew on a urine culture. *Enterococcus faecalis* also grew on the urine culture. The chills and fever receded with IV antibiotics. It was believed that the patient's problems represented postoperative complications of the herniorrhaphy.

    Discharge diagnoses: (1) Postoperative sepsis and urinary tract infection, (2) postoperative wound infection.

    Code(s):

14. **Inpatient admission:** A patient who is 50 days post stem cell transplant due to multiple myeloma that is currently in remission was admitted with fever, severe nausea and vomiting, splenomegaly, and cervical lymphadenopathy. A left inguinal lymph node needle biopsy was performed when the lymphadenopathy enlarged and spread to the inguinal area.

Discharge diagnoses: (1) Post stem cell transplant lymphoproliferative disorder, (2) multiple myeloma in remission.

Code(s):

Index

A

Abbreviations in ICD-10-CM, 16–17
    NEC (not elsewhere classified), 17, 49
    NOS (not otherwise specified), 17, 49
Abdomen, internal injuries of, 510
Abdominal aortic aneurysm repair, 449, 450*
Ablation
    endometrial, 279
    of lung, 238–239
    thermal, 479
Ablation of heart tissue, 441–442
Abnormal findings, 30–31, 137–138
Abortion, 322, 342, 342, 343, 355–364, 361
    complications associated with, 356–357
    inadvertent, 358–359
    maternal condition as reason for, 358
    missed, 364
    procedure resulting in liveborn infant, 359
    procedures, 360–361, 361
    spontaneous, 356, 359
    types of, 356
    weeks of gestation for pregnancies with abortive outcomes,
        codes for, 357
Abrasions, 511
Abuse, 173
    adult, 495–497
    alcohol, 182–183
    child, 495–497
    elder, 496
    substance, 182–185, 187–189, 188, 535
Accidents, transport and vehicle, 492
Acidosis, in newborn, 385
Acquired immunodeficiency syndrome (AIDS) infections, 153–154, 225.
        See also Human immunodeficiency virus (HIV)
Activity codes, 492
Acute metabolic complications, 163–164
Acute pulmonary edema, 223, 236
Acute respiratory distress syndrome, 235
Adhesions, 255–256
Adjustment disorders, 179
Administration Section, 15–106, 105
    root operations in, 105–106, 105, 106
Admissions/encounters
    for aftercare management, 123–124
    for anemia, management of, 474
    for complications associated with malignant neoplasm, 474–475
    to determine extent of malignancy, 476
    following medical observation, 25
    following postoperative observation, 25
    for follow-up examination, 124–125, 478
    for management of dehydration, 474
    with normal delivery, 327–328
    for observation and evaluation, 125–127
    for obstetric care other than delivery, 329–330
    for orthopedic aftercare, 508–509
    with other delivery, 328–329
    for other obstetric care, 329–330
    from outpatient surgery, 25
    for pain control/management, 209–210
    for prophylactic organ removal, 477
Admitting diagnosis, 23, 31
Adult personality and behavior, disorders of, 181–182
Adverse effects, 527–536
    codes for, 490–491
        guidelines for assignment of, 532
        location of, 530–532, 531
    late effects of, 536
    of penicillin, 291

- of therapeutic substances, 528
- unspecified, of drugs, 534

Affective disorders, 177–178
Aftercare
    complications versus, 552
    management of, admission or encounter for, 123–124
Age, relationship to codes, 369, 376–377
AHA Coding Clinic®, 4, 33, 62
Alcohol dependence and abuse, 182–183, 524
Alcohol use during pregnancy, 334–335
Alphabetic Index of Diseases and Injuries, 4, 7–9, 41, 42
    abbreviations in, 16–17
    alphabetization rules, 10
    complication codes in, locating, 539–540
    distinction between acquired and congenital conditions in, 368–369
    essential modifiers in, 18
    finding applicable Table in, 80
    format of, 7–9
    in ICD-10-PCS, 62
    locating code entry in, 42
    locating main term in, 78–79
    multiple coding in, 50–53
    punctuation marks in, 18, 50
    using both Tabular List and, 43, 48
Alteration, as root operation, 99, 99
Altered mental state, 176
Alzheimer's disease, 175, 206
American Health Information Management Association (AHIMA), 4
    developing and maintaining ICD-10-CM, 24
    Standards of Ethical Coding, 33
American Hospital Association (AHA), 4
    Coding Clinic®, 4, 33, 62
    developing and maintaining ICD-10-CM, 24
American Medical Association (AMA), *Current Procedural Terminology*
    (CPT®) of, 83, 577, 578
American Psychiatric Association, 174
Amnesia, transient global, 176
Amnioinfusion, 343–344
Amputations, 81–82, 82, 511, 512
    complications of, 548–549
    traumatic, 510, 511
Anastomosis, 251, 439
Anatomical regions body system codes, 67
Anatomical site
    of burn, 520, 520
    in classifying injuries, 4888
Ancillary procedures, 112–119
    Imaging Section, 112–114, 113, 114
    New Technology Section, 119–120, 119, 120
    Nuclear Medicine Section, 114–115, 114, 115
    Physical Rehabilitation and Diagnostic Audiology Section, 117–119,
        117, 118, 119
    Radiation Therapy Section, 115–116, 115, 116
"And," as relational term, 20, 64
Anemia, 193, 194–198
    acute blood-loss, 195
    acute posthemorrhagic, 194, 195
    admission/encounter for management of, 474
    aplastic, 196
    of chronic disease, 196
    deficiency, 194
    drug-induced
        folate deficiency, 194
        idiopathic, 196
    due to blood loss, 195
    due to chemotherapy, 196
    pancytopenia, 196
    postoperative, 540

*Page numbers in color refer to tables, figures, or illustrations.

Anemia (continued)
   of pregnancy, 194
   sickle-cell, 193, 197–198
   thalassemia, 197
Aneurysms, 410–411, 449–454
   procedures on, 449–454, 450, 451
      endovascular implantation of branching or fenestrated graft
         into aorta, 453
      endovascular repair, 449–454, 451
      open aneurysmectomy, 449, 450
      open surgical repair, via tube graft, 449, 450
      pseudoaneurysm, 452
Angina pectoris, 398–399
   postinfarction, 404
   unstable, 398–399
Angiocardiography, 426–427
Angioplasty
   of noncoronary vessels, 436
   with stent insertion, 434, 435
Animal bites, 510
Anterior lumbar interbody fusion (ALIF), 313, 307, 308
Antineoplastic drugs, 349
   extravasation of, 546
Antineoplastic therapy, 170, 196, 475–476
Anxiety disorders
   organic, 175
   phobic, 179
Aorta, congenital malformations of, 370–371
Aortic valve insufficiency, 396
Aortocoronary artery bypass, 437–440, 437
Apnea, 380
Apparent life-threatening event (ALTE), 386
Appendicitis, 257
Approach to procedure site, 61
   code characters for, 71, 72, 74–75
Aqueous misdirection, 218
ARCUATE™ XP (percutaneous vertebroplasty) procedure, 314
Arterial system, major vessels of, 394
Arthritis, 300, 302–304
Arthropathy, 300
Ascites, malignant, 477
Aspergillosis, 226
Asphyxia, 379–380
Aspiration
   fine needle, 251
   meconium, 380
Assistance, as root operation, 107, 108
Asthma, 230–231
   burns and, 524
Atelectasis, 232
Atherectomy
   of noncoronary vessels, 436
   transluminal coronary, 435–436
Atherosclerosis
   of coronary artery bypass (grafts), 405
   of extremities, 419–420
Atherosclerotic heart disease, of native coronary artery, 404
Atmospheric control, as root operation, 109
Atrial fibrillation, 441
Atrial septal defect, 377, 403
Atrophy, 305
Automatic implantable cardioverter defibrillator (AICD), 428–430
Autonomic dysreflexia, 210
Axial lumbar interbody fusion (AxiaLIF®), 313, 314, 314

B

Bacillus Calmette-Guerin (immunotherapy agent), 479
Back disorders, 300–302
Bacteremia, 143, 146, 149
Baroreflex system, 447
Battered spouse syndrome, 496
Behavioral syndromes, 181
Bell's palsy, 216
Bilateral body part values, 70, 70
Bilateral sites, coding for, 53
Biliary system, 245
   diseases of, 252–254
Biliopancreatic diversion, 259
Biofeedback, as mental health procedure, 187
Biopsies
   of breast, 280
   of bronchus, pleura, and lung, 237–238
   brush, 237, 251
   coding, 88–89

   defined, 88
   endoscopic, 237–238
   liquid, 237
   thoracoscopic, 237
   vertebral, 315
Bipolar disorders, 177, 178
Birth. See Childbirth
Bleeding. See also Hemorrhage
   in gastrointestinal tract, 246–247
   occult, 246
   rectal, 247
Blindness, 214
Blisters, 511
Blood and blood-forming organs, diseases of, 193–202
   Alzheimer's disease, 206
   anemia, 194–198
   bleeding caused by anticoagulation therapy, 198
   coagulation defects, 198–199
   disorders of immune system, 201–202
   epilepsy, 206
   headache and migraine, 207–208
   Parkinson's disease, 205–206
   platelet cells, 199
   thalassemia, 197–198
   white blood cells, 199–201
Blood brain barrier (BBB), 480
Blood brain barrier disruption (BBBD) chemotherapy, 480, 480
Blood cells, types of, 200
Blood vessels
   distinguishing between central and peripheral, 425–426
   injuries to, 510
Body layers, coding procedures in overlapping, 89
Body mass index (BMI), 38, 169
Body part
   branches of, 69–70, 425
   code characters for, 69–71, 70
   for coronary arteries, 425
   musculoskeletal guidelines for, 307
   root operations, 89–99
      to alter diameter or route of a tubular, 94–95, 94
      to take out solids/fluids/gases from a, 91–92, 91
      to take out some or all of a, 89–90, 89
      that put in/put back or move some/all of a, 93–94, 93
   vessels, distinguishing central from peripheral, 425–426
Body systems
   code characters for, 66–67, 67
   complications affecting specific, 541–543
Bone, joint versus, 300
Brachytherapy, 115, 116
Brackets, square, 19, 50
Brain, side view of, 174
Breast
   biopsies of, 280
   diseases of, 280–281
   hypertrophy of, 283
   reconstruction of, 281–283, 282
   surgery on, 280–283, 282
Brevetoxin, environmental exposure to, 532
Bronchitis, asthmatic, 231
Bronchoalveolar lavage (BAL), 237
Bronchopulmonary dysplasia, 376–377
Bronchoscopic procedures, 237
Bronchospasm, 231
Brush biopsy, 237, 251
Burns, 519–524
   anatomical site of, 520, 520
   associated injuries and illnesses, 524
   chronic bronchitis and, 524
   depth of (first-, second-, and third-degree), 521
   electrical, 524
   extent of, 522–523
   external causes of, 523
   friction, 520
   of internal organs, 521
   pre-existing conditions and, 524
   sequencing of codes for, 521–522
   seventh-character values for, 522
   sunburn, 523
   thermal, 520
Bypass
   cardiopulmonary, 449
   coronary, 398
   gastric, 259
Bypass, as root operation, 94–95, 94

C

Calculus, 245
  biliary, removal of, 254, **254**
  urinary, removal of, 274
Carcinoma
  Merkel cell, 459
  neuroendocrine, of skin, 459
  in situ, 459–460
Cardiac arrest, 409–410
Cardiac pacemakers, 430–432, **430**
  intracardiac (leadless, transcatheter), 432
Cardiac resynchronization defibrillator (CRT-D), 433
Cardiac resynchronization pacemaker without internal cardiac defibrillator
    (CRT-P), 433
Cardiac resynchronization therapy, 433
Cardiac tamponade, 408
Cardiofaciocutaneous (CFC) syndrome, 369
Cardiomyopathy, 409, 448
  hypertensive, 409
  ischemic, 409
  pregnancy associated, 339
Cardiomyoplasty, dynamic, 448
Cardiomyostimulation system, implantation of, 448
Cardiovascular disorders, burns and, 524
Carotid sinus stimulation system, implantation of, 447–448
Carryover lines, indention of, in Alphabetic Index, 8
Cataracts, 164–165, 216
Catheter, 265, 270, 271–272, 444–445, **446**
  central venous (CVC), 445–446, **446**
  hemodialysis via, 271–272
  peripherally inserted central (PICC), 445, **446**
  tunneled, 271, 444–446
Cellulitis, 294–295, 511
  of female external genital organs, 295
  pelvic, 295
Centers for Disease Control and Prevention (CDC), 4, 228, 334
Centers for Medicare & Medicaid Services (CMS), 4, 577–580
  developing and maintaining ICD-10-CM, 24
Central nervous system (CNS), 203, **204**
  inflammatory diseases of, 205
Central venous catheter (CVC), 445, **446**
Cerebral degeneration, 204
Cerebral dysfunction, 174
Cerebral infarction, 411–414
  types of, **411**
Cerebrospinal fluid leak, 213
Cerebrovascular accident (CVA), 208
Cerebrovascular diseases and disorders, 411–414, **411**
  hypertensive, 418
  sequelae of, 413–414
Cervical disc disorders, 300–302
Cervical intraepithelial neoplasia (CIN), 278–279
Cervical ripening, 343
Cesarean deliveries, 343, 346
Change, as root operation, 95–96, **95**, 103, **103**
Character function in codes, 64, **64**
Chemotherapy
  admission or encounter involving administration of, 475–476
  anemia due to, 196
  aplastic anemia and, 196, 474
  in treating neoplasms, 479, **479**
Chest, internal injuries of, 510
Chiari II malformation, 370
Child
  abandonment of, 496
  abuse, 495–497
  health supervision of, 386–387
Childbirth. *See also* Deliveries; Labor and delivery
  classification of, 377
  complications of, 321–351
  conditions complicating, 331–335
  forceps delivery, 344
  fractures due to injury in, 506
  hypertension complicating, 419
  malnutrition in, 324
  sequelae of complication of, 340
  vacuum extraction, 344
  weeks of gestation, coding for, 321, 324, 357
Chiropractic Section, 111, **111**
Cholecystectomy, 253
Cholecystitis, 252–253
Cholesterolosis, 253
Chronic conditions, 29, 54–55
Chronic giant papillary conjunctivitis, 215

Chronic ischemic heart disease, 405
Chronic kidney disease (CKD), 164, 263
  anemia in, 196
  burns and, 524
  end-stage renal disease and, 267
    diabetes mellitus and, 269
  following transplant, 548
  hypertension and, 268–269, **269**, 417
Chronic obstructive pulmonary disease (COPD), 230–231
  burns and, 524
Chronic stroke, 412
Circulatory system
  diabetic complications, 165
  diseases of, 393–454
    aneurysm, 410–411, 449–454, **450**, **451**
    angina pectoris, 398–399
    atrial fibrillation, 441
    cardiac arrest, 409–410
    cardiac tamponade, 408
    cardiomyopathy, 409
    cerebrovascular disorders, 411–414
    chronic kidney disease and, 417
    heart failure, 406–408
      compensated, decompensated, and exacerbated, 408
      hypertensive disease and, 408
    hypertension, 415–416
      chronic kidney disease and, 268–269, **269**, 417
      complicating pregnancy, childbirth, and the puerperium,
        419
      with other conditions, 418
    hypertensive heart disease, 416–417
    interior of heart, 396
    ischemic heart disease, 397–406
      chronic, 398
      chronic total occlusion, 406
      myocardial infarction, 399–402, **401**
      other acute, 403
      postmyocardial infarction syndrome, 404
  major vessels
    of arterial system, **394**
    body part values for, 425
    of venous system, **395**
  National Institutes of Health Stroke Scale (NIHSS), 38, 139
  other conditions, 423
  procedures involving, 425–444
    ablation of heart tissue (maze procedure), 441–442
    aneurysms, 449–454, **450**, **451**
    angiocardiography, 426–427
    angioplasty and atherectomy of noncoronary vessels,
      436
    body part values for, 425
    cardiac pacemaker therapy, 430–432, **430**
    cardiac resynchronization therapy, 433
    coronary artery bypass graft, 437–440, **437**
    diagnostic cardiac catheterization, 426
    electrophysiological stimulation and recording studies,
      427–428
    exclusion or excision of left atrial appendage, 441
    heart assist devices, 442–444
    heart transplantation, 448–449
    implant of automatic cardioverter defibrillator, 428–430
    implantable hemodynamic monitor, 446
    implantation of cardiomyostimulation system, 448
    implantation of carotid sinus stimulation system, 447–448
    intracardiac pacemaker, 432
    intraoperative fluorescence vascular angiography, 427
    intravascular and intra-aneurysm pressure measurement,
      446–447, **447**
    percutaneous aortic and pulmonary valve repair, 433–434
    percutaneous balloon valvuloplasty, 434
    percutaneous mitral valve repair, 433
    percutaneous transluminal coronary angioplasty, 434–435,
      435
  pulmonary embolism, 421–422
  rheumatic heart disease, 394–397
  saddle embolism, 421
  status Z codes, 424–425
  thrombosis and thrombophlebitis of veins of extremities,
    422–423
  transluminal coronary atherectomy, 435–436
  vascular access devices (VADs), 444–446
Classification system, 4
Coagulation defects, 198–199
  bleeding caused by anticoagulation therapy, 198

"Code also," 16
"Code first," 16, 51
    underlying condition, 50–51
    "use additional code" and, 16, 50
Codes. *See also* Combination codes
    activity, 492
    age relationship of, 369, 376–377
    alphanumerical, 4
    assigning
        basis for, 37–38
        combination, when available, 49–50
        to highest level of detail, 48–49
        multiple, as needed, 50–53
        residual, as appropriate, 49
    characters and their definitions, 66–76, 66
    combination, 47, 55, 144, 161
    counseling, 497
    laterality in, 53
    locating
        late effect, 56, 57
        for neoplastic disease, 462, 463
        when associated with poisoning, adverse effects, and
            underdosing, 530–532, 531
    place of occurrence, 493
    representing patient history, status, or problems, 129–130
    for residual effect, 158
    sequencing
        for burns/corrosions and related conditions, 521–522
        for external cause, 492
        of injury, 490
        of mechanical ventilation, 241
        for neoplastic diseases, 472–478
    sign/symptom, use of, 54
    for social determinants of health, 38
    in Tabular List, 4–7
    "unspecified," use of, 54
    V, 4
    verifying number, in Tabular List, 43
    W, 4
    Weeks of gestation of pregnancy, 321, 324, 357
    X, 4
    Y, 4
    Z, 4
Coding
    clinical systems of, 577–580
    demonstrations of, 44–45, 80–82, 81, 82
    discontinued procedures, 87–88
    discretionary multiple, 51–52
    ethical, 33–34
    mandatory multiple, 50–51
    multiple, 50–53, 87
        of injuries, 489–490, 499
    for reimbursement, 33–34, 577–580
Colic, infantile, 386
Colonoscopy, 247
Colons (:), meaning of, in ICD-10-CM, 19
Colostomy, complications of, 249
Coma, 176
    Glasgow coma scale, 38, 138–139
    nondiabetic hypoglycemic, 168
Combination codes, 47, 55, 144, 161
    in arthritis, 302
    assigning, when available, 49–50
    in digestive system, 252–253
    drugs and medicinal and biological substances and, 528
    in hemorrhage, 246–247
    for hemorrhoids, 246–247
    for injuries, 489–490
    for pneumonia, 224–225
    toxic effect codes as, 529
    for ulcers, 248
Communicating hydrocephalus, 210
Comparable conditions, 27
Compartment syndrome, 512
Complication codes, locating, in Alphabetic Index, 539–540
Complications, 8
    affecting specific body systems, 541–543
    aftercare versus, 552
    of artificial openings of digestive system, 249
    associated with abortion, 356–357
    associated with malignant neoplasms, admission for, 474–475
    in breast reconstruction, 282, 283
    of childbirth, 321–351
    of cystostomy, 273
    of diabetes mellitus for pregnancy, 166–167
    due to insulin pump malfunction, 166
    due to presence of internal device, implant, or graft, 546–547
    of ectopic pregnancies, 363–364
    following infusion, transfusion, and therapeutic injection, 544–546
    following myocardial infarction, 403
    of foreign body left during surgery, 551–552
    intraoperative and postprocedural, 541–543
    of labor and delivery, 335–337, 336
    manifestations and, of diabetes mellitus, 163–166
    mechanical, 539, 540, 546–547
    of molar pregnancies, 363–364
    nonmechanical, 546–547
    postoperative conditions not classified as, 540
    postpartum, 337–339
    postprocedural, 265
    post-transplant surgical, 548
    of pregnancy, 321–351
    of procedures not classified elsewhere, 550–551
    of puerperium, 321–351
    of reattachment and amputation, 548–549
    sequelae of
        of childbirth, 340
        of pregnancy, 340
        of puerperium, 340
    of surgery and medical care, 537–554
    tracheostomy, 241–242
    transplant, 547–548
Compression, as root operation, 103, 103
Concussion, 502
Congenital anomalies, 367–373
    congenital deformities versus perinatal deformities, 369–370
    congenital malformations of genital organs, 372–373
    cystic kidney disease, 372
    gastroschisis, 373
    location of terms in Alphabetic Index, 368–369
    of the great arteries, 370–371
    neurofibromatosis, 371
    newborn with congenital conditions, 369, 371
    omphalocele, 373
    relationship of age to codes, 369
Congenital conditions, 8
    newborn with, 369, 371
Congenital disorders, 305
Congestive heart failure, 397, 406–407
Conjunctivitis, 215–216
Conjunctivochalasis, 215
Connecting words, coding guidelines regarding. *See* Relational terms
Constipation, 258
Contraceptive management, services related to, 347
Contrasting/comparative diagnoses, symptom followed by, 27
Contrasting conditions, 27
Control, as root operation, 98, 98
Contusions, 511
Conversion disorder, 180
Coordination and Maintenance Process (of changing codes/code titles), 4
Coronary arteriosclerosis. *See* Ischemic heart disease
Coronary artery bypass graft (CABG), 437–440, 437
    procedures, 427
Coronary artery disease. *See* Ischemic heart disease
Coronary artery of transplanted heart with angina pectoris, 405
Coronary ischemia. *See* Ischemic heart disease
Coronavirus, *See* COVID-19
Coumadin therapy, 199
Counseling, as mental health procedure, 186, 187, 187, 188
    codes for, 497
COVID-19, 38, 52, 53, 125, 129, 143, 155–158, 228, 384
Creation, as root operation, 99, 99
Crisis intervention, as mental health procedure, 187
Critical access hospitals, 579
Crohn's disease, 247
Cross-reference notes, 17–18
    "see," 17
    "see also," 17–18
    "see category," 18
    "see condition," 18
Cross-references, 42
Croup, 229
Cryptorchidism, 372
Current illness or injury, late effect versus, 58
Cuts, 510
Cyclothymia, 178
Cystectomy, radical, 276
Cystic fibrosis, 162, 170

Cystic kidney disease, 372
Cystitis, 264
Cystoscopy, 273
Cystostomy, complications of, 273
Cytokine release syndrome, 202

D

Dash, at end of Index entry, (-), 8, 78
Deafness, 220
Debridement, 296, 506
Decompression, as root operation, 109
Dehydration, admission/encounter for management of, 474
Delirium tremens, 183
Deliveries, 342–346, 343. *See also* Labor and delivery
    admission with normal, 327–328
    cesarean, 343, 346
    with forceps, 344
    outcome of, 324–325
    principal diagnosis for, selecting, 328–329
    procedures assisting, 343–346
    vacuum extraction, 344
Dependence on drugs and alcohol, 182–184
Dermatitis
    allergic-contact, 290
    due to drugs, 290–291
Destruction, as root operation, 89, 90
Detachment, as root operation, 89, 90
    terms used for qualifiers for, 512
Detoxification, 185, 188
Devices
    code characters for, 73
    root operations that always involve, 95–96, 95
Diabetes mellitus (DM), 159, 160–166
    bronze, 160
    burns and, 524
    cataracts and, 164, 216
    chronic kidney disease with, 164, 269
    complications of, 163–166
    with conditions not classified elsewhere, 161
    eye disease and, 164–165
    gestational, 166–167, 333–334
    glaucoma in, 217–218, 218
    with hypoglycemia, 163
    ketoacidosis (DKA), 163
    manifestations of, 163–166
    maternal, neonatal conditions associated with, 167
    neonatal, 384
    in pregnancy, 166–167, 333–334
    secondary, 161, 162
    skin ulcers and, 165
    types of, 161–163
Diagnoses
    admitting, 31
    borderline, 54, 161
    coding uncertain, as if established, 53–54
    discharge, 36–39
    with no documentation supporting reportability, 28–29
    other, 28–29
        reportable, 28–31
    previous conditions stated as, 28
    principal, 24–27, 36
    reporting same, more than once, 56
    "rule out" versus "ruled out," 54
    signs and symptoms, 54, 136–137
        as additional, 137
        as principal, 136–137
    unconfirmed, of human immunodeficiency virus (HIV) infections, 153
    Z codes as principal/first-listed, 131
Diagnostic cardiac catheterization, 426, 426
Diagnostic statement of toxic effect, toxicity, or intoxication, 529
Diagnostic and Statistical Manual of Mental Disorders, Fifth Edition (DSM-5®), 174
Dialysis. *See* Renal dialysis
Diarrhea, 258
Digestive system, 246
    complications of artificial openings of, 249
    diseases of, 245–260
        adhesions, 255–256
        appendicitis, 257
        bariatric surgery, 258–260, 259
        biliary system, 252–254
        complications of artificial openings of, 249
        constipation, 258
        diarrhea, 258
        Dieulafoy lesions, 248–249
        diverticulitis and diverticulosis, 245, 247, 249–250
        esophagitis, 247–248
        gastrointestinal hemorrhage, 246–247
        hernias of abdominal cavity, 256
        liver, 253
        procedures for, 251
        ulcers of stomach and small intestine, 248
Dilation, as root operation, 94–95, 94
Dilation and curettage (D & C), 356
Direct lateral lumbar interbody fusion (DLIF), 313, 314, 314
Discectomy, 302, 315
Discharge diagnoses, 36–39
Discharge summary, 36–39
Discontinued procedures, coding, 87–88
Discretionary multiple coding, 51–52
Diseases. *See also specific*
    of biliary system, 252–254
    of blood and blood-forming organs, 193–202
    of breast, 280–281
    cerebrovascular, 411–414, 411
    of circulatory system, 393–454
    conditions that are not an integral part of process of, 30
    cystic kidney, 372
    of digestive system, 245–260
    of ear, 219–220
    endocrine, nutritional, and metabolic, 159–170
    of eye, 204, 214–218
    genetic susceptibility to, 130–131
    of genitourinary system, 263–283
    of liver, 253
    musculoskeletal system and connective tissue, 299–316
    nervous system, 203–220
    parasitic and infectious, 143–158
    respiratory system, 223–242
    skin and subcutaneous tissue, 289–297
Disorders of adult personality and behavior, 181–182
Dissociative disorders, 180
Diverticula, congenital versus acquired, 250
Diverticulitis and diverticulosis, 245, 247, 249–250
Division, as root operation, 92, 92
Dorsopathy, 300
Drainage, as root operation, 91–92, 91
Dressing, as root operation, 103, 103, 104
Drug-induced
    aplastic anemia, 196
    folate deficiency anemia, 194
    hypoglycemia without coma, 168
Drug-resistant infections, 151
Drug use during pregnancy, 335
Drugs. *See also* Medications; Table of Drugs and Chemicals
    antineoplastic, 349
    dependence and abuse of, 183–184
    dermatitis due to, 290–291
    poisoning, toxic effects, adverse effects, and underdosing of, 527–536
    unspecified adverse effect of, 535
Dry eye syndrome, 215
DSM-5®, 174
Dual classification, 50, 144
"Due to," as relational term, 11, 21, 49, 161, 215, 247
Dysplasia, of cervix, vagina, and vulva, 278–279
Dysreflexia, autonomic, 210

E

Ear, 219
    diseases of, 219–220
Eating disorders, 181
Eclampsia, 333
Eczema, 290
Edema
    acute pulmonary, 236
    gestational, 333–334
Electroconvulsive therapy, as mental health procedure, 187
Electromagnetic therapy, as root operation, 109
Electrophysiological stimulation and recording studies, 427–428
Elevated troponin, 400
Embolism
    atheroembolism, 423
    pulmonary, 421–422
    saddle, 422

INDEX

Encephalopathy, 211–212
  alcoholic, 211
  anoxic, 211
  hepatic, 211, 253
  metabolic, 211
  neonatal, 380
  toxic, 211
  unspecified, 212
  Wernicke's, 211
Encounter. *See* Admission/encounter
Endocrine, nutritional, and metabolic diseases, 159–170
  diabetes mellitus, 160–166
  hypoglycemic and insulin reactions, 168
  metabolic disorders, 170
  nutritional disorders, 169
  specific to fetus and newborn, 385
Endocrine system, major organs of, **160**
Endograft procedures, 451–454
Endometriosis, 276, 277
Endoscopic banding of esophageal varices, 248, 454
Endoscopic therapy, 274
Endovascular aneurysm repair (EVAR), 449, **451**, 452
Endovascular embolization, 454
End-stage renal disease (ESRD), 267
Enterostomy, complications of, 249
Environmental toxins, 532
Epiglottitis, acute, 229
Epilepsy, 206
Episiotomy, 344
Eponyms, guidelines for coding and, 42
Erectile dysfunction, 166
Erythema multiforme, 291–292
Esophageal varices, 245, 248, 454
Esophagitis, 245, 247
Esophagostomy, complications of, 249
Esophagus, diseases of, 247–248
Ethical coding and reporting, 33–34
Examinations
  root operations that involve only, 97–98, **97**
  screening, 128
  special investigations and, 127–128
Excision
  for graft, 90
  of left atrial appendage, 441
  of lesion, 295
  of lymph nodes, 478–479
  radical, 90
  resection versus, 90
  as root operation, 89–90
"Excludes1" note, 15
"Excludes2" note, 15–16
Exclusion notes, 14–16, 19, 49
  for injuries, 488, 491
External cause of morbidity, 487, 490–493, 529
  of burns, 523
  effects of, 513–514
  of injury classified by intent, 493
  late effects of, 493
  medical care as, 553–554
  status of, 490–493
  surgical care as, 553–554
  Z codes and, 122
Extirpation, as root operation, 91, **91**
Extracorporeal shock wave lithotripsy (ESWL), 254, 274
Extracorporeal or Systemic Assistance and Performance Section,
    107–108, **107**, 239
Extracorporeal or Systemic Therapies Section, 108–109, **108**
Extraction, as root operation, 89, **890**
Extreme lateral interbody fusion (XLIF®), 313, 314, **314**
Extremities
  atherosclerosis of, 419–420
  fractures of, 503–504
  thrombophlebitis of veins of, 422–423
  thrombosis of veins of, 422–423
Eye, **215**
  burns of, 521
  corneal injury, 214–215
  diseases of, 204, 214–218
    diabetic, 164–165

F

Factitious disorders, 181–182
Family counseling, **188**
Family planning, 347, 349

Fasciitis, 316
Female reproductive system, 278, 279
  cellulitis of external genital organs, 295
  primary organs of, 323
Fertility preservation
  counseling, 350
  procedures, 350
Fetal conditions
  affecting management of pregnancy, 330–331, **336**
  suspected, not found, 350–351
Fetal distress, 379–380
Fetal reduction, multiple gestation following, 359–360
Fetus
  endocrine and metabolic disturbances specific to newborns and,
      385
  loss of, with remaining fetus, 359
  malnutrition in, 378
  maternal conditions affecting newborn or, 384–385
  monitoring of, 346
  seventh-character codes for, 325–326
  with slow growth, 378
  surgical operation on mother and, 385
  suspected fetal conditions not found, 350–351
Fifth-character subclassifications
  for asthma, 230–231
  for chronic ischemic heart disease, 405
  for diabetes mellitus, 161–163
  for epiglottitis, 229
  for epilepsy, 206
  for identifying lymph nodes, 471
  for indicating birth weight, 378–379
  for narcolepsy, 208
  for neoplasms, 471
  for status asthmaticus, 230–231
  for supraglottitis, 229–230
Fistula, arteriovenous (AV), 272
Five-character codes, 6, 48
Fluids
  overload of, 170
  root operations to take out, from a body part, 91–92, **91**
Follow-up examinations, admission for, 124–125, 478
Foreign bodies
  complications involving, 551–552
  in injuries, 511–512
  superficial, 511–512
Four-character codes, 6, 48
Fourth-character subclassifications
  for asthma, 230–231
  for cerebrovascular disease, 413–414
  for Hodgkin lymphoma, 468–470
Fractures, 497–499, **498**
  closed, 498, **498**
  comminuted, 498–499
  compound, 498–499
  compression, 305, 505
  due to birth injury, 506
  of extremities, 503–504
  femoral, atypical, 307
  intracranial, 501–502
  malunion of, 501
  nonunion of, 310, 501
  open, 498, **498**
    Gustilo classification of, 499–500, **501**
  pathological, 305–306, 477, 505
  of pelvis, 503
  periprosthetic, 307, 505
  procedures related to, 506–507
  reduction of, 506
    internal and external fixation, 506–507
  seventh-character values for, 499–501, **500**
  skull, 501–502
  stress, 307, 505
  vertebral, 502–503
Fragmentation, as root operation, 91
Fusion
  and refusion, spinal, 310–314, **310, 311, 312, 313, 314**
  as root operation, 99, **99**
  surgeries, spinal, 310–314, **313, 314**

G

Gallbladder, strawberry, 253
Gallbladder stones, removal of, 254
Gangrene, 165, 295
Gases, root operations to take out, from a body part, 91–92, **91**

Gastric banding, 258–260, **259**
Gastroschisis, 373
Gastrostomy, complications of, 249
General notes in ICD-10-CM, 14
Genetic susceptibility to disease, 130
Genital organs, congenital malformations of, 372–373
Genital prolapse, 277–278
Genitourinary system
    cystostomy, complications of, 273
    diseases of, 263–283
        breast, 280–281
        and breast reconstruction, 281–283, **282**
        cystoscopy as operative approach to treat, 273
        dysplasia of cervix, vagina, and vulva, 278–279
        endometrial ablation to treat, 279
        endometrial hyperplasia, 278
        endometriosis, 276, **277**
        genital prolapse, 277–278
        hematuria, 265–266
        infections of tract, 264–265
        prostate, and therapy, 275–276
        removal of urinary calculus to treat, 274
        renal, 266–269
            acute kidney failure, 268
            chronic kidney disease and end-stage renal disease, 267
            kidney disease with diabetes mellitus, 269
            kidney disease with hypertension, 268–269, **269**
            renal dialysis to treat, 270–272
            urinary incontinence, 266
    hysterectomy, 279
Glasgow coma scale, 138–139
Glaucoma, 217–218, **218**
Gout, 304
Graft
    arteriovenous, 272
    complications due to presence of, 546–547
    dermal regenerative, 296–297
    endograft procedures, 449–454, **450, 451**
    excision for, 90
Gram-negative bacterial infections, 150, **150**
Gram-negative pneumonia, 226
Group counseling, **188**
Group psychotherapy, **187**
Gustilo classification of open fractures, 499–500, **501**

H

Haemophilus influenzae, type B, 229
Hand foot syndrome, 291
Headaches
    migraine, 207–208
    posttraumatic, 502
Health Insurance Portability and Accountability Act (HIPAA), 48, 83, 559, 577, 594
Healthcare Common Procedure Coding System (HCPCS), level II codes for, 577, 58
Hearing loss, 220
Heart
    congenital defects of the, 448
    exclusion or excision of left atrial appendage, 441
    interior of, 396
Heart assist devices, 442–443
    intra-aortic balloon pump (IABP), 444
    short-term external, 443–444
Heart disease
    arteriosclerotic. *See* Ischemic heart disease
    atherosclerotic, 405
    hypertensive, 408, 417–418
    ischemic, 397–406
    rheumatic, 394–397
Heart failure, 406–408
Heart revascularization, 427, 437, 440
Heart tissue, ablation of, 441–442
Heart transplantation, 448–449
Heat prostration, 496
Hematopoietic system, malignancies of, 468–471, **469**
Hematuria, 265–266
Hemiplegia/hemiparesis, 208–209
Hemodialysis, 270–272
    via arteriovenous fistula, 272
    via arteriovenous graft, 272
    via catheter, 271–272
    renal replacement therapy (RRT), 271
    single versus multiple encounters for, 271
Hemodynamic monitor, implantable, 446

Hemorrhage. *See also* Bleeding
    gastrointestinal, 246–247
    intraventricular, 382
    from tracheostomy, 241–242
Hemorrhoids, 247
Heparin locks, 445
Heparin therapy, 198
Hepatobiliary system extirpation, 254
Hermaphroditism, 373
Hernias of abdominal cavity, 256
Herniation of intervertebral disc, 301–302
Herniorrhaphy, 256
Hip resurfacing, 309
Hospital-acquired infections, 151
Human immunodeficiency virus (HIV), 153–154, 194, 235. *See also* Acquired immunodeficiency syndrome (AIDS) infections
    in newborns, 383–384
    during pregnancy, 334
    sequencing of diagnoses, 154
    serologic testing for, 153–154
    unconfirmed diagnosis of, 153
Hydrocephalus, 210–211, 370
Hypercoagulable states, 198–199
Hyperosmolarity, 163
Hyperparathyroidism, 305
Hyperplasia
    endometrial, 278
    of prostate, 275
Hypertension, 415
    benign, 416
    chronic kidney disease and, 268–269, **269**, 417
    complicating pregnancy, childbirth, and the puerperium, 419
    elevated blood pressure versus, 419
    essential (primary), 415
    gestational, 333
    kidney disease with, 268–269, **269**
    malignant, 415–416
    with other conditions, 418
    postoperative, 540–541
    postprocedural, 419
    in pregnancy, 332–333
    secondary, 415–416
    secondary pulmonary, 420–421
    uncontrolled, 416
Hypertensive heart and chronic kidney disease, 268–269, **269**, 416–417
Hyperthermia, as root operation, 109
Hypoglycemia
    diabetes with, 163
    insulin reactions and, 168
Hypopituitarism, 340
Hypospadias, 373
Hypothermia, 513
    as root operation, 109
Hypoxic-ischemic encephalopathy (HIE), 380
Hysterectomy, 279

I

ICD-10-CM (*International Classification of Diseases, Tenth Revision, Clinical Modification*). *See also* Alphabetic Index; Tabular List of Diseases and Injuries
    abbreviations in, 16–17
        NEC (not elsewhere classified), 17, 49
        NOS (not otherwise specified), 17, 49
    basic coding guidelines of, 47–58
        assigning codes
            to highest level of detail, 48–49
            combination, when available, 49–50
            multiple, as needed, 50–53
            residual, as appropriate, 49
        chronic conditions, 54–55
        impending or threatened condition, 56
        late effects, 56–58
        late effects versus current illness or injury, 58
        reporting same diagnosis code more than once, 56
        uncertain diagnoses as if established, 53–54
        using both Alphabetic Index and Tabular List, 48
    conventions in, 13–21
        "code also," 16
        "code first" and "use additional code," 16
        cross-reference notes, 17–18
            "see," 17
            "see also," 17–18

ICD-10-CM (continued)
   "see category," 18
   "see condition," 18
   instructional notes, 14–16
      exclusion, 15–16
      general notes in, 16
      inclusion, 14–15
      inclusion terms, 15
      punctuation marks, 18
      relational terms, 20–21
         "and," 20, 64
         "due to," 11, 21, 49, 161, 216, 247
         "in," 11, 20–21, 49, 217, 247
         "with," 11–12, 20–21, 49, 161, 217, 247
   dash (-), used at end of Index entries, 8, 42, 78
   development of, 4
   format, 4
   Official Guidelines for Coding and Reporting, 4, 26, 36, 48, 586, 595
   placeholder character for, 7
   in public domain, 4
   reimbursement using, 577
   table of contents from, 4, 5, 6
   three-character categories in, 6
ICD-10-PCS (*International Classification of Diseases, Tenth Revision, Procedure Coding System*)
   ancillary procedures, 112–119
      Imaging Section, 112–114, 113, 114
      New Technology Section, 119–120, 119, 120
      Nuclear Medicine Section, 114–115, 114, 115
      Physical Rehabilitation and Diagnostic Audiology Section, 117–119, 117, 118, 119
      Radiation Therapy Section, 115–116, 115, 116
   Body Part Key (Appendix C) in, 69–70
   classification of, 61–76
   code characters and their definitions, 66–76, 66
      character 1: section, 66, 66
      character 2: body system, 66–67, 67
      character 3: root operation, 68–69, 68
      character 4: body part, 69–71, 70
      character 5: approach, 71, 72, 74–75
      character 6: device, 73, 76
      character 7: qualifier, 76
   code structure, 64, 64, 65
   coding demonstrations using, 80–82, 81, 82
   development of, 4
   Device Aggregation Table (Appendix E) in, 73
      excerpt from, 76
   Device Key (Appendix D) in, 73
   digestive system procedures of, 251
   format
      Alphabetic Index, 63
      list of long and abbreviated code titles, 62
      Tables, 63, 63
   locating
      applicable Table, 80
      main term, 78–79
   medical- and surgical-related procedures, 101–111, 102
      Administration Section, 105–106, 105
      Chiropractic Section, 111, 111
      Extracorporeal or Systemic Assistance and Performance Section, 107–108, 107
      Extracorporeal or Systemic Therapies Section, 108–109, 108
      Measurement and Monitoring Section, 106, 106
      Osteopathic Section, 110, 110
      Other Procedures Section, 110–111, 111
      Placement Section, 102–104, 102, 103
   Official Coding Guidelines, 86, 345, 425, 594
   relational terms, 64
   root operation guidelines, 86–89, 84
      coding
         biopsies, 88–89
         discontinued procedures, 87–88
         multiple procedures, 87
         procedures on overlapping body layers, 89
   root operations in Medical and Surgical Section, 89–99
      to alter diameter or route of tubular body part, 94–95, 94
      involving cutting or separation only, 92–93, 92
      to take out solids/fluids/gases from a body part, 91–92, 91
      to take out some or all of a body part, 89–90, 89
      that include other objectives, 99, 99
      that include other repairs, 98, 98
      that involve examination only, 97–98, 97
      that put in/put back or move some/all of a body part, 93–94, 93

   standardized terminology in, 62
   Uniform Hospital Discharge Data Set (UHDDS) for reporting procedures, 82–83
Ill-defined conditions, 139
Illnesses. *See also specific*
   associated with burns, 524
   late effect versus current, 58
Imaging Section, 112–114, 113, 426
Immobilization, as root operation, 103, 103, 104, 104
Immune system, disorders of, 201–202
Immunodeficiency disorders, 194
Immunotherapy
   admission or encounter involving administration of, 475–476
   in treating neoplasms, 479–480
Impending condition, 56
Implantation
   of automatic cardioverter defibrillator, 428–430
   of cardiomyostimulation system, 448
   of carotid sinus stimulation system, 447–448
   complications due to presence of, 546–547
   of hemodynamic monitor, 446
   of vascular access devices, 271, 272, 444–446, 446
Impotence, organic, 166
"In," as relational term, 11, 20–21, 49, 217, 247
Inclusion notes, 19, 49
   in ICD-10-CM, 14–15
   for injuries, 488, 491
Index to External Causes, 7, 41
Index tables in Alphabetic Index, 12
Infantile colic, 386
Infants. *See also* Newborns
   abortion procedure resulting in liveborn, 359
   health supervision of, 386–387
   observation and evaluation of, 382–383
Infections, 143–158
   AIDS and HIV, 153–154
   drug-resistant, 151
   of genitourinary tract, 264–265
   gram-negative bacterial, 150, 150
   late effects, 158
   nosocomial, 151
   organism versus site or other subterm, 144
   originating during perinatal period, 383–384
   postsurgical, 548
   puerperal, 337–339
   respiratory, 224–227
   sepsis, severe sepsis, and septic shock, 146–149
   toxic shock syndrome, 149–150
   tuberculosis, 145–146
   West Nile virus fever, 145
   Zika virus, 145
Inflammatory diseases of central nervous system, 205
Influenza, 228
Infusions, complications following, 544–546
Injuries, 487–515
   admissions or encounters for orthopedic aftercare, 508–509
   amputations, 89, 90, 511, 512
   associated with burns, 524
   blood vessel, 510
   child and adult abuse, 495–497
   classification of, 488
   corneal, 214–215
   dislocations, 509–510
   early complications of trauma, 512–513
   effects of external causes, 513–514
   external cause of morbidity, 490–493
      late effects of, 493, 514–515
   fractures, 497–506, 498
   initial care for, 500
   internal, of chest, abdomen, and pelvis, 510
   intracranial, 501–502
   multiple coding of, 489–490
   nerve, 510
   open wounds, 510–511
   other, 511–512
   sequencing of codes, 490
   seventh-character values for, 488–489, 491
   subluxations, 509–510
   superficial, 511–512
Insect bites, 511
Insertion, as root operation, 95–96, 95
Inspection, as root operation, 97, 97
Intracranial hypotension, 213

Instructional notes, 6, 14–16, 175
    exclusion, 14–16
    general, 14
    inclusion, 14–16
Insulin, 161–163
Insulin pump malfunction, complications due to, 166
Insulin reactions, hypoglycemic and, 168
Intent, external cause of injury classified by, 493
Interbody fusion devices, 310–314
Internal device, complications due to presence of, 546–547
Interstitial lung diseases, 225–226
Intervertebral disc
    disorders of, 300–302
    herniation of, 301–302
Intestinal adhesions, 255
Intra-aortic balloon pump (IABP), 444–454
Intracardiac (leadless, transcatheter) pacemakers, 432
Intraoperative electron radiation therapy in treating neoplasms, 481–482, 482
Intraoperative fluorescence vascular angiography, 427
Intraoperative and postprocedural complications, 542–543
Intrauterine pressure monitor, 346
Intravascular and intra-aneurysm pressure measurement, 446–447, 447
Introduction, as root operation, 105, 105
Iron deficiency anemia secondary to blood loss (chronic), 195
Irrigation, as root operation, 105, 105
Ischemic heart disease, 397–406
    chronic, 405
    chronic total occlusion, 406
    myocardial infarction, 399–402, 401
    other acute, 403
    postmyocardial infarction syndrome, 404

J

Joint
    bone versus, 300
    dislocations and subluxations, 509–510
    replacement of, 308–309
    revision, 309

K

Kaposi's sarcoma, excision of, 295
Kennedy ulcers, 293
Ketoacidosis, 163
Kidney disease. *See* Chronic kidney disease
Kidney stones, 274
Kidneys
    acute failure of, 268
    transplant of, 267
        complications of, 547–548
Klebsiella, 150, 150
Kyphoplasty, 314–315

L

Labor and delivery, 335–337, 336. *See also* Childbirth; Deliveries
    complications of, 335–337, 336
        fetal stress, 337
        obstructed labor, 335–337, 336
    stages of, 322
    weeks of gestation, 324, 357
Laboratory reports, 36–39
Lacerations, 510
    perineal, during delivery, 345–346
        coding degrees and types of, 345
    repair of, 345–346
Laryngitis, 229–230
Laser interstitial thermal therapy in treating neoplasms, 481, 481
Late effects, 8, 56–58
    cerebrovascular disease sequelae and, 8, 413–414
    current illness or injury versus, 58
    defined, 56
    due to previous infection or parasitic infestations, 145
    of external causes, 493
    of injuries, 514–515
    locating codes, 57
    need for two codes, 57–58
    of poisoning, adverse effects, and underdosing, 536
Laterality, 53, 29300
Legionnaires' disease, 226
Leprosy, 29304
Lesions
    Dieulafoy, 248–249
    excision of, 295
Leukemias, 194, 471
Leukocytosis, 200–201

Light therapy, as mental health procedure, 187
Lithotripsy
    extracorporeal shock wave (ESWL), 254, 274
    ultrasonic, 274
Long-term care reporting, relationship of UHDDS to, 32–33
Lung
    ablation of, 238–239
    biopsies of, 237–238
Lyme disease, 205
Lymph nodes or glands
    excision/resection of, 478–479
        radical, 90
    neoplasms of, 468
Lymphatic system, 469
    malignancies of, 468–471, 469
Lymphomas
    Hodgkin, 468, 470
    non-Hodgkin, 470–471

M

Main terms, 8, 9, 42, 78–79
Malabsorptive operations, 258, 259
Male reproductive system, 276
Malignancy
    current, versus personal history of, 476
    encounter/admission to determine extent of, 476
Malnutrition, 496
    in childbirth, 324
    fetal, 378
Mammoplasty, 283
Mandatory multiple coding, 50–51
Manic-depression, 178
Manifestation codes, 16, 50–51
Manipulation, as root operation, 111, 111
Map, as root operation, 97, 97
Mastectomy, 280
Maternal conditions
    affecting fetus or newborn, 384–385
    as reason for abortion, 358
    suspected, not found, 350–351
Maze procedure, 441–442
Measurement, as root operation, 106
Mechanical complication, 539, 540, 546–547
Mechanical ventilation, 239–242
    sequencing of codes for, 241
Medicaid reimbursement methods, 33–34, 577–580
Medical record
    contents of, 36–39
    documentation of error in, 529–530
    as source document, 36–39
Medical- and surgical-related procedures, 102–109, 102
    Administration Section, 105–106, 105
    Chiropractic Section, 111, 111
    Extracorporeal or Systemic Assistance and Performance Section, 107–108, 107
    Extracorporeal or Systemic Therapies Section, 108–109, 108
    Measurement and Monitoring Section, 106, 106
    Osteopathic Section, 110, 110
    Other Procedures Section, 110–111, 111
    Placement Section, 102–104, 102, 103
Medical and Surgical Section root operations, 89–99
Medicare reimbursement methods, 33–34, 577–581
Medications. *See also* Drugs
    management of, 188
    record of, 37
Meningitis, 204, 205
    bacterial, 205
    candidal, 205
Mental disorders, 173–189
    adult personality and behavior, disorders of, 181–182
    affective, 177–178
    altered mental state, 176
    behavioral syndromes associated with physiological disturbances and physical factors, 181
    dementia in other diseases classified elsewhere, 175
    due to known physiological conditions, 174–175
    nonpsychotic, 179–181
    schizophrenic, 176–177
    substance abuse, 182–185
    transient global amnesia, 176
    treatment procedures, 186–189, 187, 188
Metabolic disorders, 170. *See also* Acute metabolic complications; Endocrine, nutritional, and metabolic diseases
Metastasis, 457, 458

Methicillin-resistant *Staphylococcus aureus* (MRSA), 144, 151
Midlevel providers, 36
Migraine, 207–208
MitraClip® implant, 433
Mitral valve
　insufficiency, 395–396, 397
　stenosis, 395
Monitoring, as root operation, 106, **106**
Monoplegia, 208
Mood (affective) disorders, 177–178
Mortality, ill-defined and unknown cause of, 139
Mother, surgical operation on, and fetus, 385
Multiple coding, 50–53
　avoiding indiscriminate, 52
　discretionary, 51–52
　of injuries, 489–490
　laterality, 53
　mandatory, 50–51
　as needed, 50–53
Multiple endocrine neoplasia (MEN) syndrome, 459
Multiple gestation, 326, 331
　following fetal reduction, 359–360
Multiple procedures, coding, 87
Muscular dystrophies, 204
Musculoskeletal system and connective tissue, diseases of, 299–316
　acute traumatic versus chronic or recurrent conditions, 300
　arthritis, 300, 302–304
　back disorders, 300–302
　bone versus joint, 300
　derangement of joints, 304–305
　fasciitis, 316
　kyphoplasty, 314–315
　musculoskeletal body part guidelines, 307
　osteoporosis, 305
　pathological fractures, 305–306
　plica syndrome, 316
　replacement of joint, 308–309
　site and laterality, 300
　spinal decompression, 315
　spinal disc prostheses, 315
　spinal fusion and refusion, 310–314, **310, 311, 312, 313, 314**
　spinal motion preservation, 315–316
　vertebroplasty, 314–315
Myasthenia gravis, 204
Myeloma, multiple, 471
Myelomeningocele/spina bifida, 370
Myelopathy, 301–302
Myocardial infarction (MI), 399–404
　acute, 399–401, **401**
　current complications following, 403
　evolving, 401–402
　postinfarction hypotension, 401
　postmyocardial infarction syndrome, 404
Myopathy, critical illness, 213

N

Narcolepsy, 208
National Center for Health Statistics (NCHS), 4
　developing and maintaining ICD-10-CM, 8, 24
National Institutes of Health Stroke Scale (NIHSS), 38, 139
National Uniform Billing Committee for inpatient reporting, 39
NEC (not elsewhere classified), 17, 49
Necrosis, 549
Necrotizing enterocolitis, 381
Neisseria, 224
Neonatal aspiration, 380
Neonatal cerebral infarction, 380
Neonatal cerebral leukomalacia, 381–382
Neonatal conditions, associated with maternal diabetes, 167
Neoplasm Table, 7, 12, 462, **463**
Neoplasms, 457–482
　associated with transplanted organ, 476
　benign, 459
　carcinoma in situ, 459–460
　coding of, of hematopoietic and lymphatic systems, 468–471
　defined, 458
　direct extension, spread by, 464
　immunoproliferative, 471
　malignant, 162, 340, 349, 458–478, **463, 469**
　　admission for complications associated with, 474–475
　　coding of solid, 464–466
　　of ectopic tissue, 459
　　types of, 463–464
　Merkel cell carcinoma, 459

　metastatic, 461, 465–466
　morphology of, 461
　multiple myeloma, 471
　neuroendocrine tumors, 458–459
　pathological fracture due to, 306, 477
　plasma cell, 471
　in pregnant patient, 476–477
　sequencing of codes for neoplastic diseases, 472–478
　　admission for complications associated with malignant, 474–475
　　admission or encounter involving administration of radiation therapy, immunotherapy, or chemotherapy, 475–476
　　coding of admissions or encounters for follow-up examinations, 478
　　current malignancy versus personal history of malignancy, 476
　　encounter for prophylactic organ removal, 477
　　encounter to determine extent of malignancy, 476
　　malignant ascites, 477
　　malignant pleural effusion, 477
　　pathologic fracture due to, 477
　　treatment directed at primary site, 473
　　treatment directed at secondary site, 473
　treatment of
　　chemotherapy, 479–480, **479**
　　immunotherapy, 479–480
　　intraoperative electron radiation therapy, 481–482, **482**
　　laser interstitial thermal therapy, 481, **481**
　　radiation therapy, 480–481, **481**
　　thermal ablation in, 479
　of uncertain behavior, 460
　of unspecified behavior, 460
　unspecified mass or lesion, 460
Neoplastic diseases
　anemia in, 196
　locating codes for, 462, 463
　sequencing of codes for, 472–478
Nephritis, 164
Nephropathy, 266–267
　diabetic, 164
Nephrosis, 164, 267
Nephrotic syndrome, 266
Nervous system, **204**
　diseases of, 203–220
Neurofibromatosis, 371, 460
New Technology Section, 119–120, **119**
Newborns. *See also* Infants
　aspiration of fetal and, 380–381
　with congenital conditions, 369
　disorders of stomach functions in, 382
　endocrine and metabolic disturbances specific to fetus and, 385
　failure to thrive in, 382
　feeding problems in, 382
　fetal distress and asphyxia in, 379–380
　hemolytic disease of, 381
　immaturity of, 375, 378–379
　infections in, 383
　low birth weight of, 375, 378–379
　maternal conditions affecting fetus or, 384–385
　　suspected, not found, 350–351
　necrotizing enterocolitis in, 381
　neonatal cerebral leukomalacia in, 381–382
　observation and evaluation of, 382–383
　other diagnoses for, 377–378
　postmaturity, 375, 378–379
　prematurity, 378–379
　routine vaccination of, 386
　sepsis in, 383
Nonessential modifiers and code assignment, 18, 42
Nonmechanical complication, 546–547
Nonproliferative diabetic retinopathy, 164
Non-ST-elevation myocardial infarction (NSTEMI), 399–400, 412
NOS (not otherwise specified), 17, 49
Nuclear Medicine Section, 114–115, **114, 115**
Numerical entries in Alphabetic Index, 10
Nurse practitioners, 36
Nutritional disorders, codes for, 169

O

Objectives, root operations that include other, **98**, 99
Observation and evaluation, admission for, 125–127
　of newborns and infants, 382–383
Obsessive-compulsive disorder, 179
Obstetrics Section
　root operations in, 341–343, **342**
　structure of codes in, 341–343, **342**
Occlusion, chronic total, 406

Occlusion, as root operation, 94–95, 94, 454
  distinguishing between restriction and, 454
Omphalocele, 373
Open aneurysmectomy, 449, 450
Open surgical aneurysm repair via tube graft, 449, 450
Organic anxiety disorder, 175
Organic brain syndrome, 175
Organic impotence, 166
Organism, site versus, 144
Orthopedic aftercare, admissions or encounters for, 508–509
Osteopathic Section, 110, 110
Osteoporosis, 305, 499
Other diagnoses, reporting guidelines for, 27–31
Other Procedures Section, 110–111, 111
Otitis, 219
Outpatient records, 38
Outpatient reporting, relationship of Uniform Hospital Discharge Data Set
  (UHDDS) to, 32
Outpatient visits
  prenatal for high-risk patients, 326–327
  routine prenatal, 326
Over-coding, 33
Over-reporting, 33
Oxytocin, 343

P

Pacemakers, 430–432
  intracardiac (leadless, transcatheter), 432
Packing, as root operation, 103, 103
Paget's disease, 305
Pain, 209–210
  disorders of, 180
  encounter/admission for controlling, 209–210
  low back, 300, 302
  postoperative, 210
Palliative care, 123
Pancytopenia, 196, 474
Parasitic diseases. See Infections
Parentheses, meaning of, in ICD-10-CM, 18
Parkinsonism, 205–206
Parkinson's disease, 29, 205–206
Patient history, status, or problems, codes representing, 129–130
Patient's reason for visit, 38
Payment policies, impact on coding, 33, 577–581
Pelvis, internal injuries of, 510
Penicillin, adverse effect of, 291
Percutaneous aortic and pulmonary valve repair, 433–434
Percutaneous balloon valvuloplasty, 434
Percutaneous mitral valve repair, 433
Percutaneous transluminal coronary angioplasty, 434–435, 435
Percutaneous vertebral augmentation, 314–315
Performance, as root operation, 107, 108
Pericardiocentesis, 408
Perinatal conditions, 375–387, 506
  apparent life-threatening event, 386
  classification of births, 377
  disorders of stomach function and feeding problems, 382
  endocrine and metabolic disturbances specific to fetus and
    newborn, 385
  fetal distress and asphyxia, 379–380
  fetal and newborn aspiration, 380–381
  general perinatal guidelines, 376
  health supervision of infant or child, 386–387
  hemolytic disease of newborn, 381
  infantile colic, 386
  infections originating during perinatal period, 383–384
  locating codes for perinatal conditions in Alphabetic Index, 376
  maternal, affecting fetus or newborn, 384–385
  necrotizing enterocolitis, 381
  neonatal cerebral leukomalacia, 381–382
  observation and evaluation of newborns and infants, 382–383
  other diagnoses for newborns, 377–378
  prematurity, low birth weight, and postmaturity, 378–379
  relationship of age to codes, 376–377
  routine vaccination of newborns, 386
  surgical operation on mother and fetus, 385
Perinatal deformities, congenital deformities versus, 369–370
Perineal lacerations during delivery, 345–346
Peripheral nervous system (PNS), 203, 204
  disorders of, 212
Peripherally inserted central catheter (PICC), 445, 446
Periventricular leukomalacia, 381–382
Persistent vegetative state, 176
Phantom limb syndrome, 549

Pharmacotherapy, 188
Pheresis, as root operation, 109, 109
Phototherapy, as root operation, 109
Physical Rehabilitation and Diagnostic Audiology Section, 117–119, 117
Physician assistants, 36
Physician query, 37–38
Physicians' orders, 36
Pickwickian syndrome, 169
Pitocin, 343
Place of occurrence, 493
Placeholder character, 7, 48, 488
Placement Section, 102–104, 102, 103
  codes in, 102–104
  root operations in, 102–104
Planar nuclear medicine imaging, 114
Platelet cells, diseases of, 199
Pleural effusion, 223, 232–233
  malignant, 233, 477
Pleurodesis, 238–239
Plica syndrome, 316
Pneumocystis carinii, 154, 225, 610
Pneumocystosis, 225
Pneumonia, 224–227
  aspiration, 227
  gram-negative, 226
  interstitial, 225–226
  lobar, 225
  lymphoid interstitial, 226
  multilobar, 225
  ventilator-associated, 227
Poisoning, 527
  codes for, 488, 490–492, 514, 528–532, 531
  due to substance abuse or dependence, 535
  guidelines for assignment of codes for, 532
  late effects of, 536
  by penicillin, 291
Poliomyelitis, acute, 205
Polyneuropathy, 204, 213
Polyps, colon, 250–251
Positron emission tomographic (PET) imaging, 114, 115
Postcholecystectomy syndrome, 253
Postconcussional syndrome, 175, 502
Posterior lumbar interbody fusion (PLIF), 313, 314, 314
Postinfarction hypotension, 401
Postlaminectomy syndrome, 540
Postoperative conditions, not classified as complications, 540–541
Postoperative drains, 73, 123, 552
Postpartum, complications of, 337–339, 357, 363
Postprocedural complications, 265
Postprocedural infection, sepsis due to, 148
Post-transplant lymphoproliferative disorders, 548
Post-transplant surgical complications, 548
Posttraumatic stress disorder (PTSD), 179
Preeclampsia, 333
Pregnancy
  alcohol, tobacco, and drug use during, 334–335
  anemia of, 194
  biochemical, 362
  cardiomyopathy and, 339
  complications of, 321–335, 356
  diabetes in, 166–167, 333–334
  ectopic, 362–364
  failed attempted termination of, 356
  fetal conditions affecting management of, 330–331
    suspected maternal and fetal conditions not found, 350–351
  HIV infection during, 334
  hypertension in, 332–333, 419
  malignant neoplasms in, 476–477
  molar, 362–364
  prenatal outpatient visits, 326
  procedures for termination of, 360–361, 361
  sequelae of complication of, 340
  supervision of high-risk, 326–327
  trimesters of, 322–324
  tubal, 362, 363
  weeks of gestation of, 321, 324, 357
Prematurity, 378–379
Presbycusis, 220
Present on admission (POA) indicator, 39, 585–588
  definition, 585
  documentation, 585–586
  guidelines, 586
  reporting options, 586–588
Pressure measurement, intravascular and intra-aneurysm, 446–447, 447

Previous conditions, stated as diagnoses, 28
Primary cerebral dysfunction, 174
Primary site, treatment directed at, 473
Principal diagnosis, 24–27, 36
    for obstetric deliveries, 328–329
    selection of first-listed and, 326–330
    signs and symptoms as, 54, 136–137
    two or more diagnoses that equally meet definition for, 26–27
    Z codes as, 131
Principal procedure, 77
    designating, 83
Procedural risk, 82
Procedures
    coding
        for digestive system, 251
        multiple, 87
        on overlapping body layers, 89
    discontinued or incomplete, 87–88
    failed, 88
    mental health and substance abuse treatment, 186–189, 187
    not classified elsewhere, complications of, 550–551, 552
    obstetric, 341–343, 342
    Uniform Hospital Discharge Data Set (UHDDS) requirements for
        reporting, 32, 83
Procreative management, 349–350
Progress notes, 36
Prolapse, 277–278
Prolonged prothrombin time, 199
Prolonged reversible ischemic neurological deficit (PRIND), 414
Prophylactic organ removal, encounter/admission for, 477
Prostaglandin gel, 343
Prostate
    disease and therapy, 275
    hyperplasia of, 275
Prostatectomy, radical, 276
Prostheses, 315
Proteinuria, gestational, 333
Pseudarthrosis, 310
Pseudoaneurysm, 452
Pseudohermaphroditism, 373
Psychoactive substance use, 184
Psychological tests, as mental health procedure, 187
Psychotherapy, as mental health procedure, 187
Puerperium, complications of, 321–351
    sequelae of, 340
Pulmonary artery anomalies, 371
Pulmonary collapse, 232
Pulseless electrical activity (PEA), 410
Punctuation marks, meaning of, in ICD-10-CM
    colons, 19
    parentheses, 18
    square brackets, 19, 50

Q
Qualifiers, 61
    code characters for, 76
    common fusion and refusion ICD-10-PCS, 314

R
Radiation therapy, 115–116, 115, 116, 349, 475–476
    admission or encounter involving administration of, 475
    in treating neoplasms, 480–481, 481
Radiculopathy, 300, 302
Raynaud's phenomenon, 398
Reattachment, as root operation, 93, 93
    complications of, 548–549
Reconstruction, breast, 281–283, 282
Rehabilitation for control of drug use, 185
Reimbursement models, 577–581
    for commercial payers, 581
    for home health agencies, 579–580
    for hospice, 580
    for hospitals, 577–579
        acute inpatient, 578
        critical access, 579
        long-term care, 579
        outpatient, 578
        rehabilitation, 579
        psychiatric, 578–579
    for physicians and nonhospital providers, 577
    for skilled nursing facilities, 580
Relational terms, 20–21
    "and," 20, 64
    "due to," 11, 21, 49, 161, 215, 247

"in," 11, 20–21, 49, 216, 247
"with," 11–12, 20–21, 49, 161, 216, 247
Release, as root operation, 92, 92
Removal, as root operation, 95–96, 95, 103, 103, 104
    of biliary calculi, 254, 254
    prophylactic organ, 477
    of urinary calculus, 274
Renal complications of diabetes, 164
Renal dialysis, 270–272
    hemodialysis, 270–272
        via arteriovenous fistula, 272
        via arteriovenous graft, 272
        via catheter, 271–272
        single versus multiple encounters for, 270
    peritoneal dialysis, 270
Renal disease, 266–269
    chronic kidney disease and end-stage renal disease, 267
        acute, 268
        with diabetes mellitus, 269
        with hypertension, 268–269, 269
Renal failure, 268
Renal insufficiency, 268
Repair, as root operation, 98, 98
Replacement, as root operation, 96, 95
Reposition, as root operation, 93–94, 93
Reproductive system
    female, 278–283, 278
    male, 275–278, 276
Resection, excision versus, as root operation, 89, 90
    radical, 90
Residual codes, assigning, as appropriate, 49
Residual effect, code for, 158
Respiratory failure, 233–235
Respiratory infection, 224–225
Respiratory syncytial virus (RSV), 379
Respiratory system, 223, 224
    diseases of, 223–242
        ablation of lung, 238–239
        acute pulmonary edema, 236
        acute respiratory distress syndrome, 235
        asthma, 230–231
        atelectasis, 232
        bronchospasm, 231
        chronic obstructive pulmonary disease, 230–231
        influenza, 228
        laryngitis, 229–230
        pleural effusion, 232–233
        pleurodesis, 238–239
        pneumonia, 224–227
        respiratory failure, 233–235
        surgical procedures involving, 237
        tracheitis, 229–230
        tracheostomy complications, 241–242
Restoration, as root operation, 107, 108
Restriction, as root operation, 94–95, 94
    distinguishing between occlusion and, 454
Retinopathy, 164
    hypertensive, 418
    proliferative diabetic, 164
Reversible ischemic neurological deficit (RIND), 414
Revision, as root operation, 95–96, 95
Rheumatic heart disease, 394–397
Roman numerals, alphabetization rules and, 10
Root operations, 61, 68–69, 68, 78
    in Administration Section, 105, 105
    to alter diameter or route of tubular body part, 94–95, 94
    that always involve device, 95–96, 95
    in Chiropractic Section, 111, 111
    code characters for, 68–69, 68
    for digestive system procedures, 251
    in Extracorporeal or Systemic Assistance and Performance Section,
        107–108, 107
    in Extracorporeal or Systemic Therapies Section, 108–109, 108
    involving cutting or separation only, 92–93, 93
    in Measurement and Monitoring Section, 106, 106
    in Medical and Surgical Section, 85–99
        to take out solids/fluids/gases from body part, 91–92, 91
        to take out some or all of body part, 89–90, 89
        that always involve a device, 95–96, 95
        that include other objectives, 99, 99
        that include other repairs, 98, 98
        that involve examination only, 97–98, 97
        that put in/put back or move some/all of body part, 93–94, 93
    in Obstetrics Section, 343

in Osteopathic Section, 110, 110
in Other Procedures Section, 110–111, 111
in Placement Section, 102–104, 102, 103
Rule of nines, 519, 523
"Rule out" versus "ruled out," 54

S

Salter-Harris classification, 503
Sarcoidosis, 201–202
Schizophrenic disorders, 176–177
Schwannomas, 371, 460
Sclerotherapy, 248
Screening examinations, 128
Secondary hypercoagulable states, 199
Secondary site, treatment directed at, 473
Section, code characters for, 66, 66
Section X codes. See New Technology Section
"See," 17
"See also," 17–18
"See category," 18
"See condition," 18
Seizures, grand mal, 206
Sense organs, diseases of, 214–220
Sensorineural hearing loss, 203
Sepsis, 146–149
    associated with noninfectious process, 148–149
    bacterial, in newborns, 383
    due to postprocedural infection, 148, 149
    with localized infection, 148
    puerperal, 337–339
    severe, 146–149
    streptococcal, 146, 149
    viral, 146
Septic shock, 146–149
Sequelae. See Late effects
Sequencing
    of external cause codes, 492
    of injury codes, 490
    of mechanical ventilation codes, 241
Serologic testing for human immunodeficiency virus (HIV) infection, 153–154
Seventh-character subclassifications, 6, 48
    assigning codes to, 48–49
    for burns, 522
    for fetus, 325–326
    for fractures, 499–501, 500, 503
    for initial encounter, 500, 538
    for injuries, 488–489
    for new technology, 119–120
    for pathological fractures, 306
    placeholder character and, 7, 48
Sexual dysfunction, 181
Shaken infant syndrome, 495, 496
Sheehan's syndrome, 340
Shock
    anaphylactic, 514
    septic, 146–147
    traumatic, 524
Shock wave therapy, as root operation, 109, 109
Sick sinus syndrome, 425
Sickle-cell anemia, 193, 197–198
Sickle-cell thalassemia, 197–198
Sickle-cell trait, 193, 197
Signs and symptoms, 54, 136–137
    as additional diagnoses, 137
    as principal diagnoses, 136–137
Sites, 300
    bilateral, 53
    organism versus, 144
Sixth-character subclassifications, 6, 7, 48
    for angina pectoris, 405
    for diabetes mellitus, 161
Skeleton, human, 301
Skin and subcutaneous tissue, 291, 520. See also Burns
    diseases of, 289–297
        cellulitis of, 294–295
        debridement, 296
        dermal regenerative graft, 296–297
        dermatitis due to drugs, 290–291
        erythema multiforme, 291–292
        excision of lesion, 295
        ulcers of, 292–294
Sleep disorders, 181
Smoke inhalation, 522, 524
Social determinants of health codes, 38

Somatoform disorders, 180–181
Somnolence, 176
Source document, medical record as, 35–39
Special investigations and examinations, 127–128
Spina bifida, 370
Spinal column, 303, 310, 311, 312, 313
Spinal decompression, 315
Spinal disc prostheses, 315
Spinal fusion and refusion, 310–314, 310, 311, 312, 313, 314
    surgeries, 310–314, 313, 314
Spinal motion preservation, 315–316
Spondylosis of intervertebral disc, 301, 303
Square brackets ([ ]), 19, 50–51
Staphylococcus aureus, 150, 151
Status asthmaticus, 230–231
Status post, 553
ST-elevation myocardial infarction (STEMI), 399–400, 412
Stenosis, aortic valve, 396–397
Sterilization, 348
Stoma reversal surgery, 251
Stomach
    disorders of, in newborns, 382
    ulcers of, 248
Streptococcus, 146, 224
Stress
    incontinence, 266
    reactions, acute, 179
Stroke Scale scores, National Institutes of Health (NIHSS), 38, 139
Subcutaneous cardioverter/defibrillators, 429
Subcutaneous tissue. See Skin and subcutaneous tissue
Subsequent care for injuries, 500–501
Substance abuse and dependence
    disorders, 182–185
    poisoning due to, 535
    therapy for, 185, 187–189, 188
Subterms, 8, 10–12, 42
Sudden idiopathic hearing loss, 220
Sudden infant death syndrome (SIDS), 335, 386
Sunburn, 520, 523
Supplement, as root operation, 95–96, 95
Supraglottitis, 229
Surgeries
    admissions from outpatient, 25
    bariatric, 258, 259, 260
    on breast, 280–283, 282
    complications of, 537–554
    on mother and fetus, 385
    on respiratory system, 237
    spinal fusion, 310–314, 311, 313
    stoma reversal, 251
    in utero, 331, 385
Surgical care as external cause, 553–554
Suspected maternal and fetal conditions not found, 350–351
Symptom code, 125, 127, 135, 136, 137
Symptoms, 54, 135. See also Signs and symptoms
    as additional diagnoses, 137
    followed by contrasting/comparative diagnoses, 27
    as principal diagnoses, 136–137
Synonyms, guidelines for coding and, 42
Systemic inflammatory response syndrome (SIRS), 147, 149, 213
Systemic nuclear medicine therapy, 115

T

Table of Drugs and Chemicals, 7, 12, 528, 530–531, 531
Table, Neoplasm, 7, 12, 462, 463
Tables in ICD-10-PCS, 63, 63
    finding applicable, 80
Tabular List of Diseases and Injuries, 4–7
    codes in, 6
    discrepancy between Index entry and, 43
    placeholder character, 7
    table of contents of, 5
    using both Alphabetic Index and, 48
    verifying code number in, 43
Tachypnea, 381
Terrorism, injuries as result of, 491–493
Thalassemia, 197–198
Therapeutic injection, complications following, 544–546
Thoracoscopic procedures, 237
Threatened condition, 56
Three-character categories, 6
    for fractures, 497
Three-character codes, 6, 48
Thrombocytopenia, 193, 199

Thrombolytic agent, 403, 434, 436
Thrombophlebitis of veins, 393, 422–423
Thrombosis
    of atrium, 403
    of auricular appendage, 403
    of veins, 393, 422–423
    of ventricles, 403
Tissue expander, insertion of, 281
Tobacco use during pregnancy, 334–335
Tomographic (tomo) nuclear medicine imaging, 114
Torticollis, ocular-induced, 214
Toxic effects, 527, 529
    guidelines for assignment of codes for, 532
    of substances, 528, 532
Toxic shock syndrome, 149–150
Tracheitis, 229–230
Tracheostomy, complications of, 241–242
Traction, as root operation, 103, 103, 104, 104
Transcatheter aortic and pulmonary valve replacement, 433
Transfer, as root operation, 93, 93
Transforaminal lumbar interbody fusion (TLIF), 313, 314, 314
Transfusion, as root operation, 105, 106
    complications following, 544–546
Transient alteration of awareness, 176
Transmyocardial revascularization (TMR), 427, 440
Transplantation
    complications from, 547–548
    heart, 448–449
    kidney, 267
    malignant neoplasm associated with, 476
    as root operation, 93, 93
Trauma
    early complications of, 512–513
    compartment syndrome, 512–513
Treatment, as root operation, 110, 110
Treatment plan, original, not carried out, 27
Troponin, elevated, 400
Tubal ligation, 348
Tuberculosis, 145–146
    pleural effusion due to, 233
Tuboplasty, 348
Tumor lysis syndrome (TLS), 170, 475–476
Tumors
    ablation, 238–239
    carcinoid, 458–459
    neuroendocrine, 458–459
    registry, 461

U

Ulcerative colitis, 247
    burns and, 524
Ulcers
    diabetic foot, 165
    diabetic skin, 165
    duodenal, 248
    gastric, 248
    Kennedy, 293
    peptic, 248, 524
    pressure, 38, 292–293
    of skin, 292–294
    stasis, 293–294
    of stomach and small intestine, 248
Ultrasound therapy, as root operation, 109
Ultraviolet light therapy, as root operation, 109
Uncertain diagnoses, coding, as if established, 53–54
    borderline diagnoses, 54, 161
    "rule out" versus "ruled out," 54
Underdosing, 527, 529
    codes for, 490, 530
        guidelines for assignment of, 532
        location of codes associated with, 530–532, 531
    late effects of, 536
Uniform Hospital Discharge Data Set (UHDDS), 23–34, 77
    data items, 24
        other diagnoses, 27–31
        principal diagnosis, 24–27
    ethical coding and reporting, 33–34
    exceptions to guidelines, 377
    guidelines for reportable diagnoses, 36
    procedures, 32
    relationship of, to long-term care reporting, 32–33
    relationship of, to outpatient reporting, 32
    reporting guidelines for other diagnoses, 28–31
    for reporting procedures, 82–83
    severe sepsis in, 147–148
"Unspecified" codes, use of, 54
Unspecified mass or lesion, 460
Ureter, 264, 274
Ureteroscopy, 273, 274
Urethritis, 264
Urinary incontinence, 266
Urinary system, 264
Urinary tract infection (UTI), 264–265
"Use additional code," 16, 275
Uterine atony, 338–339
Uterine myomas, 459
Uterus, prolapse of, 277–278

V

V codes, 4
Vaccinations, routine, of newborns, 386
Vaginal enterocele, 277–278
Vaginal intraepithelial neoplasia (VAIN), 279
Value of a code character, 61, 64
Valvular insufficiency, 398
Vaping-related disorder, 229
Varicose veins, 293
Vascular access devices (VADs), 271, 272, 444–446, 446
    totally implantable, 271, 444–446
    tunneled, 271, 444–446
Vascular dementia, 175
Vasoplasty, 348
Venous system, major vessels of, 395
Ventricular fibrillation (VF), 427–428
Ventricular septal defect, 403
Vertical banded gastroplasty, 258, 259
Viadur (leuprolide acetate) implant, 480
Visual impairment, 214
Vulvar intraepithelial neoplasia (VIN), 279

W

W codes, 4
West Nile virus infection, 145
Wheezing, 230, 231, 381
White blood cells, diseases of, 199, 200–201
Whole lung lavage, 238
"With," as relational term, 11–12, 20–21, 49, 161, 216, 247
Work-related activity, 491
World Health Organization (WHO) ICD-10, 4
Wounds
    dehiscence, 550
    open, 498, 510
    puncture, 510

X

X codes, 4

Y

Y codes, 4

Z

Z codes, 4, 121–131
    admission
        for aftercare management, 123–124
        for follow-up examination, 124–125
        for observation and evaluation, 125–127
    aftercare, 552
    for burns, 522
    external cause of morbidity codes and, 122
    genetic susceptibility to disease, 130–131
    for health status related to circulatory system, 424–425
    locating, and external cause of morbidity codes, 122
    for orthopedic aftercare, 508–509
    as principal/first-listed diagnosis, 131
    representing patient history, status, or problems, 129–130
    screening examinations, 128
    special investigations and examinations, 127–128
    Tabular List for, 122
Zika virus, 145